Clinical Handbook of Mindfulness

Clinical Handbook
of Mindfulness

Fabrizio Didonna

Editor

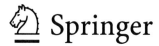 Springer

Editor
Dr. Fabrizio Didonna
Coord. Unit for Mood & Anxiety Disorders
Department of Psychiatry
Casa di Cura Villa Margherita
Arcugnano, Vicenza - Italy
fabdidon@libero.it

ISBN: 978-0-387-09592-9   e-ISBN: 978-0-387-09593-6
DOI 10.1007/978-0-387-09593-6

Library of Congress Control Number: 2008938818

Printed on acid-free paper

springer.com

To my wife Rachele, For her love, support and understanding. May she be always safe, happy, healthy and free from inner and outer harm

F. D.

Contents

Acknowledgments

I wish to acknowledge my indebtedness to a number of people.

First and foremost, I wish to acknowledge the influence of many teachers and mentors: I am profoundly grateful to Jon Kabat-Zinn for his precious and invaluable teaching throughout the past years, for his extraordinary and contagious enthusiasm and wise example in transmitting and embodying the deep meanings and principles of mindfulness. My warmest thanks to him also for his precious help, support and feedback during the final stage of this project, for helping me to expand the list of mindfulness centres and groups in Appendix B and last, but not least, for his kind and thorough foreword to this book.

My heartfelt thanks goes to Thich Nath Hanh and Thomas Trobe, who have allowed me to see new paths over the years to improve professionally and grow personally and to effectively integrate mindfulness and meditation into my understanding and treating of psychological suffering in clinical practice.

A special and nostalgic acknowledgement goes to Ma Yoga Sudha, who left us a few months ago. She personally taught me the precious and healing value of compassion, disidentification and free emotional expression in psychotherapy through meditation.

I am also grateful to Giovanni Liotti who illuminated me with many wise ideas and helped me learn how to understand and treat challenging and complex psychiatric patients.

I also want to offer my sincere and warm thanks to Mark Williams, Marsha Linehan and Jeffrey Young for their kind comments and support to the book.

I am extremely grateful to Thomas Bien, Sarah Guth and Jeffrey Brantley for their valuable, thorough and helpful feedback and review on chapters 8, 11 and 24.

A Special thanks goes to Zindel Segal for sharing his advice and clinical insights and for supporting me in this wonderful project right from the start.

I am very grateful to all the authors who have contributed to this book and who have put so much work into helping bring this project to fruition. I also thank them for their enthusiasm and collaborative way of accompanying me throughout this fascinating, but also laborious, journey and lastly for their precious and invaluable contribution to the field. Each has furnished many new insights for me personally.

I am most grateful to the staff of Springer Publisher, in particular Executive Editor Sharon Pannulla, and Editorial Assistant Jennifer Hadley, for their kind assistance, advice, and support and for their flexible approach throughout the process of putting this book together. Many thanks also to the Project Manager Sasikala Rajesh.

I am also very indebted to my patients, who have taught me most of what I know about clinical work with their efforts, perseverance and trust in the therapy, and, in the end, their love of life.

Finally, I wish to offer my heartfelt thanks to my wife Rachele for her love and patience as I toiled long hours and was often absent while editing and writing this manual. To her this book is dedicated.

F. D.

About the Editor

Fabrizio Didonna, Psy D, is a Clinical Psychologist and Cognitive Behaviour Psychotherapist. He is a founder and President of the *Istituto Italiano per la Mindfulness (IS.I.MIND)*. He is a Coordinator of the Unit for Mood and Anxiety Disorders, and he also works at the Unit for Borderline Personality Disorders in the Department of Psychiatry at the *Casa di Cura Villa Margherita* in Vicenza, Italy. He is a teacher and trainer at the School of Cognitive Therapy in Bologna, at the School of Cognitive and Forensic Psychotherapy in Reggio Emilia and at the Institute for Cognitive Science in Grosseto, Italy. He is an experienced instructor of mindfulness groups both in inpatient and outpatient settings and was one of the first therapists who planned and used mindfulness training with patients with severe disorders in inpatient treatment programs. He has given workshops worldwide in the field of CBT for obsessive compulsive disorder, depression, anxiety disorders and mindfulness-based training, has presented scientific papers at conferences in Italy and Europe, and published many articles, several chapters and two books. He is Vice-President of the Italian Association for Obsessive–Compulsive Disorder and also the Representative of the Regional Section of SITCC, the Italian Society for Cognitive and Behaviour Therapy. He has been practicing and teaching meditation for many years and gives training retreats in MBCT and mindfulness-based interventions in Italy and in many countries in Europe.

Contributors

Baer Ruth is Professor of Psychology at the University of Kentucky. Her research interests include mindfulness and acceptance-based interventions, assessment and conceptualization of mindfulness, cognitive-behavioral interventions, and psychological assessment. She is the editor of *Mindfulness-Based Treatment Approaches: Clinician's Guide to Evidence Base and Applications* (Academic Press, 2006).

Barnhofer Thorsten is a post-doctoral clinical research psychologist working in a Wellcome Trust funded team led by Professor Mark Williams at the University of Oxford. He teaches MBCT classes and trainings as part of ongoing research into the effects and mechanisms of mindfulness meditation, most recently, in collaboration with Dr Catherine Crane, a study funded by a Franciso J Varela Research Award from the Mind & Life Institute examining the effects of MBCT in chronically depressed patients with a history of suicidality.

Battista Susan completed her Master's work with Dr. Nancy Kocovski at Wilfrid Laurier University where she was involved with research on mindfulness and social anxiety. Susan is now at Dalhousie University completing a doctoral degree in clinical psychology.

Best Jennifer L., Ph.D. is a clinical health psychologist and Assistant Professor of Psychology at the University of North Carolina at Charlotte. Prior to this position she pursued post-doctoral research training with Duke Integrative Medicine in applying mindfulness-based approaches to the regulation of weight, eating and metabolism in eating disorders and obesity. She also has experience developing and leading mindfulness-based groups for the management of stress and for reducing symptoms of anxiety and depression with community samples. Dr. Best is published in the area of mindfulness and glucose metabolism among obese binge eaters. Her current research examines how mindfulness may be a useful skill for improving appetite regulation among overweight individuals seeking to maintain weight loss.

Bien Thomas, Ph.D. is an author and practicing psychologist in Albuquerque, New Mexico, where he teaches mindfulness and meditation. In addition to his doctorate in psychology from the University of New Mexico, he also holds a master's degree in theology from Princeton Theological Seminary. He presents nationally and internationally. His work is at the forefront of integrating mindfulness into the practice of psychotherapy. He is author of: *Mindful Therapy: A Guide for Therapists and Helping Professionals* (Wisdom, 2006), *Mindful Recovery: A Spiritual Path to Healing From Addiction* (Wiley, 2002), and *Finding the Center Within: The Healing Way of Mindfulness Meditation* (Wiley, 2003), and co-editor of the Guilford volume, *Mindfulness and the Therapeutic Relationship* (2008).

Birnie Kathryn received her BA (Hons) Psychology from the University of Calgary in 2007. Under the direction of Dr. Linda Carlson, Kathryn studied the impact of the MBSR program for patients with cancer and their partners. In particular, her thesis focused on examining changes in symptoms of stress, mood disturbance, and social support in this group. For this work, Kathryn received an honorable mention for the Research Award for outstanding undergraduate research. Kathryns personal interest in yoga and meditation prompted her to study abroad in India at the University of Pune, as well as complete a minor in religious studies. She plans to continue a focus on psychosocial oncology in her graduate studies.

Brantley Jeffrey, M.D., is a Board-Certified psychiatrist and has practiced mindfulness meditation for over 25 years. He is a founding faculty member of Duke Integrative Medicine, and is the founder and director of the Mindfulness-Based Stress Reduction Program at Duke Integrative Medicine. Dr. Brantley is the author *"Calming Your Anxious Mind: how mindfulness and compassion can free you from anxiety, fear, and panic"*, 2nd edition, (New Harbinger Publications, 2007). He is also the co-author of a popular book series, *Five Good Minutes* (New Harbinger Publications, 2005, 2006, 2007) and has contributed to book chapters, and numerous articles focused on applications of mindfulness to enhance health and well-being in daily life.

Carlson Linda is a Clinical Psychologist and Associate Professor in Psychosocial Oncology in the Department of Oncology, Faculty of Medicine at the University of Calgary, and the holder of the Enbridge Endowed Research Chair in Psychosocial Oncology. She also holds an Adjunct Associate Professor appointment in the Department of Psychology. Dr. Carlson has been studying MBSR since 1997 and published papers on its effects in cancer patients in peer-reviewed journals including *Psychosomatic Medicine, Psychoneuroendocrinology*, and *Brain, Behavior and Immunity*. Her group has shown its efficacy for decreasing symptoms of stress, improving mood, sleep and quality of life, and altering stress hormone and immune function in cancer patients. She has published almost 80 book chapters and research papers in peer-reviewed journals, holds several millions of dollars in grant funding and regularly presents her work at international conferences.

Cordon Shari, MA, is a Doctoral candidate in Social Psychology at Virginia Commonwealth University. Ms. Cordon's research focuses on the role of mindfulness in interpersonal contexts. Conducted in both laboratory and intervention settings, her studies investigate the effects of trait and state mindfulness on relationship formation, satisfaction, and psychological well-being correlates.

Crane Catherine is a post-doctoral research psychologist working in a Wellcome Trust funded team led by Professor Mark Williams at the University of Oxford. In collaboration with Dr. Thorsten Barnhofer she is currently conducting a study funded by a Fransisco J Varela Research Award from the Mind & Life Institute, examining the feasibility and immediate effects of mindfulness-based cognitive therapy for patients who are chronically depressed and suicidal. Catherine has a personal interest in mindfulness meditation and a number of publications on the role of mindfulness-relevant psychological processes in depression and suicidal behaviour.

Didonna Fabrizio (see *about the editor*)

Dimidjian Sona, Ph.D., is an assistant professor in the department of psychology at the University of Colorado, Boulder. Her research focuses on the treatment and prevention of depression. She has a strong interest in the clinical application of mindfulness, including both Dialectical Behavior Therapy and Mindfulness-Based Cognitive Therapy, and a longstanding personal mindfulness and yoga practice.

Drossel Claudia received her doctoral degree in experimental psychology from Temple University. She is currently pursuing a doctoral degree in clinical psychology at the University of Nevada, Reno, where she encountered the concepts of acceptance and mindfulness through Dialectical Behavior Therapy and Acceptance and Commitment Therapy. Claudia views acceptance and mindfulness as complex cognitive-behavioral skill sets that require extensive practice, permeate all aspects of inter and intra personal relationships, and are not teachable with words alone. Daily life provides the practicing ground for acceptance and mindfulness. Claudia engages in formal practice by studying yoga.

Follette Victoria M., PhD, is a Professor of Psychology and Chair of the Department of Psychology at the University of Nevada, Reno. She was named Distinguished Alumna by the Department of Psychology at the University of Memphis, Tennessee where she completed her graduate work. Dr. Follette heads the Trauma Research Institute of Nevada, which utilizes a contextual behavioral approach to understanding the sequelae of trauma. Her areas of interest include the empirical study of applied treatment and mindfulness-based approaches to treatment and she had published extensively in these areas.

Fulton Paul R., Ed.D. is a founding member and President of the Institute for Meditation and Psychotherapy. He is a clinical psychologist, having received his doctorate from Harvard University's Laboratory for Human Development. Paul received lay ordination in Zen Buddhism in 1972. He is currently Director of Mental Health for Tufts Health Plan in Massachusetts, and in private psychotherapy practice. He is on the board of directors of the Barre Center for Buddhist Studies in Barre, Massachusetts. Paul has taught applications of Buddhist psychology to mental health professionals internationally, and is co-author and co-editor of *Mindfulness and Psychotherapy*, Guildford, 2005.

Gardner-Nix Jackie graduated from London University, UK as an MBBS (British equivalent of M.D.) and Ph.D. (biochemistry), and obtained membership in the Royal College of Physicians of UK in Internal Medicine. Currently, she is a Chronic Pain Consultant in the Departments of Anaesthesia's Pain Clinics at St Michael's Hospital and Sunnybrook Health Sciences Centre, Toronto, and an Assistant Professor at University of Toronto. She has given many workshops and presentations on pain management and specialized in medications for pain, but in the last six years has focused on developing and researching mindfulness-based meditation courses for pain sufferers based on Jon-Kabat-Zinn's MBSR work. Her courses are taught through telemedicine as well as on site to patients throughout Ontario, Canada.

Garland Sheila. Under the supervision of Dr. Linda Carlson, Sheila Garland has been investigating the use of MBSR in individuals with cancer since 2003. Specifically, her interest has been the potential application of mindfulness meditation to reduce insomnia symptoms and improve sleep quality. Sheila Garland previously published pilot work demonstrating that participants reported improved sleep quality after participation in the MBSR program. In addition, she has published a comparison of the MBSR program to another psychosocial intervention on measures of spirituality and post-traumatic growth. Finally, she has contributed to work exploring the experience of partners and support persons taking part in the program.

Germer Christopher K., PhD is a clinical psychologist in private practice, specializing in mindfulness-based treatment of anxiety and panic, and couples therapy. He has been integrating meditation and mindfulness principles into psychotherapy since 1978. His special interest is the cultivation of self-compassion in psychotherapy. Dr. Germer is a founding faculty member of the Institute for Meditation and Psychotherapy, a Clinical Instructor in Psychology, Harvard Medical School, and co-editor, *Mindfulness and Psychotherapy* (Guilford Press).

Gilbert Paul is Professor of Clinical Psychology at the University of Derby and Consultant Psychologist at Derbyshire Mental Health Services NHS Trust. He has a visiting Professorship at the University of Fribourg (Switzerland) and Coimbra (Portugal). He has been a Fellow of the British Psychological Society since 1993 published over 100 papers and book chapters and 14 books. He has a special interest in the the role of shame in psychopathology and its treatment with compassion focused therapy.

Goodman Trudy, Ed.M., is the Founder of InsightLA, a non-profit organization that offers mindfulness meditation courses, sitting groups and retreats. She has trained and taught extensively in Zen and Vipassana meditation, psychotherapy, and Mindfulness-Based Stress Reduction. Trudy teaches with Jack Kornfield and others worldwide. She co-founded the first Institute for Meditation and Psychotherapy in Cambridge, MA, in 1995, and Growing Spirit, a family mindfulness program in Los Angeles, with Susan Kaiser Greenland, in 2002.

Greeson Jeffrey, Ph.D., is a clinical health psychologist with a Master's degree in Biomedical Chemistry. He has practiced and researched mindfulness meditation for over 10 years. He is an Assistant Professor in the Department of Psychiatry and Behavioral Sciences at the Duke University School of Medicine and a scientist-practitioner at Duke Integrative Medicine. Dr. Greeson has investigated the psychological and physiological benefits of Mindfulness-Based Stress Reduction and other mindfulness-based clinical interventions since 1998, and he has published several peer-reviewed papers in the field. He is especially interested in the measurement, neuroscience, and molecular biology of mindfulness as a core self-regulation skill.

Hayes Steven C. is Nevada Foundation Professor at the Department of Psychology at the University of Nevada. An author of 32 books and nearly 400 scientific articles, his career has focused on an analysis of the nature of human language and cognition and the application of this to the understanding and alleviation of human suffering. He is the originator of Acceptance and Commitment Therapy, which is one of the family of new acceptance and mindfulness therapies emerging within cognitive behavior therapy. Along with Victoria Follette and Marsha Linehan he edited the 2004 book *Mindfulness and acceptance: Expanding the cognitive behavioral tradition.* (New York: Guilford) and is co-editor of the upcoming book *"Mindfulness and acceptance in children."* His work has been recognized by the Exemplary Contributions to Basic Behavioral Research and Its Applications from Division 25 of APA, the Impact of Science on Application award from the Society for the Advancement of Behavior Analysis, and the Lifetime Achievement Award from the Association for Behavioral and Cognitive Therapy.

Hutchins Marion completed her undergraduate honors thesis at the University of Calgary in 2007, under the supervision of Dr. Linda Carlson. Marion's thesis examined the effects of MBSR on spirituality, post-traumatic growth, and social support in cancer patients and their partners. She co-presented her findings at the Canadian Psychological Association conference in 2007. Marion is a strong proponent of mindfulness meditation and its use in maintaining physical, emotional, and spiritual well-being.

Kaiser Greenland Susan JD, co-founder and executive director of InnerKids Foundation develops mindful awareness curriculum for and teaches programs to children as well as educators, parents, therapists and health care professionals. Susan is a member of the clinical team of the Pediatric Pain Clinic at UCLA's Mattel's Children's Hospital, Co-Investigator on MARC's MAPs in pre-k and elementary education research studies, and Collaborator on a UCSF research study looking at the impact of mindful eating on children and families. In 2006, Susan was named a 'Champion of Children' by First 5 LA. She speaks at universities, medical centers and professional programs throughout the country and consults with various organizations on teaching mindful awareness in an age-appropriate and secular manner. Susan is currently writing a book on mindfulness and children for Free Press.

Kocovski Nancy, PhD is an Assistant Professor in the Department of Psychology at Wilfrid Laurier University where she conducts research on mindfulness and social anxiety. She also has an affiliation as a Research Scientist at the Centre for Addiction and Mental Health where she conducts research on the use of mindfulness in the treatment of Social Anxiety Disorder.

Labelle E. Laura is a doctoral student in clinical psychology, co-supervised by Dr. Linda Carlson and Dr. Tavis Campbell. Laura Labelle has been evaluating the effects of MBSR on physiological and psychological outcomes in cancer patients. She is currently conducting a waitlist-controlled trial examining the impact of MBSR on blood pressure, acute neuroendocrine and cardiovascular stress responses, and psychological functioning in women with cancer. Her doctoral dissertation will evaluate whether increased mindfulness and improved emotion regulation mediate the impact of MBSR on psychological functioning, in cancer survivors.

Lazar Sara W., PhD is a scientist in the Psychiatry Department at Massachusetts General Hospital and an Instructor in Psychology at Harvard Medical School. The focus of her research is to elucidate the neural mechanisms underlying meditation, both in clinical settings and to promote and preserve health and well-being in healthy individuals. She has been practicing yoga and mindfulness meditation since 1994, and is a Board member of the Institute for Meditation and Psychotherapy.

Lykins Emily is a doctoral student in clinical psychology at the University of Kentucky. Her research interests center on positive psychology, with a focus on mindfulness, acceptance, and psychological well-being.

McBee Lucia, LCSW, MPH, is a geriatric social worker who has worked with elders and their caregivers for 27 years. For the past 13 years she has integrated mindfulness and other complementary therapies into her practice with frail elders in the nursing home and those who are homebound; elders with cognitive and physical challenges; patients at the end of life; and their formal and informal caregivers. Her work has been published in peer reviewed journals and presented at national and international conferences. She has just completed a book on her practice with elders: Mindfulness-Based Elder Care, scheduled for a March 2008 release by Springer Publishers.

Olendzki Andrew, PhD, Executive Director and Resident Scholar at the Barre Center for Buddhist Studies (www.dharma.org) in Barre Massachusetts, an educational center focusing on the integration of scholarly understanding and meditative insight. A scholar of Pali literature and early Buddhist thought, he has taught at numerous New England colleges, including Harvard and Brandeis, is on the faculty of the Institute of Meditation and Psychotherapy, and is the editor of the Insight Journal.

Pinto Antonio, is a Medical Doctor, psychiatrist and cognitive behavioural therapist. He's been lecturer of Psychotherapy at University of L'Aquila

(Italy). He's ordinary membership and teacher of the SITCC, and one of the italian representatives of the EABCT (European Association Behavioural and Cognitive Therapy). He leads regularly trainings and workshops in CBT of Psychosis, and has published on this topic the results of a Randomized Controlled Trial. He is a EMDR supervisor and, at the moment he is leading researches about the application of mindfulness protocol on complex psychiatric diseases. He takes part in an International research group leaded by Prof. A.T. Beck for the application of new psychotherapeutic findings with psychotic patients. He's membership of IEPA (International Early Psychosis Association). At the present time he works as psychiatrist in a Department of Mental Health in Naples (Italy).

Quillian Wolever Ruth, PhD is a clinical health psychologist and the Research Director of Duke Integrative Medicine at the Duke University School of Medicine in Durham, NC, USA. She specializes in behavioral change, treatment of stress-related problems and mind-body health. Her clinical practice and research focus on utilizing the mind-body connection to improve health. Her research explores 1) the application of mindfulness to improve eating patterns, lifestyle change and weight; 2) the emerging role of health coaching in mainstream medicine; and 3) the efficacy of integrative approaches to health. She and her husband Mark are active in educating the public on Rett Syndrome.

Rizvi Shireen L., Ph.D., is an assistant professor in the department of psychology at the New School for Social Research in New York City. Her research focuses on treatment development for chronic and severe mental health problems, as well as the emotion of shame and its relation to the development and maintenance of psychopathology. Dr. Rizvi has written and presented numerous theoretical and research papers on BPD, DBT, and trauma. She also maintains a small private practice in New York.

Rosillo Gonzalez Yolanda is a clinical psychologist and a cognitive-behavioural psychoterapist. She works as a private practitioner in a Medical Center for Eating Disorders connected with Villa Margherita Clinic in Vicenza, Italy. She practice mindfulness meditation for many years and has been trained by M. Williams, J. Kabat-Zinn and F. Didonna. She conducted, as a co-leader, for several years mindfulness-based groups in inpatient and outpatient setting for patients affected by severe anxiety, mood and personality disorders.

Schwartz Jeffrey M., M.D. is Research Psychiatrist at UCLA School of Medicine and a seminal thinker and researcher in the field of self-directed neuroplasticity. He has been a devoted practitioner of mindfulness meditation in the Pali Theravada Buddhist tradition for over thirty years. His primary research goal has been to develop a theoretically grounded scientific account for the finding that mindful awareness systematically affects how the brain works. He is co-author of the book. The Mind and The Brain: Neuroplasticity and the Power of Mental Force (2002). New York: Harper Collins.

Segal Zindel, PhD, is the Morgan Firestone Chair in Psychotherapy in the Department of Psychiatry at the University of Toronto. He is Head of the Cognitive Behaviour Therapy Unit at the Centre for Addiction and Mental Health and is a Professor in the Departments of Psychiatry and Psychology at the University of Toronto. Dr. Segal is the author of *Mindfulness-based Cognitive Therapy for Depression: A new approach for preventing relapse* and*The Mindful Way Through Depression*. His research has helped to characterize psychological markers of relapse vulnerability to affective disorder and he continues to advocate for the relevance of mindfulness-based clinical care in psychiatry and mental health.

Shaw Welch Stacy, Ph.D is a clinical psychologist at the Evidence-Based Treatment Centers of Seattle, which includes a Dialectical Behavior Therapy treatment program. In addition to her work in DBT, she directs a center devoted to the treatment of anxiety. She has a longstanding interest in the use of mindfulness in DBT as well as in possible applications of mindfulness in the treatment of anxiety disorders.

Siegel Ronald D., PsyD is an Assistant Clinical Professor of Psychology at Harvard Medical School, where he has taught for over 20 years. He is a long time student of mindfulness meditation and serves on the Board of Directors and faculty of the Institute for Meditation and Psychotherapy. Dr. Siegel teaches throughout the United States about mindfulness and psychotherapy and mind/body treatment, while maintaining a private clinical practice in Lincoln, Massachusetts. He is coeditor of *Mindfulness and Psychotherapy* (Guilford Press) and coauthor of *Back Sense: A Revolutionary Approach to Halting the Cycle of Chronic Back Pain* (Broadway Books).

Smalley Susan L., Ph.D. is a Professor of Psychiatry, Founder and Director of the Mindful Awareness Research Center in the Semel Institute at UCLA, investigates the genetic basis of childhood-onset psychiatric disorders, such as ADHD, and the role of mindful awareness (and other tools of self-regulation) to influence gene/environmental interactions to enhance health and well-being. Her research includes studies of biological mechanisms, longitudinal course, intervention, and dissemination of mindful awareness practices (MAPs) across the lifespan, from Pre-K to the elderly. http://www.adhd.ucla.edu and http://www.marc.ucla.edu.

Tirch Dennis PhD is the Director of Education at the American Institute For Cognitive Therapy in Manhattan. He serves as an Adjunct Associate Professor at Albert Einstein Medical School, an Instructor to psychiatric residents in CBT at New York Medical College, and is a Fellow of The Academy of Cognitive Therapy. Dr. Tirch is a long time student and practitioner of Japanese Tendai and other Buddhist meditation methods. He has co-authored several articles and chapters regarding meditation and CBT, and is currently developing methods of integrating mindfulness and compassionate mind training into psychotherapy supervision.

Treadway Michael is a PhD student in the Clinical Science program at the Graduate School of Arts and Sciences at Vanderbilt University. Mr. Treadways research focuses on the behavioral and neurobiological mechanisms of emotion regulation among healthy individuals and individuals with depression. He is especially interested in understanding how the utility of different emotion regulation strategies may vary according to context.

Varra Alethea A. is a Mental Illness Research, Education, and Clinical Center (MIRECC) Postdoctoral Psychology Fellow in Post Traumatic Stress Disorder (PTSD) at the VA Puget Sound Health Care System in Seattle, WA, USA. Her primary clinical and research interests involve the application of acceptance and mindfulness-based therapies to the treatment of individuals with post-traumatic sequalea including PTSD and substance abuse disorders. She is the author of several chapters and research articles concerning the application and conceptualization of Acceptance and Commitment Therapy.

Vijay Aditi is a graduate student in the Clinical Psychology doctoral program at the University of Nevada, Reno. Her research interests are in the area of interpersonal violence and the impact and prevention of sexual revictimization. Ms. Vijay's clinical interests and in the applications of mindfulness based treatments for trauma survivors.

Walsh Erin is a doctoral student in clinical psychology at the University of Kentucky. Her current research examines how particular ways of emotional responding (acceptance vs. avoidance) influence psychological and physiological states. Other interests include investigating the psychological and physiological mechanisms of change associated with mindfulness-based practices, as well as exploring the transdiagnostic utility of such practices.

Warren Brown Kirk, PhD, completed graduate training in Psychology at McGill University and post-doctoral training at the University of Rochester. He is currently an Assistant Professor of Psychology at Virginia Commonwealth University. His research centers on the role of attention to and awareness of internal states and behavior in self-regulation and well-being. He has a particular interest in the nature of mindfulness, and the role of mindfulness and mindfulness-based interventions in affect regulation, behavior regulation, and mental health in healthy and clinical populations. He has authored numerous journal articles and chapters on these topics. His research is funded, in part, by the National Institutes of Health.

Woods Susan, M.S.W., L.I.C.S.W. is a psychotherapist who has practiced meditation and yoga for 25 years. Ms. Woods has been a long time teacher of Mindfulness-Based Stress Reduction (MBSR) and more recently Mindfulness-Based Cognitive Therapy (MBCT). She is certified as an MBSR teacher by the Center for Mindfulness in Medicine, Health Care, and Society, University of Massachusetts Medical School, Worcester, Massachusetts, USA and has taught there. Ms. Woods trains health care professionals in mindfulness-based interventions and teaches a MBCT professional training program with Zindel Segal, PhD. Ms. Woods co-designed and leads an Advanced Teaching and Study professional training program for experienced MBCT teachers.

Zylowska Lidia, M.D, adult psychiatrist, is a Co-founder of and the Assistant Clinical Professor at Mindful Awareness Research Center in the Semel Institute at UCLA. Her research investigates the use of the Mindful Awareness Practices (MAPs) for ADHD adults and teens. In her work, Dr. Zylowska promotes integration of conventional psychiatric treatment with mindfulness training and other self-regulation tools to enhance psychological well-being across the lifespan. http://www.marc.ucla.edu and http://www.lidiazylowska.com.

Foreword

Anytime a handbook such as this one appears, we know from experience that it represents a kind of pause in the head-long momentum of research, inquiry, and application within a field; a moment in which we can individually and collectively stop and reflect, take a breath so to speak, and consider where we are at. In twenty years, if it does its job, many of the details herein might be obsolete, or perhaps seen as naïve or preliminary; even as, in the broad-brush strokes of the field and its inevitable links to, if not, hopefully, embeddedness within the dharma, many aspects of these pages and findings will always be germane, perhaps even timeless and wise. In twenty years, this book might, as most handbooks do, take on a new role as an historical object in its own right, a marker of a creative moment in the history of an emerging field, still in its infancy.

But in this here and this now, this handbook is a marvelous vehicle for gathering from far and wide a range of different current views and efforts. It offers the contributors an opportunity to say to the world and to each other: "This is what we have been thinking," "This is what we have tried," "This is what we have seen," "This is what we suspect is going on," "This is what we have learned." It is also an occasion to say with a degree of openness and candor: This is where we have not succeeded, or were surprised, or disappointed." "This is what we feel is missing. "This is what we don't know." Or even, "This is what we suspect we don't even know we don't know." Most of the presentations in this book do just that, and the authors are to be congratulated for their openness and courage in this regard. As a result, this handbook presents a rich treasure trove of important issues for contemplation, deep inquiry, and study, as well as a hearty invitation to come to it all with a broad and an open-minded skepticism, renewing hopefully, over and over again, our commitment to keep a beginner's mind, in Suzuki Roshi's immortal phrase [1].

A volume such as this one is a potentially powerful resource for actually educating ourselves to the nature of possibly new dimensions embedded within our own work and the work of others ... orthogonal ways of thinking and seeing that can reveal and open up new dimensions of clinical understanding and care as well as new dimensions of basic research into questions such as the nature of what we call *mind*, and how it relates to emotion, thinking, consciousness, awareness, attention, perception, the brain, the body as a whole, and what we call "the self."

As so many of the contributors point out, none of us should imagine that we fully understand mindfulness, nor its implications in regard to these or other questions. Nor should we fall into the conceit that we come even close to fully embodying it in our lives or work, whatever that would mean, even as we speak of the importance of doing so. It is very important that we neither idealize nor reify whatever we mean when we speak of mindfulness. Really, we are all beginners, and when we are truthful about it, we also cannot but be humbled by the enormity of the undertaking. This is a very healthy framework to adopt. Happily, it is palpable in the work presented here by the many different authors and groups. The editor, Dr. Didonna is to be congratulated for taking on such an ambitious and challenging project and shepherding it to completion.

It is also important to keep in mind that, as deep and broad as the author list is for this handbook, there are many more colleagues out there, literally around the world, who are doing important work under the umbrella of mindfulness and its clinical applications who have not contributed to this volume. Their contributions as individuals and groups to the overall conversation, inquiry, and forward momentum of the field are immense. No doubt many will study these presentations in some detail, perhaps agreeing with or arguing with particular formulations or findings, recommending the handbook to their students, and possibly here or there making particularly creative use of some of the nuggets lying within to stimulate their own thinking.

So while a handbook such of this cannot in the end be all-inclusive, it can nonetheless serve as a catalyst within the entire field (and, dare I say, *sangha* of clinicians and investigators and practitioners, hopefully overlapping in the majority of people?) in pausing in the way I have just suggested, reflecting on where things are now in their fullness and their incompleteness, and then participating in both the inner and the outer conversations (through, respectively, silence for the former, and speech, deep listening, and writing for the latter), asking the deep questions and trusting our deepest intuitions about what is called for now, given the scope of the conditions, challenges, and promises inherent in psychology and psychotherapy, medicine and health care, neuroscience and phenomenology, and indeed, in the world – domains in which we are all agents of creativity, wonder, and caring.

The welcome advent of this volume [2] is diagnostic of a remarkable phenomenon that has been unfolding in both medicine and psychology over the past five years or so, and promises to continue long into the future in ways that may be profoundly transformative of both disciplines and of our understanding, in both scientific and poetic terms, of what it means to be human, and of our intrinsic capacity to embody the full potential of our species – to which we have accorded the name *homo sapiens sapiens* – for wakefulness, clarity, and wisdom. This intrinsically self-reflective nomenclature and the implicit promise or potential it carries brings to mind the rejoinder of Gandhi when asked by a reporter what he thought of Western Civilization, to wit: "I think it would be a very good idea [3]." The same might be said of our species' name.

For *homo sapiens sapiens* really means *the species that knows and knows that it knows*, from the Latin verb *sapere* (to taste or to know). To *know* invokes awareness and meta-awareness, certainly one of the core mysterious elements, along with language, cognition, compassion, and music that together constitute the final common pathway, one might say, of what it means to be fully human. I prefer *awareness* and *meta-awareness* to *cognition* and *meta-cognition*, as the latter formulation unavoidably privileges conceptualization. Any direct first-person introspective examination of the human repertoire from the perspective of experience itself requires a much larger container, one that distinguishes between thinking and awareness, and differentiates wisdom from knowledge and information; one that includes a capacity to embody what is known in ways that round out and complete the full potential of that human repertoire. One might say that the fate of the earth and of the species itself hangs in the balance. The challenge may come down to whether or not, and to what degree we can embody and enact the qualities that this appellation is pointing to. Mindfulness may be the key to this awakening to the full potential of our nature as human beings, both individually and as a species.

If one charts the number of scientific papers over the past twenty-five years or so with the word *mindfulness* in the title, one sees the phenomenon depicted in Fig. 1 [4].

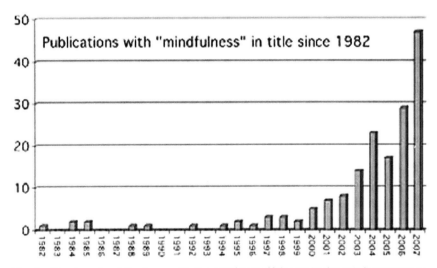

Fig. 1. Number of publications with the word "mindfulness" in the title by year since 1982.

It is immediately apparent that the field is growing exponentially. As suggested above, this volume both in number of contributors and in its shear size represents a watershed in this process. It allows us to drink in the vast range of interest and potentially useful applications of mindfulness in the disciplines of psychology, psychiatry, and psychotherapy and the breadth and depth in the quality of the work and the thought and effort behind it.

The book itself will also very likely serve as a catalyst to amplify even further the phenomenon depicted in Figure 1, as it both legitimates academic and scholarly interest and invites students and young investigators and clinicians to consider whether this emerging exploration of mindfulness resonates in some deep way with their calling in both professional and personal terms. My hope is that it will also germinate a whole new generation of research investigations that bring together the emerging fields of what is now being called *contemplative neuroscience* or neuro-phenomenology on both the cognitive and affective sides, with practical high-quality mindfulness-based clinical applications that may be of benefit to large numbers of people who are experiencing pain and suffering in their lives, both from outright illness and disease, and also from what could be termed "dis-ease," the stress and intrinsic unsatisfactoriness of a life that is always seeking some other state or condition in which to feel fulfilled, complete, and happy – what the Buddha was pointing to in his articulation of the first of the four noble truths: in the Pali language, the actuality of *dukkha* [5].

Interestingly, the Four Noble Truths were articulated by the Buddha in a medical framework, beginning with a specific diagnosis, dukkha itself: then a clearly stated etiology, that the dis-ease or dukkha has a specific cause, namely craving: a salutary prognosis, namely the possibility of a cure of the dis-ease through what he called cessation: and fourth, a practical treatment plan for bringing about liberation from suffering, termed *The Noble Eightfold Path*. This is all recounted in Chapters 1 [Siegel, Germer, and Olendzky] and Chapter 2 [Olendzky], where it is made abundantly clear that right or wise mindfulness is one but only one of the eight path factors. However, as a number of authors here and elsewhere point out, the term *mindfulness* (in Pali, *sati*) has a range of different meanings that are hotly debated to this day among Buddhist scholars, and even among scholars who share specializing in a particular Buddhist tradition.

Perhaps it is important to state explicitly at this point that in my own work and that of my colleagues in the Center for Mindfulness, from the very beginning we have consciously used the term mindfulness in several complementary ways: one, as an operationally defined regulation of attention (see below); and two, as an umbrella term that subsumes all of the other elements of the Eightfold Noble Path, and indeed, of the dharma itself, at least in implicit form. We never limit our use of mindfulness to its most narrow technical sense of whether the attention is or is not fully on the chosen object of one's attention in any given moment. As noted, there is a considerable range of definitions of mindfulness even among Buddhist scholars who specialize in the subject. I offered an *operational* definition for the sake of clarifying what we mean when we speak of cultivating mindfulness through both formal and informal meditative practices, namely, the awareness that arises through paying attention on purpose in the present moment, nonjudgmentally. It was meant to be just that – an operational definition. This approach leaves the full dimensionality and impact of mindfulness or mindful awareness implicit and available for ongoing inquiry and investigation, and indeed, it has recently become the subject of much interest and inquiry, in the many attempts by researchers to develop with some degree of validity and precision various scales to "measure" mindfulness [see Chapters by Brown and Cordon; and Baer, Walsh and Lykins]. Along with these attempts come many attendant problems that are also well-recognized in these pages and elsewhere [6].

The choice to have the word *mindfulness* does double-duty as a comprehensive but tacit umbrella term that included other essential aspects of dharma, was made as a potential skillful means to facilitate introducing what

Nyanaponika Thera referred to as *the heart of Buddhist meditation* into the mainstream of medicine and more broadly, health care and the wider society in a wholly universal rather than Buddhist formulation and vocabulary. I felt that Nyanaponika Thera's inclusive and non-dual formulation offered both validation and permission to trust and act on my own direct experience of the meditation practice and the dharma teachings I had received over the course of my life, even if technically speaking, it was glossing over important elements of Buddhist psychology (as outlined in the Abbidharma, and in Zen and Vajrayana teachings) that I felt could be differentiated and clarified later, once it was recognized that *mindfulness*, based on our operational definition, however, it was construed or contextualized in detail, might contribute profoundly to clinical care and to our understanding of the nature of the mind itself in a Western mainstream medical and scientific setting. In Nyanaponka's words, mindfulness is

> the unfailing master key for *knowing* the mind and is thus the starting point; the perfect tool for shaping the mind, and is the focal point; and the lofty manifestation of the achieved *freedom* of the mind, and is thus the culminating point.[7]

That means that mindfulness is the aim, the methods or practices, and the outcome or consequences all wrapped up together, wholly fitting for a non-dual orientation that emphasizes nowhere to go, nothing to do, and nothing to attain [8]. Together with the words of the Buddha in his most explicit teaching on mindfulness, found in the Mahasattipathana Sutra, or great sutra on mindfulness

> this is the direct path for the purification of beings,
> for the surmounting of sorrow and lamentation,
> for the disappearance of pain and grief,
> for the attainment of the true way,
> for the realization of liberation –
> namely, the four foundations of mindfulness

it seemed like an appropriate choice to feature mindfulness as the unifying factor and name under whose umbrella the work of the stress reduction clinic, later known as *mindfulness-based stress reduction*, or MBSR, could unfold. Now we have our first clinical handbook of mindfulness, which includes a broad range of perspectives on this veritable koan, the nature of mindfulness, its myriad applications, and potential impacts.

To make matters even more interesting, since in all Asian languages the word for mind and the word for heart are the same word, it feels important to remind ourselves that unless we hear "heartfulness" when we are using or hearing "mindfulness," we may be missing the mark in a fundamental way that could have unfortunate consequences both for how mindfulness-based interventions are constructed and delivered, and for how we approach relevant research issues. Many of the authors here are very strong on this point in the discussion of their work. For me, the dimension of heartfulness reinforces the core Hippocratic injunction: *primum non nocere* – first, do no harm, to which we all need to accord continual present-moment attention in relationship to those who come to us with untold vulnerabilities.

One last word on the subject of mindfulness and its definitions: a small group of meditation teachers and Buddhist scholars recently developed a collective articulation/definition of *mindfulness* that may contribute to the conversation and perhaps amplify some of these issues as explicitly addressed in this volume. In part, it states:

> .... Many contemporary Buddhist teachers use the term mindfulness in a more comprehensive way than simply "remembering" or lacking confusion. According to John Dunne, Buddhist scholar at Emory University, the components of mindfulness as it is more broadly construed might include not only *sati*, but also *sampajanna* (meaning clear comprehension) and *appamada*, (meaning heedfulness). Clear comprehension includes both the ability to perceive phenomena unclouded by distorting mental states (such as moods and emotions) and the meta-cognitive capacity to monitor the quality of attention. Heedfulness in this context can be understood as bringing to bear during meditation what has been learned in the past about which thoughts, choices and actions lead to happiness and which lead to suffering.
>
> Though the contexts and interpretations of these terms may vary, scholars and meditation teachers would probably agree on the factors of *sati, sampajanna* and *appamada* as foundational to the development of mind. Moreover, as both Buddhist and secular mindfulness programs proliferate in the west, this broader use of mindfulness has become a culturally meaningful and accessible "umbrella" term for the vast majority of practitioners unversed in the intricacies of translating Sanskrit or Pali.[9]

As interest in mindfulness proliferates in both clinical and research environments, it is critical to keep in mind and communicate to others that mindfulness; however, it is construed cognitively and conceptually, is a *practice*, not merely a good idea. To my mind, one of the greatest risks we face in this growing field is that mindfulness will be grasped and understood in a limited way, simply as a concept. Unless we stress the element of embodied practice and the vibrant paradox of a non-striving orientation, unless we live it in our own lives as best we can, and allow it to inform both our research designs and our clinical work, it may be that many people yet to come into the field might imagine that they already understand what mindfulness is, and insist, naively but sincerely, perhaps, that they already live in the present moment and know how to be non-judgmental – and wonder what all the fuss is about. What is the big deal? Without grounding our concepts, intuitions, and assumptions, however deep or superficial they may be, in actual practice, the true depths of the meditation practice cannot be experienced directly. Mindfulness as a living practice, as a way of being, makes available to us to the full extent of our first-person experience, itself a huge mystery worthy of scientific and philosophical inquiry and investigation [10] This has important implications for how mindfulness-based interventions are taught, and for basic teacher-readiness and competency standards (see point # 8 below) [11].

To mistake the concept of mindfulness for the actuality would be a betrayal of what the lawfulness of dharma is offering us at this moment of confluence between contemplative and scientific/medical disciplines. It would potentially collapse the hidden dimensions that lie at the heart of authentic meditative experience and eudaemonia [12,13] and thus deny both medicine and psychology the possibility of investigating on a much deeper level our understanding of human nature, the nature of the mind itself, and of the mind/body connection, with its potential practical implications for health and disease across the lifespan. All this and more could be lost in a denaturing of the essence of mindfulness if divorced from a non-dual perspective, wisdom, and practice. This cautionary note must be kept in mind or our inveterate habits of unawareness may ironically obviate this most precious and most rare of opportunities for true creativity and healing. To that end, it is obvious that engaging in periodic mindfulness meditation retreats led by highly developed and competent teachers is essential for all those who would bring the practice of mindfulness into their work, whether it is on the clinical side, the research side, or both. There is simply no substitute for using one's own body, mind, and life as the ultimate laboratory for investigating and refining mindfulness. This perspective is implicit or explicitly emphasized by many of the contributors.

The dharma as it is described in this volume, and in the huge literature on the subject, ancient and contemporary, emphasizes that it is a living, evolving understanding, not a fixed dogma relegated to a museum honoring a culturally constrained past. As the Dalai Lama has stated on many occasions, the framework of the dharma welcomes being put to empirical test, and would need to change if it is found to be inadequate in some fundamental way according to well-accepted criteria of scientific investigation and epistemology. Now, as the glaciers of science and contemplative practices melt into each other (due to another kind of global warming) and move ever-faster in tandem to carve out new understandings of the most fundamental questions of what makes us human, the nature of mind and consciousness, and the sources of empathy, compassion, and kindness within us, this kind of open empiricism is more important than ever. While the dharma, in its most universal articulation, cannot and should not dictate how things should be explored, it is important, if not critical, for clinicians and researchers to know what they are dealing with from first-person experience before being able to authentically test the utility, efficacy, and potential of training in mindfulness and its sisters, loving-kindness and compassion, in the secular coordinate system of healing and knowing within psychology, psychiatry, psychotherapy, and medicine.

Fruitful areas for future dialogue and investigation, all eloquently addressed or pointed to in this volume, include: (1) whether mindfulness is best characterized as a state, a trait, or a way of being in relationship to any state or trait, or put otherwise, a way of seeing/knowing/being that is continually deepening and changing; (2) differentiating between thinking and awareness; and refining the clinical utility of both without confusing them; (3) elucidating the various dimensions of the experience of "self" and its neural correlates, as per the work of Farb et al. [14] and the skillful understanding and clinical utility of the experience and embodiment of anata (not self); (4) investigation of possible biological pathways via which mindfulness might exert the various effects that are now being elucidated; (5) the need for much more creative control groups to differentiate between mindfulness-specific and general enthusiasm/attention-based outcomes; (6) how we continue to remind ourselves that the deepest insights relevant to both clinical applications and also study design and interesting research questions may come out of our own direct experience of mindfulness practice as clinicians and researchers; (7) on-going conversations about skillful ways to avoid reifying mindfulness into a concept or a "thing" as it becomes increasingly well known; (8) developing well-considered and appropriate standards for training and assessing mindfulness instructors, recognizing that the particular background, first-person experience with formal mindfulness meditation practice, and attendant skill sets required to teach mindfulness-based interventions are not readily amenable to the customary manualized approach to delivery of psychological interventions; (9) effective ways to train clinically based mindfulness instructors in the practice itself and in specific curricula for specific mindfulness-based interventions without losing the essence and simplicity of the practice or collapsing its multiple-dimensionality; and (10) a continual raising of the challenges involved in taking on the work of mindfulness in clinical settings, the occupational hazards associated with professional roles and callings, and the recognition of increasingly skillful ways to catch ourselves getting caught up in ambition-driven striving or mere endless doing, and losing track of the domain of being, and of awareness itself.

In this vein, I couldn't help noticing and delighting in the fact that the words "wise" and "wisdom" were not shied away from in appropriate contexts in many of the chapters of this book. To me, this is a positive indicator that the practice itself is shifting the vocabulary we use to think and talk about effective clinical interventions and outcomes, and is elevating the ways in which we hold those who come to us who are sorely suffering and in need of being seen and met wholly and wholeheartedly (as we need to do for ourselves and each other as well). I will single out only one sentence from one chapter because it states a perspective that is often tragically missing in the clinical setting in both medicine and psychology: "In DBT, it is assumed that all people have innate access to wisdom [15]."

The heart of mindfulness-based interventions lies in a deep silence, stillness and openheartedness that is native to pure awareness and can be experienced directly both personally and interpersonally. The consequences of such cultivation (Pali: *bhavana*) may go far beyond symptom reduction and conventional coping adjustments, defining new ways of being in the body and in the world that are orthogonal to the conventional perspective on both health and well-being. Indeed, perhaps the collective efforts in this emerging field, as represented here, are defining new ways of being and knowing that express the wisdom and beauty inherent in being human - as well as new ways to measure its biological and psychological consequences. It is my hope that this volume, and the flowering of present and future research and clinical practices that it represents, be a major catalyst in our deepening understanding of the human psyche and its capacity for, and yearning for experiencing the wholeness that is its intrinsic nature.

Jon Kabat-Zinn, Ph.D.

Worcester, Massachusetts
September 15, 2008

References

1. Suzuki, S. *Zen Mind, Beginner's Mind*, Weatherhill, NY, 1970.
2. Coupled with another Handbook on the subject which appeared in German in 2004: Heidenreich T and Michalak J. Aksamkeit und Akzeptanz in der Psychotherapie: Ein Handbuch dvgt-Verlag, Tübingen, 2004.

3. Ghandi, M. http://www.quotationspage.com/quotes/Mahatma_Gandhi/

4. Ludwig, D. personal communication, June, 2008.

5. Bodhi, B. *The Noble Eightfold Path: Way to the End of Suffering*, Buddhist Publication Society Pariyatti, Onalaska, WA, 1994.

6. Grossman, P. On measuring mindfulness in psychosomatic and psychological research, *Journal of Psychosomatic Research 64*:405–408, 2008.

7. Thera, N. *The Heart of Buddhist Meditation*, Samuel Weiser, NY, 1962.

8. See *The Heart of Understanding: Commentaries on the Prajnaparamita Heart Sutra* Hanh TN Parallax Press, Berkeley 1988; also Kabat-Zinn J *Coming to Our Senses*, Hyperion, NY, 2005, pp.172-183.

9. Cullen, M. Mindfulness: A Working Definition In: *Emotional Awareness: Overcoming the Obsatacles to Psychological Balance and Compassion*, The Dalai Lama and Paul Ekman, Henry Holt, New York, 2008. pp.61–63

10. See for example, Varela FJ, Thompson E, Roach E. *The Embodied Mind: Cognitive Science and Human Experience*, MIT Press, Cambridge, 1991 ; and Thompson, E. Mind in Life: Biology, Phenomenology, and the Sciences of Mind. Belknap Harvard University Press, Cambridge, 2007; Depraz N, Varela F, Vermersch P. The Gesture of Awareness: An Account of its Structural Dynamics. In: *Investigating Phenomenal Consciousness*. Velmans M (ed.), John Benjamins Publishing, Amsterdam, 2000.

11. Santorelli, SF. CFM Guidelines for Assessing the Qualifications of MBSR Providers, 2004. In: *MBSR Professional Training Manual*, Santorelli SF and Kabat-Zinn, J (Eds), CFM UMass Medical School Worcester, MA.

12. Wallace, A. *Genuine Happiness: Meditation as the Path to Fulfillment* Wiley, Hoboken, NJ 2005.

13. Ricard, M. *Happiness: A Guide to Developing Life's Most Important Skill* Little Brown, NY 2006.

14. Farb NAS, Segal ZV, Mayberg, H et al. Attending to the present: mindfulness meditation reveals distinct neural modes of self-reference. *Social Cognitive and Affective Neuroscience Advance Access*, August 13, 2007.

15. Rizvi, SL, Welch, SS, Dimidjian S. *Mindfulness and Borderline Personality Disorder* (Chapter 13, this volume).

Introduction: Where New and Old Paths to Dealing with Suffering Meet

Fabrizio Didonna

All humanity's miseries derive from not being able to sit quietly in a room alone.
– Blaise Pascal, Seventeenth-century French philosopher

Over the last 2 decades there has been growing interest in the possible effectiveness of Eastern psychology in a clinical setting and in particular, those techniques based on practices of Buddhist origin. Numerous studies have attempted to investigate the possible clinical implications of these approaches and their application in the treatment of psychological disorders. In a spontaneous manner and through the independent work and studies of many researchers and therapists, this has given rise to a trans-epistemological approach, leading to experimentation and the application in clinical settings of principles and methods deeply rooted in Eastern psychology.

Interest in these approaches stems from an awareness that despite the importance of scientific methodology, which aims at ensuring rigorous procedure and seeks to further evidence-based knowledge, there appears to be a considerable need to combine these practices with the innate components of human nature that are decisive in influencing an individual's interpretation of events and his/her emotional attitudes and behavior. These components can be found in the *acceptance of experience* (Hahn, 1998; Hayes, Strosahl, & Wilson, 1999), a *compassionate attitude* toward one's own and other people's suffering (Gilbert, 2005), the *capacity to observe oneself without judging* (Kabat-Zinn, 1990), and the idea that the mind can observe itself and understand its own nature (Dalai Lama, Benson, Thurman, Goleman, & Gardner, 1991). They are also found in the capacity to direct attention toward the emotional sphere and the relationship of interdependence and reciprocal influence existing between the mind and the body (Goleman, 1991) and in more general terms in a harmonizing and normalizing attitude toward intrapersonal and interpersonal variables.

All of these components can be summed up in the concept of *mindfulness*.

As is well explained in the first part of this book, mindfulness is the "heart," or the core teaching, of Buddhist psychology (Kabat-Zinn, 2003), and it is inherently a state of consciousness that involves consciously attending to

1

one's moment-to-moment experience (Brown & Ryan, 2003). This state is cultivated and developed through meditation practice (Kabat-Zinn, 2005), which offers a method by which we can become less reactive to what is happening to us in the present moment. It is a way of relating to our entire experience (be it positive, negative, or neutral), which provides us with a means by which we may reduce our general level of suffering and increase our level of well-being (Germer, Siegel, & Fulton, 2005).

A crucial aspect of most mindfulness practices is a sense of heightened but detached awareness of sensory and thought experience and, as Wolinsky (1991) argues, mindfulness is actually the way out of the everyday trances we live at the mercy of through unconscious, habitual, automatic patterns of conditioning. Understanding the therapeutic value of these processes may represent a particularly important integration of Eastern and Western psychologies (Walsh, 1996).

The ever-growing integration between mindfulness and psychotherapy is justified by the fact that mindfulness can be considered a trans-theoretical construct that has been used and integrated into different Western theoretical and therapeutic approaches that up to only two decades ago had few, if any, points of contact and dialogue. Today, different therapeutic models (cognitive-behavior therapy, constructivism, evolutionary psychology, humanist psychology, psychoanalysis, brain science, traumatology, positive psychology) now seem to have found a unifying factor and significant shared element that will make it possible, in the future, to better understand and develop the therapeutic factors common to all effective psychological treatments. Indeed, it can be argued that the mechanisms of change that form the basis of mindfulness meditation can be found in most Western psychotherapeutic perspectives.

Mindfulness-based approaches also pay particular attention to the importance of personal resources and potential and to the capacity of an individual's "system" to heal itself (or healing from within). By doing so, individuals spontaneously reach a point (especially when properly guided and oriented) at which they may pass from a state of imbalance and distress to a state of greater harmony and serenity with respect to themselves with a consequent enhanced subjective perception of well-being. Mindfulness practice (and all of the therapeutic possibilities that may stem from its use and application) is a discipline that unites all of the above "healing" components and provides a point of convergence in the fertile dialogue that has arisen over the last two decades between the East and West within the sphere of psychological science.

The Dialogue Between Western and Eastern Psychologies

Eastern meditative traditions and Western psychology have both aspects in common as well as significant differences. In order to better integrate the differing scientific approaches and methods of investigation, these similarities and differences must be fully understood. Western science has historically focused on the observer-independent physical world that can be studied objectively, using empirical facts and excluding subjective experience. Western psychology, and especially neuroscience, tends to view the mind from a mechanistic perspective, in which an often used metaphor is that of the mind as machine. From this perspective, it has been suggested that meditation works through such psychological mechanisms as relaxation, exposure, desensitization, dehypnosis, deautomatization, catharsis, and decounterconditioning (Murphy & Donovan, 1997). Other suggestions of cognitive mechanisms include insight, self-monitoring, self-acceptance, and self-understanding (Baer, 2003). Potential physiological mechanisms include decreased arousal, changes in autonomic nervous system activity, stress immunization, and hemispheric synchronization and laterality shifts (e.g., Cahn & Polich, 2006). Some of these mechanisms have often been misinterpreted in a reductionistic way, leading to a limited understanding of the processes of meditation (Wilber, 2000b). On the contrary, Eastern meditative disciplines have a very different view of the mind. These traditions, and Buddhism in particular, have focused primarily on the human mind and consciousness as the primary subjects of introspective investigation, which they see as the source of human joy and suffering, and, in general, as the source of all phenomena (Walsh & Shapiro, 2006) to the degree that they are considered to have a tremendous impact on the understanding of the rest of the world (Wallace, 1999).

Buddhist tradition maintains that, in the words attributed to the Buddha, "All phenomena are preceded by the mind. When the mind is comprehended, all phenomena are comprehended," and "by bringing the mind under control, all things are brought under control" (Santideva, 1961, p. 68, as cited in Wallace, 1999). This perspective differs from that of Western modern science, which assumes that the mechanistic control of the environment, particularly the body and the brain, can alter one's sense of well-being, comfort, and distress.

Another important point is that Western culture tends to be monophasic, meaning that it is centered on, and conceptualized within, the usual waking state of consciousness, whereas the culture of meditative traditions (both Eastern and Western) is polyphasic and multistage, drawing on multiple states of consciousness and multiple adult developmental stages (Laughlin, McManus, & Shearer, 1992; Wilber, 2000a). As meditative practices are studied using a Western scientific paradigm, there is a danger of "degeneracy," in which multiple dimensions are simplified into fewer ones, resulting in a loss of complexity and multidimensionality (Tart, 1992).

According to Thurman (1991), scientists have more often than not considered reality to be something external to the world of human thought in as much as reality is part of the physical world. They have thought that the environment must be tamed, controlled, and modified in order to be adapted to human needs. In order to understand the outside world, Western science has without a doubt made extraordinary efforts and achieved excellent results. Examples of this are the use of chemistry, pharmacology, and surgery to cure illness, both physical and psychological. However, Western science has focused solely on the study of potential cures outside the self, introducing them into ourselves via highly advanced technologies. And yet by doing so, it has given less importance to the positive and therapeutic potential that each one of us has within ourselves. Buddhist tradition, on the contrary, focuses on the importance of internal science and considers the science of the mind to be the most important to the internal sciences, the king of all sciences. These beliefs have developed, thanks to the intense and antique tradition based on the practice of meditation.

Another important difference between the two psychologies lies in the methods and the means for obtaining mental health. Both systems of belief have their own theories, but there is room for fruitful and effective collaboration between the two. Western psychotherapy tends to focus mainly on *the content* of the consciousness and does not try to achieve the more radical transformation proposed by Buddhist psychology, which focuses on the process of the consciousness. The aim is to free individuals from negative mental states by altering the perceptive and cognitive processes.

Westerners that have tried to understand and adopt these meditative practices have had the opportunity to try them out on themselves involving their own very intense and profound sensations and emotions. Thanks to these experiences, they have been able to develop positive psychological competences, for example, managing "destructive emotions" such as anger, mental agitation, and attachment. In this process, they have managed to cultivate a lifestyle that enables them to prevent what Western culture would consider to be "mental illness".

In the past few decades, rigorous scientific studies based on Western technologies have demonstrated that meditation practiced by experts such as Buddhist monks can modify cerebral activity and have a positive influence on individual's health, both mental and physical.

The aim is to open up dialogue on the issue of therapy for mental health between these two cultures, which differ significantly from technological, scientific, and ideological points of view. At the same time, they both focus on the search for human well-being in all of its components and for ways to overcome suffering. As Engler has stated (Wilber, Engler & Brown, 1986), when the two psychologies are combined, the result is a much more complete diagram of human development. This combination makes it possible to trace the developments that have been well founded and well studied in Western psychology and to see, therefore, how they can be improved by integrating the techniques of Eastern psychologies.

In many ways this book is the fruit of this fertile dialogue between the two cultures, the two sciences, and the two psychologies that has taken place over the past decades. It exemplifies the result of a synthesis, translated into conceptual models and therapeutic interventions, that is the expression of the integration of Eastern psychology with its rigorous principles dating back thousands of years and the ability to translate scientific progress and theoretical advances into operational models and therapeutic techniques that can be scientifically verified and belong, therefore, to Western psychological cultures.

Unity of the Mind and Body

An important aspect to be emphasized in mindfulness approaches is the considerable relevance attributed to the *unity of the mind and body*, whereby the identification and description of bodily sensations and perceptions open up a channel of information with respect to the cognitive-emotional sphere. It should be noted that in mindfulness interventions, the conception of an individual's relationship with the body is substantially different from that normally adopted in Western culture and, more specifically, with respect to psychotherapy, in standard cognitive-behavioral approaches (which make little effort to contemplate the physical dimension), but also in other psychotherapeutic models that may even involve physical contact with the patient. While these latter models lead patients to experience bodily sensations and/or emotions evoked by external stimuli, the practice of mindfulness allows patients to explore the dimension of their own physicality in an autonomous, spontaneous, and decentered manner. This aspect is found to be all the more useful if one considers that a number of patients have difficulty expressing their thoughts and emotions through verbal communication and would rather make use of the body as a metaphor of their experiences.

This fundamental unity of mind and body has basically been lost in Western culture. In meditative practice this union is a crucial assumption: The two entities communicate in an active and continuous way leading to a concept of, a whole living being that continuously interacts with its internal world. Behind this main difference between the two cultures are a very different understanding of the concept of mind and a different mental representation of the idea of health and illness. The point of view of Eastern psychology stimulates the emergence of a wider vision compared to the Western view in as much as it recognizes this basic unity of mind and body.

The basis of this difference is a significant dichotomy that has characterized Western thought since the seventeenth century when Descartes introduced the subdivision of the whole being into separate entities: the body and the mind. According to Kabat-Zinn (1990), this is, at one level, an efficient simplification, but what we often tend to forget is that the mind and the body are only separated abstractly, from the point of view of thought. This Cartesian dualism of mind and body has permeated Western culture to the point that it has nearly eliminated the entire sphere of body–mind interactions as a legitimate field of scientific research. We can no longer think of health and illness as entities that belong separately to the body or the mind because they are extremely interconnected. Only recently, as the weak points of the dualistic paradigm have become more evident, has this tendency started to be turned upside down.

The Concept of Illness in Eastern and Western Cultures

Modern Western medicine has never given great importance to developing an understanding of the experiences of the internal functioning of individuals focusing almost exclusively on external appearances (the symptom) and concentrating, therefore, on eliminating the external manifestation rather than the latent cause in the organism, that is, the root of the problem. Therefore, the fact that Westerners tend to ignore the inside of the body and its processes comes first of all from our approach to illness: The "miracle medicines" that were developed and widely diffused in the 1930s and 1940s, thanks to the discovery of antibiotics, took over the public imagination, and within a very short amount of time, it was assumed that in the end science would be able to demonstrate that every physical problem had its cause in invasive microorganisms and germs.

This way of dealing with health problems was even extended to mental illness. This is demonstrated by the often overuse of pharmaceuticals that influence the mind and emotions. Attention was taken away from internal states to focus on the external world. As Thurman (1991) states, in the West our ability to influence the external reality has by far surpassed the power we have over ourselves. Today we are at a point at which illness is seen as something that invades us and as such must be fought against using external means that are often, unfortunately, just as invasive.

As Goleman (2003) has clearly pointed out, in the West, medicines have become the most common solution to dealing with destructive emotions, that is, those that create significant suffering for ourselves and others. Without questioning the fact that pharmaceuticals that alter and stabilize mood have helped millions of persons, it is possible to point out alternative ways to control the mind. Differently from modern science, which has concentrated on developing ingenious chemical compounds to help people overcome the most intoxicating emotions, Buddhist psychology offers more difficult paths to recover involving a series of methods aimed at training the mind through the practice of meditation.

From a Western point of view, mental health is defined by defect as absence of psychiatric pathologies, that is, in the West normalcy is the aim. However, in Buddhist psychology, for example, normalcy is only the starting point for practicing the principles that lead to freedom from suffering and mental uneasiness.

Tibetan Buddhism has a very refined psychology that has been practiced for more than 2,000 years as well as a model of well-being that extends our concept of mental health. Buddhist psychology has developed an elaborate model of the mind that, as is the case for every complete psychological system, describes how perception, motivation, cognition, and emotions work in detail and analyzes both the causes of human suffering (etiology) and the ways out of this suffering (therapy). It has developed its own representation of the mind and how it works as well as its own definition of mental health. Over the centuries, it has defined a precise map of how changes in the mind and body have a reciprocal influence on one another and has developed a series of techniques aimed a voluntarily controlling these changes.

This psychology allows Westerners to have a complementary vision and perspective with regard to some of the more central questions of modern psychology: the possibility to cultivate mental health, the nature of the mind, the limits of the growth potential of human beings, and the tools and methods needed to enact changes on the psyche.

Negative and Positive Mental Factors

In the Buddhist model of the mind and mental health, the measurement used is a single moment of the mind characterized by several mental factors. The concept of "mental factor" partially corresponds to the Western concept of "emotion," but this is not the appropriate term since some of the factors are cognitive or perceptive (Goleman, 1991).

Every mental factor has unique properties that influence our perception of reality and our subjective experience moment after moment. For this reason, the primary cause of changes in experience should not be attributed to external realities, to objects, but rather to the properties of that specific moment in our mind and conscience. It is also well known in Western psychology that any fact in our life can be considered pleasant or unpleasant depending on the situation we find ourselves in and the "lenses" we wear to examine it. Every mental state, every moment of the mind, is made up of a changeable variety of properties that can be combined in order to determine a particular mental state and its tone (Goleman, 1991). Abidharma, one of the branches of Buddhist psychology, takes about 50 mental factors into consideration, half of which are considered to be negative or harmful in as much as they distort one's perception of reality, and the others are considered to be positive and beneficial. The rule of mental health in this system is very "simple" and direct because it is based on experience: Negative or harmful states are those that do not lead to calmness, tranquillity, balance, and meditation. This is the basic rule in this psychological system: If a mental factor supports and promotes balance, then it is to be considered positive and beneficial (Goleman, 1991).

The basic negative mental factors are *illusion* or *ignorance, attachment* or *desire*, and *aversion* or *hostility. Illusion* or *ignorance* is to be understood as a perceptive defect, a fogging up of the mind that inhibits individuals from seeing things clearly and without making any sort of judgment. *Attachment* or *desire* is expressed as a selfish longing for gratification, which tends to overestimate the quality of what one is desiring (idealization) and distorts reality in as much as it leads the person to remain anchored to an object or thought, creating a sort of fixation that is difficult to break away from. *Aversion* and *hostility* are to be understood as intense anger that leads to a distortion of reality, but in the opposite direction of attachment, and that makes a person see everything in a negative way (see also Chapters 1 and 2 of this volume). Combinations of these factors lead to various types of distress. For example, anger can lead to fury, revenge, contempt, and envy, while attachment brings about phenomena such as avarice, futility, various forms of dependency and addictions, excitement, and mental agitation. According to the Abidharma, excitement often influences people's mind because it sets the mind up for uncontrollable and useless fantasies. Basically we prefer the flow of awareness: a normal and habitual condition of excitement and agitation. It is this very agitated and destructive "mental state," which disrupts a person's overall well-being, that meditation aims to relax and heal (Goleman, 1991).

Each negative mental factor is countered by a health factor that is diametrically opposed to it and that can replace it through a mechanism similar to "reciprocal inhibition," which is used in systematic desensitization in cognitive-behavioral techniques. For example, relaxation inhibits its physiological opposite, which is tension (Goleman, 1988). In other words, for every negative mental factor, there is a corresponding positive one that can dominate it (e.g., penetration, mindfulness, non-attachment, impartiality), and when a positive health factor is present in a mental state, the harmful one it is suppressing cannot reappear.

When one factor or a group of specific factors frequently inhabit the mental state of an individual, it becomes one of that individual's personality traits: The sum total of a person's mental factors determines his/her type of personality.

The issue of motivation is closely related to mental factors. Mental states are what push a person to look for one thing and avoid another. If a mind is dominated by greed, this will become the predominant motivational factor and the individual's behavior will be influenced as a consequence, that is, by seeking to conquer the object of his/her desire.

Mindfulness Meditation, Cognitive Processes, and Mental Suffering

One of the main factors that causes and maintains mental suffering (e.g., depression, anxiety) is the relationship that people have learned to activate in relation to their own private experience. An important aspect of this relationship is people's tendency to let themselves be overcome and dominated by thoughts that start from far away, deep in our minds, and slowly spread out to a point in which they can no longer be controlled and taken over. During meditation the same thing happens and we become aware of it. People become aware, maybe for the first time, of the fact that we are continuously immersed in an uninterrupted flow of thoughts that come regardless of our will to have them or not, one after the other, in very rapid succession. Indeed this is simply the nature of our mind, intrinsically transient and fluctuating. Therefore, the problem is not to eliminate the thoughts that are generated, but rather to disidentify oneself from them. One of the most valuable teachings and principles mindfulness-based programmes are based on (e.g., MBSR, Kabat-Zinn, 1990, and MBCT, Segal, Williams & Teasdale, 2002) is this idea of *not being your own thoughts*.

Patanjali (1989) speaks about this "process of identification," but broadens the concept as it is understood by modern psychology, which maintains that the ego identifies itself in objects and people, that is, stimuli coming from the outside world. Patanjali suggests that there is something that lies beneath even the smallest thought, and this is when we identify with this, without being aware of it, that we believe we are the thoughts we are thinking. Patanjali claims something that is radically different from the Western concept of "I think, therefore I am," basically assuming that we are different from our thoughts. As the mind becomes less and less identified with the content of our thoughts, the greater our ability to concentrate and the greater the resulting sense of calm.

Meditation seems to function not by changing the contents of our mind, but rather our identification with these contents through a "seeing" that is more accepting, intuitive, and immediate, thanks to which the coercive power of some cognitive-affective contents progressively decreases until it eventually disappears. Consequently, the central theme of psychopathology seems to focus on automating our cognitive and emotional processes, and crystallizing thought configurations, memories, emotions, and bodily reactions that become automatic beyond our awareness of them and will to control them (Segal, Williams & Teasdale, 2002). In some ways mindfulness works in the opposite direction. As will be carefully explained in various chapters in this book, the processes of *decentering* and *disidentification*, which in standard cognitive therapy are considered a means for achieving the end (i.e., changing the contents of a though), are actually the end itself of therapy based on mindfulness. Non-attachment and non-identification with what we take to be real is the basis of mindfulness-based approaches.

Rumination is one of the major cognitive processes in many psychological illnesses. When people worry or ruminate about their problems, even if it seems to them that they are facing the difficulty, they are actually moving further away from a direct perception of the nature of the difficulty. This happens because ruminating always involves making a judgment about the experience. Meditation techniques based on mindfulness work in exactly the opposite direction favoring a "letting-go" attitude toward one's own thoughts. This is an indispensable skill for people's psychological and physical health since it helps them avoid getting stuck once again in harmful vicious cycles. The worst damage caused by depressive rumination is the fact that the ruminative thought feeds itself continuously. This process generates thoughts and, therefore, emotions that become more and more intense and far from the actual situation, such that over time it becomes more and more difficult to differentiate reality from one's judgment of it. For this reason, according to mindfulness, it is extremely important that patients learn how to disidentify themselves from their thoughts.

Mindfulness-based programs seem to be able to directly intervene on several aspects of ruminative thoughts by exploiting the repetitive way these thoughts work. The possibility to disidentify ourselves from our own thoughts can free us up from one of the strongest and most deeply rooted attachments: the attachment to thinking for the sake of thinking, that is, being dependent on the incessant mental conversation that goes on in our minds. There seems to be a unique fascination with this attachment since we only feel normal when our minds are thinking a lot and since we think that the solution to all of our problems can come solely from thoughts as if we had a sort of blind faith in the presumed magical power of thinking and re-thinking. Mindfulness offers a passage through which thoughts can be stripped of the importance we attribute to them. When we realize that our thoughts are non-concrete and have no substance, that their true nature does not necessarily have anything to do with reality, we have overcome the obstacle of attachment and the possibility that it will degenerate into the negative effects of rumination.

Through diligently practicing the ability to detach ourselves from our own thoughts, our consciousness gradually evolves. The consistent practice of meditation leads to the intentional suspension of every judgment and evaluation we make regarding what happens around us and inside us. This allows us to observe and accept, without wanting to change, the processes of thought and our emotional reactions in all areas of experience. Therefore, the main aim of mindfulness-based programs is to help individuals make a transformation at the root of their relationship with their thoughts, feelings, and physical sensations that contribute to activating and maintaining psychopathological states.

The issues that have been discussed demonstrate why and how, especially in the last 20 years, there has been a natural and fruitful synthesis between mindfulness meditation and cognitive-behavioral approaches. This synthesis has made significant integrations between the two perspectives possible, many of which will be illustrated in this handbook.

The Clinical Relevance of Mindfulness-Based Treatment

There are an estimated 10 million practitioners of meditation in the United States and hundreds of millions worldwide. The widespread use of meditation in all the major world religions is based on the experience of many that meditation aids several processes related to personal development. Deurr (2004) points out that meditation is one of the most widely used, lasting, and researched psychological disciplines worldwide. In the last 20 years, there has been a dramatic increase in clinical interventions that use meditation skills, especially in the form of mindfulness. Salmon, Santorelli, and Kabat-Zinn (1998) have reported that over 240 hospitals and clinics internationally were offering mindfulness-based stress-reduction trainings as of 1997. This number has certainly significantly increased today.

One of the most significant problems psychology has had in drawing upon the practices of Eastern and Buddhist cultures is that until 15–20 years ago, the word "meditation" was considered by many to be suspect and associated with images of fraudulent mysticism (Kabat-Zinn, 1990). Meditation was almost demonized and considered solely as an esoteric aspect. In part this was due to cultural and conceptual ignorance regarding these techniques, which have only recently started to be considered in scientific research in psychology and neurology. This led some authors (Benson & Proctor, 1984), especially in the 1990s, to recommend separating meditation from its Eastern roots in order to make this practice more appealing and acceptable within Western psychotherapy practice (Carrington, 1998; Shapiro & Walsh, 1984) and in order to overcome suspiciousness and prejudices. However, leaving out the spiritual aspect of meditation practice may limit a complete understanding of the potential of this practice (Kabat-Zinn, 1990).

Eastern roots need to be manifested in a universal way and language as skillful means, so that people who are suffering can understand why meditation might be helpful to them without all the cultural and ideological baggage that invariably accompanies the whole Eastern gestalt, and for that matter, spirituality as it is often spoken about (Jon Kabat-Zinn, personnal communication, 2008).

The clinical areas of use of mindfulness-based treatment today are extremely broad, and various outcome studies have highlighted the clinical relevance of these forms of treatment with respect to a variety of disorders. Mindfulness is a key component of several standardized therapy models, most of which are included in the cognitive-behavioral approach as will be widely illustrated in this handbook: the Mindfulness-Based Stress Reduction (MBSR) protocol (Kabat-Zinn, 1990), perhaps the first model involving a clinical application of mindfulness, which has been found to be effective in the treatment of various anxiety disorders, especially GAD, panic disorder, and social phobia (Kabat-Zinn et al., 1992; Borkovec & Sharpless, 2004; Miller, Fletcher, & Kabat-Zinn, 1995); the Mindfulness-Based Cognitive Therapy (MBCT) model (Segal et al., 2002), an integration of cognitive therapy and MBSR, which has been found to be effective in significantly reducing the relapse rate in major depression; the integration between evolutionary psychology and compassion in psychotherapy by Paul Gilbert (2005); Marsha Linehan's Dialectical-Behavioral Dialectrical-Behavioral Theraphy (DBT) model, which comprises an important mindfulness-based treatment component and which has demonstrated significant effectiveness in reducing multi-impulsive and suicidal behaviors in patients suffering from borderline personality disorder (Linehan, 1993a, b); and the Acceptance and Commitment Therapy (ACT; Hayes et al., 1999), which is consistent with mindfulness approaches though it does not explicitly include mindfulness or meditation training. In this last therapy method, patients learn to recognize an observing self able to see their own thoughts, emotions, and body sensations and view them as separate from themselves. In addition to these, as will be well described in Parts 3 and 4 of the handbook, there are at this moment several other relevant application of mindfulness-based approaches for many different psychological disorders in various clinical settings and across diverse populations.

Regarding the state of the art (see also Chapter 3 of this volume), Baer's (2003) judgment after reviewing the empirical literature is that "mindfulness-based interventions can be rigorously operationalized, conceptualized, and empirically evaluated" (p. 140) and that at present they meet the American Psychological Association Division 12 designation as "probably efficacious." Studies of the effectiveness of these approaches are encouraging, but further investigation with more randomized and controlled studies is still required. It would be important to conduct methodologically sound empirical evaluations of the effects of mindfulness interventions for a range of problems, both in comparison to other well-established interventions and as a component of treatment packages.

We also need to better understand which mindfulness-based interventions work and for whom, and which strategies work best for particular patients and conditions. It will be possible to reach these goals by developing valid and reliable measures of mindfulness (see Chapter 9 of this volume), allowing measurement of mindfulness and its components and the associations between them and clinical change.

Another central issue to be investigated in working with psychological problems is whether or not there are particular brain processes associated with specific clinical conditions that mindfulness practice either augments or reduces. We also have to improve our understanding of the cognitive, emotional, behavioral, biochemical, and neurological factors that contribute to the state of mindfulness and investigate what mechanisms of action of mindfulness training actually lead to clinical change (exposure, relaxation, cognitive, and behavior change). In order to reach these goals we need to stimulate and increase the dialogue between mindfulness-based perspectives, Eastern traditions, and neuroscience.

Outline and Aims of the Book

One of the major stimuli behind the development of this project was the need to bring together, in an operative, pragmatic, and easily accessible form, the ever-increasing amount of knowledge and experience now available from research and practice about mindfulness and its clinical application. This book illustrates the links between theory, science, and the therapeutic application of mindfulness for psychological and physical problems, highlighting the connections of these themes with Eastern tradition. The book is divided into four parts.

Part 1 (Chapters 1–4) covers theoretical issues and includes chapters on the origin and conceptualization, phenomenology and state of the art of research on the constructs of mindfulness and meditation. This part provides an important theoretical framework and rationale for the clinical sections of the book.

Part 2 (Chapters 5–9) addresses the relationships between mindfulness and clinical problems, especially regarding psychopathology, explaining the rationale of the use of mindfulness practice for mental diseases. Several relevant clinical and phenomenological issues are also discussed, such as the use of compassion and metaphor in psychotherapy, and the feeling of emptiness. The possibilities to assess and measure mindfulness components and the possible effects of mindfulness-based interventions for non-clinical and clinical populations are also illustrated.

Part 3 (Chapters 10–20) illustrates several mindfulness-based interventions for a wide range of psychological disorders, but also for some severe medical problems (cancer, chronic pain), for which this kind of approach has shown clinical relevance and effectiveness. The chapters include a clear explanation of the rationale for using mindfulness-based therapy with the specific diseases discussed, illustrations of case studies, and descriptions of the limitations and obstacles of the interventions as well as the strategies and techniques that can be used to deal with problems and to implement mindfulness interventions.

Part 4 (Chapters 21–25) shows how it is possible to implement and provide mindfulness-based interventions for specific populations (children, the elderly) and in specific clinical settings (individual, inpatient treatment). The last chapter in this part illustrates and explores some of the implications for clinicians wishing to use mindfulness-based approaches in terms of the training that they need to be able to competently deliver the clinical intervention.

Appendix A illustrates some classic mindfulness exercises that can help readers both to more thoroughly understand mindfulness-based approaches as well as to start developing their own meditation practice. Appendix B lists a number of resources in several countries helpful for readers who wish to train themselves in mindfulness-based approaches or maintain and deepen their own meditation practice.

All the chapters were written by well-known experts and leaders in several fields of mindfulness-based approaches and by clinical researchers with extensive experience in the implementation of this kind of treatment with their respective population and in their respective setting.

This book will hopefully provide readers with a comprehensive and integrated volume that illustrates the current development and evolution of *third wave approach* in cognitive-behavioral therapy, as well as a practical and valuable tool for practitioners interested in applying mindfulness in a wide range of clinical settings. I hope and wish that this book will serve as a helpful source of information for clinicians, researchers, and scholars from a wide range of disciplines, in particular psychology, psychiatry, and the social sciences, who wish to learn and/or more thoroughly understand mindfulness and its clinical applications. The handbook can also serve as a reference text for university students and for trainees in psychology, psychiatry, social work, psychiatric nursing, counseling, and in general for all mental health professionals.

I sincerely hope that this book will inspire future creative and novel applications of mindfulness-based approaches on the part of clinical practitioners, as well as stimulate further research that investigates the effectiveness and power of mindfulness practice in achieving clinical change. This could favor the opening of at least some of the many "closed doors" in the complex understanding of mental functioning and human suffering.

The true value of a human being is determined primarily by the measure and sense in which he has attained liberation from the self. We shall require a substantially new manner of thinking if humanity is to survive.
                    Albert Einstein (From The World as I see it, 1934)

References

Baer, R. A. (2003). Mindfulness training as a clinical intervention: A conceptual and empirical review. *Clinical Psychology: Science and Practice, 10*(2), 125–143.

Benson, H., & Proctor, W. (1984). *Beyond the relaxation response*. New York: Putnam/Berkeley.

Borkovec, T. D., & Sharpless, B. (2004). Generalized anxiety disorder: Bringing cognitive-behavioral therapy into the valued present. In S. C. Hayes, V. M. Follette, M. M. Linehan, (Eds.), *Mindfulness and acceptance*. New York: Guilford Press.

Brown, K. W., & Ryan, R. M. (2003). The benefits of being present: Mindfulness and its role in psychological well-being. *Journal of Personality and Social Psychology, 84*(4), 822–848.

Cahn, B. R., & Polich, J. (2006). Meditation States and Traits: EEG, ERP, and Neuroimaging Studies. *Psychological Bulletin, 132*(2), 180–211.

Carrington, P. (1998). *The book of meditation*. Boston: Element Books.

Dalai Lama, Benson, H., Thurman, F., Goleman, D., Gardner, H. (1991). *MindScience, an East-West dialogue*. Boston: Wisdom Publications.

Deurr, M. (2004). *A powerful silence: The role of meditation and other contemplative practices in American life and work*. Northampton, MA: Center for Contemplative Mind in Society.

Germer, C., Siegel, R., & Fulton, P. (Eds.) (2005). *Mindfulness and psychotherapy*. New York: Guilford Press.

Gilbert, P. (2005). *Compassion*. New York: Routledge.

Goldstein, J., & Kornfield, J. (1987). *Seeking the heart of wisdom: The path of insight meditation*. Boston: Shambhala.

Goleman, D. (1988). *The meditative mind*. Los Angeles: JP Tarcher.

Goleman, D. (1991). The Tibetan and Western models of mental health. In R. Thurman, & Goleman, D. (Eds.), *Mind science, East and West*. Boston: Wisdom Publications.

Goleman, D. (2003). *Destructive emotions*. New York: Bantam Books.

Hahn, T. N. (1998). *The heart of Buddha's teaching: Transforming suffering into peace, joy and liberation*. Berkeley, CA: Parallax.

Hayes, S. C., Strosahl, K., & Wilson, K. G. (1999). *Acceptance and commitment therapy*. New York: Guilford Press.

Kabat-Zinn, J. (1990). *Full catastrophe living*. New York: Delacorte

Kabat-Zinn, J., Massion, A. O., Kristeller, J., Peterson, L. G., Fletcher, K. E., & Pbert, L. (1992). Effectiveness of a meditation-based stress reduction program in the treatment of anxiety disorders. *American Journal of Psychiatry, 149*, 936-943.

Kabat-Zinn, J. (2003). Mindfulness-based interventions in context: Past, present, and future. *Clinical Psychology: Science and Practice, 10*, 144-156.

Kabat-Zinn, J. (2005). *Coming to our senses*. London: Piatkus Books Ltd.

Linehan, M. (1993a). *Cognitive-behavioral therapy of borderline personality disorder*. New York: Guilford Press.

Linehan, M. (1993b). *Skills training manual for treating borderline personality disorder*. New York: Guilford Press.

Laughlin, C., McManus, J., & Shearer, J. (1992). *Brain, symbol and experience*. New York: Columbia University Press.

Miller, J., Fletcher, K, & Kabat-Zinn, J. (1995). Three year follow-up and clinical implications of a mindfulness meditation-based stress reduction intervention in the treatment of anxiety disorders. *General Hospital Psychiatry, 17*, 192-200.

Murphy, M., & Donovan, S. (1997). *The physical and psychological effects of meditation* (2nd ed.). Sausalito, CA: Institute of Noetic Sciences.

Patanjali (Feuerstein, G. trans.) (1989). The Yoga-Sutra of Patanjali: A New Translation and Commentary. Inner Traditions.

Salmon, P. G., Santorelli, S. F., & Kabat-Zinn, J. (1998). *Intervention elements promoting adherence to mindfulness-based stress reduction programs in the clinical behavioural medicine setting*. New York: Springer.

Segal, Z. V., Williams, M. G., & Teasdale, J. D. (2002). *Mindfulness-based cognitive therapy for depression: A new approach to preventing relapse*. New York: Guilford Press.

Shapiro, D. H., Jr., & Walsh, R. N. (Eds.). (1984). *Meditation*: Classic *and con-*tem*porary perspectives*. New York: Aldine.

Tart, C. E. (1992). *Transpersonal psychologies* (3rd ed.). New York: HarperCollins.

Thurman, R. (1991). Tibetan psychology: Sophisticated software for the human biocomputer. In R. Thurman & D. Goleman (Eds.), *Mind science, East and West*. Boston: Wisdom Publications.

Wilber, K. (2000a). *The collected works of Ken Wilber, Vol 5-8*. Boston, MA: Shambhala.

Wilber, K. (2000b). *Integral psychology: Consciousness, spirit, psychology, therapy*. Boston: Shambhala.

Wilber, K., Engler, J., & Brown, D. (1986). *Transformation of consciousness*. Boston: Shambala.

Wallace, B. A. (1999). The buddhist tradition of samatha: Methods for refining and examining consciousness. *Journal of Consciousness Studies, 6*(2), 175-187.

Walsh, R. (1996). Toward a synthesis of Eastern and Western psychologies. In A. A. Sheikh & K. S. Sheikh (Eds.), *Healing East and West* (pp. 542-555). New York: Wiley.

Walsh, R., & Shapiro, S. L. (2006). The meeting of meditative disciplines and western psychology: A mutually enriching dialogue. *American Psychologist, 61*(3), 227-239.

Wolinsky, S. (1991). *Trances people live, healing approaches in quantum psychology*. Falls Village: CT: The Bramble Company.

Part 1

Theory, Conceptualization, and Phenomenology

Mindfulness: What Is It? Where Did It Come From?

Ronald D. Siegel, Christopher K. Germer, and Andrew Olendzki

We can make our minds so like still water that beings gather about us, that they may see, it may be, their own images, and so live for a moment with a clearer, perhaps even with a fiercer life because of our quiet.

William Butler Yeats

Throughout history, human beings have sought to discover the causes of suffering and the means to alleviate it. Sooner or later, we all ask the same questions: "Why am I not feeling better?" "What can I do about it?" Inhabiting a physical body inevitably exposes us to pain associated with sickness, old age, and death. We also struggle emotionally when confronted with adverse circumstances or with benign circumstances that we see as adverse. Even when our lives are relatively easy, we suffer when we don't get what we want, when we lose what we once had, and when we have to deal with what we do *not* want. From birth until death, we are relentlessly trying to feel better.

As this book will show, mindfulness is a deceptively simple way of relating to all experience that can reduce suffering and set the stage for positive personal transformation. It is a core psychological process that can alter how we respond to the unavoidable difficulties in life—not only to everyday existential challenges, but also to severe psychological problems such as suicidal ideation (Linehan, 1993), chronic depression (Segal, Williams, & Teasdale 2002), and psychotic delusions (Bach & Hayes, 2002).

Mindfulness is not new. It's part of what makes us human—the capacity to be fully conscious and aware. Unfortunately, we are usually only in this state for brief periods of time and are soon reabsorbed into familiar daydreams and personal narratives. The capacity for *sustained* moment-to-moment awareness, especially in the midst of emotional turmoil, is a special skill. Fortunately, it is a skill that can be learned.

Mindfulness is an elusive, yet central, aspect of the 2,500-year-old tradition of Buddhist psychology. We can talk about mindfulness or write at length about it, but to truly understand mindfulness, we have to experience it directly. This is because mindfulness points to something intuitive and preconceptual. With committed practice, every person can gradually figure out how to become more and more mindful in life, even in the face of significant suffering. Cultivating mindfulness is, and has always been, a deeply personal journey of discovery.

The Ancient Meaning of Mindfulness

"Mindfulness," as used in ancient texts, is an English translation of the Pali word, *sati*, which connotes *awareness, attention,* and *remembering.* (Pali is the language in which the teachings of the Buddha were originally recorded.) The first dictionary translation of *sati* into "mindfulness" dates to 1921 (Davids & Stede 1921/2001). As we shall see, the definition of "mindfulness" has been somewhat modified for its use in psychotherapy, and it now encompasses a broad range of ideas and practices.

Awareness is inherently powerful, and attention, which is focused awareness, is still more powerful. Just by becoming aware of what is occurring within and around us, we can begin to untangle ourselves from mental preoccupations and difficult emotions. Sometimes this can be quite simple, as in the case of a mentally retarded man who managed his anger outbursts by shifting his attention to the "soles of the feet" whenever he noticed he was angry (Singh, Wahler, Adkins, & Myers, 2003). By redirecting attention, rather than trying to control or suppress intense emotions, we can regulate how we feel.

Another aspect of mindfulness is "remembering." This does not refer to memory of past events. Rather, it means remembering to be aware and pay attention, highlighting the importance of *intention* in mindfulness practice. Each moment we remind ourselves: "Remember—be aware!"

But "mindfulness" means more than being *passively* aware or being aware for awareness' sake. The Buddhist scholar, John Dunne (2007), has pointed out that awareness, attention, and remembering (*sati*) are present when a sniper, with malice in his heart, aims at an innocent victim. Obviously this is not what we're trying to cultivate as psychotherapists, nor is it the goal of Buddhist psychology. Rather, the purpose of mindfulness in its ancient context is to eliminate needless suffering by cultivating insight into the workings of the mind and the nature of the material world. The mindfulness practitioner is actively working with states of mind in order to abide peacefully in the midst of whatever happens.

Through mindfulness, we develop "street smarts" to manage the mind (Bhikkhu, 2007). It helps us to recognize when we also need to cultivate other mental qualities—such as alertness, concentration, lovingkindness, and effort—to skillfully alleviate suffering. For example, if in meditation we are being self-critical, we may want to add a dose of compassion; if we are feeling lazy, we might want to try to raise the level of energy in the mind or body. Mindfulness alone is not sufficient to attain happiness, but it provides a solid foundation for the other necessary factors (Rapgay & Bystrisky 2007). In the classical literature, mindfulness was usually discussed in terms of its *function*, not as a goal in itself. Mindfulness is ultimately part of a project designed to uproot entrenched habits of mind that cause unhappiness, such as the afflictive emotions of anger, envy, or greed, or behaviors that harm ourselves and others.

The recent focus on mindful awareness in psychotherapy is a strategic correction to some modern treatment trends. Many well-intentioned therapists prematurely attempt to "fix" a patient's problems, unwittingly bypassing self-acceptance and self-understanding. As will be demonstrated throughout this volume, our emotional and behavioral problems can be amplified by our instinctive efforts to avoid discomfort by propelling ourselves into change-seeking activity. The approach of the new, mindfulness-oriented agenda is "awareness and acceptance first, change second."

Therapeutic Mindfulness

As mindfulness is adopted by Western psychotherapy and migrates away from its ancient roots, its meaning is expanding. Most notably, mental qualities beyond *sati* (awareness, attention, and remembering) are being included in "mindfulness" as we adapt it to alleviate clinical conditions. These qualities include *nonjudgment, acceptance*, and *compassion*

Jon Kabat-Zinn, the foremost pioneer in the therapeutic application of mindfulness, defines it as "the awareness that emerges through paying attention on purpose, in the present moment, and nonjudgmentally to the unfolding of experience moment to moment" (Kabat-Zinn 2003, p. 145). In 2004, Bishop et al. (2004) offered a consensus paper on the definition of mindfulness: Mindfulness is "self-regulation of attention so that it is maintained on immediate experience, thereby allowing for increased recognition of mental events in the present moment" and "adopting a particular orientation toward one's experience that is characterized by curiosity, openness, and acceptance" (p. 232). The second part of this definition captures an essential emotional or intentional attitude of mindfulness in clinical settings.

A stripped-down definition of "therapeutic mindfulness" that we and our colleagues at the Institute for Meditation and Psychotherapy find useful is *awareness, of present experience, with acceptance* (Germer, Siegel, & Fulton, 2005). These three elements can be found in most modern psychological literature on mindfulness. Although the "acceptance" component is implied in the classical Buddhist texts, it helps to make it explicit for clinical application. Other related shorthand expressions we might use for therapeutic mindfulness include "affectionate awareness," "mindful acceptance," "openhearted presence," and "mindful compassion."

The explicit addition of acceptance to the mindfulness formula makes sense to most psychotherapists. This is especially the case when our patients are confronted with overwhelming traumatic circumstances. Awareness without acceptance can be like looking at a scary scene under a bright floodlight. Sometimes we need softer light—like a candle—to approach difficult experience. The more intensely we suffer, it seems, the more we need acceptance and compassion to be able to work with what is occurring in our lives. Conversely, kindness without clear awareness can lead to sugar coating the difficulties of life that need to be addressed. *Sans* awareness, acceptance could become a form of defensive avoidance.

When patients come to psychotherapy, they are often in dire distress, seeking a person who will take the time to understand who they are and why they suffer. They desperately want a strategy for relief. Compassion is the invisible matrix that holds the entire enterprise. The word "compassion" comes from the Latin roots *com pati*, meaning to "suffer with." That's how we really come to understand what our patients are going through—we suffer *with* them. If we offer helpful advice to a patient without first providing acceptance and compassion, he or she simply feels misunderstood.

Similarly, in the *intra*personal, therapeutic relationship—the one we have with ourselves—compassion is also important. Self-compassion and self-acceptance are "skillful means" for being aware under trying circumstances. We need an open heart to have open eyes. When we practice mindfulness by ourselves, self-acceptance is hopefully part of our emotional landscape; in the therapy relationship, acceptance and compassion are essential for the process to be effective.

Mind*ful*ness and Mind*less*ness

A psychotherapist needs to experience mindfulness in order to integrate it into his or her clinical practice. Learning meditation from an experienced teacher is the best way to begin and is strongly recommended. Psychotherapists also benefit from a conceptual road map to guide their work. To this end, we suggest using the definition of mindfulness just mentioned: (1) *awareness*, (2) *of present experience*, and (3) *with acceptance* (Germer et al., 2005). A moment of mindfulness contains these three intertwined elements. The mindfulness-oriented therapist may ask, moment to moment, "How do I cultivate awareness of present experience with acceptance, for myself and my patient?" This can be a touchstone for practice.

While its definition is easy to remember, the direct experience of mindfulness is more elusive. Sometimes mindfulness is easiest to understand by examining its opposite. Even casual self-examination reveals that our typical mental state is remarkably mindless. We spend most of our time lost in memories of the past and fantasies of the future. More often than not, we operate on "autopilot," where our minds are in one place and our bodies are in another.

An embarrassing example of this happened to one of us recently while driving to present a workshop on mindfulness and psychotherapy:

> I was in a rush and running late. Suddenly, a few minutes into my drive, I realized that I was heading in the wrong direction on the Massachusetts Turnpike— a toll road on which the exits can seem as though they are 50 miles apart. I wondered, "Who was driving the car?" "Who decided to head west? My mind was busy preparing my presentation, while my body was steering the car automatically, skillfully heading in the wrong direction.

Similar examples abound. Consider the leading cause of emergency room visits to New York hospitals on Sunday mornings: bagel-cutting accidents. While interacting with family members on the weekend, many people are so distracted by interpersonal events that their bodies cut bagels automatically—and their bodies aren't very good at this without guidance from the conscious mind.

Another less painful example of everyday mindlessness occurs in restaurants. Have you noticed how much restaurant conversation revolves around where you ate in the past or where you might eat in the future? Only occasionally do we actually taste the food that we're eating.

And then there are our *deliberate* efforts to escape the present moment— trying to get to the "good stuff." Do you ever find yourself rushing through the dishes to get to your cup of tea, book, or television program? Have you ever had the thought, perhaps 10 minutes, into a psychotherapy session with a frustrating patient, "Darn, forty minutes to go!" When we reflect honestly, we notice that we're rushing through, or trying to get rid of, much of our life experience.

You may notice this even in the present moment: As you read these sentences, where has your mind gone? Have you had thoughts such as, "I wonder if this book is going to be worthwhile?," "Maybe I should've gotten another one," or "This is pretty interesting, I hope the rest of it is good too." Perhaps your mind has left the book entirely, and you're thinking about what you'll do later or what happened earlier today.

The pervasiveness of everyday mindlessness is particularly striking when we inquire into what really matters in our lives. Take a few seconds to recall a moment in your life that you really valued. (Really, stop reading for a moment and think of one.) Perhaps it was a special time with someone you love or a magical experience in nature. During this moment, where was your mind? Was it focused on recalling the past or imagining the future? Most people find that the moments they value the most are those in which they're fully present, noticing what is happening here and now.

These are moments of mindfulness. We notice the positions of our hands and the sensations of holding a knife and bagel. We are aware of our bodies sitting in the car when we drive, and we notice the other cars, the road, and the scenery. We taste the food we eat, and we actually experience the sight, sound, and emotional presence of our patients during psychotherapy. Right now, try noticing the position of your hands as you hold this book, the physical experience of sitting or lying down, and how your mind reacts to these words. Mindfulness involves being present to our lives.

While notoriously difficult to convey with words, the Zen Haiku tradition endeavors to capture moments of mindfulness. Here is a classic example from Matsuo Basho, a wandering Japanese poet of the seventeenth century:

> *An old pond!*
> *A frog jumps in —*
> *The sound of water.*

> (Toyomasu, 2001)

Mindfulness Practice

While it can be disturbing to notice how frequently we are mindless, and how much of our lives we wish away, there is also good news: Mindfulness can be cultivated. Just as we can improve physical fitness through regular physical exercise, we can develop mindfulness through deliberate mental practices.

Mindfulness practices all involve some form of meditation. Especially in the West, misconceptions about meditation practice abound. It may therefore be helpful to examine some of the most common misunderstandings.

Not having a blank mind: While some concentration practices are designed to empty the mind of thought, this is not an aim of mindfulness practice. Nor do we wish to become stupid or lose our analytical abilities. Instead, mindfulness practice involves training the mind to be aware of what it is doing at all times, including being aware that we are thinking when we think.

Not becoming emotionless: Many people secretly hope that mindfulness practice will relieve them of the burden of emotion. Especially when in distress, the fantasy of becoming emotionless can be quite appealing. In reality, mindfulness practice often has quite the opposite effect. Because we practice noticing the contents of the mind, we come to notice our emotions *more* fully and vividly. Our ability to recognize how we feel increases as we relinquish normal defenses, such as distracting ourselves from discomfort with entertainment or eating.

Not withdrawing from life: Because most meditation practices were originally refined by monks, nuns, and hermits, people often assume that they involve withdrawing from living a full, interpersonally rich life. While there are certainly benefits to be derived from practicing mindfulness in a simplified environment, even in these settings, one isn't exactly withdrawing. Instead, the vicissitudes of life are experienced more vividly, because we're taking the time to pay attention to our moment-to-moment experience.

Not seeking bliss: The image of the spiritual master blissfully smiling while the rest of us struggle with existential reality is very appealing. Early in their meditation careers, many people become distressed when they find that their minds wander and they feel agitated or unsettled. While exceptionally pleasant states of mind do occur, in mindfulness meditation we allow them to arise and pass—not clinging to blissful states nor rejecting unpleasant ones.

Not escaping pain: Rather than escaping pain, mindfulness practice helps us to increase our capacity to bear it. We deliberately abstain from automatic actions designed to make ourselves feel better. For example, if we are meditating and an itch arises, a typical instruction is to observe the itch and notice any impulses that arise (such as the urge to scratch)—but to not act on the urge. As a result, we actually experience pain and discomfort more vividly. This extends beyond itches and physical pain to include the full spectrum of emotional discomfort as well. As we explore and accept these unpleasant experiences, our capacity to bear them increases. We also discover that painful sensations are distinct from the suffering that accompanies them. We see that suffering arises when we react to pain with resistance, protest, or avoidance rather than moment-to-moment acceptance.

Forms of Practice

There are many ways to cultivate awareness of current experience with acceptance. Not surprisingly, all of them involve repeated practice. If we want to improve our cardiovascular fitness, we might begin by integrating physical exercise into our everyday routine—taking the stairs instead of the elevator or riding a bicycle instead of driving to work. If we want to become even more physically fit, we might set aside time to exercise formally, perhaps at a gym or health club. To really accelerate the process, we might go on a fitness-oriented vacation in which much of the day is spent in vigorous exercise. Similar options are available for cultivating mindfulness.

Everyday mindfulness: This involves reminding ourselves throughout the day to pay attention to what is happening in the moment without radically altering our routines. It means noticing the sensations of walking when we walk, the taste of our food when we eat, and the appearance of our surroundings as we pass through them. The Vietnamese Zen teacher Thich Nhat Hahn suggests a number of techniques to enhance everyday mindfulness. For example, when the telephone rings, try just listening at first, attending to the tone and rhythm of the sound as one might listen to a musical instrument. Or while driving, when the red tail lights of another vehicle appear, try appreciating their color and texture as one might do in looking at a beautiful sunset.

Formal meditation practice: This involves setting aside time to go to the mental "gym." We regularly dedicate a certain period to sit quietly in meditation. There are many types of meditation that can cultivate mindfulness. Most involve initially choosing an object of attention, such as the breath, and returning our attention to that object each time the mind wanders. This develops a degree of calmness which, in turn, enables us to better focus the mind on the chosen object. Once some concentration is established, mindfulness meditation entails directing the mind to whatever begins to predominate in the mind—usually centering on how the event is experienced in the body. These objects of attention can be physical sensations such as an itch, an ache, or a sound, or emotional experiences as they manifest in the body, such as the tightness in the chest associated with anger or the lump in the throat that comes with sadness. Regardless of the chosen object of attention, we practice being aware of our present experience with acceptance.

Retreat practice: This is the "vacation" that is dedicated entirely to cultivating mindfulness. There are many styles of meditation retreats. Most involve extended periods of formal practice, often alternating sitting meditation with walking meditation. They are usually conducted in silence, with very little interpersonal interaction, except for occasional interviews with teachers. All of the activities of the day—getting up, showering, brushing teeth, eating, doing chores—are done in silence and used as opportunities to practice mindfulness. As one observer put it, the first few days of a retreat are "a lot like being trapped in a phone booth with a lunatic." We discover how difficult it is to be fully present. The mind is often alarmingly active and restless, spinning stories about how well we're doing and how we compare to others. Memories of undigested emotional events enter, along with elaborate fantasies about the future. We get to vividly see how our minds create suffering in an environment where all of our needs are tended to. Many people find that the insights that occur—during even a single week-long intensive meditation retreat—are life transforming.

The effects of mindfulness practice seem to be dose related. If one does a little bit of everyday practice, a little bit of mindfulness is cultivated. If one does more everyday practice, and adds to this regular formal practice and retreat practice, the effects are more dramatic. While this has long been evident to meditators, it is beginning to be documented through scientific research (Lazar et al., 2005).

Why Mindfulness Now?

We are currently witnessing an explosion of interest in mindfulness among mental health professionals. In a recent survey of psychotherapists in the United States (Simon, 2007), the percentage of therapists who said that they do "mindfulness therapy" at least some of the time was 41.4%. In comparison, cognitive–behavioral therapy was the most popular model (68.8%), and psychodynamic/psychoanalytic therapy trailed mindfulness at 35.4%. Three years ago, we speculated that mindfulness could eventually become a model of psychotherapy in its own right (Germer et al., 2005). That time is rapidly approaching.

Why? One explanation is that the young people who were spiritual seekers and meditators in the 1960s and 1970s are now senior clinical researchers and practitioners in the mental health field. They have been benefiting personally from mindfulness practice for many years and finally have the courage to share it with their patients.

Another explanation is that mindfulness may be a core perceptual process underlying all effective psychotherapy—a *transtheoretical* construct. Clinicians of all stripes are applying mindfulness to their work, whether they are psychodynamic psychotherapists who primarily work relationally; cognitive–behavioral therapists who are developing new, more effective, and structured interventions; or humanistic psychotherapists encouraging their patients to enter deeply into their "felt experience." The common therapeutic question is, "How can I help the patient to be more accepting and aware of his or her experience in the present moment?"

Perhaps the strongest argument for the newfound popularity of mindfulness is that science is catching up with practice—the soft science of contemplative practice is being validated by "hard" scientific research. Meditation is now one of the most widely studied psychotherapeutic methods (Walsh & Shapiro, 2006)—although, admittedly, many of the studies have design limitations (Agency for Healthcare Research and Quality, 2007). Between 1994 and 2004, the preponderance of the research on meditation has switched from studies of concentration meditation (such as transcendental meditation and the relaxation response) to mindfulness meditation (Smith, 2004).

We are currently in a "third wave" of behavior therapy interventions (Hayes, Follette, & Linehan, 2004). The first wave focused on stimulus and response in classical and operant conditioning. The second wave was *cognitive–behavior therapy*, which works to change the content of our thoughts to alter how we feel. The current "third wave" is *mindfulness- and acceptance-based therapy*. Researchers such as Steven Hayes, the founder of Acceptance and Commitment Therapy, discovered mindfulness- and acceptance-based treatment strategies while looking for novel solutions to intractable clinical dilemmas. Others, such as Marsha Linehan, who developed Dialectical Behavior Therapy, had a personal interest in Zen Buddhism and sought to integrate principles and techniques from that tradition into clinical practice. We are now in the midst of a fertile convergence of modern scientific psychology with the ancient Buddhist psychological tradition.

In the new mindfulness and acceptance-based approach, therapists help patients shift their *relationship* to personal experience rather than directly challenging maladaptive patterns of thought, feeling, or behavior. When patients come to therapy, they typically have an aversion to what they are feeling or how they are behaving—they want *less* anxiety or *less* depression, or want to drink or eat *less*. The therapist reshapes the patient's relationship to the problem by cultivating curiosity and moment-to-moment acceptance of uncomfortable experience.

For example, a panic patient, Kaitlin, spent the previous 5 years white-knuckling the steering wheel of her car while driving to work. She was doing all the traditional behavioral strategies: She exposed herself to high-ways and bridges, she practiced relaxation, and she could effectively talk herself out of her fear of dying from a heart attack. Still, Kaitlin wondered aloud, "Why the heck do I still suffer from panic?" The answer is that Kaitlin never learned to really *tolerate anxiety itself*. She was always running away from it. She needed the missing link that the third generation of behavior therapies addresses—learning to accept inevitable discomfort as we live our lives in a meaningful way.

Another arena of research that is fueling interest in mindfulness is brain imaging and neuroplasticity. We know that "neurons that fire together, wire together" (Hebb, 1949, in Siegel, 2007) and that the mental activity of medi-tation activates specific regions of the brain. Sara Lazar et al. (2005) demon-strated that brain areas associated with introspection and attention enlarge with years of meditation practice. Davidson et al. (2003) found increased activity in the left prefrontal cortex following only 8 weeks of mindfulness training. The left prefrontal cortex is associated with feelings of well-being. Increased activity in this part of the brain also correlated with the strength of immune response to a flu vaccine. More dramatic changes could be found in the brains of Tibetan monks who had between 10,000 and 50,000 hours of meditation practice (Lutz, Grelschar, Rawlings, Richard, & Davidson, 2004).

The evidence from scientific studies is validating what meditators have long suspected, namely that training the mind changes the brain (Begley, 2007). We are now beginning to see *where* and *how much* change is possible. Furthermore, the changes that occur in the brain when we are emotionally attuned to our own internal states in meditation seem to correlate with those brain areas that are active when we are feeling connected to others (Siegel, 2007)—suggesting that therapists can train their brains to be more effective therapeutically by practicing mindfulness meditation.

Practical Applications for Psychotherapy

Psychotherapists are incorporating mindfulness into their work in many ways. We might imagine these on a continuum, from implicit to explicit applications—from those hidden from view to those that are obvious to the patient.

On the most implicit end is the *practicing therapist*. As just mentioned, when a therapist begins personally practicing mindfulness, his or her capac-ity for emotional attunement seems to increase. Regardless of theoretical ori-entation, models of psychopathology, or modes of intervention, the therapist seems to be able to more carefully attend to and empathize with a patient's experience. The therapist's need to "fix" problems diminishes as he or she cultivates the capacity to be with another's pain. Therapists feel closer to their patients, developing compassion both by becoming aware of the universality of suffering and by seeing more clearly their interconnection with others. Research in this area is just beginning (Grepmair, Mitterlehner, Loew, & Nickel, 2006; Grepmair, Mitterlehner et al., 2007).

Next along the continuum is the practice of *mindfulness-informed* psychotherapy (Germer et al., 2005). This is treatment informed by the insights that derive from Buddhist psychology and mindfulness practice. The therapist's understanding of psychopathology and the causes of human suffering change as a result of observing his or her own mind in meditation practice. Insights such as understanding the arbitrary and conditioned nature of thought, seeing the counterproductive effects of trying to avoid difficult experience, and noticing the painful consequences of trying to buttress our sense of separate self, all have an impact on how we approach our patients' problems.

Finally, the most explicit application of mindfulness to psychotherapy is *mindfulness-based* psychotherapy (Germer et al., 2005). Mindfulness-based therapists actually teach mindfulness practices to patients to help them work with their psychological difficulties. A host of mindfulness-based interventions are currently being developed for a wide range of clinical problems. Sometimes the patient is taught a traditional meditation practice, and other times that practice is customized for the patient's particular diagnosis, personality style, or life circumstances.

Untangling Terminology

As "mindfulness" is absorbed into modern psychology and Western culture, there is growing confusion about the term. It has come to cover a lot of ground. At least some of the confusion could be eliminated if we used Pali, rather than English, words. (The reader is referred to *Mindfulness in Plain English* by Bhante Gunaratana (2002) for a remarkably lucid exposition of Pali terms and how they relate to mindfulness practice.)

The following is an effort to tease apart the different meanings of mindfulness currently used in modern psychology.

Classical concept

As discussed earlier, the Pali term *sati*, which is often translated as "mindfulness," denotes "awareness," "attention," and "remembering." In the Buddhist tradition, *sati* is cultivated as a tool for observing how the mind creates suffering moment by moment. It is practiced to develop wisdom and insight, which ultimately alleviates suffering.

Psychological process

Process definitions have an *instructional* aspect—they indicate what we should *do* with our awareness. Two process definitions of mindfulness in clinical settings are "moment-to-moment, nonjudgmental awareness" (Kabat-Zinn, 1990, 2006) and "awareness, of present experience, with acceptance" (Germer, et al., 2005). These process definitions suggest, "Look at your moment-to-moment experience, and try to do it with a spirit of acceptance."

Another process definition of therapeutic mindfulness, "attentional control" (Teasdale, Segal, & Williams, 1995), suggests redirecting attention to manage emotional distress.

Process definitions are especially valuable because they identify *processes of change* or *mechanisms of action* that may help particular patients. In therapy, "mindfulness" in general is considered a change process and so are the individual elements that constitute therapeutic mindfulness—acceptance, present experience, and awareness. Different patients might require more emphasis on one element or another. For example, self-critical persons might benefit most from "acceptance," obsessive patients might be helped by focusing on "present moment sensations," and people with impulse control disorders might benefit most from greater "awareness"—observing the precursors to problem behaviors such as drinking, gambling, or overeating.

We can break down the processes even further to fine-tune treatment for particular individuals. For example, there are different styles of awareness that can benefit certain patients: *metacognitive* awareness ("thoughts are not facts") helps chronically depressed people disentangle from depressive ruminations (Teasdale et al., 2002), while people with a schizoid or detached style of relating to their feelings might benefit from a more *participatory* observational style—intimately observing feelings as they arise in the body.

Meditation practice: When someone says, "I practice mindfulness meditation," what is he or she actually doing? There are three key meditation skills often subsumed under the heading of "mindfulness meditation."

Concentration meditation: This technique has a focal object, such as the breath or a mantra. The instruction is, "When you notice that your mind has wandered, gently bring it back to [the object]." Concentration meditation produces a feeling of calmness. The Pali word most associated with concentration practice is *samatha*, while the traditional word for meditation is *bhavana*, which means "developing." "Concentration meditation" is a translation of *samatha bhavana*, the cultivation of concentration. The "relaxation response" (Benson & Klipper, 2000) is a well-known example of this meditation approach.

Mindfulness meditation

The instruction for mindfulness meditation is, "Notice whatever predominates in awareness, moment to moment." Here the intention is *not to choose* a single object of focus, but rather to explore changing experience. The skill of mindfulness cultivates insight into the nature of one's personal conditioning (e.g., "fear of disapproval," "anger at authority") and the nature of mental reality ("it's changing," "it's often unsatisfactory," "the 'self' is fluid").

This is primarily what distinguishes "mindfulness meditation" from other forms of meditation, such as concentration meditation and various forms of visualization meditation, and it is a unique contribution of Buddhist psychology. The Pali words for mindfulness meditation are *vipassana bhavana*, which translates well as the cultivation of insight or "insight meditation." Western researchers and clinicians usually use the expression "mindfulness meditation" to refer to this practice.

Making matters a bit more complicated, *sati* is actually cultivated by, and necessary for, both concentration and mindfulness meditation techniques.

That is, we need to know where the mind is to concentrate on either a single object or many arising objects. Since the mind is actively engaged with a wider range of experiences during mindfulness meditation, it can be said that *sati* is more deliberately developed in this particular practice.

During mindfulness or insight meditation, the meditator can always return to concentration practice to stabilize attention if he or she becomes lost in daydreams and discursive thinking. In this regard, concentration practice (*samatha*) facilitates mindfulness or insight (*vipassana*) practice.

Lovingkindness meditation: Lovingkindness is the *emotional* quality associated with mindfulness. Translated from the Pali word, *metta*, lovingkindness meditation can be a form of concentration meditation. The practitioner returns attention again and again to phrases such as "May I and all beings be safe, happy, healthy, and live with ease." This technique allows the person to soften into and allow arising experience to be just as it is. It is cultivating the *intention* to be loving and kind, rather than superimposing warm feelings on our moment-to-moment experience. The emotional flavor of affectionate awareness typically follows our kindly intentions. Lovingkindness (feeling safe, peaceful, healthy, and free from suffering) keeps the *function* of mindfulness practice clear in the mind of the practitioner. It is a quality of mind that ideally pervades the other meditation practices. Therefore, while practicing concentration meditation, we work to receive mental distractions with openheartedness rather than sternness; when practicing mindfulness or insight meditation, we greet all mental contents like welcome visitors.

When our *sati* (mindfulness) is strong, we can choose to switch fluidly among *metta* (lovingkindness), *samatha* (concentration), or *vipassana* (mindfulness or insight) practices, as needed, even in a single sitting of meditation. For example, if dealing with psychological trauma, we can notice when we are overwhelmed and can choose to redirect attention to the breath or external sights and sounds (*samatha*). We can also add some lovingkindness (*metta*) to our experience to reestablish a measure of calmness. When we feel more stable, we can open up the field of awareness again to observe how the trauma memories are experienced in the mind and body (*vipassana*). In other words, the three skills—concentration, mindfulness, and lovingkindness—can be selectively emphasized in meditation and daily life to reduce suffering and increase happiness.

Common usage

To make matters even more confusing, the general public in Western culture uses the term "mindfulness" loosely to refer to every variety of formal and informal secular Buddhist practice. Under this label, we have not only the different meditation skills just mentioned—lovingkindness, concentration, and mindfulness or insight—but also visualization techniques and innumerable, informal meditation strategies to deal with everyday life. Visualization meditations include practices that cultivate equanimity, such as imagining oneself as a solid mountain unaffected by the wind and weather or as a deep pond unperturbed by the waves.

As mindfulness is incorporated into diverse fields such as health care, education, and business, the term will probably continue to accrue an increasing array of meanings. Within clinical psychology, "mindfulness" is already used interchangeably with "acceptance" to describe the third wave of behavioral treatments. In the field of education, Ellen Langer (1989) describes "mindfulness" as a cognitive process that implies openness, curiosity, and awareness of more than one perspective. In the business world, Richard Boyatzis and Annie McKee (2005) encourage "mindfulness practice" to "observe emotional reality" (p. 124) in an organization and "avoid narrow focus and constant multitasking" (p. 131).

Despite the recent proliferation of interest in mindfulness and its multiplying meanings, the various uses of the term still have much in common. Only time will tell what happens to "mindfulness" as the theory and practices that began in Buddhist psychology move into new, heretofore unimaginable domains.

Radical Roots

The cultivation of mindfulness in a rigorous way comes from a tradition with ancient roots and lofty goals. These origins are important to understand so that modern clinicians don't inadvertently miss its profound potential for psychological transformation.

As far back as 4,000 years ago, we find images of yogis in ancient India sitting cross-legged in meditation, gazing inward with eyes half closed. Training the mind was understood as the principle means of achieving mental and physical health, emotional equanimity and for perfecting the human condition.

Mindfulness, as we are coming to know it in the West, was most clearly described in ancient times in the teachings of the historical Buddha. According to tradition, he was born a prince some 2,500 years ago. At the age of 29, he renounced a life of comfort and privilege to undertake rigorous mental and physical disciplines for 7 years. Finally, at age 36, he experienced a breakthrough of understanding that profoundly reordered his mind. He wandered from place to place for the next 45 years, exhibiting behaviors devoid of the usual human propensities toward attachment, aversion, or delusion. The psychological teachings he left behind—including how to cultivate mindfulness—are still accessible to us today.

For the Buddha, the mind and body are seen as the product of material causes, lacking the divine essence that was assumed by the Indo-European religions of his time. Nonetheless, in the Buddha's view the body and mind can be the vehicle for a profound experience of transcendence. Rather than breaking through to something divine, however, this experience results from a radical transformation of the mind. Consciousness itself, though conditioned, can be purified to such an extent that it entirely understands itself and its conditioning. The result is not only a deep sense of personal well-being, but also the possibility of a more evolved way of being human.

The primary interest of this tradition is the quality of consciousness in the present moment. How exactly is the mind and body manifesting here and now? Consciousness arises from a whole network of interdependent factors, including all of the details of our genetic makeup and personal history. Each moment of consciousness, in turn, has an impact upon our subsequent beliefs, feelings, and behaviors. Knowing both the causes and the effects of a moment of consciousness allows us to participate intentionally in the process of living, to steer a course away from suffering and toward healthier states.

What the Buddha saw with great lucidity on the night of his awakening was the workings of his own mind. His insights have profound implications for modern psychotherapy, as they reveal how our minds construct our experience moment by moment and how these constructions can lead to suffering. The following description is not for the faint hearted—it is a radically new psychology for many readers, and somewhat complicated, so we encourage you to consider it slowly.

How We Construct Our Experience

The Buddha saw that all experience involves a process in which the raw data streaming into the mind through the sensory organs or "sense doors" is compiled and synthesized into a virtual world of meaning. There are six sense doors in all: eye, ear, nose, tongue, body, with the mind itself viewed as the sixth. There are also five primary categories, or systems, whereby the information flowing through these sense doors is processed.

The first category is *material form*, which acknowledges that the mind and body have a material, biological foundation. The next is *consciousness*, or the act of becoming aware of an object by means of one of the six sense organs (again with the mind as the sixth organ). At this stage the eye sees, the ear hears, the tongue tastes, and so on. The third and fourth systems, which shape how consciousness manifests, are *perception* and *feeling*. Perception identifies *what* is experienced through a series of associations, interpreting incoming data in the light of historically learned patterns of recognition. For example, you can recognize just two dots and a curved line to be a face ☺ or identify the object in your hands to be a book. "Feeling" provides an affect tone for each moment of cognition, *pleasant, unpleasant*, or *neutral*. This is a hedonic assessment of each object's value to the organism. In every moment, we like, dislike, or aren't interested in what we perceive.

The fifth and final component of the construction of experience is called *formations* and reflects the intentional stance we take toward all objects that we perceive and toward which we have feelings. Volition or intention is the executive function of the mind which initiates conscious or unconscious choices. Whereas the first four systems yield a sense of *what* is happening at any given moment, the fifth decides what we are going to *do* about it.

How do these processes unfold together? Imagine that you're hungry, and you open the refrigerator door. The eye *sees* patterns of light, dark, and color in the visual field, which are quickly organized by the brain and *perceived* as a freshly made sandwich. Instantaneously, a positive *feeling* toward the sandwich arises, and an *intention* forms to pick it up and eat it. This is soon followed by the *behavior* of actually taking a bite. Consciousness creates and responds to our reality so quickly that the process is usually unconscious.

Intentions and the behaviors that follow from them tend to become habitual and turn into *dispositions*. Dispositions are the residue of previous decisions, stored in memory as habits, learned behaviors, personality traits, etc., and provide historical precedents for how to respond to each newly arising moment. Feedback loops develop, whereby one's present response to any situation is both shaped by previous experience and goes on to mold the dispositions that will influence future responses. If we enjoyed this and other sandwiches in the past, we may develop the habit of reflexively picking up and eating sandwiches, even when we're not really hungry.

Putting this all together, the six sense doors and five systems interact simultaneously to form a dynamic interdependently arising process of mind and body, constructing meaning from an ever-changing barrage of environmental information. In each moment, which can be measured in milliseconds, all this arises concurrently, organizes around a particular bit of data, and then passes away.

One unique feature of Buddhist psychology is that consciousness is regarded as an unfolding *process*, or an occurring *event*, rather than as an existing entity. Nothing permanent abides (and there is no enduring "me" to be found) because every "thing" is a series of interrelated events. The everyday sense that we (and other beings) have separate existence comes from the fact that each moment of cognition is followed by another moment of cognition, yielding the subjective sense of a stream of consciousness. We have simply learned to connect the snapshots together into a coherent narrative. This is like the illusion of continuous action that our minds create out of separate frames in a movie. Among the great insights of the Buddhist tradition is not only that this is all happening below the threshold of ordinary awareness, but also that this process can unfold in either healthy or unhealthy ways, depending on the skills of its handler.

This analysis of human experience has important and radical clinical implications. It suggests that our reality, including the sense of "self" around which so much personal psychology is centered, is based on a fundamental misunderstanding. It is as though we believed that a powerful automobile like a Ferrari was a living being—until we saw it disassembled on the floor of a workshop. When we know the component parts and how they're put together, we can never look at a Ferrari in quite the same way. Similarly, seeing the way the "self" is constructed can help both us and our patients loosen our identification with the changing kaleidoscope of thoughts and feelings that arise in the mind, allowing us to live more flexible, adaptive, happier, and productive lives.

A Physician of the Mind

The Buddha sometimes referred to himself as a physician, and to his teaching as a kind of medicine. The illness he treated was the fact that consciousness is continually influenced by patterns of conditioning that inevitably result in unhappiness, frustration, and disappointment. This is certainly an observation familiar to the modern psychotherapist. Rather than changing brain chemistry by pharmaceuticals or probing past traumas arresting normal development, however, the Buddha's approach was to help the patient gain direct insight into the nature of experience. This takes many forms.

One track is to notice the extent to which the patterns of conditioning we acquire, through learned behaviors, conditioned responses, or cultural osmosis, are for the most part built upon certain *illusions* or even *delusions*. Foremost of these are our remarkably robust habit of taking what is impermanent and subject to change to be stable or reliable; believing that the satisfaction or gratification of desires is sustainable for longer than a few moments when, because of the former point, it is not; and projecting again and again onto the field of experience the notion of a person or agent that owns, controls, or consists of what is happening. In other words, we continuously delude ourselves into believing that we can hold onto what we want and get rid of what we don't want, despite considerable evidence to the contrary. And on top of this, we delude ourselves into believing that a stable, independent "I" or "me" is running this show. To the extent these misperceptions can be gradually uncovered and corrected, considerable healing can occur.

For example, there is the story of a monk who complained to his Zen teacher that he was an angry person. The teacher said, "Show me." Since the student was not angry at the moment, he could not show it, whereupon the teacher said, "See, you are not an angry person because you are not angry all the time." Such insight into the fluidity of experience and insubstantiality of identity can be enormously helpful to patients who have core beliefs about being unworthy, unlovable, unintelligent, and so forth.

Another approach is to recognize the fact that behavior is *driven by desire*, both conscious and unconscious, and to use that knowledge to diminish and eventually eliminate the role of desire in the moment-to-moment functioning of mind and body. The impulse to like some things and dislike others leads to pulling some objects of experience closer and pushing others farther away from a sense of self that sets itself apart from what is actually happening. Ironically, say the Buddhists, the very strategies we employ to overcome the perceived shortcomings of the world as we find it—embracing what offers pleasure and rejecting what brings pain—have the result of causing and perpetuating greater suffering. The solution is to practice letting go of desire itself, which can be replaced by an attitude of equanimity or acceptance. In clinical practice, we see countless examples that "what we resist persists" and how patients suffer terribly from wishing that things would be other than they are, that is, from not facing "reality."

The underlying tendencies of both delusion and desire are deeply embedded in human nature, but can be successfully diminished and even eliminated. The word "Buddha" actually means "awake," and the historical Buddha was a man who undertook a program of transformation that resulted in his "awakening" from the misconceptions of delusion and the addictions of desire.

Bottom-Up Versus Top-Down Processing

Modern cognitive scientists distinguish between bottom-up and top-down information processing (Eysenck & Keane, 2000). At the heart of mindfulness meditation is an emphasis on bottom-up, rather than top-down, functions of the mind. That is to say, mindfulness seeks to bring attention directly to the stream of sensory data entering experience through each of the sense doors—the visual forms, sounds, smells, tastes, and bodily sensations—as well as to the arising of thoughts and images in the mind. In doing so, it steers attention away from the many "upper level" schemas, narratives, beliefs, and other conceptual maps we normally use to guide our way through a day's experience. This is cognitive–behavioral therapy on steroids—bringing attention to subtle sensory experience, and in so doing, coming to see all thoughts and their associated feelings as arbitrary, conditioned events. While ordinary consciousness tends to overlook the details of sensory experience (usually we are just trying to extract from it what is of interest to achieve our goals), mindfulness practice instead focuses on the sensory data itself, for its own sake, and invites the practitioner to consistently abandon conceptual judgments and narrative stories. Such a method has the effect of depriving the mind of much of the energy that fuels its stories and delusions, and transfers our awareness to the areas that will directly reveal the transient, constructed, and selfless nature of experience.

Mindfulness in Context

As mentioned earlier, mindfulness is part of a project designed to uproot harmful habits of mind. In the traditional Buddhist context, mindfulness is embedded in an eight-fold path to alleviate suffering; mindfulness is guided and directed by seven other factors. They are as follows: (1) the *view* one has of what is real, important, valuable, and useful; (2) how *intention* is used to initiate and sustain action in skillful ways; (3) the nature of *speech* that can be either harmful or beneficial; (4) the quality of *action* as it relates to ethical principles; (5) one's means of sustaining oneself in the world as *livelihood*; (6) the degree and quality of *effort* employed to bring about change; and (7) *concentration* as a focusing and supporting factor to mindfulness. When mindfulness is taken out of this broader context, its power may be limited. For example, it is difficult to sustain mindful awareness if we are causing harm to ourselves or others, or if we do not have the concentration and beneficial intentions to focus our efforts. In other words, it's hard to have a good meditation session after a busy day of cheating, stealing, and killing.

The Buddhist tradition has focused on universal challenges in human life, such as the problem of suffering in general. Many aspects of Buddhist psychology are therefore as applicable today as they were in ancient India. As this book demonstrates, psychotherapy is harnessing the power of mindfulness and acceptance to bring relief to intractable psychological conditions. However, the proposed outcome of dedicated Buddhist practice is radically different: *the complete cessation of suffering*. In modern terms, this means envisioning a life without a trace of psychological symptoms found in our diagnostic manuals. Such an "awakened" person lives naturally, with a full range of physical, emotional, and intellectual capacities, but without needing events to be other than what they are in order to feel fulfilled. By practicing mindfulness, we can learn to lead a peaceful, balanced, and loving life, all the while working for the benefit of others. There is no need to wait for another time, place, or condition for this to occur—we can begin where we are, therapists and patients alike.

References

Agency for Healthcare Research and Quality (2007). Meditation practices for health: State of the research. *U.S. Department of Health and Human Services, Evidence Report/Technology Assessment, Number 155.*

Bach, P., & Hayes, S. (2002) The use of acceptance and commitment therapy to prevent the rehospitalization of psychotic patients: A randomized controlled trial. *Journal of Consulting and Clinical Psychology, 70*(5), 1129-1139.

Begley, S. (2007). *Train you mind, change your brain.* New York: Ballantine Books.

Benson, H., & Klipper, M. (2000). *The relaxation response.* New York: Avon Books.

Bhikkhu, T. (2007). *Mindfulness defined.* Retrieved November 30, 2007, from http://www.dhammatalks.org/Archive/Writings/CrossIndexed/Uncollected/MiscEssays/Mindfulness%20Defined.pdf

Bishop, S., Lau, M., Shapiro, S., Carlson, L., Anderson, N., Carmody, J., et al. (2004). Mindfulness: A proposed operational definition. *Clinical Psychology: Science and practice, 11*(3), 230-241.

Boyatzis, R. & McKee, A. (2005). *Resonant leadership: Renewing yourself and connecting with others through mindfulness, hope, and compassion.* Boston, MA: Harvard Business School Press.

Davids, T. & Stede, W. (Eds.) (1921/2001). *Pali-english dictionary.* New Delhi, India: Munshiram Manoharlal Publishers Pvt, Ltd.

Davidson, R. J., Kabat-Zinn, J., Schumacher, J., Rosenkranz, M., Muller, D., Santorelli, S., et al. (2003). Alterations in brain and immune function produced by mindfulness meditation. *Psychosomatic Medicine, 65*(4), 564-570.

Dunne, J. D. (2007, March). *Mindfulness & Buddhist contemplative theory.* Poster presented at the 2007 annual conference, Integrating Mindfulness-Based Approaches & Interventions into Medicine, Health Care, and Society, Worcester, MA.

Eysenck, M.W., Keane, M. T. (2000). *Cognitive psychology: A student's handbook.* New York: Psychology Press.

Germer, C., Siegel, R., & Fulton, P. (Eds.) (2005). *Mindfulness and psychotherapy.* New York: Guilford Press.

Grepmair, L., Mitterlehner, F., Loew, T., & Nickel, M. (2006) Promotion of mindfulness in psychotherapists in training and treatment results of their patients. *Journal of Psychosomatic Research 60*(6), 649-650.

Grepmair, L., Mitterlehner, F., Loew, T., & Nickel, M. (2007) Promotion of mindfulness in psychotherapists in training: preliminary study. *European Psychiatry, 22*, 485-489.

Gunaratana, B. (2002). *Mindfulness in plain english.* Somerville, MA: Wisdom Publications.

Hayes, S., Follette, V., & Linehan, M. (Eds.). (2004). *Mindfulness and acceptance: Expanding the cognitive-behavioral tradition.* New York: Guilford Press.

Hebb, D. (1949). *The organization of behavior: A neuropsychological theory.* New York: Bantam Books.

Kabat-Zinn, J. (1990). *Full catastrophe living.* New York: Delacorte Press.

Kabat-Zinn, J. (2003). Mindfulness-based interventions in context: Past, present, and future. *Clinical Psychology: Science and Practice, 10*(2), 144-156.

Kabat-Zinn, J. (2006, June 10). Some clinical applications of mindfulness in medical and mental health practice. In *Meditation in Psychotherapy.* Conference conducted by Harvard Medical School, Boston, MA.

Langer, E. (1989). *Mindfulness.* Cambridge, MA: Da Capo Press.

Lazar, S., Kerr, C., Wasserman, R., Gray, J., Greve, D., Treadway, M., et al. (2005). Meditation experience is associated with increased cortical thinkness. *NeuroReport, 16*(17), 1893-1897.

Linehan, M. (1993). *Cognitive-behavioral treatment of borderline personality disorder.* New York: Guilford Press.

Lutz, A., Grelschar, L., Rawlings, N., Richard, M., & Davidson, R. (2004). Long-term meditators self-induce high-amplitude gamma synchrony during mental practice. *Proceedings of the National Academy of Sciences, 101*(46), 16369-16373.

Rapgay, L. & Bystrisky, A. (in Press). Classical mindfulness: An introduction to its theory and practice for clinical application. In Longevity and Optimal Health: Integrating Eastern and Western perspectives. *Annals of the New York Academy of Sciences.*

Segal, Z., Williams, J., & Teasdale, J. (2002). *Mindfulness-based cognitive therapy for depression: A new approach to preventing relapse.* New York: Guilford Press.

Siegel, D. (2007). *The mindful brain.* New York: W.W. Norton.

Simon, R. (2007). The top ten. *Psychotherapy Networker*, March/April, pp. 24, 25, 37.

Singh, N., Wahler, R., Adkins, A., & Myers, R. (2003). Soles of the feet: a mindfulness-based self-control intervention for aggression by an individual with mild mental retardation and mental illness. *Research in Developmental Disabilities, 24*(3), 158–169.

Smith, J. (2004). Alterations in brain and immune function produced by mindfulness meditation: three caveats. *Psychosomatic Medicine, 66*, 148–152.

Teasdale, J., Moore, R., Hayhurst, H., Pope, M., Williams, S., & Segal, Z. (2002). Metacognitive awareness and prevention of relapse in depression: Empirical evidence. *Journal of Consulting and Clinical Psychology, 70*(2), 275–287.

Teasdale, J., Segal, Z., & Williams, J. (1995). How does cognitive therapy prevent depressive relapse and why should attentional control (mindfulness) training help? *Behaviour Research and Therapy, 33*, 25–39.

Toyomasu, K. G. (2001, January 10). Haiku for People. Retrieved July 20, 2007 from http://www.toyomasu.com/haiku/#basho

Walsh, R. & Shapiro, S. (2006). The meeting of meditative disciplines and western psychology: A mutually enriching dialogue. *American Psychologist, 61*(3), 227–239.

2

Mindfulness and Meditation

Andrew Olendzki

> *What should be done for his followers by a teacher with compassion and care for their welfare, that I have done for you. Here are the roots of trees. Here are empty places. Meditate! Do not be lazy. Do not be ones who later have regrets. This is my instruction to you.*
>
> Buddha (Majjhima Nikāya 8)

As words become more widely used, and especially as they become fashionable, they may often become more difficult to understand. One might think it would be the other way around, but this obfuscation of meaning has generally been the rule with the popularization of Buddhist vocabulary. While each had a precise technical meaning in its original context, terms like zen, yoga, karma, and nirvana can mean almost anything the modern writer wants them to mean. A similar trend may well be underway with *mindfulness*, and perhaps even with the more general word *meditation*. Understanding the sense in which these words are used in their original setting should prove to be a worthwhile undertaking as we see them applied in the current creative encounter between psychology and Buddhist thought.

What Is Meditation?

The traditional sense of meditation in Western culture, before significant encounter with Asian practices, involves sustained consideration or thought upon a subject. Originating from the Indo-European root $\sqrt{med}$, primarily meaning "to measure," it suggests a discourse upon a subject (as in the title of Descartes' famous work) or calm thought upon some subject (as with structured religious prayers). As such, it is always an exercise of ordered conceptual contemplation, involving the systematic and disciplined use of language, symbol, and concept. As we shall see, this is exactly what one is *not* doing in mindfulness meditation. While such a structured exploration of a conceptual landscape can be important to some forms of psychotherapy that focus on reframing the narrative of one's prior experience, most forms of Buddhist meditation are working in the other direction, toward less conceptual modes of consciousness.

The most common word for meditation in the classical languages of Buddhism (Sanskrit and Pali) is *samādhi*. The etymology of this term suggests gathering (*sam-*) the mind and placing ($\sqrt{dh\bar{a}}$) it upon (*-ā-*) an object. In this broad sense, its meaning seems similar enough to English usage, but there is a subtle and crucial difference between the Western and Buddhist understanding of how the mind operates. As mentioned in the previous chapter, experience ensues from the confluence of three things: consciousness, an organ, and an object. An organ cognizes an object; an object is cognized by an organ; consciousness of an object arises by means of an organ—these are three ways of describing the same event. What we consider conceptual thinking is only one of six modes of the mind, the other five being sensory, so meditation may or may not involve conceptual thought. Placing the mind upon a sensory object is just as much meditation as placing the mind upon a conceptual object, and it is not possible to do both at once. The point here is that while in Western usage meditation generally assumes the exercise of "thinking about" something, in Buddhism it may mean this, but more often refers to placing the mind upon physical sensations, upon raw sights or sounds, or upon the tangible objects of smell and taste. This gives it a wider range of meaning, and this difference will become important.

The primary characteristic of meditation, and the term most often used to define it, is *ekaggatā*, which literally means one (*ek-*) pointed (*-agga-*) ness (*tā*). Meditation is about focusing the mind to a single point, unifying it, and placing it upon a particular object. To some extent this happens naturally every mind moment, and it if did not, there would be a serious lack of cohesion to mental experience. According to Buddhist models of mind, consciousness takes a single object at a time and organizes various supporting mental functions around it. This can be construed as a single episode of consciousness, which is essentially an event that takes place rather than something that exists. The knowing of a particular object by means of a particular organ arises in response to a stimulus, persists for only a very brief moment, and then passes away almost immediately. Another mind moment arises right away in response to another stimulus, and this too immediately ceases. Subjective experience presents itself to us as a stream on conscious moments; the sense of continuity, and of subject and object stability, is projected onto the stream much as a narrative is constructed from rapidly presented frames of a movie. One-pointedness is a factor in every frame, for each moment has a single focus, but concentration meditation has to do with extending this singularity of focus over multiple ensuing mind moments. Using the cinema image further, concentration meditation is like holding the video camera steady for a long time—one takes multiple pictures of the same scene.

This is something that does not come easily to the human mind and must be practiced diligently if the skill is to be learned. We have evolved to stay alert to all significant changes to our environment, and attention is naturally drawn to sensory data that is out of the ordinary or that presents in sudden or unexpected ways. Like a bird or chipmunk, rapidly casting around in all directions to check for danger, our mind is habituated to lurching rapidly from one sense object to another, or from one thought to another. As anyone who has practiced meditation can attest, or as you can discover for yourself in a few moments, holding the mind steady on a single object, such as the breath or a repeated word, is exceedingly difficult to do. But like so many other things, it is a skill that can be learned through patient and diligent practice. Much of Buddhist meditation is a process of placing the mind on a particular object, often called the primary object, and then noticing (sooner or later) that it has wandered off that object. When one notices this, one gently and forgivingly abandons the train of thought the mind has boarded and returns the attention once again to the primary object. This process is then repeated again and again: The mind is placed on a particular object; it wanders off on trails of association, reverie, recollection, judgment, planning, verbalizing, conceptualizing, calculation, commentary, fantasy, and daydream, only to be carefully and patiently retrieved from its adventuring and settled back upon the primary object.

Obstacles to Meditation

As with every other learned skill, people have differing aptitudes for meditation; make progress in an apparently endless series of breakthroughs, plateaus, and reversals; and can experience repeated episodes of triumph and failure in rapid succession. Any given meditation session might be influenced by how comfortable the body is, how much sleep one has had recently, the overall state of health, the temperature in the room, whether one has a problem on the mind or is working through some emotional issues—all sorts of factors. An interesting feature of the traditional Buddhist understanding of meditation is that it is always influenced by one's overall ethical behavior. The ability of the mind to concentrate is directly hampered by such acts as deliberately harming living creatures, taking what has not been given, speaking untruthfully or harshly, misbehaving sexually, or taking intoxicants of various kinds. Thus, the ethical precepts of Buddhism are a matter of great practical importance, rather than mere moral injunction. But if one is relatively free of the remorse and emotional turmoil that can come from unhealthy behavior, it is reasonable to expect significant progress in the enterprise of unifying and concentrating the mind such that it can remain steadily upon a single object over multiple mind moments.

Buddhist psychology identifies five primary obstacles to meditation, known appropriately as the five hindrances. The first of these is *sense desire*, or the impulse of the senses to seek out their objects. It is as if the eye wants to see forms, the ear is eager to hear sounds, and so on for the other senses, including the mind liking to think the thoughts that please it in one way or another. We are so used to having our senses connect with their corresponding object that a considerable habit energy is present in any given moment inclining the mind to "lean toward" or be attracted to their habitual forms of stimulation. This pull of the senses, including mind as the sixth sense, is subtle but can be viscerally discerned as the mind gets more sensitive. The second hindrance is *ill-will*, a corresponding propensity to shy away or withdraw from those objects of experience that do not please us or are painful in some way. These first two hindrances act as a matched pair of polar opposites, pulling and pushing the mind and senses from one object to another in ways that make it difficult to settle down. The third and fourth hindrances also work together as an opposed pair, *restlessness* and *sluggishness*. Restlessness is a matter of too much energy, driving the mind relentlessly from one object to another, while sluggishness is too little energy, bogging the mind down in slothful, sleepy, or lazy states. The antidote for restlessness is to relax and tranquilize the mind, while the remedy for sluggishness is to arouse greater interest and enthusiasm. Paradoxically, the goal is to reach a state that is simultaneously tranquil and alert. The mind should be calm without being sluggish and alert without being restless. The final hindrance is *doubt*, often manifest as recurring thoughts of self-doubt, doubt about making progress, or doubt about the entire enterprise of learning such a daunting thing as meditation. As long as any of these five states or factors is arising in the mind, it will be difficult or impossible to focus the mind and hold it steady upon a particular object. But they can, with patient practice, be temporarily put aside or abandoned. They are likened to wind-blown waves on the surface of water, and when they quiet down, the mind, like water, becomes limpid and clear.

Deepening Meditation

Although at first the attention has an almost irresistible propensity to be drawn to sounds, physical sensations, or stray thoughts—wherever the action is—it eventually gets less and less diverted by random stimuli. At some point the momentum shifts, and it becomes more compelling to remain with the primary object than to pursue the shallow stimulation of some novel input. It is not that the object itself is of particular interest, but rather the quality of mind with which the object is cognized becomes more intriguing as it gains in power, depth, and lucidity. Under the scrutiny of a concentrated mind, everything becomes fascinating. If this process of steadying the mind on a single object is allowed to mature, it will eventually reach a stage called *absorption*, or *jhāna* in Pali (the same word is rendered *dhyāna* in Sanskrit, *ch'an* in Chinese, and *zen* in Japanese). In this state the mind is so thoroughly attending to a particular object that it is no longer aware of other objects that might present themselves at a sense door. A bird might sing and the sound waves will reach the ear and may even be processed by subliminal sensory systems, but it will not enter conscious awareness since "the line is busy" as it is absorbed by the primary object of awareness. This is a state most resembling a trance to the outside observer and is the target of considerable caricature of meditation in popular culture. But while the mind may appear non-functioning from the outside, it has reached a state of remarkable capability when regarded from the practitioner's subjective standpoint.

The classical meditation literature of the Buddhist tradition describes a systematic (and repeatable) four-stage process by which the mind becomes gradually purified of its distractions as it becomes increasingly focused and potent. Nothing significant happens until the mind has at least temporarily abandoned the five hindrances mentioned above, and any progress is immediately canceled if any sort of harmful or unethical impulse arises in the stream of consciousness. Again, this is not so much a proscription as it is a description of the natural qualities of the mind, which can only achieve an advanced state of concentration if its thoughts and intentions remain ethically wholesome. The first stage of absorption meditation is accompanied by intense physical pleasure and mental joy, more a state of deep well-being permeating the body than of sensory titillation. This stage also involves the normal conceptual or discursive functions of the mind. One can feel very focused while retaining the ability to verbalize and direct thought at will. In the second stage these discursive functions cease, while the joy that comes naturally with concentration persists. It is not that the mind has stopped functioning, rather certain functions of the mind, those that direct and sustain deliberative conceptual thought, come to rest. In Buddhist understanding the more profound levels of mind, characterized by a strong inner clarity, are only reached when the chatter of verbalization and symbol manipulation ceases. The third stage of absorption sees the diminishing of the intensive joy permeating the first two stages into a more subtle sense of happiness and well-being. With the fourth and final stage, all pleasure is replaced with equanimity, a deep evenness of mind that regards phenomena with compete objectivity. The usual attraction toward what is pleasing and avoidance of what is displeasing, both attitudes of mind that prevent us from seeing clearly, are surmounted by equanimity. At this point the concentrated mind is said to be purified, bright, and steady. Moreover, like gold purified in a crucible, it becomes malleable and can be turned with great effect to a number of non-ordinary modes of functioning.

The civilization into which the Buddha was born had been adept at the contemplative arts for centuries. The world he inhabited was filled with a marvelous diversity of spiritual teachers and teachings, and he learned many meditation practices from others. The *yogis* of his day, those disciplined practitioners of the meditative arts, were influenced considerably by ancient shamanic practices and used deep mental training in the service of universal religious pursuits such as gaining magical powers, traveling to other dimensions of reality, and interacting with non-human beings. Many operated in traditional Hindu contexts, employing meditative practices in the mystical pursuit of realizing and uniting with god in various ways. The Buddha seemed to have a very different set of interests, however, and both discouraged the development of magical abilities and repudiated the theistic assumptions of his day. He fully embraced the science of purifying and training the mind, but directed it to the goal of understanding the nature of human experience. In particular, he was interested in investigating the moment-to-moment functioning of mind and body, the synthetic construction of experience, and the specific ways in which both suffering and well-being are conditioned by interdependent factors. He saw humanity as being in an existentially challenging situation, given the ubiquity of change and the inevitability of aging, sickness, and death. He also saw that human beings have deep instincts for personal survival, which manifest as a whole array of afflictive emotional responses rooted in greed, hatred, and delusion. The bulk of our difficulties, he discerned, come not from the existential challenges themselves, but from internally generated maladaptive responses activated by the relentless and unreflective pursuit of pleasure and avoidance of pain. Through the example of his own awakening and a subsequent life devoted to training others, the Buddha demonstrated that these internal causes of suffering can be seen, understood, and healed. His approach is basically psychological, his methods are mostly empirical, and his goal is ultimately therapeutic, which is why his teachings are of growing interest to modern psychologists.

Mindfulness Meditation

The primary tool for bringing about the radical transformation from reflexive suffering to profound well-being is meditation, but the one-pointed concentration meditations described so far are of only limited usefulness. The discipline and focus they bring to the mind are indispensible, but insight into the workings of the complex mind requires a more agile meditative tool. That tool is *mindfulness*. Called *sati* in Pali, mindfulness derives from a root (√*smṛt*) meaning memory or recollection and refers to the cultivation of a certain presence of mind that remembers to attend with persistent clarity to the objects of present experience. Like meditation in general, it involves placing attention deliberately upon an object and sustaining it over time, but unlike one-pointedness and absorption, mindfulness tends to open to a broader range of phenomena rather than restricting the focus to a singular object. Like a floodlight rather than a spotlight, mindfulness illuminates a more fluid phenomenological field of ever-changing experience rather than isolating a particular object for intensive scrutiny. This alternative mode of observation is necessary because mindfulness practice is more about investigating a *process* than about examining an object. All mindfulness meditation requires a certain degree of concentration in order to gather and focus the powers of the mind, but the concentrated mind is then directed to a moving target—the flowing stream of consciousness—rather than being allowed to stabilize on a single point. Whereas concentration practice involves returning the mind again and again to the primary object of meditation, mindfulness practice allows the mind to follow whatever is arising in experience. There is less a sense of controlling *what* the awareness is resting upon and more care given to *how* awareness is manifesting.

In classical Buddhist psychology, mindfulness is regarded as a mental state, one of the 52 functions of the mind that can arise in various combinations to assist the cognizing of an object by consciousness. These mental factors are similar to what are often called intentions, attitudes, or qualities of mind. Among the mental states are found certain functions that are universal to all mind moments, such as perception, feeling, volition, and attention, some that may or may not arise in any given mind moment, such as decisiveness, energy, or joy, and some that occur only in unwholesome states of mind such as conceit, envy, or avarice. Mindfulness is among a list of factors that are considered wholesome, and these serve as antidotes and alternatives to the unwholesome factors. Mindfulness is always accompanied by such complementary mental factors as trust, equanimity, and kindness, along with factors that contribute to the mind's tranquility, malleability, and proficiency. This system thus maps out a rather precise definition of mindfulness, which says as much about what it is not as what it is. Mindfulness is not mere attentiveness to experience; nor is it the deliberate turning of the mind toward a particular object and the sustaining of attention upon that object; nor can mindfulness ever co-arise with restlessness or any of the mental states rooted in greed, hatred, or delusion. Mindfulness consists of a quality of attention that is at once confident, benevolent, generous, and equanimous. It is a manner of being aware, an attitude of mind toward experience, and a mode of awareness that is paradoxically both intimately close and objectively removed (Olendzki, 2008).

One more classical word for meditation that should be considered in this context is *bhāvana*. It is based on the causative construction of the verb "to be" and is thus literally "causing to be"; it is generally translated as *development*. One of the important functions of meditation is the development of those qualities of mind that are beneficial to a path of transformation. There are meditations that develop concentration, there are those that develop mindfulness, and there are those that develop other specific qualities such as kindness, compassion, appreciative joy, and equanimity. The idea, as it is stated in an early text, is that "Whatever a person frequently thinks and ponders upon, that will become the inclination of his mind" (*Majjhima* 19) (Nanamoli & Bodhi, 1995). In a model where each mind moment arises and passes away in serial progression, with each moment taking a single object and each object being regarded with either a wholesome or an unwholesome attitude, the quality of each mind moment becomes a matter of great concern. In a moment of anger, for example, kindness cannot simultaneously manifest. In a moment of confusions, there can be no mindfulness. Psychological cultivation thus involves abandoning the unwholesome states as they naturally arise in the mind and encouraging or developing the wholesome states that arise. Mindfulness is the mental factor of most benefit to those seeking mental well-being, so the development of mindfulness is a universally healthy thing to do. Much of Buddhist meditation consists of the cultivation of mindfulness, and this can only be done with great patience and perseverance. Putting aside an hour or two each day or attending a full-immersion retreat setting from time to time is among the ways to practice being mindful. The *content* of experience in this pursuit is almost irrelevant—one can be mindful of breathing, of walking, of eating, or of almost any ordinary activity. What is of most importance is the *quality of attention* brought to these pursuits.

Summary

What we have outlined above can be seen as a continuum that appears at this point to have returned to its beginning. We start with the workings of the ordinary mind, which takes anything that happens to appear in the mind or senses as an object of awareness, but in an undisciplined and apparently random way. According to Buddhist thought, nothing is truly random in the human mind and body, however, so what appears to be the spontaneously attentive mind is actually a mind reacting to phenomena with host of unconscious habits, reflexes, and attitudes. To the extent these subliminal conditioning factors are rooted in greed, hatred, and delusion, our behavior will continually incline toward more suffering for ourselves and others. To counter this tendency, we might embark upon the enterprise of deliberately controlling and disciplining the mind to return to a primary object of awareness during sessions of sustained concentration practice. To some extent this involves countering the mind's natural inclination to turn away to something else, and like any form of discipline, it can seem onerous at first. But as the mind concentrates it accesses considerable power, and one can chooses to direct that power either to explore the deeper reaches of altered states of consciousness or to investigate more carefully the flow of ordinary experience. When, in mindfulness meditation, awareness is encouraged to roam freely over the phenomena of experience, it does so with qualitatively more clarity and continuity than is accessible in ordinary states of mind.

The benefits of this heightened capability of awareness are manifold, both within and outside the Buddhist context. Traditionally, mindfulness was seen as a tool to be used for gaining wisdom, which consists of the direct, experiential understanding of the impermanence, selflessness, unsatisfactoriness, and interdependence of all phenomena. This might not seem like much at first glance, but the implications of these insights are far reaching, leading to no less than the thorough purification of human nature of its inherited toxins and the complete emancipation of consciousness from its hedonic conditioning. The usefulness of mindfulness to the modern psychotherapist and researcher is being discovered and creatively explored in ever new ways each day, as will be amply demonstrated in the rest of this book.

References

Nanamoli, B., & Bodhi, B. (1995). *The middle length discourses of the Buddha.* Boston: Wisdom Publications, p. 208.

Olendzki, Andrew. (2008). *The real practice of mindfulness.* Buddhadharma, The Practitioner's Quarterly. Fall 2008, p. 50.

3

The Neurobiology of Mindfulness

Michael T. Treadway and Sara W. Lazar

The mind precedes all things, the mind dominates all things, the mind creates all things.

Buddha

As Western culture has become more aware of Eastern spiritual traditions, scientists have been increasingly interested in verifying the anecdotal claims from expert meditators regarding mindfulness practice. For almost 50 years, the practice of meditation and mindfulness has been studied by Western neuroscientists looking to better understand its phenomenology, neurobiology, and clinical effects. In this chapter, we provide an overview of current neurobiological research on mindfulness and meditation practices, including key findings, methodological issues, and clinical implications. It is not our intent to provide a complete review of this vast and diverse body of work; for extensive reviews of the neurobiological literature, please see Cahn and Polich (2006), Austin (1998, 1998), and Murphy, Donovan, and Taylor (1997); for reviews of the clinical literature, see Lazar (2005) or Baer (2006). The goal of this chapter is to review the most recent literature and orient the reader to this developing research area and its implications for mindfulness-based interventions.

Although all forms of meditation increase one's capacity to be mindful, the Buddhist traditions place a particular emphasis on cultivating mindfulness. Therefore, it is these traditions that have served as the primary source for the mindfulness techniques that are now incorporated into Western psychotherapeutic practices such as DBT, ACT, and MBCT (mindfulness-based cognitive therapy). As the focus of this chapter is mindfulness, the term "meditation" in this chapter will be used to denote the Buddhist meditation practices that cultivate mindfulness, unless otherwise specified.

Studying Mindfulness

The goal of the neuroscientific investigation of mindfulness meditation is to understand the neural systems that are utilized to achieve meditative states and also to determine the effects that regular practice of mindfulness has on brain function and structure. Meditation is associated with both state and trait-like effects. State effects refer to changes that occur in individuals while they actively meditate. In contrast, trait-like changes occur gradually over time as a consequence of sustained meditation practice and persist throughout the day. Trait-like effects are thought to result from stable, long-term transformations in brain activity and structure. When studying trait-like versus state effects, scientists can ask different questions, all of which may have clinical applications. Understanding state effects will help elucidate why mindfulness may be useful within a therapy session when dealing with painful memories or sudden bursts of emotion. Conversely, understanding the long-term effects will help identify why mindfulness is useful for treating chronic conditions such as depression and general anxiety (see Chapters 10 and 12).

One primary challenge of studying the state effects of meditation is the complexity of meditation itself (see also Chapter 2). Typically, when scientists want to investigate the neural systems that underlie a certain skill, they use tasks that are very simple, repetitive, and easy to monitor, such as reaction times to stimuli. By keeping tasks simple, it is easier to isolate specific areas of the brain that are involved in task performance. In contrast, meditation is highly complex and variable from moment to moment. In one instance a person may be concentrating deeply on the breath, and in the next they suddenly recall an errand to run; a few moments later they may become mindful of having just been distracted and then return focus to the breath, but then a few moments later an image from their childhood suddenly pops up and so forth. Focusing on the breath, remembering an errand, recognizing that you have become distracted, and seeing an image from the past, all involve discrete brain systems. Should all of those systems be considered part of the "meditative state?" Or should the term "meditative state" include only those brain regions that are active when we are focused on the breath? How can scientists tease apart those moments of clear focus from those moments of being distracted? Our experimental technology is not yet capable of determining when the mind switches between these mental events.

In the sections that follow, we review recent findings on neurobiological studies of mindfulness mediation. The first two sections summarize the primary findings regarding the effects of meditation on attentional ability, cognitive and emotional processing, and brain function and structure. The third section addresses some recent studies pointing toward possible mechanisms of action involved in meditation, and the final section addresses the possible ramifications of these findings for clinical interventions.

Cognitive and Behavioral Effects of Mindfulness

According to the claims of experienced meditation practitioners, increased levels of practice are accompanied by a heightened sense of awareness and enhanced capacity for deep concentration both during meditative states and throughout the day. Scientists have therefore reasoned that experienced meditators should show better performance on high cognitive-demand attention and concentration tasks than individuals without meditation and mindfulness training. In this section, we summarize several key findings regarding the cognitive and behavioral effects of mindfulness meditation training.

Studies of Attention

Drawing from the self-reported claims of meditation practitioners, changes in attentional resources have been the focus of several recent studies. In the cognitive psychology literature, "attention" is a blanket term that may be used to describe all or some of a set of discrete sub-processes that collectively underlie our ability to attend to different stimuli. Examples of these sub-processes include alerting (becoming aware of a stimulus, such as to a car horn honking), sustained attention, and conflict monitoring (remaining focused on a stimulus despite the presence of a distracting/conflicting stimulus). In one recent study, Jha et al. (2007) sought to compare these three attentional sub-processes across three participant groups: a group of experienced meditation practitioners before and after an intensive 1-month retreat, a group of novice meditators before and after an 8-week MBSR course, and a control group tested 8 weeks apart. They found that both the retreat and MBSR groups showed improvements on the sustained attention task over the course of the intervention, relative to the control group. The other two types of attention did not change, showing the specificity of the results.

Another recent longitudinal study sought to investigate whether intense meditation practice during a 3-month silent retreat would increase an individual's attentional capacity. When two stimuli are presented in quick succession, people generally have trouble identifying the second stimulus, a phenomenon known as "attentional blink." This reduced ability to process two stimuli in close temporal proximity is thought to be an index of stimuli competition for limited attentional resources (Shapiro, Arnell, & Raymond, 1997). Researchers found that meditators showed less of an attentional blink response after the 3-month retreat. In addition, there was a group by time point interaction, confirming the hypothesis that meditators improved more during the 3 months than the non-meditating controls. Consistent with theses behavioral findings, simultaneously recorded electroencephalography (EEG) signals showed that individuals who performed best on the attentional blink task also exhibited the least amount of brain activity at the onset of the first stimulus. This suggests that these individuals were effectively able to reserve attentional resources for the second stimulus (Slagter et al., 2007).

Finally, in an earlier study, Valentine and Sweet (1999) sought to directly compare the effects of mindfulness and concentration meditation on sustained attention in both novice and experienced practitioners of Zen meditation. In traditional Buddhist practice, novice meditators are first instructed to concentrate on observing the breath. Over time, as a mediator's ability to sustain attention on breath increases, he or she is gradually instructed to broaden his or her attention to other external and internal stimuli. For this study, Valentine and Sweet classified all subjects as either mindfulness- or concentration-style meditators depending on self-report as to their mental focus during meditation. Meditation subjects and a control group were compared on a task in which they had to count rapidly-presented beeps, which is a measure of sustained attention. All meditators were significantly better than controls in their ability to detect all stimuli, suggesting that both groups had developed heightened attention as a result of their practice. However, the mindfulness meditators were significantly better in their ability to detect unexpected stimuli (tones with different repetition frequencies) compared to the concentration group, consistent with the intention of each practice. It should be noted, however, that the sample sizes were quite small (9–10 subjects per group), so this finding should be interpreted cautiously. Finally, when the two meditation groups were subdivided based on total number of years they had practiced, there were striking and significant differences between novice and experienced subjects in their ability to detect the stimuli, with subjects having *more* than 2 years of practice able to detect approximately 5% more of the stimuli than the subjects with less than 2 years of practice, regardless of meditation style. This last finding strongly suggests that the differences between the meditators and controls were due to practice effects and not due to personality differences between groups.

Habituation

An additional claim of experienced meditators is that increased open awareness to all internal and external stimuli will result in a decreased tendency toward habituation. Habituation is the tendency to exhibit reduced neural activity in response to a given stimulus if the stimulus has been repeated multiple times. A decreased tendency toward habituation is therefore reflective of what the Buddhist tradition calls "beginner's mind." An early study by Kasamatsu and Hirai (1973) with four highly experienced Zen masters demonstrated that their EEG patterns failed to habituate to repeated clicking sounds, while the pattern of non-meditating controls did habituate. Becker and Shapiro failed to replicate these findings 15 years later (Becker & Shapiro, 1981) using three groups of meditators and two control groups—one control group was instructed to attend to the sound closely and one to ignore it. However, the subjects in the different groups were not matched for age (Zen, 37.8 years old; yoga, 31.5 years old; TM, 28.7 years old; two control groups, 26.5 and 29.5 years old). Furthermore, the sound characteristics and method in which the clicks were presented in the two studies differed, which might account for the differences. In the Kasamatsu study the sounds were presented through stereo speakers, while in the Becker study the subjects wore headphones. The physical sensations associated with the headphones would likely draw more attention to the ears and make all subjects more attentive to the clicks. Also, neither study reported the magnitude of the tones, so it is possible that in the second study the sounds were louder or more intrusive, overcoming the subtle effects observed in the first study.

These studies provide support for two central claims reported by experienced meditators regarding the effects of their practice: Meditation practice does appear to increase an individual's attentional capacity and to decrease habituation. As we will discuss later in this chapter, these effects may contribute to the observed clinical benefits that accrue from mindfulness-based interventions.

Effects of Mindfulness on Neural Activity

EEG Studies of Meditative States

Early in the history of the neuroscience of mindfulness and meditation, researchers were primarily interested in determining the extent to which meditative states represented a unique form of conscious experience. In the first of these studies, scientists focused on evaluating physiological and psychological changes that occurred during meditation (Cahn & Polich, 2006). It was not until the late 1960s, however, that scientists began using EEG to examine changes in brain activity during the act of meditation. An EEG recording measures changes in electrical activity within the brain and can distinguish between different frequencies of electrical signals, which are associated with different types of brain activity.

Despite a large number of studies, EEG findings have been inconsistent. These differences are in part due to differences in the type of meditation studied, as well as methodological differences. Therefore, a clear, concise summary of EEG findings remains elusive (Cahn & Polich, 2006). Long-term meditators appear to have higher baseline levels of alpha and theta band activity, which is associated with sleep and rest (Aftanas & Golocheikine, 2005; Andresen, 2000; J. M. Davidson, 1976; Delmonte 1984; Jevning, Wallace, & Beidebach, 1992; Schuman, 1980; West, 1979; Woolfolk, 1975). Some studies have reported that increases in alpha band power are associated with entering a meditative state (Banquet, 1973; Hirai, 1974; Kasamatsu & Hirai, 1966; Taneli & Krahne, 1987), while some have reported decreases of alpha band (G.D. Jacobs & Lubar, 1989; Pagano & Warrenburg, 1983), and still other have reported no difference between meditation and non-meditation within the same subjects (Cuthbert, Kriteller, Simons, Hodes, Lang, 1981; Delmonte, 1985). Increases in theta power during meditative practice have also been widely reported and are somewhat more consistent (Cahn & Polich, 2006).

Lehmann et al. (2001) studied a highly advanced Buddhist lama while he practiced five distinct exercises. Although all the exercises were of the concentration type, the study clearly showed in a single subject that different meditation practices elicit different patterns of brain activity. Furthermore, the regions activated were consistent with what was known about the functions of those regions (i.e., use of mantra-activated language areas and imagery-activated visual areas), which helps verify that the subject's neural activity was consistent with his subjective report.

One possible explanation of the discrepant results of EEG studies is that different meditation styles may produce unique patterns of activity. Meditation practices that emphasize deep physical relaxation are more likely to produce higher theta and delta activity (which are more closely associated with deep sleep), while practices that focus more on intensive concentration and mindfulness will likely have higher alpha and beta power. This hypothesis has not been thoroughly tested, as few studies have endeavored to compare different meditation styles directly, a phenomenon likely due to the bias in favor of studying expert mediators, who have significant experience in one particular style of meditation. However, one study using non-expert mediators was able to contrast relaxation, concentration, and mindfulness meditation styles. These researchers found that baseline relaxation was associated with higher delta and theta increases as compared to both the concentration and mindfulness meditation styles, but that the two different meditation conditions resulted in increased alpha and beta 1 power. Interestingly, mindfulness meditation was associated with higher alpha and beta 1 increases as compared to concentration meditation (Dunn, Hartigan, & Mikulas, 1999). This study supports the interpretation that different meditation styles may significantly affect the resulting EEG data, despite the fact that most, if not all, meditation practices utilize overlapping techniques.

Finally, one recent study comparing Tibetan Buddhist monks to normal controls reported that the ratio of gamma band activity as compared to slow oscillatory activity was initially higher for the monks during the resting baseline. This difference increased sharply once the monks began a loving-kindness meditation. The authors concluded that these data support the possibility that meditation may promote short-term and long-term changes in neural functioning (Lutz et al., 2004).

Neuroimaging Studies of Meditative States

As both earlier EEG studies and more recent behavioral studies have confirmed, meditation and mindfulness appear to represent unique patterns of neural functioning. Although EEG allows scientists to see rapid changes in types of brain activity, the major drawback of this technique is the extremely limited spatial information it provides. One cannot assert with much confidence where in the brain the observed activity is emanating from.

Conversely, two neuroimaging techniques developed over the last 10 or 15 years, fMRI and PET, have excellent spatial resolution but give no information as to different types of neuron firing. The wealth of information these tools provide concerning specific brain regions has revolutionized neuroscience, allowing scientists to identify activity inside the brain during a wide variety of tasks. Following the growing interest in mindfulness techniques, a handful of studies using these tools to investigate meditation have been published.

As with the earlier EEG studies, neuroimaging studies have varied significantly in their design and the type of meditation studied, and therefore often present conflicting results. However, several consistent findings have emerged. The first is the activation of the dorsolateral prefrontal cortex (DLPFC), an area that has been associated with executive decision-making and attention. This area was activated in 5 of the 14 studies and appeared across a range of meditation styles, including Kundalini yoga (Lazar et al., 2000), mindfulness meditation (Baerentsen, 2001), Tibetan Buddhist imagery meditation (Newberg et al., 2001), Psalm recitation (Azari et al., 2001), and Zen meditation (Ritskes, Ritskes-Hoitinga, Stodkilde-Jorgensen, Baerentsen, & Hartman, 2003). Our lab has found trait-like changes of increased cortical thickness in this area, consistent with increased usage (Lazar, 2005). Taken together, these findings suggest that meditation produces state changes of increased activation in the DLPFC.

Another frequent finding is that meditation leads to increased activation in the cingulate cortex, particularly the anterior subdivision (ACC). The ACC has been described as playing a primary role in the integration of attention, motivation, and motor control (Paus, 2001). A functional subdivision of the ACC into dorsal and rostral areas has also been proposed, in which the rostral portion is more activated by emotionally charged tasks, and the dorsal portion is more activated by cognitive tasks (Bush, Luu, & Posner, 2000). As the ACC is often associated with directing attention, it might be expected that more experienced meditators would show greater activation than novice meditators. Alternatively, as more experienced meditators often report that they can sustain periods of uninterrupted attention longer than novice meditators, it may result in less need for ACC activity. This was recently reported in a study by Brefczynski-Lewis et al. in 2007. In this study, novice meditators were also found to show more activity in the ACC as compared to Buddhist monks (Brefczynski-Lewis, Lutz, Schaefer, Levinson, & Davidson, 2007). However, when Hölzel et al. attempted to replicate these results using experienced insight (mindfulness) practitioners, they instead found that these participants showed *more* activity in the ACC as compared to non-meditators (Hölzel et al., 2007). This discrepancy may result from the fact that Brefczynski-Lewis et al. utilized highly trained monks, while Hölzel et al. utilized experienced lay practitioners, whose ability to sustain attention is undoubtedly less developed than in the monks.

Finally, the insula has also been shown to activate during meditation (Brefczynski-Lewis et al., 2007). The insula is associated with interoception, which is the sum of visceral and "gut" feelings that we experience at any given moment, and has also been proposed as a key region involved in processing transient bodily sensations, thereby contributing to our experience of "selfness" (Craig, 2004). One hypothesis for the increased activation of the insula during meditation is that it reflects the mediator's careful attention to the rising and falling of internal sensations. The sub-region of insula identified in these studies is also strongly implicated in several psychopathologies (Phillips, Drevets, Rauch, & Lane, 2003). The gray matter in this region is significantly smaller among schizophrenic patients as compared to controls (Crespo-Facorro et al., 2000; Wright et al., 2000). Insular activity has also been found among depressed and healthy subjects during the induction of sad mood (Liotti, Mayberg, McGinnis, Brannan, & Jerabek, 2002), experience of pain (Casey, Minoshima, Morrow, & Koeppe, 1996) or disgust (Wright, He, Shapira, Goodman, & Liu, 2004). Studies have also highlighted the role of the insula in internally generated emotions (Reiman, Lane, Ahern, & Scwartz, 1997) as well as during guilt (Shin et al., 2000). These findings suggest that abnormalities in insular function may play a critical role in various psychiatric disorders.

In addition to brain regions that become active during meditation, neuroimaging techniques can also be used to identify specific differences in brain structure. In 2005, our group published a study that strongly supports the hypothesis that mindfulness practice has long-term effects on brain structure. Twenty long-term mindfulness meditators and 15 controls participated in a comparison of cortical thickness using high-resolution MRI images. Meditators and controls were matched for gender, age, race, and years of education. It was found that long-term meditators had increased cortical thickness in the anterior insula, sensory cortex, and prefrontal cortex. Given the emphasis on observing internal sensations that occurs during meditation, thickening in these regions is consistent with reports of mindfulness practice (Lazar et al., 2005). A more recent study confirmed and extended the results from our group, reporting increased gray matter density in the right anterior insula, as well as the hippocampus and left temporal gyrus among mindfulness meditators as compared to non-meditators (Hözel et al., 2008).

Mechanisms of Action

As more information regarding the underlying neural networks involved in meditation have been published, researchers are now beginning to investigate the neural mechanisms that may explain how these networks promote the reported behavioral and clinical effects of mindfulness practice. In so doing, scientists hope to better understand mindfulness by exploring how it is related to other types of mental activities.

Although this work is very much in its nascent stages, two recent studies deserve special note. The first study examined how MBSR training may impact neural networks involved in self-referential experience. Self-reference has historically been divided into two distinct forms: momentary self-awareness focused on present experience, and extended self-reference in terms of enduring characteristics (e.g., I am tall, I am generally upbeat, etc.). Farb et al. (2007) hypothesized that mindfulness training may help individuals to better discriminate between these two forms of self-reference. Using fMRI, the authors investigated the neural networks that became active during an experiential focus condition in which subjects focused on present-moment experiences as compared to a narrative focus condition in which subjects considered their personality traits. Farb et al. found that while the control group showed significant overlap in brain regions that activated between the experiential and narrative focus conditions, the mindfulness group did not. This data suggests that one possible mechanism of action for mindfulness meditation is a decoupling of two self-referential neural networks that are normally integrated, and a strengthening of the experiential network, consistent with the goals of MBSR training.

A second study explored the relationship between self-reported mindfulness and identifying emotions expressed in facial stimuli in healthy college students who were non-meditators (Creswell, Way, Eisenberger, & Lieberman, 2007). This study is unique, in that it focused on mindfulness as a skill/trait outside of the context of meditation practice. The authors found that trait mindfulness as measured by self-report was correlated with increases in activity in the medial prefrontal cortex (mPFC) as well as simultaneous decreases in activity in the amygdala during an affect-labeling task. The authors propose that mindfulness may therefore be associated with improved prefrontal regulation of limbic responses and may help explain part of why mindfulness is a useful component of therapy.

While these studies are encouraging, they are preliminary. Significantly more research will be required to elucidate the means by which mindfulness practices may provide its putative cognitive, emotional, and psychological benefits. In the final section, we will briefly touch on some of the clinical implications of the studies that have thus far been reviewed.

Clinical Implications

The goal of this section is not to review the clinical literature of mindfulness-based interventions. Rather, we wish to explore how recent neurobiological studies of meditation and mindfulness may be relevant to clinical applications. A summary of important clinical findings is provided below.

Increased time "Living in the Moment"

One of the hallmarks of expert meditators is their ability to experience negative emotions without necessarily "getting caught up" in them. This skill has significant implications for the treatment of common forms of psychopathology, particularly mood and anxiety disorders. Both families of disorders involve excessive forms of rumination on negative thoughts. Mindfulness training incorporates a set of techniques that helps individuals reduce their tendency to ruminate (Jain et al., 2007). If mindfulness can indeed help individuals decouple their present moment experience from their long-term sense of narrative self as suggested by Farb et al. (2007), then this may explain how it helps individuals focus on their current experience rather than negative thoughts relating to past experiences or future worries.

Increased Positive Affect

Although many long-term practitioners have reported high levels of equanimity and contentment as a result of their meditation practice, objective measurement of the tantalizing link between mindfulness and positive affect is difficult to quantify. However, a few studies have offered some hints that mindfulness practices may help to foment positive affect, inclusive of clinical populations.

Richard Davidson and colleagues measured resting EEG patterns in healthy subjects before and after an 8-week MBSR intervention as compared to a control group (Davidson et al., 2003). Davidson had previously shown that patients suffering from depression and anxiety have increased EEG power in the right half of the brain while resting quietly, while psychologically healthy subjects have greater activity on the left. Although the study was small, the results indicated that a leftward shift in resting EEG patterns could be detected after 8 weeks of practice and persisted for 3 months following the study completion. More importantly, the observed changes were correlated with improved immune function.

Additionally, a recent EEG study of MBCT using a group of 22 acutely suicidal patients found that positive affective style as measured by EEG activity increased significantly in the MBCT condition as compared to treatment as usual. This suggests that the success of MBCT may in part be attributable to helping individuals to maintain an emotionally stable pattern of brain activity (Barhofer et al., 2007).

Reduced Stress Reactivity

Cultivation of equanimity increases the practitioner's ability to experience negative events with less reactivity. Goleman and Schwartz (1976) hypothesized that meditators should demonstrate less physiological reactivity to unpleasant stimuli compared to controls. To test this hypothesis, they measured skin conductance responses (SCR) from meditators and controls while the subjects viewed re-enacted wood-shop accidents. SCR measure the amount of sweat produced as an indicator of autonomic arousal. Compared to controls, the meditation subjects experienced a slightly larger initial increase in SCR, but then returned to baseline levels more quickly, indicating that the meditation subjects had heightened responses to the negative images, but were then able to quickly "let go" of the images and return to a state of mental calm and equilibrium. Presumably these subjects are less engaged in ruminative thoughts that would prolong their autonomic arousal.

Enhanced Cognitive Vitality

Another potentially important benefit of regular meditation is the protection against cortical thinning that normally occurs in old age. In our 2005 study, it was found that among meditators, one small region of prefrontal cortex appeared to be spared from normal age-related cortical thinning. This suggests that meditation may protect against cortical thinning that is typically associated with aging. A similar recent study comparing the cortical thickness of a group of Zen practitioners with non-meditators also found that age was correlated with decreased cortical thickness in the control group but not for the meditator group (Pagnoni, personal communication) 2007. Future studies will be required to verify whether this is indeed the case. If so, meditation could be a potentially powerful intervention against some of the age-dependent cognitive declines in older adults.

Summary

The purpose of this chapter has been to provide an overview of the recent neurobiological literature on mindfulness meditation, as well as some of the clinical applications of this work. We now possess sufficient evidence to demonstrate that meditation is a unique mental state—distinct from resting states—and that it appears to promote long-term structural and functional changes in brain regions important for performing clinically relevant functions. By identifying these neurobiological changes and connecting them to behavioral and clinical benefits, we will be able to better understand how meditation and mindfulness practice work at the brain level, which may help validate their use and help identify those conditions that are more likely to respond favorably to mindfulness-based interventions.

Given the heterogeneity of meditation techniques, future comparative studies are needed to elucidate both common mechanisms and differential effects that are associated with different styles of meditation practice. Particularly when working with a clinical population, we are likely to find that different forms of meditation are more or less well-suited to help individuals with a specific type of disorder. Learning how to select the right form of meditation practice to best match an individual patient is a critical next step in the clinical application of mindfulness-based treatment. Of crucial importance in this effort will be the use of longitudinal study designs, in which scientists can compare clinical and neurobiological changes in individuals at pre- and post-treatment time points.

Overall, clinicians should be encouraged by the results of the neurobiological research on meditation. While there is still much that we have yet to understand, research findings generally support the use of meditation as a powerful technique in clinical practice.

References

Aftanas, L. I., & Golocheikine, S. A. (2005). Impact of regular meditation practice on EEG activity at rest and during evoked negative emotions. *International Journal of Neuroscience, 115*, 893–909.

Andresen, J. (2000). Meditation meets behavioral medicine: The story of experimental research on meditation. *Journal of consciousness Studies, 7*, 17–73.

Austin, J. H. (1998). *Zen and the Brain: Toward an understanding of meditation and consciousness*. Cambridge, MA: MIT Press.

Azari, N. P., Nickel, J., Wunderlich, G., Niedeggen, M., Hefter, H., Tellmann, L., et al. (2001). Neural correlates of religious experience. *European Journal of Neuroscience, 13*, 1649–1652.

Baerentsen, K. B. (2001). Onset of meditation explored with fMRI. *Neuroimage, 13*, S297.

Baer, R. A. (Ed). (2006). *Mindfulness-based treatment approaches: Clinician's guide to evidence base and applications*. San Diego, CA: Elsevier Academic Press.

Banquet, J. P. (1973). Spectral analysis of the EEG in meditation. *Electroencephalography and Clinical Neurophysiology, 35*, 143–151.

Barnhofer, T., Duggan, D., Crane, C., Hepburn, S., Fennell, M. J., & Williams, J. M. (2007). Effects of meditation on frontal alpha-asymmetry in previously suicidal individuals. *Neuroreport, 18(7)*, 709–812.

Becker, D. E., & Shapiro, D. (1981). Physiological responses to clicks during zen, yoga, and TM meditation. *Psychophysiology, 18(6)*, 694–699.

Brefczynski-Lewis, J. A., Lutz, A., Schaefer, H. S., Levinson, D. B., & Davidson, R. J. (2007). Neural correlates of attentional expertise in long-term meditation practitioners. *Proceedings of the National Academy of Sciences of the USA, 104(27)*, 11483–11488.

Bush, G., Luu, P., & Posner, M. I. (2000). Cognitive and emotional influences in anterior cingulate cortex. *Trends in Cognitive Sciences, 4(6)*, 215–222.

Cahn, B. R., & Polich, J. (2006). Meditation states and traits: Eeg, erp, and neuroimaging studies. *Psychological Bulletin, 132(2)*, 180–211.

Casey, K. L., Minoshima, S., Morrow, T. J., & Koeppe, R. A. (1996). Comparison of human cerebral activation pattern during cutaneous warmth, heat pain, and deep cold pain. *Journal of Neurophysiology, 76(1)*, 571–581.

Craig, A. D., (2004). Human feelings: Why are some more aware than others? *Trends in Cognitive Sciences, 8(6)*, 231–241.

Crespo-Facorro, B., Kim, J., Andreasen, N. C., O'Leary, D. S., Bockholt, H. J., & Magnotta, V. (2000). Insular cortex abnormalities in schizophrenia: A structural magnetic resonance imaging study of first-episode patients. *Schizophrenia Research, 46(1)*, 35–43.

Creswell, J. D., Way, B. M., Eisenberger, N. I., & Lieberman, M. D. (2007). Neural correlates of dispositional mindfulness during affect labeling. *Psychosomatic Medicine, 69(6)*, 560–565.

Cuthbert, B., Kriteller, J., Simons, R., Hodes, R., & Lang, P. J. (1981). Strategies of arousal control: Biofeedback, meditation, and motivation. *Journal of Experimental Psychology: General, 110*, 518–546.

Davidson, J. M. (1976). The physiology of meditation and mystical states of consciousness. *Perspectives in Biology and Medicine, 19*, 345–379.

Davidson, R. J., Kabat-Zinn, J., Schumacher, J., Rosenkranz, M., Muller, D., Santorelli, S. F., et al. (2003). Alterations in brain and immune function produced by mindfulness meditation. *Psychosomatic Medicine, 65(4)*, 564–570.

Delmonte, M. M. (1984). Physiological responses during meditation and rest. *Biofeedback and Self Regulation, 9*, 181–200.

Delmonte, M. M. (1985). Effects of expectancy on physiological responsivity in novice meditators. *Biological Psychology, 21*, 107–121.

Dunn, B. R., Hartigan, J. A., & Mikulas, W. L. (1999). Concentration and mindfulness meditations: Unique forms of consciousness? *Applied Psychophysiology and Biofeedback, 24*(3), 147-165.

Farb, N. A. S., Segal, Z. V., Mayberg, H. M., Bean, J., McKeon, D., Fatima, Z., & Anderson, A. K. (2007). Attending to the present: mindfulness reveals distinct neural modes of self-reference. *Social Cognitive and Affective Neuroscience, 2(4),* 313-322.

Goleman, D. J., & Schwartz, G. E. (1976). Meditation as an intervention in stress reactivity. *Journal of Consulting and Clinical Psychology, 44*(3), 456-466.

Hirai, T. (1974). *Psychophysiology of Zen.* Tokyo: Igaku Shoin.

Holzel, B. K., Ott, U., Hempel, H., Hackl, A., Wolf, K., Stark, R., et al. (2007). Differential engagement of anterior cingulate and adjacent medial frontal cortex in adept meditators and non-meditators. *Neuroscience Letters, 421*(1), 16-21.

Jacobs, G.D., & Lubar, J. F. (1989). Spectral analysis of the central nervous system effects of the relaxation response elicited by autogenic training. *Behavioral Medicine, 15,* 125-132.

Jain, S., Shapiro, S. L., Swanick, S., Roesch, S. C., Mills, P. J., Bell, I., et al. (2007). A randomized controlled trial of mindfulness meditation versus relaxation training: Effects on distress, positive states of mind, rumination, and distraction. *Annals of Behavioral Medicine, 33*(1), 11-21.

Jevning, R., Wallace, R. K., & Beidebach, M. (1992). The physiology of meditation: A review. A wakeful hypometabolic integrated response. *Neuroscience and Biobehavioral Reviews, 16,* 415-424.

Jha, A. P., Krompinger, J., & Baime, M. J. (2007). Mindfulness training modifies subsystems of attention. *Cognitive Affective and Behavioral Neurosciences, 7(2),* 109-119.

Kasamatsu, A., & Hirai, T. (1966). An electroencephalographic study on the Zen meditation (zazen). *Folia Psychiatrica et Neurologica Japonica, 20,* 315-336.

Kasamatsu, A., & Hirai, T. (1973). An electroencephalographic study on the Zen meditation (zazen). *Journal of the American Institute of Hypnosis, 14,* 107-114.

Lazar, S. W., Bush, G., Gollub, R. L., Fricchione, G. L., Khalsa, G., & Benson, H. (2000). Functional brain mapping of the relaxation response and meditation. *NeuroReport, 11,* 1581-1585.

Lazar, S. W. (2005). Mindfulness research. In R. D. Siegel, P. R. Fulton, (Eds.), *Mindfulness and psychotherapy* (pp. 220-238) New York, NY, US: Guilford Press.

Lazar, S. W., Kerr, C., Wasserman, R. J., Gray, J. R., Greve D., Treadway, M. T. et al., (2005). Meditation experience is associated with increased cortical thickness. *Neuroreport* 16(17):1893-1897.

Lehmann, D., Faber, P. L., Achermann, P., Jeanmonod, D., Gianotti, L. R., & Pizzagalli, D. (2001). Brain sources of EEG gamma frequency during volitionally meditation-induced, altered states of consciousness, and experience of the self. *Psychiatry Research, 108*(2), 111-121.

Liotti, M., Mayberg, H. S., McGinnis, S., Brannan, S. L., & Jerabek, P. (2002). Unmasking disease-specific cerebral blood flow abnormalities: Mood challenge in patients with remitted unipolar depression. *American Journal of Psychiatry, 159*(11), 1830-1840.

Lutz, A., Greischar, L. L., Rawlings, N. B., Ricard, M., & Davidson, R. J. (2004). Long-term meditators self-induce high-amplitude gamma synchrony during mental practice. *Proceeding of the National Academy of Sciences of the USA, 101*(46), 16369-16373.

Murphy, M., Donovan, S., & Taylor, E. (1997). The physical and psychological effects of meditation: A review of contemporary research 1991-1996. Petaluma, CA: Institute of Noetic Sciences.

Newberg, A., Alavi, A., Baime, M., Pourdehnad, M., Santanna, J., & d'Aquili, E. (2001). The measurement of regional cerebral blood flow during the complex cognitive task of meditation: a preliminary SPECT study. *Psychiatry Research, 106(2)*, 113-122.

Pagano, R. R., & Warrenburg, S. (1983). Meditation: In search of a unique effect. In R. J. Davidson, G. E. Schwartz, & D. Shapiro (Eds.), *Consciousness and self-regulation* (Vol. 3, pp. 152-210). New York: Plenum Press.

Pagnoni, G., & Cekic M. (2007) Age effects on gray matter volume and attentional performance in Zen meditation. *Neurobiol Aging , 28(10)*,1623-7.

Paus, T. (2001). Primate anterior cingulate cortex: Where motor control, drive and cognition interface. *Nature Reviews Neuroscience, 2(6)*, 417-424.

Phillips, M. L., Drevets, W. C., Rauch, S. L., & Lane, R. (2003). Neurobiology of emotion perception ii: Implications for major psychiatric disorders. *Biological Psychiatry, 54(5)*, 515-528.

Reiman, E. M., Lane, R. D, Ahern, G. L., & Scwartz, G. E. (1997). Neuroanatomical correlates of externally and internally generated human emotion. *American Journal of Psychiatry, 154*, 918-925.

Ritskes, R., Ritskes-Hoitinga, M., Stodkilde-Jorgensen, H., Baerentsen, K., & Hartman, T. (2003). MRI scanning during Zen meditation: The picture of enlightenment? *Constructivism in the Human Sciences, 8*, 85-90.

Schuman, M. (1980). The psychophysiological model of meditation and altered states of consciousness: A critical review. In J. M. Davidson & R. J. Davidson (Eds.), *The psychobiology of consciousness* (pp. 333-378). New York: Plenum Press.

Shapiro, K. L., Arnell, K. A., & Raymond, J. E. (1997). The attentional blink. *Trends in Cognitive Sciences, 1*, 291-296.

Shin, L. M., Dougherty, D. D., Orr, S. P., Pitman, R. K., Lasko, M., Macklin, M. L., et al. (2000). Activation of anterior paralimbic structures during guilt-related script-driven imagery. *-Biological Psychiatry, 48(1)*, 43-50.

Slagter, H. A., Lutz, A., Greischar, L. L., Francis, A. D., Nieuwenhuis, S., Davis, J. M., et al. (2007). Mental training affects distribution of limited brain resources. *PLoS Biology, 5(6)*, e138.

Taneli, B., & Krahne, W. (1987). EEG change of transcendental meditation practitioners. *Advances in Biological Psychiatry, 16*, 41-71.

Valentine, E. R., & Sweet, P. L. G. (1999) Meditation and attention: a comparison of the effects of concentrative and mindfulness meditation on sustained attention. *Mental Health, Religion & Culture, 2(1)*, 59-70.

West, M. A. (1979). Meditation. *British Journal of Psychiatry, 135*, 457-467.

Woolfolk, R. L. (1975). Psychophysiological correlates of meditation. *Archives of General Psychiatry, 32*, 1326-1333.

Wright, I.C., Rabe-Hesketh, S., Woodruff, P.W.R., David, A.S., Murray, R.M., Bullmore, E.T. (2000). Regional brain structure in schizophrenia: A meta-analysis of volumetric MRI studies. *American Journal of Psychiatry, 157*, 16-25.

Wright, P., He, G., Shapira, N. A., Goodman, W. K., & Liu, Y. (2004). Disgust and the insula: fMRI responses to pictures of mutilation and contamination. *Neuroreport, 15(15)*, 2347-2351.

4

Toward a Phenomenology of Mindfulness: Subjective Experience and Emotional Correlates

Kirk Warren Brown and Shari Cordon

Natural objects ... must be experienced before any theorizing about them can occur.

Husserl E. (1981)

Since its introduction to the behavioral science research community 25 years ago, interest in mindfulness has burgeoned. Much of that interest has been among clinical researchers testing the efficacy of mindfulness-based or mindfulness-integrated interventions for a variety of conditions and populations, and this volume is testament to the vitality of investigation and diversity of applied knowledge that now exist in the field. In the last 5 years or so, researchers have also become interested in describing and operationalizing the mindfulness construct itself. This more recent line of work is important for four reasons: The first concerns the basic scientific principle that a phenomenon can be studied only if it can be properly defined and measured. Second, investigation of mindfulness creates opportunities to investigate the *specific* role of this quality in subjective experience and behavior through methodologies derived from basic science that can complement applied, intervention research. Third and relatedly, it is assumed that the efficacy of mindfulness interventions is due, in large part, to the enhancement of mindful capacities through training; but only with clear definitions and operationalizations of mindfulness can this claim be tested. Fourth, and more fundamentally, the study of mindfulness can help to widen the window into the study of human consciousness and its modes of processing experience. In this way, the study of mindfulness can help to inform about the nature of consciousness, its fundamental role in human functioning, and how its processes can be refined to enhance that functioning.

This chapter has two primary, related aims designed to highlight the value of research on mindfulness itself. First, we attempt to situate mindfulness within a long-standing scholarly discussion of conscious processing to better

---

Portions of this chapter were drawn from Brown, Ryan, and Creswell (2007).

understand the nature of the phenomenon. This effort is important, we believe, because the concept of mindfulness is not well understood within contemporary behavioral science, likely due in part to its relative novelty as a topic of scientific study. Conversely, the annals of philosophical and psychological discourse are replete with discussions of consciousness that can help to inform the construction of a well-specified theory about the meaning and functional consequences of mindfulness. A second aim of this chapter is to highlight the findings of recent research on those functional consequences of mindfulness, particularly as they pertain to emotional states and well-being. The study of emotion in the context of consciousness is important for several reasons, including the fact that emotions are a primary, ongoing feature of day-to-day consciousness and, as we will argue, the valence, duration, and other aspects of emotion are dependent on the modes through which events and experiences are processed. Also, emotions can significantly influence cognitive experience and behavior, and not coincidentally in view of its impact on human functioning, emotion is the domain in which much of the extant research on the mindfulness construct has been conducted.

The Nature of Mindfulness

Central to the scientific enterprise of describing the nature and effects of mindfulness is a clear definition of the phenomenon. In contemporary behavioral science discourse, the term is often used in an unclear, even confusing way (Brown, Ryan, & Creswell, 2007; Lutz, Dunne, & Davidson, 2007). There is general agreement in both historical and contemporary philosophical and psychological discourse that mindfulness is rooted in the fundamental capacities of consciousness, namely, attention and (meta-) awareness. Yet consciousness is a challenging area of study, thus making a firm understanding of mindfulness more difficult. In this chapter we attempt to clarify the nature of mindfulness by drawing on scholarship that has devoted considerable study to its experiential nature. In particular, we discuss work that has attempted to deconstruct human consciousness into its primary modes of processing. Viewing mindfulness through such a lens may facilitate an understanding of mindfulness as a basic human capacity (e.g., Goldstein, 2002; Kabat-Zinn, 2003) and not simply as a therapeutic practice. In so doing, the task of understanding mindfulness per se, apart from the attitudes and techniques used to cultivate it in clinical and other practices, may be simplified considerably (cf. Olendzki, 2005). This will also aid the advancement of the science of mindfulness, insofar as it aims to de-confound mindfulness from its antecedents, consequences, and particular uses in clinical practice and research.

In this discussion we draw on two rich traditions of historical and contemporary scholarship, namely phenomenology, particularly with the Husserlian school, and Buddhism, especially within the Theravadin tradition, which has and continues to have intense interest in mindfulness. We begin with Husserlian phenomenology. This vital philosophical tradition offers a rich analysis of subjective states of mind that can inform our understanding of the Buddhist psychology on mindfulness. Indeed, the various points of inter-section between these schools of thought may help to show what features of conscious experience that are relevant to mindfulness extend beyond the specific cultural and practice traditions of Buddhism. Such dialogue may facilitate the scientific investigation of mindfulness and related conscious states. Given space constraints, we will not attempt a detailed analysis of such descriptive parallels, but will simply indicate basic points of connection that, recent theory and research suggest, may be generative for further investigation.

A Phenomenological Perspective

While the concept of mindfulness appears to have been first described in Asia, its phenomenological nature is strikingly familiar to Western philosophical and psychological schools of thought. Phenomenology, particularly in the Husserlian school (e.g., Husserl, 1999), has a considerable literature of relevance to the experiential nature of mindfulness. Buddhist psychology and phenomenology naturally converge in their interest in discovering the operation of the mind through first-person experience, specifically by closely observing our subjective and sensory experiences (Dreyfus & Thompson, 2007). Phenomenology, and more recently cognitive science, propose that there are two primary modes of conscious processing. Husserl called these the natural attitude and the phenomenological attitude. The *natural attitude* – the default mode of processing – is an orientation toward ourselves, others, and the world in which events and experiences are treated as objects upon which cognitive operations are made. In this mode, what comes into awareness through the senses or the mind is both subjectively experienced as a sense impression, image, feeling, and so on and filtered through cognitive operations, typically of a habitual nature – evaluation of it, rumination about it, for example – all designed to disclose the content of what we experience, and in particular what it represents (or could represent) *to me* or *for me*. This mode of processing has a variety of expressions. A common one is a rapid presumption of truth about some phenomenon in which the discursive mind makes cognitive commitments that say, in effect, "I know what this is" or "I know what's going on" without careful observation, or sometimes without more than a glance (cf. Langer, 2002). In this conceptual mode or attitude, similar to what has been called second-order processing (Lambie & Marcel, 2002) and propositional processing (Teasdale, 1999), our reality takes mental representational form; that is, our experience becomes what we *conceptualize* it to be.

Contemporary cognitive and social cognitive science has lent support to the phenomenological claim that the natural attitude can be considered a default mode of conscious processing because what comes into awareness is often held in focal attention only briefly, if at all, before some cognitive and emotional reaction to it occurs. These rapid perceptual reactions have several characteristics of relevance to subjective experience and functioning: First, they are often of an evaluative nature, in which a primary appraisal of the object is made as, most basically, "good," "bad," or "neutral," usually in reference to the self and usually with an affective tone of, most basically, pleasantness or unpleasantness. Second, they are usually conditioned by past experience of the sensory object or other objects of sufficient similarity to evoke an association in memory. Third, perceptual experience is easily assimilated or, through further cognitive operations upon the object, made to assimilate into existing cognitive schemas.

The psychological consequence of such processing is that concepts, labels, ideas, and judgments are often imposed, often automatically, on everything that is encountered (e.g., Bargh & Chartrand, 1999). This is not to imply that humans simply process the world passively, however, because cognitive schemas, beliefs, and opinions also channel our attention and subsequent cognitive processing of what is attended to (Leary, 2004; 2005). This mode of processing does have adaptive benefits, including the establishment and maintenance of order upon events and experience of relevance to the self, and the facilitation of goal pursuit and attainment. However, it also means that we do not experience reality impartially, as it truly is, but rather through cognitive filters that are frequently of a habitual, conditioned nature. These filters can furnish superficial, incomplete, or distorted views of reality, and they lend themselves to particular emotional colorings. For example, an optimistic view or bias may conduce to hope or excitement; a pessimistic view may result in frustration, fear, or sadness.

Husserl called the second mode of processing the *phenomenological attitude* in which our attention is turned toward reality simply as it appears or is given to us, that is, simply as a flow of phenomena or appearances. Husserl termed the means to do so *phenomenological reduction*. This does not mean a replacement or an elimination of our typical cognitive operations upon reality but rather a "stepping back" from our usual way of processing in order to receive experience as it manifests itself to us. In this way, everything – sense impressions, feelings, images, and thoughts – remain but are perceived in a different way, that is, strictly as they appear (Thompson & Zahavi, 2007). In this stepping out of the natural attitude, through a "suspension" or "bracketing" of our habitually conceptual mode of processing, the mind discloses how reality is "constituted" in the present moment and within the structure of our conscious minds.

This mode of processing, similar to first-order processing (Lambie & Marcel, 2002) and buffered implicational processing (Teasdale, 1999), involves a receptive state of mind, wherein attention is kept to a bare registering of the facts observed. That this is possible is suggested by a simple illustration (Kriegel, 2007): An individual looks at the sky with a particular shade of blue that we will call $blue_{17}$. But when later presented with two shades of blue, $blue_{17}$ and $blue_{18}$, he is unable to recognize which shade of blue he saw before. This suggests that he lacks the concept of $blue_{17}$ and that his experience of that color is non-conceptual. Another illustration to help make the distinction between the natural and phenomenological attitudes comes from Varela and Depraz (2003, p. 205):

> When I am perceiving a pear tree in the garden and its gradual blossoming during early spring, the tree is here in front of me. I can touch it if I stretch out my hand, I can sense its perfume and listen to the noise of the wind in its branches. I am attending to the whole situation in flesh and bone, directly and concretely. If, on the contrary, I close my eyes and try to get a mental image of

the tree and its surroundings, I might be able to accurately describe the just-lived scene if I have been quite attentive to its developing. But most probably I will forget some features of the experience and will add some others.

At this point, it may be apparent that if one were not fully attending to the scene in the first place, both the subjective quality of the experience and one's memory of it would be quite different than if one were giving full attention. When attention is used to make bare or direct contact with the world, the basic capacities of consciousness – attention and awareness – permit the individual to "be present" to reality as it is rather than to habitually react to it. Even the usual psychological reactions that may occur when our attention is engaged – thoughts, images, verbalizations, emotions, impulses to act, and so on – can be observed as part of the ongoing stream of consciousness. For example, in the moment-to-moment experience of anger or some other emotion, it can be known in its cognitive, affective, somatic, and conative manifestations.

It is important to note that the suspension of the second-order mode of processing described here does not imply an objectification of, or disso-ciation from, our experience; in fact, the process is exactly the opposite. When cognitive elaborations are set aside, the phenomenological attitude creates an intimacy with conscious experience, a "view from within" the world (Varela & Shear, 1999) rather than set apart from it as an indepen-dent perceiver (Legrand, 2007; Thompson & Zahavi, 2007). Indeed, as noted above, from this intimate perspective not only external events but also inter-nal experiences, including the operations of the mind, can be experienced attentively.

This opens the question of who is doing the looking or, said differently, who is the self simply attending to what is? A number of philosophical tra-ditions propose that there are two selves that correspond to the modes of processing outlined here (e.g., Gallagher, 2000). The "narrative self" is that coherent set of cognitive activities that establish and maintain an ongoing narrative or set of stories about ourselves and our place in the world. This conceptual model of self and the world forms a powerful cognitive filter through which second-order processing can take place; so powerful that Dennett (1992) termed it "the center of narrative gravity." In contrast, the "minimal self" is our basic, immediate experience of reality; it is that feature of consciousness that constitutes our experience of "what it feels like" to see our friend approaching, feel joy or sadness, receive a creative insight, and otherwise be an active recipient of what conscious awareness brings to our attention (Legrand, 2007).

To speak of being an active recipient of experience is to suggest that the phenomenological attitude has both active and passive aspects. Husserl pointed out that consciousness is intentional, in that it aims toward or intends something beyond itself; it is not self-enclosed (Thompson & Zahavi, 2007). This is not to be confused with the more familiar usage of the term that implies goal directedness. For Husserl, our most fundamental intentional activity is to be actively receptive to reality, to take notice by giving attention to that which affects us. By speaking of "that which affects us" is to recognize that attention is subject to influence; it tends to turn toward what is salient at a given time or, said differently, toward stimuli that are sufficiently strong to engage the conscious mind. Thus, in this mode we are actively receptive to that which engages the mind, and this dynamic forms our fundamental way of being open to reality (Thompson & Zahavi, 2007).[2]

A Basic Phenomenology of Mindfulness

Husserl's detailed analysis of the natural attitude and the phenomenological attitude offers considerable insight into how mindfulness can be understood, particularly as it operates in a day-to-day life context. Indeed, the study of the nature of mindfulness is inherently phenomenological, as it concerns the subjective nature and uses of the conscious mind. Further, mindfulness bears several striking similarities to the phenomenological attitude that Husserl described, as we hope to make clear in our effort to characterize mindfulness.

Much historical and contemporary scholarship uses the term mindfulness (*sati* in Pali) to refer to heightened attention and specifically the sustained focusing of the mind upon an object or experience (e.g., Lutz et al., 2007; Wallace, 1999). As contemporary Theravadin scholars Analayo (2003) and Bodhi (2000) note, mindfulness, in its simplest form, is *bare attention*, or full attention to the present. As Nyanaponika (1973) first used that expression, attention is bare when undisturbed by, or captured by, the mind's usual discriminative thought and language – evaluations, conceptual elaborations, and so on. In this way, mindfulness is intended to *lay bare* events and experiences as clearly as possible (Bodhi, 2000; cf. Dreyfus & Thompson, 2007). Thus, for example, thoughts and emotions are experienced as psychological and somatic events, not as episodes in a narrative or personal drama (Bodhi, 2000). Even though attention may shift from one event or experience to another, mindful attention is given to each.

Focused attention is the traditional, core meaning given to mindfulness. However, Theravadin thought, like contemporary cognitive science, recognizes that attention and awareness are intertwined in daily life. That is, attention regularly pulls "figures" out of the "background" of sensory and internal stimuli that come into awareness. In traditional mindfulness training, once a student has a certain familiarity with focused attention, it is supplemented by meta-awareness (Pali: *sampajanna*). This term has multiple meanings: The simplest meaning is knowing the state of the mind at a given moment, including the quality of one's attention. A deeper meaning is insight or clear seeing into the nature of the phenomena that are given attention. Such insight comes as refined attention brings the field of experience into ever finer focus, allowing for a deepening discovery of the elements that constitute experience – for example, the fact that thoughts, emotions, and other mental events are in constant flux (Analayo, 2003; Bodhi, 2000, 2006).

Sati and *sampajanna*, though often discussed separately in scholarship, can operate together in practice (Pali: *satisampajanna*; Analayo, 2003). For example, in MBSR and other mindfulness-based treatment approaches,

---

[2] It is important to note that an active–passive dynamic also occurs in object-oriented, second-order processing, but in that case, the activity is not about opening to what is, but rather concerns evaluation, discrimination, and other cognitive activities that attention has been affectively turned to.

the student is encouraged to take a kinesthetic experience as an object of focused attention – most commonly, the breath. When awareness arises that the mind has strayed from this object, attention is gently brought back to its focus. In this way, attention is refined while awareness is made more sensitive to what is occurring at any given moment, both of which are key, interrelated skills to be translated into day-to-day life. For example, one can be aware of all that is currently salient and can use that meta-awareness to bring a focus of attention toward some stimulus or phenomenon (Kornfield, 1993). In this way, mindfulness involves a voluntary, fluid regulation of attention. This mindful mode of processing may have particular value for mental and physical health maintenance and treatment, wherein a more sensitive awareness can lead to the uncovering of (perhaps challenging) psychological or somatic realities that can be given focused attention as a means to investigate, more fully process, and thereby better regulate or transcend them.

Nyaniponika (1973) noted that when both attention and meta-awareness work together in this way, mindfulness achieves its intended purpose.[3] Bodhi (2006) has called this conjoining of attention and awareness "integrated wise attention." The subjective experience of this refinement of the basic capacities of consciousness is *presence* (Bodhi, 2006; Tsoknyi, 1998; Uchiyama, 2004) – an immediacy of experience as it occurs. As we have noted elsewhere (Brown et al., 2007), the mind is adept at "time-traveling" into memories of the past, fantasies about the future and, in general, away from the realities of the present. This time travel can serve the important regulatory purpose of protecting, maintaining, and enhancing the self in, for example, the pursuit of goals (Sheldon & Vansteenkiste, 2005), but it is easily forgotten that we and our thoughts exist only in the present moment, with no direct experience of either past or future. With consciousness dwelling in current reality as it actually offers itself, rather than caught up in thought-generated accounts about the past, present, and future, reality is more likely to be seen objectively, as it is, rather than ignored or conceptually controlled, and thereby only partially experienced. Indeed, in this experiential mode of processing, thoughts of past, present, and future can be attentively engaged in the same way that other phenomena are – that is, without the loss of psychological autonomy that presence of mind confers.

This discussion suggests that the Buddhist concept of mindfulness has several broad points of connection to Husserl's phenomenological attitude: First, in both traditions the experience of what is occurring in the present becomes of paramount interest, whether that experience arises from within the body-mind or through the senses. Second, both propose that this presence is entered through a suspension of the habitual or automatized way of processing experience in favor of an open attentiveness that simply processes what is occurring moment by moment. In both traditions, two activities are involved in this – a suspension of inattentive immersion in

---

[3] It is this integration of attention and meta-awareness that helps to distinguish mindfulness from concentration. As Georges Dreyfus (personal communication, October 17, 2007) notes, attention may become focused on an object but without sufficient clarity or presence to retain that focus. That is, the mind may become concentrated, but without meta-awareness to help preserve that focused attentiveness, it would be lacking in mindfulness.

experience that meta-awareness allows and a turning of attention to the manner in which things appear. Both traditions claim that this flexibility of attention helps to bring a freshness and clarity to subjective experience (Thompson, 2007; Varela & Depraz, 2003). Third and relatedly, as an experiential state, this attention is actively receptive to what enters the mind rather than placed in the service of cognitive manipulation of that mental content. Fourth, both systems of thought propose that presence can be cultivated (lengthened, deepened, etc.) through practice, although historically, these traditions have differed in their emphasis on the practical application of attention to investigate first-person experience. Recently, phenomenologists have sought to more explicitly delineate pragmatic approaches to the study of conscious experience from a first-person perspective (Depraz, 1999; Thompson & Zahavi, 2007), but mindfulness and other attentional practices have been foundational to informing Buddhist philosophy and psychology for centuries.

Historically, these traditions have also received different degrees of attention from scientists interested in the benefits of the experiential mode of processing and the way of being in the world, perhaps in part due to the differing focus on practical application. Recently, phenomenologically informed researchers have begun to examine the neural correlates and perceptual effects of attentional stability and other features of the experiential stance described here (see Thompson, 2007, for a review). In contrast, mindfulness researchers have, to date, emphasized the study of the purported mental and physical health-relevant consequences of this state. The vast majority of this research has been conducted using the mindfulness-based and mindfulness-integrated interventions described in other chapters of this volume. But there has been increasing interest in the study of the nature and effects of the phenomenon itself. In the remainder of this chapter, we outline recent findings from this recent research on the emotional correlates and consequences of mindfulness, both as an induced state of mind, typically conducted in laboratory settings (state mindfulness), and as a disposition toward day-to-day experience (trait mindfulness). As we have suggested here, the two modes of processing outlined herein have differing implications for emotional experience, and research on state and trait mindfulness has begun to offer support for that claim. Before discussing that evidence, we first briefly outline developments in the operationalization of the mindfulness construct.

Operationalizations of Mindfulness

While the capacity for mindful presence is inherent to the human organism, this experience can vary considerably, from heightened states of clarity and sensitivity to low levels, as in habitual, automatic, mindless, or blunted thought or action (Wallace, 1999). This suggests both that individuals may differ in the frequency with which mindful capacities are deployed, due to inherent capability, inclination, or discipline, and also that there are intra-individual variations in mindfulness. This research thus investigates mindfulness as an attribute that varies both between and within persons, and examines the significance of both kinds of variation for emotional and other correlates and consequences.

Trait and State Mindfulness

The study of individual differences in mindfulness is based on a current scientific consensus that "trait mindfulness" reflects a more frequent abiding in the experiential state described earlier. Several self-report measures have been recently published in attempts to assess dispositional mindfulness and mindfulness practice skills, a number of which are reviewed by Baer in this volume.[4] Self-report measures of momentary mindful states have also been developed (Brown & Ryan, 2003; Lau et al., 2006), though to date these have not been subjected to much study. Most study of the mindful state has been conducted using brief, laboratory-based experimental inductions of mindfulness to examine its short-term effects on the regulation of mental health-relevant behavior, particularly affect. Most induction research has used guided instruction designed to bring attention to, and deepen awareness of, moment-to-moment physical, emotional, and cognitive experiences. The induction exercises used to date, usually 5–10 minutes in duration, are designed to facilitate close observation of current events and experiences so that present realities can be seen clearly and without cognitive interference. A variant of this induction strategy is the use of very brief instructions (2–3 sentences) that simply cue individuals to enter an experiential state of presence akin to mindfulness. This induction approach permits investigation of the manifestations and effects of experiential processing in real time.

Mindfulness and Emotional Experience

Emotional experience and its regulation is, of course, central to mental health and intimately bound up with mental health-relevant cognition and behavior. Thus, research addressing how mindful traits and states explain variance in emotion and emotion regulation can contribute to our understanding of how mindfulness may foster mental health more broadly.

Elements of Emotional Experience

Emotion can be understood in terms of both its content – what is felt – and its underlying neurobiological processes or causes (Barrett, Mesquita, Ochsner, & Gross, 2007). At its core, emotional content concerns subjective feelings of pleasure or displeasure. This is termed *core affect*. There is now considerable evidence that people represent emotions in these terms (e.g., Posner, Russell, & Peterson, 2005; Russell, 1980). But as Barrett et al. (2007) note, the experience of emotion is typically *about* something, as well; that is, it is an intentional state that is dependent on level of arousal, relational meaning, and situational meaning that all help to create psychologically distinct experiences of joy, calm, fear, sadness, anger, and many others. It is in the meaning assigned to situations (i.e., cognitive appraisals) through

---

[4] We refer to "mindfulness practice skills" as the variety of practice-based supports for the expression of mindful attention, including an attitude of acceptance toward experience, discursive description of subjective experiences as they arise (e.g., labeling), and so on.

which the study of emotional content and emotion regulation has been commonly conducted.

Barrett et al. (2007) note that most influential theories of emotion assume that experiences of emotion – like other mental events – are rooted in (though not necessarily reducible to) neurological processes. In its current state, neuroscience cannot pinpoint particular brain regions or types of neural activity that instantiate specific emotional contents, but it has been able to show what parts of the brain are active during core affective experiences of pleasant and unpleasant emotion and in the experience of particular emotions. Neuroscience research has also begun to hone in on those brain regions that appear important to the regulation of core affect, particularly unpleasant emotion.

Why Should Mindfulness Be Associated with Emotional Well-Being?

From the foregoing discussion of the subjective or phenomenological nature of mindfulness, there are several reasons to propose that this quality should have distinctive emotional content and regulatory correlates, all of which center on the experiential nature of this manner of processing. First, because mindfulness involves a disengagement from habitually evaluative conceptual processing, it should conduce to more balanced states of core affect. That is, it should be related to less unpleasant affect and perhaps less pleasant affect as well, although a freshness and immediacy of contact with experience may, in some circumstances, add a pleasant affective overlay to it (as in the Varela & Depraz (2003) example given earlier; see also Brown & Ryan, 2003; Csikszentmihalyi, 1990; Deci & Ryan, 1985). Second, with the clearer objective perception that mindfulness is thought to afford, potentially challenging events and experiences are less likely to be distorted by cognitive biases or misinterpretations that can generate unpleasant emotional responses. So, for example, mild breathlessness can simply be "seen" as is, rather than anxiously construed as a panic attack. A selfish or lustful thought is observed as it is – a thought – rather than taken as depressing evidence of personal unworthiness (Claxton, 1999). Thus, this movement of the "cursor of consciousness" (Claxton, 1999) back to a more immediate, less elaborated state should not only help to diminish core, unpleasant affective experience but also inhibit emotional reactivity to challenging stimuli. Third, the quality of attention is known to influence emotion regulatory outcomes (e.g., Gross & Thompson, 2007), and because mindfulness concerns a sustained, open attentiveness to internal and external phenomena as they are, it should discourage maladaptive emotion regulatory tendencies like rumination and thought suppression that involve cognitive entanglement and also encourage voluntary exposure to unpleasant or challenging events and experiences that has been shown to promote adaptive emotion regulation (e.g., Felder, Zvolensky, Eifert, & Spira, 2003; Levitt, Brown, Orsillo, & Barlow, 2004; Sloan, 2004).

Research has begun to show that both trait and state mindfulness are related to emotional content, particularly core affect, and emotion regulation. The empirical evidence on mindfulness and emotional content comes from the use of cross-sectional, experience sampling, induction-based, and intervention methods. A fundamental question for such research has been: Is mindfulness associated with a more balanced or positive affective tone (less unpleasant and more pleasant affect)? Cross-sectional and experience sampling methods have primarily been used to address the role of trait mindfulness in the experience of core affect. Both cross-sectional and induction-based research has also begun to disclose how both mindful traits and states alter the primary appraisal and regulation of emotionally laden events and experiences. Finally, mindfulness-based intervention research has begun to show whether core affective experience and its regulation can be changed. Research addressing affective processes is still incipient, but studies of both mindful traits and states have begun to uncover neural substrates for both the subjective experience and the regulation of emotion that may accrue with mindfulness. We review research on each of these areas in turn.

Mindfulness, Affect, and Emotional Content

Core affect. Trait measures of mindfulness have been shown to correlate with a variety of affective (and cognitive) indicators of mental health and well-being in college student, community adult, and clinical samples. For example, the various extant measures of mindfulness and mindfulness practice skills have been associated with higher pleasant affect, lower unpleasant affect, and lower levels of emotional disturbance (e.g., depressive symptoms, anxiety, and stress), along with other, related mental health indicators including satisfaction with life and eudaimonic well-being (e.g., vitality, self-actualization) (e.g., Baer, Smith, Hopkins, Krietemeyer, & Toney, 2006; Beitel, Ferrer. & Cecero, 2004; Brown & Ryan, 2003; Cardaciotto, Herbert, Forman, Moitra, & Farrow, 2008; Carlson & Brown, 2005; Feldman, Hayes, Kumar, Greeson, & Laurenceau, 2007; Frewen, Evans, Maraj, Dozois, & Partridge, in press; McKee, Zvolensky, Solomon, Bernstein, & Leen-Feldner, 2007; Walach, Buchheld, Buttenmuller, Kleinknecht, & Schmidt, 2006). There is indication that relations between dispositional mindfulness (as measured by the mindful attention awareness scale [MAAS; Brown & Ryan, 2003]) and various emotional and other mental health indicators cannot be explained away by social desirability biases or by shared variance with global personality traits that have known impacts on emotional well-being, such as neuroticism and extroversion (Brown & Ryan, 2003; Wupperman, Neumann, & Axelrod, in press).

This correlational research is suggestive in revealing a possible wide range of influence that dispositional mindfulness may have on emotional experience, but there are known limitations to global self-reports, including their retrospective nature, which introduces room for memory biases and other errors in reporting subjective experience (e.g., Brown & Moskowitz, 1998; Stone & Shiffman, 1994). Self-reports also tend to engage semantic knowledge or beliefs about thoughts, emotions, and other subjective experiences, so it is not clear whether they accurately reflect the actual content of those experiences in real time (Barrett et al., 2007; Barrett, 1997; Robinson & Clore, 2002).

Such real-time or lived experiences can be assessed through experience sampling and related ecological momentary assessment techniques designed to capture subjective and overt behavioral experience as it occurs, typically in individuals' natural environments and over periods of days or weeks. Two studies have shown that MAAS-assessed trait mindfulness predicts core affective experience (Brown & Ryan, 2003). A 3-week-long experience sampling study with community adults, in which participants were asked to record the presence and intensity of their affective experience several times a day on a quasi-random schedule when a pager signal was received, found that trait MAAS predicted lower day-to-day unpleasant affect (but not pleasant affect). Parallel results were found in a 2-week-long experience sampling study with college students. This latter study also found that being in a mindful state (as assessed by the state MAAS) was associated with higher pleasant affect and lower unpleasant affect after controlling for variance attributable to the trait MAAS. These effects were independent, suggesting that the benefits of mindfulness may not be limited to those with a general disposition toward mindfulness. However, this research also found that those higher in trait mindfulness were more likely to report higher states of mindfulness on a day-to-day basis.

Experimental research exploring the effect of a mindful state on core affective experience has also been conducted. In a study contrasting the effects of mindful, distracted, and no-instruction control states on reading task-related subjective experience and performance, Brown and Ryan (2007) found that those randomly assigned to the induced mindfulness condition reported greater interest and enjoyment of the task relative to those in both the distraction and the no-induction conditions, after controlling for interest and enjoyment in a baseline (pre-induction) reading task.

Emotion regulation. While emotions, both pleasant and unpleasant, can serve a number of adaptive purposes, they do not always do so, and optimal emotional responding often requires regulation of the experience or expression of emotion (Barrett & Gross, 2001). This is most frequently the case for unpleasant emotions, and the regulation of negative emotional states is important to mental health (Barrett, Gross, Christensen, & Benvenuto, 2001; Gross & Munoz, 1995; Ryan, 2005). Barrett and Gross (2001) argue that effective emotion regulation requires two major skills: accurately tracking ongoing emotional states and knowing when and how to intervene to alter those states as needed. There are considerable inter-individual differences in such skills, and such differences have consequences for adaptive psychological and social functioning.

There is some evidence that mindfulness may promote the effective use of both of these skills. For example, trait mindfulness has been positively associated with measures tapping clarity about emotional experience (e.g., Baer et al., 2006; Brown & Ryan, 2003). Research has also found that mindfulness may be related to greater emotional self-awareness, as measured by indicators of implicit and explicit emotional self-concept. Implicit emotional self-concept refers to (typically) nonconscious emotional dispositions that develop through repeated learning experiences. There is considerable debate about whether and how individuals can be aware of implicit emotions and other processes (Wilson, Lindsey, & Schooler, 2000), one manifestation of which may be represented by concordance between implicit and self-reported associations of emotions with the self. Brown and Ryan (2003) found that, in general, people showed little or no concordance between explicit (self-) reports of their pleasant and unpleasant emotional self-concept on the one hand and their implicit emotional self-concept on the other. However, those higher in MAAS-assessed mindfulness showed a stronger concordance between explicit and implicit emotional self-concept, suggesting that these individuals may have greater emotional self-awareness. This finding is consistent with the phenomenological nature of mindfulness discussed earlier, but the research is still preliminary, and replication and extension are needed before it can be concluded that mindfulness fosters emotional awareness.

There is more research addressing the other primary emotion regulatory skill, namely, the alteration of emotional responses. First, trait mindfulness and mindfulness practice skills have been associated with less thought suppression, rumination, impulsivity, and passivity, all maladaptive forms of regulation linked with poorer mental health (Baer et al., 2006; Brown & Ryan, 2003; Cardaciotto et al., 2008; Chambers, Lo, & Allen, 2008; Feldman et al., 2007; Frewen et al., in press; McKee et al., 2007; Shapiro, Brown, & Biegel, 2007; Wupperman et al., in press). Conversely, mindfulness and mindfulness skills have been positively associated with adaptive regulatory strategies, including acceptance and letting go of negative thoughts (e.g., Baer et al., 2006; Brown & Ryan, 2003; Frewen et al., in press). The adaptive nature of acceptance of emotional and other subjective experiences is consistent with the notion that it is sometimes more adaptive to experience or express an emotion than to alter its trajectory (Barrett & Gross, 2001).

Beyond such preliminary investigations of dispositional emotion regulatory tendencies, several trait-based studies have tested the efficacy of mindfulness to attenuate the experience of negative emotion in emotionally provocative situations. Among the most emotionally charged situations that individuals find themselves in are those involving interpersonal conflict. It has been argued (Goleman, 2006) that the receptive attentiveness that characterizes mindfulness may promote a greater ability or willingness to take interest in a communication partner's thoughts and emotions and may also enhance an ability to attend to the content of a partner's communication while also being aware of the partner's (sometimes subtle) affective tone and nonverbal behavior. At the same time, such a person may be more aware of their own cognitive, emotional, and verbal responses to the communication. Boorstein (1996) has argued that mindfulness promotes an ability to witness thought and emotion so as not to react impulsively and destructively to them. Initial research guided by this theorizing has been conducted in the realm of romantic relationships, in which studies have addressed whether mindfulness may affect the emotional tone of romantic partner conflicts and, perhaps relatedly, enhance the communication that happens within those relationships.

Barnes, Brown, Krusemark, Campbell, and Rogge (2007) and Wachs and Cordova (2007) found that higher MAAS-measured trait mindfulness predicted higher relationship satisfaction and greater capacities to respond constructively to relationship stress among non-distressed dating couples and married couples. In the second study in their series with dating couples, Barnes et al. (2007) tested the reliability of those findings in the heat of a relationship conflict. Using a well-validated paradigm (e.g., Gottman, Coan, Carrere, & Swanson, 1998), higher trait MAAS scores predicted lower emotional stress responses to conflict (anxiety and anger hostility), and this effect was explained by lower emotional stress before the discussion. This corroborates other cross-sectional and experience sampling research, noted already, showing that those more dispositionally mindful are less susceptible to negative emotional states in general, and suggests that this lower susceptibility extends into the specific context of romantic couple interactions. Interestingly, Barnes et al.'s (2007) results showed that rather than buffering the effects of emotional arousal during conflict, mindfulness helped to inoculate against such arousal. The capacity of mindfulness to inhibit reactivity to conflict was also evident in the cognitive judgments that each partner made; those higher in trait mindfulness showed a more positive (or less negative) pre–post conflict change in their perception of the partner and the relationship. This study also supported the importance of bringing a mindful state into challenging exchanges, in that self-reported state mindfulness was related to better communication quality, as assessed by objective raters of the videotaped conflicts.

Whether mindfulness influences affective appraisals has also been tested experimentally in two studies using state inductions of mindfulness. Arch and Craske (2006) used a focused breathing exercise to induce a mindful state, while two experimental control groups received inductions of unfocused attention and worrying. Relative to experimental controls, those receiving a mindfulness induction showed less negative reactivity and emotional volatility in response to affectively valenced picture slides and a greater willingness to maintain visual contact with aversive slides. This latter finding suggests evidence for one process theorized to explain the salutary effects of mindfulness on emotion regulation and mental health, namely, willing exposure to threatening information. Interestingly, this study also found that those receiving mindfulness instructions maintained consistent, moderately positive responses to neutral picture slides, while the groups induced by unfocused attention and worry responded more negatively to neutral slides, providing some basis for the claim that mindfulness helps to protect against negatively biased processing of experience.

The Barnes et al. (2007), Wachs and Cordova (2007), and Arch and Craske (2006) findings suggest that mindfulness may influence emotional content by altering situational meaning through a primary appraisal process, in particular by reducing negative emotional reactivity to challenging stimuli. Other evidence suggests that a mindful state may alter the time course of emotion by facilitating recovery following a provocative event. Broderick (2005) found that, in comparison to those in distraction and rumination conditions, individuals in a mindful induction condition showed quicker emotional recovery from an induced sad mood. Though preliminary, these findings on reduced reactivity and speeding the recovery from unpleasant emotional experiences offer support for the hypothesized consequences of the receptive, non-evaluative mode of processing that characterizes mindfulness, and also offer promise for clinical research by suggesting a means to cope with difficult emotions when they arise (Broderick, 2005).

Dynamic relations between mindfulness and emotional content and regulation. As other chapters in this volume attest, a growing body of research indicates that mindfulness-based interventions can have positive impacts on mental health. Mindfulness interventions are purported to increase participants' mindfulness, and this is believed to be responsible for the positive effects of the interventions on cognitive, emotional, and behavioral indicators of mental health. Yet to date little research has examined whether mindfulness itself is enhanced through such multi-modal treatments and whether such enhancements are related to emotional content, emotion regulation, and other mental health outcomes observed. Such research can not only help to address basic questions about the role of mindfulness in mental health, but can also inform study of the processes by which mindfulness interventions achieve their beneficial effects. In large part, the lack of attention to such questions is because measures of the mindfulness construct have developed only recently, but since then, intervention studies have begun to test the dynamic relation between change in mindfulness and changes in emotional and cognitive indicators of mental health in healthy, healthy stressed, and clinical populations.

Several uncontrolled studies have shown scores on dispositional mindfulness and mindfulness practice skills to increase significantly over the course of MBSR and related interventions with healthy and distressed samples (e.g., Carmody & Baer, 2008; Cohen-Katz et al., 2005; Frewen et al., in press; Forman, Herbert, Moitra, Yeomans, & Geller, 2007). In a study of healthy adults participating in a 10-day intensive mindfulness training, Chambers et al. (2008) found that, relative to matched control participants, trained participants reported significant increases in MAAS mindfulness from pre- to post-training and significant reductions in negative affect, reflective rumination, and depressive symptoms. Increases in mindfulness over the study period were associated with declines in anxiety, depressive symptoms, and reflective rumination, and increases in positive affect and working memory.

Other intervention studies testing these dynamic associations have focused on health-care professionals, and professionals in training, whose occupations can put them at risk for a range of stress-related conditions, including depression, anxiety, emotional exhaustion, and occupational burnout (Sherwin et al., 1992; Tyssen, Vaglum, Gronvold, & Ekeberg, 2001). In a matched-control MBSR study of psychotherapists in training, Shapiro et al. (2007) found that intervention participants reported significant increases in MAAS-assessed mindfulness over 8 weeks, as well as increases in positive affect and declines in perceived stress, negative affect, state and trait anxiety, and rumination relative to controls. Further, enhanced mindfulness was associated with declines in anxiety and distress and a reduced tendency to use rumination to regulate emotion. Research has also begun to test such associations in clinical populations. In an uncontrolled MBSR study with cancer patients, Brown and Ryan (2003) found that increases in MAAS-assessed trait mindfulness were related to declines in stress as well as anxiety, depressive symptoms, and other indicators of mood disturbance (cf. Carlson & Brown, 2005).

In sum, preliminary trait-based research suggests that mindfulness is associated with a variety of affective (and cognitive) indicators of well-being, while both trait- and state-based research suggests that mindfulness is associated with more pleasant affect and, in particular, less unpleasant affective experience. Those higher in dispositional and state mindfulness appear to experience unpleasant affect less intensely on a day-to-day basis, and when in a mindful state, individuals react less intensely to emotionally provocative stimulation. This lower reactivity, combined with initial evidence for quicker recovery from induced unpleasant (sad) moods, suggests that mindfulness promotes more efficient emotion regulation, which may help to explain the more positive emotional states associated with mindfulness. In turn, this research also offers support for a variety of theories emphasizing the importance of attentional sensitivity to psychological and other cues for self-regulated functioning (e.g., Baumeister, Heatherton & Tice, 1994; Carver & Scheier, 1998; Deci & Ryan, 1985).

Mindfulness and Affective Processes

Research on the affective processes underlying the apparent salutary emotional correlates of mindfulness is even more recent than that focused on core affect, specific emotional content, and cognitive appraisals, but the few available studies are worth noting, particularly because they help to corroborate the research on mindfulness and subjective emotional experiences described already as well as suggest neural substrates for them.

Emotional processes involve an array of diverse, correlated neurological processes (Anderson, 2007), but two areas of the brain – the amygdala and the prefrontal cortex (PFC) – appear to be important to both the experience and the regulation of emotion. There is indication that amygdala activation is associated with negative emotional experience (particularly fear), perhaps by increasing perceptual sensitivity to negative stimuli (Barrett, Bliss-Moreau, Duncan, Rauch, & Wright, 2007). Activation in the PFC, particularly in lateral and dorsal regions, has been associated with both decreased amygdala activation and the deliberate diminishment of negative emotional responses (i.e., emotion regulation), perhaps via ventral and medial PFC regions (Phelps, 2006; Urry et al., 2006). Together, analysis of amygdala and PFC regions provides a window into the processes of emotional reactivity and regulation, thereby opening opportunities to study the neural correlates of mindful processing of emotionally provocative stimuli.

In a study addressing this topic, Creswell, Way, Eisenberger, and Lieberman (2007) examined whether more mindful individuals would show less reactivity to emotionally threatening (negative) picture stimuli, as measured by fMRI-assessed amygdala activation and stronger regulation of emotional responses through prefrontal cortical mechanisms. The study found that, relative to those lower in mindfulness, higher MAAS scorers were less reactive to threatening emotional stimuli, as indicated by an attenuated bilateral amygdala response and greater prefrontal cortical activation (in dorsomedial, left and right ventrolateral, medial, and right dorsolateral PFC) while labeling those stimuli. Also, a stronger inverse association between these areas of the PFC and the right amygdala was found among higher MAAS scorers. This latter result suggesting a greater emotion regulatory capacity through mindfulness may come through enhanced prefrontal cortical inhibition of amygdala responses. Ochsner, Bunge, and Gross (2002) have suggested that this pattern of activations may be associated with a "turning down" of evaluation processes, thus switching from an emotional mode of stimulus analysis to an unemotional one. This is consistent with the receptive, non-evaluative phenomenology of mindfulness described already, in which objects and events in focal attention are simply observed, without attempts to alter or analyze them.

There is also initial evidence that mindfulness can diminish reactivity to threat and subsequent distress in social situations, and in particular that which commonly arises when connectedness is lost due to social exclusion, an experience that people are highly motivated to avoid (e.g., Allen & Knight, 2005). Creswell, Eisenberger, and Lieberman (2007) tested whether mindful attention incurred protective benefit against distress when facing exclusion by members of a peer group and whether this greater equanimity in the face of exclusion was due to reduced reactivity to this form of social threat, measured by brain imaging of regions known to be implicated in the experience of social pain and distress.

Undergraduates participated in a virtual ball-tossing game with two other "participants" (actually a computer) while undergoing fMRI. In the first task block, each participant was included in the ball-tossing game, while in the second block, the participant was excluded during the majority of the throws. After the task, participants reported their perceptions of social rejection during exclusion. Results showed that MAAS-assessed mindfulness predicted lower perceived rejection. Further, this association was partially mediated by reduced activity in the dorsal anterior cingulate cortex (dACC), a region activated during social distress (Eisenberger, Lieberman, & Williams, 2003). These findings are consistent with the study of romantic couple conflict described already, in suggesting that mindfulness predicts a more subdued response to social threat, in this case, apparent rejection by peers, and that this attenuated response is due, in part, to reduced evaluative reactivity to that threat.

The findings also provide a window into the role of mindfulness in altering the expression of self in social contexts. Theory and research suggest that personal identity, or the self-concept, is strongly influenced by the opinions and reactions of others, and negative evaluative reactions to rejection occur because the individual's sense of self-worth is invested in, or contingent upon, validation by others (e.g., Leary, 2004). However, if a sense of self that is grounded in experiential processing is operational, events like rejection that impinge upon the self-concept may be less threatening than they otherwise might be (Brown, Ryan, Creswell, & Niemiec, 2008).

While this notion requires further study, there is initial evidence that the experiential focus (EF) described by both mindfulness scholars and phenomenologists has neural referents that are distinct from the narrative, conceptual focus that is commonly the default mode of processing. Farb et al. (2007) conducted an induction-based study with both MBSR graduates and novices trained to use two types of attentional focus upon positive and negative personality trait stimuli designed to arouse self-reference. The EF entailed a present-centered, non-conceptual attention to thoughts, feelings, and bodily states, using meta-awareness to return attention to present experience when distracted by thoughts or memories (i.e., mindfulness). A narrative focus (NF) was characterized by analysis of the meaning of the trait words and their application to self in an ongoing stream of thoughts that is also characteristic of rumination, mind wandering, and resting attention. Among other findings, the study found that EF yielded reductions in midline cortical region activity associated with NF in both novices and mindfulness trainees, particularly the medial PFC (mPFC). These mPFC reductions were more marked and pervasive among those previously trained in mindfulness.

While still nascent, this neural process-based research converges with subjective report-based research reviewed above in suggesting that the phenomenological or mindful mode of processing is associated with diminished emotional reactivity to negative stimuli and enhanced regulation of emotional response, perhaps through an engagement of attention upon immediate experience that permits a disentanglement from the conceptual networks that link subjective experiences across time to promote anxiety, regret, sadness, and other unpleasant, self-referential emotions. This process research also offers a glimpse into the neural mechanisms that may underlie the more equanimous subjective experience that mindfulness is theorized to foster (e.g., Analayo, 2003; Brown & Ryan, 2003).

Conclusions and Future Directions

This chapter had two primary aims: First, we sought to clarify the nature of mindfulness by taking a "view from within" the conscious mind's dual modes of processing experience. Husserlian phenomenology and Buddhist theories were shown to converge on several points in the description of a phenomenology of experience within which the subjective nature of mindfulness may be better understood. Second, we sought to describe the implications of this experiential approach to life for a key feature of subjective experience, namely, emotions. Findings from recent research using trait measures and state inductions of mindfulness are convergent in showing that this quality of presence is associated with more balanced emotional content, particularly a relative paucity of unpleasant emotional experience. Mindfulness also appears to promote less reactivity to events that can provoke emotional distress and more efficient regulation of that distress when it occurs. Studies using neural imaging have begun to offer clues about the cortical and subcortical substrates for the more sanguine subjective experiences that more mindful individuals report.

These studies of emotional content and process provide insight into the mechanisms by which mindfulness foster emotional well-being, and by implication, mental health. Mindfulness is believed to promote emotional well-being through multiple means (e.g., Baer, 2003; Brown et al., 2007; Shapiro et al., 2007), and the present review suggests support for the claim that mindfulness is associated with diminished evaluation of stimuli (or what has also been called acceptance and non-judgment), perhaps through an immediacy of contact with them. Another explanation for the emotional benefits of mindfulness is the receptive, non-defensive processing of experiences that present emotional challenges. Studies reviewed here suggest that willing exposure, a greater willingness to tolerate or remain experientially present to unpleasant stimuli without cognitive reactivity, may help to explain the role of mindfulness in producing greater emotional balance and more effective emotion regulation in the face of emotionally challenging events and experiences.

These descriptive and explanatory conclusions must be considered provisional, however, because studies of mindful traits and states are still relatively few, existing samples are comparatively small, and most studies have used correlational designs – all factors that limit the ability to make causal conclusions about mindfulness and emotional experience and well-being. As the field of mindfulness research matures, opportunities for building a firmer foundation of knowledge are numerous. Two are briefly noted here. First, better assessment of mindful traits is needed to more accurately reflect the scholarly descriptions of this mode of processing. In this endeavor, scholarship on both conscious states and cognitive science will be invaluable for detailing the subjective quality of experience that mindfulness involves. Second, the advent of experimental research to study mindful states offers excellent opportunities to observe the nature and outcomes of mindful, or experiential processing in real time. The value of such research lies not only in disclosing the nature and functional significance of mindfulness, but also in helping to address fundamental questions about how the conscious mind processes experience and how such processing may be optimized to enhance emotional experience and human welfare in general.

Acknowledgements: Preparation of this chapter was supported in part by NIH grant R01 AG025474-02 to the first author. We thank Melissa Glennie, Laura Kiken, Jonathan Shear, and Evan Thompson for helpful comments and suggestions on a previous draft.

References

Arch, J. J., & Craske, M. G. (2006). Mechanisms of mindfulness: Emotion regulation following a focused breathing induction. *Behavior Research and Therapy, 44,* 1849–1858.

Allen, N. B., & Knight, W. (2005). Mindfulness, compassion for self, and compassion for others. In P. Gilbert (Ed.), *Compassion: Conceptualizations, research, and use in psychotherapy* (pp. 239–262). New York: Routledge.

Analayo, B. (2003). Satipatthana: The direct path to realization. Birmingham, UK: Windhorse.

Anderson, A. K. (2007). Feeling emotional: The amygdala links emotional perception and experience. *Social Cognitive and Affective Neuroscience, 2,* 71–72.

Baer, R.A. (2003). Mindfulness training as a clinical intervention: A conceptual and empirical review. *Clinical Psychology: Science and Practice, 10,* 125–143.

Baer, R. A., Smith, G. T., Hopkins, J., Krietemeyer, J., & Toney, L. (2006). Using self-report assessment methods to explore facets of mindfulness. *Assessment, 13,* 27–45.

Bargh, J. A., & Chartrand, T. L. (1999). The unbearable automaticity of being. *American Psychologist, 54,* 462–479.

Barnes, S., Brown, K. W., Krusemark, E., Campbell, W. K., & Rogge, R. D. (2007). The role of mindfulness in romantic relationship satisfaction and responses to relationship stress. *Journal of Marital and Family Therapy, 33,* 482–500.

Barrett, L. F. (1997). The relationship among momentary emotional experiences, personality descriptions, and retrospective ratings of emotion. *Personality and Social Psychology Bulletin, 23,* 1100–1110.

Barrett, L. F., Bliss-Moreau, E., Duncan, S. L., Rauch, S. L., & Wright, C. I. (2007). The amygdala and the experience of affect. *Social Cognitive and Affective Neuroscience, 2,* 73–83.

Barrett, L. F., & Gross, J. J. (2001). Emotion representation and regulation: A process model of emotional intelligence. In T. Mayne & G. Bonnano (Eds.), *Emotion: Current issues and future directions* (pp. 286-310). New York: Guilford.

Barrett, L. F., Gross, J., Chistensen, T. C., & Benvenuto, M. (2001). Knowing what you're feeling and knowing what to do about it: Mapping the relation between emotion differentiation and emotion regulation. *Cognition & Emotion, 15,* 713-724.

Barrett, L. F., Mesquita, B., Ochsner, K. N., & Gross, J. J. (2007). The experience of emotion. *Annual Review of Psychology, 58,* 373-403.

Baumeister, R. F., Heatherton, T. F. & Tice, D. M. (1994). *Losing control: How and why people fail at self-regulation.* San Diego, CA: Academic Press.

Beitel, M., Ferrer, E., & Cecero, J. J. (2004). Psychological mindedness and awareness of self and others. *Journal of Clinical Psychology, 61,* 739-750.

Bodhi, B. (2000). *The connected discourses of the Buddha.* Boston, MA: Wisdom Publications.

Bodhi, B. (2006). In B.A. Wallace (Ed.), The nature of mindfulness and its role in Buddhist meditation: A correspondence between B. Alan Wallace and the Venerable Bhikkhu Bodhi. Unpublished manuscript, Santa Barbara Institute for Consciousness Studies, Santa Barbara, CA.

Boorstein, S. (1996). Transpersonal psychotherapy. Albany, NY: State University of New York Press.

Broderick, P. C. (2005). Mindfulness and coping with dysphoric mood: Contrasts with rumination and distraction. *Cognitive Therapy and Research, 29,* 501-510.

Brown, K. W., & Moskowitz, D. S. (1998). It's a function of time: A review of the process approach to behavioral medicine research. *Annals of Behavioral Medicine, 20,* 1-11.

Brown, K. W., & Ryan, R. M. (2003). The benefits of being present: Mindfulness and its role in psychological well-being. *Journal of Personality and Social Psychology, 84,* 822-848.

Brown, K. W., & Ryan, R. M. (2007). The effects of mindfulness on task engagement, performance, and subjective experience. Unpublished manuscript, Virginia Commonwealth University.

Brown, K. W., Ryan, R. M., & Creswell, J. D. (2007). Mindfulness: Theoretical foundations and evidence for its salutary effects. *Psychological Inquiry, 18,* 272-281.

Brown, K. W., Ryan, R. M., Creswell, J. D., & Niemiec, C.P. (2008). Beyond Me: Mindful responses to social threat. In H. A. Wayment & J. J. Bauer (Eds.), *Transcending self-interest: Psychological explorations of the quiet ego* (pp. 75-84). Washington, DC: American Psychological Association.

Cardaciotto, L., Herbert, J. D., Forman, E. M., Moitra, E., & Farrow, V. (2008). The assessment of present-moment awareness and acceptance: The Philadelphia Mindfulness Scale. *Assessment, 15,* 204-223.

Carlson, L. E., & Brown, K. W. (2005). Validation of the Mindful Attention Awareness Scale in a cancer population. *Journal of Psychosomatic Research, 58,* 29-33.

Carmody, J., & Baer, R. A. (2008). Relationships between mindfulness practice and levels of mindfulness, medical and psychological symptoms, and well-being in a mindfulness-based stress reduction program. *Journal of Behavioral Medicine, 31,* 23-33.

Carver, C. S., & Scheier, M. F. (1998). *On the self-regulation of behavior.* New York: Cambridge University Press.

Chambers, R., Lo, B. C., & Allen, N. B. (2008). The impact of intensive mindfulness training on attentional control, cognitive style, and affect. *Cognitive Therapy and Research, 33,* 302-322.

Claxton, G. (1999). Moving the cursor of consciousness: Cognitive science and human welfare. In F. J. Varela & J. Shear (Eds.), *The view from within: First-person approaches to the study of consciousness* (pp. 219-222). Bowling Green, OH: Imprint Academic.

Cohen-Katz, J., Wiley, S. D., Capuano, T., Baker, D.M., Kimmel, S., & Shapiro, S. (2005). The effects of mindfulness-based stress reduction on nurse stress and burnout, Part II: A quantitative and qualitative study. *Holistic Nursing Practice, 19*, 26-35.

Creswell, J. D., Eisenberger, N. I., & Lieberman, M. D. (2007). Neurobehavioral correlates of mindfulness during social exclusion. Unpublished manuscript, University of California, Los Angeles.

Creswell, J. D., Way, B. M., Eisenberger, N. I., & Lieberman, M. D. (2007). Neural correlates of mindfulness during affect labeling. *Psychosomatic Medicine, 69*, 560-565.

Csikszentmihalyi, M. (1990). *Flow: The psychology of optimal experience*. New York: Harper/Collins.

Deci, E. L. & Ryan, R. M. (1985). *Intrinsic motivation and self-determination in human behavior*. New York: Plenum.

Dennett, D. C. (1992) The self as a center of narrative gravity. In F. Kessel, P. Cole and D. Johnson (Eds.), *Self and consciousness: Multiple perspectives*. Hillsdale, NJ: Erlbaum.

Depraz, N. (1999). The phenomenological reduction as praxis. *Journal of Consciousness Studies, 6*, 95-110.

Dreyfus, G. & Thompson, E. (2007). Asian perspectives: Indian theories of mind. In P. D. Zelazo, M. Moscovitch, & E. Thompson (Eds.), *The Cambridge handbook of consciousness* (pp. 89-114). New York: Cambridge University Press.

Eisenberger, N. I., Lieberman, M. D., & Williams, K. D. (2003). Does rejection hurt? An fMRI study of social exclusion. *Science, 302*, 290-292.

Farb, N. A. S., Segal, Z. V., Mayberg, H., Bean, J., McKeon, D., Fatima, Z., & Anderson, A. K. (2007). Attending to the present: mindfulness meditation reveals distinct neural modes of self-reference. *Social Cognitive and Affective Neuroscience, 2*, 313-322.

Feldman, G., Hayes, A., Kumar, S., Greeson, J., & Laurenceau, J. (2007). Mindfulness and emotion regulation: The development and initial validation of the Cognitive and Affective Mindfulness Scale-Revised (CAMS-R). *Journal of Psychopathology and Behavioral Assessment, 29*, 177-190.

Felder, M. T., Zvolensky, M. J., Eifert, G. H., & Spira, A. P. (2003). Emotional avoidance: An experimental test of individual differences and response suppression using biological challenge. *Behaviour Research and Therapy, 41*, 403-411.

Frewen, P. A. Evans, E. M., Maraj, N., Dozois, D. J., & Partridge, K. (in press). Letting go: Mindfulness and negative automatic thinking. *Cognitive Therapy and Research*.

Forman, E. M., Herbert, J. D., Moitra, E., Yeomans, P. D., & Geller, P. A. (2007). A randomized controlled effectiveness trial of acceptance and commitment therapy and cognitive therapy for anxiety and depression. *Behavior Modification, 31*, 772-799.

Gallagher, S. (2000). Philosophical conceptions of the self: Implications for cognitive science. *Trends in Cognitive Sciences, 4*, 14-21.

Goldstein, J. (2002). *One Dharma: The emerging western Buddhism*. New York, NY: Harper San Francisco.

Goleman, D. (2006). Social intelligence: The new science of human relationships. New York: Bantam.

Gottman, J. M., Coan, J., Carrere, S., & Swanson, C. (1998). Predicting marital happiness and stability from newlywed interactions. *Journal of Marriage and the Family, 60*, 5-22.

Gross, J. J., & Munoz, R. F. (1995). Emotion regulation and mental health. *Clinical Psychology: Science and Practice, 2*, 151-164.

Gross, J. J., & Thompson, R. A. (2007). Emotion regulation: Conceptual foundations. In J. J. Gross (Ed.), *Handbook of emotion regulation* (pp. 3-24). New York: Guilford.

Husserl, E. (1981). In P. McCormick & F. A. Elliston (Eds.), *Husserl: Shorter works*. Notre Dame, IN: University of Notre Dame Press.

Husserl, E. (1999). *The essential Husserl: Basic writings in transcendental phenomenology* (D. Welton, Ed.). Bloomington, IN: Indiana University Press.

Kabat-Zinn, J. (2003). Mindfulness-based interventions in context: Past, present, and future. *Clinical Psychology: Science and Practice, 10*, 144–156.

Kornfield, J. (1993). *A path with heart*. New York: Bantam.

Kriegel, U. (2007). Philosophical theories of consciousness: Contemporary Western perspectives. In P. D. Zelazo, M. Moscovitch, & E. Thompson (Eds.), *The Cambridge handbook of consciousness* (pp. 35–66). New York: Cambridge University Press.

Lambie, J. A., & Marcel, A. J. (2002). Consciousness and the varieties of emotion experience: A theoretical framework. *Psychological Review, 109*, 219–259.

Langer, E. (2002). Well-being: Mindfulness versus positive evaluation. In C. R. Snyder & S. J. Lopez (Eds.), *Handbook of positive psychology* (pp. 214–230). New York: Oxford University Press.

Lau, M. A., Bishop, S. R., Segal, Z. V., Buis, T., Anderson, N. D., Carlson, L., et al. (2006). The Toronto Mindfulness Scale: Development and validation. *Journal of Clinical Psychology, 62*, 1445–1467.

Leary, M. R. (2004). *The curse of the self: Self-awareness, egotism, and the quality of human life*. NY: Oxford University Press.

Leary, M. R. (2005). Nuggets of social psychological wisdom. *Psychological Inquiry, 16*, 176–179.

Legrand, D. (2007). Pre-reflective self-as-subject from experiential and empirical perspectives. *Consciousness and Cognition, 16*, 583–599.

Levitt, J. T., Brown, T. A., Orsillo, S. M., & Barlow, D. H. (2004). The effects of acceptance versus suppression of emotion on subjective and psychophysiological response to carbon dioxide challenge in patients with panic disorder, *Behavior Therapy, 35*, 747–766.

Lutz, A., Dunne, J. D., & Davidson, R. J. (2007). Meditation and the neuroscience of consciousness: An introduction. In P. D. Zelazo, M. Moscovitch, & E. Thompson (Eds.), *The Cambridge handbook of consciousness* (pp. 499–551). New York: Cambridge University Press.

McKee, L., Zvolensky, M. J., Solomon, S. E., Bernstein, A., & Leen-Feldner, E. (2007). Emotional-vulnerability and mindfulness: A preliminary test of associations among negative affectivity, anxiety sensitivity, and mindfulness skills. *Cognitive Behaviour Therapy, 36*, 91–100.

Nyaniponika (1973). *The heart of Buddhist meditation*. New York: Weiser Books.

Ochsner, K. N., Bunge, S. A., & Gross, J.J. (2002). Rethinking feelings: An fMRI study of the cognitive regulation of emotion. *Journal of Cognitive Neuroscience, 14*, 1215–1229.

Olendzki, A. (2005). The roots of mindfulness. In Germer, C. K., Siegel, R. D., & Fulton, P. R. (Eds.), *Mindfulness and psychotherapy* (pp. 241–261). New York: Guilford.

Phelps, E. A. (2006). Emotion and cognition: Insights from studies of the human amygdala. *Annual Review of Psychology, 57*, 27–53.

Posner, J., Russell, J.A., & Peterson, B.S. (2005). The circumplex model of affect: An integrative approach to affective neuroscience, cognitive development, and psychopathology. *Development and Psychopathology, 17*, 715–734.

Robinson M. & Clore, G.L. (2002). Episodic and semantic knowledge in emotional self-report: Evidence for two judgment processes. *Journal of Personality and Social Psychology, 83*, 198–215.

Russell, J. A. (1980). A circumplex model of affect. *Journal of Personality and Social Psychology, 39*, 1161–1178.

Ryan, R. M. (2005). The developmental line of autonomy in the etiology, dynamics, and treatment of borderline personality disorders. *Development and Psychopathology, 17*, 987–1006.

Shapiro, S. L., Brown, K.W., & Biegel, G. (2007). Teaching self-care to caregivers: The effects of Mindfulness-Based Stress Reduction on the mental health of therapists in training. *Training and Education in Professional Psychology, 1*, 105-115.

Sheldon, K. M., & Vansteenkiste, M. (2005). Personal goals and time travel: How are future places visited, and is it worth it? In A. Strathman, & J. Joreman, (Eds.), *Understanding behavior in the context of time: Theory, research, and application* (pp.143-163). Mahwah, NJ: Lawrence Erlbaum.

Sherwin, E., Elliott, T., Rybarczyk, B., Frank, R., Hanson, S., Hoffman, M. (1992). Negotiating the reality of caregiving: hope, burnout, and nursing. *Journal of Social and Clinical Psychology, 11*, 129-139.

Sloan, D. M. (2004). Emotion regulation in action: Emotional reactivity in experiential avoidance. *Behaviour Research and Therapy, 42*, 1257-1270.

Stone, A. A. & Shiffman, S. (1994). Ecological momentary assessment (EMA) in behavioral medicine. *Annals of Behavioral Medicine, 16*, 199-202.

Teasdale, J. D. (1999). Emotional processing, three modes of mind and the prevention of relapse in depression. *Behaviour Research and Therapy, 37*, 53-77.

Thompson, E. (2007). *Mind in life: Biology, phenomenology, and the sciences of mind*. Cambridge, MA: Belknap Press.

Thompson, E. & Zahavi, D. (2007). Philosophical issues: Phenomenology. In P. D. Zelazo, M. Moscovitch, & E. Thompson (Eds.), *The Cambridge handbook of consciousness* (pp. 67-87). New York: Cambridge University Press.

Tsoknyi, D. (1998). *Carefree dignity: Discourses on training in the nature of mind*. Hong Kong: Rangjung Yeshe Publications.

Tyssen, R., Vaglum, P., Gronvold, N. T., & Ekeberg, O. (2001). Factors in medical school that predict postgraduate mental health problems in need of treatment. A nationwide and longitudinal study. *Medical Education, 35*, 110-120.

Uchiyama, K. (2004). *Opening the hand of thought*. Somerville, MA: Wisdom Publications.

Urry, H. L., van Reekum, C. M., Johnstone, T., Kalin, N. H., Thurow, M. E., Schaefer, H. S., et al. (2006). Amygdala and ventromedial prefrontal cortex are inversely coupled during regulation of negative affect and predict the diurnal pattern of cortisol secretion among older adults. *Journal of Neuroscience, 26*, 4415-4425.

Varela, F. J. & Depraz, N. (2003). Imagining: Embodiment, phenomenology, and transformation. In B.A. Wallace (Ed.), *Buddhism and science: Breaking new ground* (pp. 195-232). New York: Columbia University Press.

Varela, F. J. & Shear, J. (1999). *The view from within: First-person approaches to the study of consciousness*. Bowling Green, OH: Imprint Academic.

Wachs, K. & Cordova, J. V. (2007). Mindful relating: Exploring mindfulness and emotion repertoires in intimate relationships. *Journal of Marital and Family Therapy, 33*, 464-481.

Walach, H., Buchheld, N., Buttenmuller, V., Kleinknecht, N., & Schmidt, S. (2006). Measuring mindfulness: The Freiburg Mindfulness Inventory (FMI). *Personality and Individual Differences, 40*, 1543-1555.

Wallace, B. A. (1999). The Buddhist tradition of *Samatha*: Methods for refining and examining consciousness. In F. J. Varela & J. Shear (Eds.), *The view from within: First-person approaches to the study of consciousness* (pp. 175-187). Bowling Green, OH: Imprint Academic.

Wilson, T. D., Lindsey, S., & Schooler, T. Y. (2000). A model of dual attitudes. *Psychological Review, 107*, 101-126.

Wupperman, P., Neumann, C.S., & Axelrod, S.R. (in press). Do deficits in mindfulness underlie Borderline Personality features and core difficulties? *Journal of Personality Disorders*.

Part 2

Clinical Applications: General Issues, Rationale, and Phenomenology

5

Mindfulness and Psychopathology: Problem Formulation

Nancy L. Kocovski, Zindel V. Segal, and Susan R. Battista

There is no greater impediment to progress in the sciences than the desire to see it take place too quickly.

Georg Christoph Lichtenberg (1742–1799)

Mindfulness-based interventions are currently being used with a variety of populations to treat a wide range of physical and psychological disorders. For example, Mindfulness-Based Stress Reduction (MBSR; Kabat-Zinn, 1990) has been used to treat chronic pain and anxiety, among other conditions. Mindfulness-Based Cognitive Therapy (MBCT; Segal, Williams, & Teasdale, 2002) has been used for the prevention of relapse in depression. Acceptance and Commitment Therapy (ACT; Hayes, Strosahl, & Wilson, 1999) includes elements of mindfulness and has been used with a wide variety of patients. Finally, Dialectical Behavior Therapy (DBT; Linehan, 1993) incorporates mindfulness as a core skill in the treatment of borderline personality disorder.

With the growing number of mindfulness-based interventions, and the growing evidence supporting the use of some of these interventions, clinicians are understandably interested in continuing to apply mindfulness to a wide variety of concerns. However, the danger of over-applying mindfulness as a treatment for psychopathology exists. Additionally, the application of a generic mindfulness program to a wide variety of complaints may not be as efficacious as tailoring the mindfulness intervention to a specific problem. In addition to tailoring a mindfulness intervention to a specific complaint, an integrative approach, one in which evidence-based interventions are retained and mindfulness is incorporated in a theoretically consistent manner, may lead to the most favorable outcomes.

The primary goal of this chapter is to highlight the importance of taking a problem formulation approach in the development and use of mindfulness interventions. Related to this, a secondary aim of this chapter is to review current theory and research on mechanisms of change of mindfulness interventions in the reduction of psychological distress and also to encourage further research in this area. A clear understanding of how mindfulness interventions lead to positive outcomes is essential for therapists, as it will enhance problem formulation.

Problem Formulation

The evidence supporting the efficacy of mindfulness interventions across a wide variety of populations might lead some to conclude that mindfulness groups are a cost-effective "general-purpose therapeutic technology" (Teasdale, Segal, & Williams, 2003, p. 157). Teasdale and colleagues posit that while there have been favorable findings for mindfulness interventions, often these studies have had instructors who "embodied, sometimes implicitly, quite specific views of the nature of emotional distress and ways to reduce that distress" (p. 157). They further argue that for mindfulness interventions to be successful, it is necessary for practitioners to have a clear formulation of the disorder being treated and how a mindfulness intervention may be helpful for that disorder. We further believe that understanding mechanisms of change is necessary for a problem formulation approach to the use of mindfulness interventions.

Teasdale et al. (2003) outlined six considerations related to mindfulness that require further investigation. Many of these considerations involve or would be enhanced by an understanding of the mechanisms of change of mindfulness interventions for a particular disorder. First, mindfulness training can be unhelpful. There are some conditions that may not benefit from mindfulness meditation or may worsen. For example, early research on the use of meditation in patients with psychotic disorders was not promising (e.g., Walsh & Roche, 1979); however, later research using ACT for psychosis found lower rehospitalization rates compared to a control group (Bach & Hayes, 2002). The Melbourne Academic Mindfulness Interest Group (2006) reviewed other adverse effects that have been reported in the literature; typically these adverse effects have been found with transcendental meditation (TM) and longer-term meditation retreats, and they include an increase in depressive and anxious symptoms. Relatedly, mindfulness interventions can be a significant time investment, often involving a two-hour group meeting weekly for at least eight weeks, possibly involving significant travel time to and from the group meetings, and a significant homework commitment (i.e., 45 minutes per day). Some programs also include a full day of mindfulness practice as a group. This large time commitment can be considered an adverse consequence if a patient has not benefited from the intervention (Melbourne Academic Mindfulness Interest Group, 2006).

Second, sharing a clear formulation with clients is important, and this involves having an understanding of how mindfulness might lead to change for that particular client's problem. Some clients may have preconceived notions of what mindfulness entails and may judge it as an unsuitable approach. A discussion of how mindfulness may be an appropriate intervention may help to counteract these preconceived notions.

The third consideration relates to the apparent simplicity of mindfulness. Mindfulness appears to be a simple procedure, but the style is as important as the technique. Understanding mechanisms of change for a particular problem can inform the specific mindfulness exercises chosen for the intervention, the style of delivery, and the emphasis for the inquiry.

Fourth, mindfulness was originally developed as part of a multifaceted approach, not as an end in and of itself. Often there are well researched and supported techniques for a particular disorder that can be integrated with mindfulness interventions. However, leaving out previously established techniques in favor of a pure mindfulness approach may result in a disservice to patients. Often there are traditional cognitive and behavioral therapies that are empirically supported for specific populations. One of the challenges of integrating mindfulness with these interventions is that the acceptance-based underpinnings of mindfulness can be at odds with the change-based focus of traditional cognitive and behavioral interventions (see Lau & McMain, 2005, for a review). However, this challenge can and has been met (e.g., MBCT; Segal et al., 2002), highlighting that, while it may seem difficult, it is possible to achieve theoretical integration with seemingly very different approaches. Therefore, rather than abandoning empirically supported treatments in favor of a pure mindfulness intervention, integration may be the most effective approach. Additionally, understanding the mechanisms of change will enhance the development of multifaceted approaches that include mindfulness interventions.

Fifth, some components of mindfulness training may be more relevant for some conditions than for others. Understanding mechanisms of change for a particular disorder will inform which components of mindfulness are most relevant for that disorder.

The sixth and final consideration outlined by Teasdale et al. (2003) is that while mindfulness training may affect processes common to many disorders, indiscriminate application of mindfulness techniques across disorders is not optimal. There is still room for specificity even if the process is similar across several disorders.

MBCT as an Example of the Problem Formulation Approach

The development of MBCT (Segal et al., 2002) is an example of the problem formulation approach. Segal and colleagues sought out to develop a program to target the recurrent nature of depression. Patients who have one episode of depression have a 50% probability of becoming depressed a second time, and those who have had two episodes of depression have a 70–80% probability of having a third episode. Segal and colleagues developed MBCT, an eight-week group intervention, for patients who have been depressed but are currently well. They integrated aspects of cognitive therapy for depression with mindfulness training, following a clear rationale of what they expected would be helpful, given current data on depression and mindfulness. The emphasis in MBCT is on changing the relationship with thinking, rather than changing the content of thought.

MBCT has been found to help patients with three or more episodes of depression, but not those who only had two depressive episodes (Teasdale, Segal, Williams, Ridgeway, Soulsby, & Lau, 2000; Ma & Teasdale, 2004). Ma and Teasdale found that those with a history of only two episodes reported a later onset of depression and less childhood abuse in their histories, suggesting that they may have represented a unique population, compared to those who had a greater number of depressive episodes. This illustrates the need to study exactly how mindfulness techniques work in specific populations as they may not be beneficial in all cases (Teasdale et al., 2003). Additionally, while MBCT was developed for formerly depressed patients who are currently well, there is growing evidence that MBCT can be effective for actively depressed and anxious patients in a primary-care setting (Finucane & Mercer, 2006) and for treatment-resistant actively depressed patients (Kenny & Williams, 2007).

Other Examples of the Problem Formulation Approach

Further examples of how mindfulness components have been incorporated into existing treatments following a problem formulation approach include the following: the mindfulness component in DBT for borderline personality disorder (Linehan, 1993), Acceptance-based behavior therapy for generalized anxiety disorder (Roemer & Orsillo, 2007), mindfulness-based CBT for co-occurring addictive and mood disorders (Hoppes, 2006), and Mindfulness- and Acceptance-based Group Therapy (MAGT) for social anxiety disorder (Kocovski, Fleming, & Rector, 2007).

Looking more closely at generalized social anxiety disorder, Koszycki, Benger, Shlik, and Bradwejn (2007) conducted a randomized controlled trial comparing MBSR and Cognitive Behavioral Group Therapy (CBGT; Heimberg & Becker, 2002). They found that CBGT, the current gold standard group intervention for social anxiety disorder, was superior to MBSR on a number of outcome variables. However, they did find MBSR to be helpful, resulting in medium to large effects. They provided a rationale for using MBSR with this patient population. However, the MBSR program was not adapted for patients with social anxiety disorder, and it was administered by an instructor who typically delivers mindfulness training to the public. Although positive effects were obtained with MBSR, the usual standard of care was found to be superior and therefore should remain the first-line psychological group intervention. Alternatively, an attempt at integrating MBSR and CBGT might prove fruitful. Kocovski et al. (2007) have incorporated mindfulness techniques along with acceptance- and exposure-based strategies using a problem formulation approach. Pilot groups have demonstrated that this approach is feasible and acceptable to patients, and there is preliminary evidence in support of its effectiveness. A trial comparing this treatment (i.e., MAGT) to CBGT is underway. Additionally, Bögels, Sijbers, and Voncken (2006) report positive results from a small pilot study where they integrated MBCT and another intervention, task concentration training, for the treatment of social anxiety disorder.

Overall, although there are many positive findings regarding mindfulness techniques (Baer, 2003), it is important to study exactly how mindfulness works for each disorder. This can be helpful in terms of the development of a problem formulation for a particular disorder or support for an existing problem formulation. Hence, the next section outlines the specific mechanisms of change that have been theorized and/or empirically supported.

Mechanisms of Change: Biological Factors

Research examining the physical benefits of meditation has been extensive (e.g., Aftanas & Golosheykin, 2005; Hankey, 2006; Orme-Johnson, Schneider, Son, Nidich, & Cho, 2006; Travis & Arenander, 2006). However, this research has often focused on experienced meditators who have had many years of training. For example, Travis and Arenander (2006) examined a sample of individuals who had been practicing TM for an average of 22 years. These highly experienced groups have then been compared to individuals who have had no experience with meditation. A number of positive findings have emerged from studies of this nature. Travis and Arenander found experienced meditators to have higher frontal alpha asymmetry and greater electroencephalogram (EEG) coherence than non-meditators. Frontal alpha asymmetry has been associated with affective responding (Davidson & Irwin, 1999) with particular patterns of asymmetry found in individuals with depression (Gotlib, Ranganath, & Rosenfeld, 1998). EEG coherence is indicative of brain coordination and has been linked to intelligence (Cranson et al., 1991), creativity (Orme-Johnson & Haynes, 1981), and mental health (Travis & Arenander). There is also support from EEG findings that long-term meditation leads to a better capability of moderating the intensity of emotional arousal (Aftanas & Golosheykin, 2005). Furthermore, in a second study, Travis and Arenander found that EEG coherence increased over one year as individuals practiced TM, indicating that even minimal meditative experience can lead to improved brain functioning.

Other physical outcomes that have been observed in experienced meditators include the following: decreased hypertension (Orme-Johnson & Walton, 1998), increased sensory acuity (Carter et al., 2005), decreased systolic blood pressure (Wallace, Dillbeck, Jacobe, & Harrington, 1982), and decreased brain responses to pain (Orme-Johnson et al., 2006). A complete review of research in this area is beyond the scope of this chapter (see Cahn & Polich, 2006, for a review of EEG, ERP, and neuroimaging studies across various forms of meditation; see Newberg & Iversen, 2003, for a model integrating data on neurotransmitter and neurochemical substrates that may underlie meditation). In sum, there is evidence that intensive meditation practice is physically beneficial across a variety of domains. It is important to question, however, whether these benefits are unique to very experienced meditators or whether these benefits are also evident in individuals who undergo more short-term forms of meditation (i.e., mindfulness training programs such as MBSR or MBCT).

Studies that have specifically examined how mindfulness techniques affect the brain are limited. Davidson et al. (2003) investigated brain and immune changes in participants who were randomly assigned to receive MBSR (Kabat-Zinn, 1990) or a wait-list control group. Compared to the wait-list control condition, participants who received MBSR showed greater left-anterior activation immediately after the mindfulness training intervention was completed and at a four-month follow-up assessment. In addition, the group that received MBSR also showed greater left-anterior activation after they wrote about positive and negative life experiences. Greater left-anterior activation is associated with positive emotions (Davidson, 1992), both dispositionally and during positive mood inductions. It is also associated with adaptive responding to negative or stressful events (Davidson, 2000), which may explain why individuals in the mindfulness group had increased left-anterior activation even after writing about negative life events. This study also investigated how mindfulness training affected immune functioning. All participants were given an influenza vaccine after the completion of mindfulness training (or lack of training in the control condition), and antibody levels were measured at two time points. Results revealed a significantly greater increase in antibodies from time one to time two for the mindfulness group as compared with the control group. This study provides initial support for the idea that even short-term mindfulness training can have widespread physical benefits for individuals. However, it should be noted that the sample used by Davidson and colleagues was not comprised of individuals seeking treatment for any clinical disorder, but rather, they likely represented a healthy population.

Given that mindfulness techniques are currently being used within clinical samples to treat a variety of disorders, it is important to examine the biological mechanisms of change that are specific to the problem undergoing treatment. Barnhofer et al. (2007) recruited a sample of individuals who had a history of suicidal depression, and randomly assigned them to receive MBCT (Segal et al., 2002) or treatment as usual. EEG readings were taken before and after the treatment period, which lasted eight weeks. Changes in prefrontal asymmetry were not found in the group that received MBCT. However, the group that received treatment as usual showed decreased levels of prefrontal asymmetry at the eight-week reading. The researchers concluded that the MBCT group had developed a more balanced pattern of prefrontal activation, whereas the treatment-as-usual group experienced more right-sided activation, a pattern associated with avoidance. The researchers suggested that developing a more balanced pattern of prefrontal activation, and hence a more balanced affective response style, may help to prevent depression relapse by decreasing the likelihood that one will fall back into a negative cognitive style. This study provides preliminary insight into potential biological changes that are the result of a specific mindfulness intervention and how such biological factors can be connected with the specific disorder that one is suffering from. Hopefully, future research will follow this path, namely, that of investigating a particular mindfulness intervention and the biological changes that occur compared to a control group, and perhaps going one step further by having a competing empirically supported intervention as the comparison group. Finally, with respect to biological mechanisms of change, there is recent research examining the brain regions involved in the tendency of minds to wander, which may help with this type of research (Mason et al., 2007).

Mechanisms of Change: Psychological Factors

There is growing evidence indicating that mindfulness has a number of positive effects on well-being. Although it is difficult to pinpoint exactly how mindfulness leads to these positive outcomes, a number of psychological mechanisms are likely responsible. At this point in time, many of the proposed mechanisms have not been empirically studied, but rather, remain theoretical. It is of utmost importance that future research focus on experimentally examining each psychological mechanism and link supported mechanisms to specific disorders. Additionally, for a variable to be considered a mediator of treatment outcome in a randomized controlled trial, it is important to show that the variable is affected by treatment before changes occur in the outcome variable (Kraemer, Stice, Kazdin, Offord, & Kupfer, 2001). At present, even the variables that have been investigated empirically do not meet this temporal requirement. This section will briefly outline psychological mechanisms that have received empirical attention, and meet some of the criteria supporting mediation, as well as those that are currently theoretical and warrant further investigation.

Increased Metacognitive Awareness, *Decentering, Reperceiving, and Defusion*

Metacognitive awareness (Teasdale et al., 2002), decentering, reperceiving (Shapiro, Carlson, Astin, & Freedman, 2006), and defusion (Hayes et al., 1999) are terms that describe a similar concept in mindfulness training. Essentially, these refer to the extent to which individuals can view their thoughts as being passing mental events as opposed to being true reflections of reality (Teasdale et al., 2002). Shapiro et al. (2006) theorized that mindfulness practice would provide training in how to shift one's perspective so that thoughts and experiences could be viewed more objectively. There is some evidence that increases in metacognitive awareness, decentering, reperceiving, and/or defusion are associated with positive outcomes in mindfulness training. For example, Teasdale and colleagues examined the effects of MBCT on a sample of individuals who had a history of recurrent major depression. It was found that those who underwent MBCT experienced an increase in metacognitive awareness and were less likely to relapse compared to those who received treatment as usual. It is unknown, however, whether increases in metacognitive awareness were directly responsible for reduced relapse rates.

Decreased Rumination

Rumination is the extent to which one dwells on the emotional consequences of an event and has been implicated as a contributing factor in both depression and anxiety (Nolen-Hoeksema, 1991; Kocovski & Rector, 2007). Jain et al. (2007) compared distressed students who had undergone a mindfulness meditation program with those who had undergone a relaxation training program on a number of variables. Results revealed that both programs reduced distress and increased positive mood compared to a control condition. However, only the meditation group demonstrated significantly reduced rumination compared to the control condition. Additionally, it was found that decreases in rumination mediated the relationship between condition (mindfulness meditation or control) and reduced distress, such that the mindfulness meditation group reported less distress at the end of treatment, partially due to a reduction in levels of rumination. As the authors point out, they only assessed rumination pre- and post-intervention, and therefore they were unable to test whether changes in rumination occurred prior to changes in distress. Thus, further research is necessary to determine if rumination is a true mediator. A prior study by Ramel, Goldin, Carmona, and McQuaid (2004) also presented data supportive of the hypothesis that mindfulness has its effect at least partially through a reduction in rumination. They examined previously depressed individuals before and after undergoing MBSR

(Kabat-Zinn, 1982) and found that MBSR led to decreases in rumination and that these decreases in rumination accounted for reductions in depressive and anxious symptoms. Additionally, compared to a control group, Chambers, Lo, and Allen (in press) found that a group of non-clinical novice meditators reported significant improvements in a number of variables including rumination.

In the area of anxiety, there is some support in favor of continuing to examine rumination as a mechanism of change. Patients with social anxiety disorder who took part in MAGT demonstrated significant reductions in levels of rumination from baseline to mid-treatment, post-treatment, and follow-up (Kocovski et al., 2007). However, the intervention consisted of elements in addition to mindfulness training; there was no control group, and a mediation model was not tested. As an aside, these variables were investigated in a student sample cross-sectionally, and there was support for a mediation model, such that rumination partially mediated the relationship between social anxiety and mindfulness (Kocovski, Vorstenbosch, & Rogojanski, 2007). Additionally, self-focused attention was also examined with this student sample and also found to partially mediate the relationship between social anxiety and mindfulness. In both cases, lower levels of mindfulness were associated with increased levels of the mediator (rumination, self-focused attention), which were in turn associated with increased levels of social anxiety. These results need to be replicated in a clinical sample that has undergone a mindfulness intervention.

Attentional Control

Mindfulness training inherently requires that individuals alter their attention to be more present-moment focused. Chambers and colleagues (in press) specifically investigated how a 10-day mindfulness meditation retreat affected sustained attention in non-clinical, novice meditators. Participants exhibited decreased reaction times when they performed an attention task after attending the meditation retreat compared to their baseline times. This decrease was not found in the control group of participants who did not undergo mindfulness training. Furthermore, decreases in reaction times were significantly correlated with decreases in depression scores, indicating that improvements in cognitive functioning may be associated with improved mood. Mindfulness training, however, did not lead to improved performance on an attention-switching task, and mediation models were not tested. Jha, Krompinger, and Baime (2007) also investigated the effect of mindfulness training on attention. They compared meditators who were attending a retreat, participants in an MBSR course with no previous meditation experience, and a control group. At baseline, participants with past mindfulness training (i.e., those in the retreat group) demonstrated better conflict-monitoring performance compared to the other two groups. At the second assessment point, participants who had completed MBSR improved in their ability to orient their attention compared to the other two groups, while those who attended the retreat improved on exogenous alerting compared to the other two groups. Therefore, various subcomponents of attention may be affected differentially depending on the type of meditation and perhaps the length of meditation experience.

Increased Acceptance

Mindfulness treatments strongly emphasize acceptance of symptoms rather than avoidance or suppression of symptoms (Baer, 2003; Brown & Ryan, 2003; Hayes et al., 1999). For example, ACT (Hayes et al., 1999) is strongly rooted in the belief that with increased acceptance, one can experience greater psychological health. There are studies showing that mindfulness- and acceptance-based therapies are in fact leading to increased acceptance. For example, Roemer and Orsillo (2007) administered the Acceptance and Action Questionnaire (AAQ) pre- and post-intervention as one measure of a proposed mechanism of change for their acceptance-based behavior therapy for generalized anxiety disorder and found lower levels of experiential avoidance (i.e., higher levels of acceptance) for patients following treatment. When looking at pain tolerance tasks, there are a number of studies to support that using acceptance strategies leads to increased pain tolerance (Hayes, Bissett et al., 1999) and greater willingness to persist at the task (Gutierrez, Luciano, & Fink, 2004) compared to more control-based strategies. Levitt, Brown, Orsillo, and Barlow (2004) randomly assigned individuals with panic disorder to a short acceptance, suppression, or distraction intervention. Individuals were then exposed to air enriched with carbon dioxide. It was found that those who received the acceptance intervention were more willing to take part in the task and reported lower levels of anxiety compared with those who received the suppression or distraction intervention. Overall, it appears that levels of acceptance are increasing following treatment, and there are laboratory studies that have manipulated acceptance and found less distress and greater willingness in the acceptance condition.

Other Psychological Mechanisms: Values Clarification, Exposure, Decreased Anxiety and Increased Emotional Stability, and Increased Psychological Flexibility

There are a number of other possible mechanisms of change that have little, if any, empirical support at this time. One such possible mechanism of action of mindfulness training is the ability to carefully make decisions that are reflective of one's true values (Shapiro et al., 2006). Often when individuals operate on automatic pilot, they make quick decisions that may not be in line with their needs and/or values. Through mindfulness training, one can adopt a more objective perspective and make choices that are more congruent with one's values. In support of this potential mechanism of change, Brown and Ryan (2003) found that individuals who scored higher on a measure of state mindfulness also reported engaging in more valued behaviors and interests. Second, mindfulness may promote exposure. Exposure has been outlined as a key component in mindfulness training (Baer, 2003; Kabat-Zinn, 1982). By having individuals focus their awareness on emotional symptoms in a nonjudgmental manner, mindfulness can help to prevent avoidance or escape. When individuals fully experience their feared emotional symptoms, they can properly observe the consequences of their emotional symptoms and formulate more effective coping strategies. In this way, mindfulness may play a role in the extinction of the fear response (Baer, 2003). Third, in conjunction with biological differences between meditators and non-meditators, Travis and Arenander (2006) found that those with meditation experience also had significantly lower levels of both state and trait anxiety compared to those without meditation experience. Experienced meditators were also more emotionally stable than non-meditators. A final mechanism of action may be that mindfulness promotes the adoption of an overall more flexible cognitive, emotional, and behavioral style (Shapiro et al., 2006), or increased overall psychological flexibility (Hayes et al., 1999).

Mechanisms of Change: Considerations and Limitations

There are several limitations and considerations in this area of research. It is important that a distinction be made between mindfulness and relaxation techniques, and only some studies have sought to do this (e.g., Jain et al., 2007). Further, clear definitions and descriptions of the particular mindfulness interventions used are essential in examining mechanisms of change (Dimidjian & Linehan, 2003). There are many different forms of meditation, and the actual results that are found may depend on the technique that is used (Hankey, 2006). Therefore, it would be beneficial to examine the specific components of meditation and how they lead to various outcomes. Additionally, mindfulness techniques are often not studied independent of the other components involved in the treatment, which does not allow for conclusions to be drawn about what is specifically helpful about mindfulness (Dimidjian & Linehan, 2003). It is important to keep in mind that while some of the research in this area does test for mechanisms of action, most research studies show that mindfulness interventions lead to a decrease or increase in a variable, but have not tested that variable as a mediator of change. Even research that does test for mechanisms of change is often not meeting the criteria for a stringent test, namely, showing that there is a change in the mediator prior to a change in the outcome variable (Kraemer et al., 2001).

As noted by Teasdale et al. (2003), mindfulness may target processes that affect many disorders (sixth consideration). Rather than taking this to mean that mindfulness can be applied indiscriminately as a treatment for many disorders, there is still room for specificity; the exact nature of each component will likely differ depending on the disorder. For example, rumination is common in both depressed and socially anxious patients. However, the content of the rumination can be different (e.g., dwelling on depressive symptoms versus dwelling on social inadequacies) and the consequences may also be different (e.g., relapse versus avoidance or increased anxiety). Therefore, knowing that rumination may be reduced via mindfulness interventions can be a starting place. However, the exact problem formulation can still vary across disorders that might have rumination as a process to be targeted.

Beyond Mechanisms of Change

In addition to understanding the mechanisms of change of mindfulness interventions for specific disorders, other factors require attention. Personality factors may also play a role in understanding which patients might benefit from a mindfulness treatment approach. For example, in our social anxiety work, our first MAGT patients had already received CBT and were still experiencing clinically significant symptoms and were interested in further treatment. They made significant gains with our mindfulness and acceptance approach; these particular patients may have been better suited for this approach. In contrast, other clients have not been interested in listening to mindfulness CDs or tapes outside of the group sessions and are not particularly open to this type of intervention. There is a paucity of research examining personality as a predictor of treatment outcome for mindfulness interventions and, as such, it is an important direction for future research.

Conclusion

Mindfulness is an old technique that has recently gained considerable attention within psychological research, and there has been a promising level of empirical support. However, as we have argued, it is important to be cautious in its application and not to expect it to be a cure-all intervention on its own. We advocate for the following basic steps for clinicians considering the use of mindfulness in their practice: (1) careful consideration of the population being served, and the current understanding with respect to etiology and maintenance of the particular condition being treated, (2) determination of how mindfulness might be helpful with this population, making reference to the mechanisms of change research, (3) evaluation of whether mindfulness training can be integrated with other empirically supported interventions, and (4) inclusion of a rationale to patients for the mindfulness components. The recent research empirically evaluating mindfulness interventions and the early research on the identification of mediators of change are exciting. Certainly, there is a need for the continued empirical evaluation of the integration of mindfulness components with other interventions. Additionally, as reviewed above, much of the research on mediators has only provided partial support for certain variables, as complete tests of mediation have been rare thus far. Hopefully, future research evaluating possible mediators will be more stringent. Overall, mindfulness interventions are gaining prominence, and with continued research on how they work and the most beneficial ways to incorporate them, this trend will continue with promising results.

References

Aftanas, L., & Golosheykin, S. (2005). Impact of regular meditation practice on EEG activity at rest and during evoked negative emotions. *International Journal of Neuroscience, 115*, 893–909.

Bach, P., & Hayes, S. C. (2002). The use of acceptance and commitment therapy to prevent the rehospitalization of psychotic patients: A randomized controlled trial. *Journal of Consulting and Clinical Psychology, 70*, 1129–1139.

Baer, R. A. (2003). Mindfulness training as a clinical intervention: A conceptual and empirical review. *Clinical Psychology: Science and Practice, 10*, 125–143.

Barnhofer, T., Duggan, D., Crane, C., Hepburn, S., Fennell, M. J. V., & Williams, J. M.G. (2007). Effects of meditation on frontal α-asymmetry in previously suicidal individuals. *Neuroreport, 18*, 709–712.

Bögels, S. M., Sijbers, G. F., & Voncken, M. (2006). Mindfulness and task concentration training for social phobia: A pilot study. *Journal of Cognitive Psychotherapy, 20*, 33–44.

Brown, K. W., & Ryan, R. M. (2003). The benefits of being present: Mindfulness and its role in psychological well-being. *Journal of Personality and Social Psychology, 84,* 822-848.

Cahn, B. R., & Polich, J. (2006). Meditation states and traits: EEG, ERP, and neuroimaging studies. *Psychological Bulletin, 132,* 180-211.

Carter, O. L., Presti, D. E., Callistemon, A., Ungerer, Y., Lui. G. B., & Pettigrew, J. D. (2005). Meditation alters perceptual rivalry in Tibetan Buddhist monks. *Current Biology, 15,* 412-413.

Chambers, R., Lo, B. C., & Allen, N. B. (2008).The impact of intensive mindfulness training on attentional control, cognitive style and affect. *Cognitive Therapy and Research,.*

Cranson, R. W., Orme-Johnson, D. W., Gackenbach, J., Dillbeck, M. C., Jones, C. H., & Alexander, C.N. (1991). Transcendental Meditation and improved performance on intelligence related measures: A longitudinal study. *Personality and Individual Differences 12,* 1105-1116.

Davidson, R. J. (1992). Emotion and affective style: Hemispheric substrates. *Psychological Science, 3,* 39-43.

Davidson, R. J. (2000). Affective style, psychopathology, and resilience: brain mechanisms and plasticity. *American Psychologist, 55,* 1196-1214.

Davidson, R. J., & Irwin, W. (1999). The functional neuroanatomy of emotion and affective style. *Trends in Cognitive Neuroscience, 3,* 11-21.

Davidson, R. J., Kabat-Zinn, J., Schumacher, J., Rosenkranz, M., Muller, D., Saki, F., et al. (2003). Alterations in brain and immune function produced by mindfulness meditation. *Psychosomatic Medicine, 65,* 564-570.

Dimidjian, S., & Linehan, M. M. (2003). Defining an agenda for future research on the clinical application of mindfulness practice. *Clinical Psychology: Science and Practice, 10,* 166-171.

Finucane, A, & Mercer, S. W. (2006). An exploratory mixed methods study of the acceptability and effectiveness of mindfulness-based cognitive therapy for patients with active depression and anxiety in primary care. *BMC Psychiatry, 6:14.*

Gotlib, I. H., Ranganath, C., & Rosenfeld, J, P. (1998). Frontal EEG alpha asymmetry, depression, and cognitive functioning. *Cognition and Emotion, 12,* 449-478.

Gutierrez, O., Luciano, C., & Fink, B.C. (2004). Comparison between an acceptance-based and a cognitive-control-based protocol for coping with pain. *Behavior Therapy, 35,* 767-784.

Hankey, A. (2006). Studies of advanced stages of meditation in the Tibetan Buddhist and vedic traditions. I: A comparison of general changes. *Complementary and Alternative Medicine, 3,* 513-521.

Hayes, S. C., Bissett, R. T., Korn, Z., Zettle, R. D., Rosenfarb, I. S., Cooper, L. D., et al. (1999). The impact of acceptance versus control rationales on pain tolerance. *The Psychological Record, 49,* 33-47.

Hayes, S. C., Strosahl, K., & Wilson, K. G. (1999). *Acceptance and commitment therapy*. New York: Guilford.

Heimberg, R. G., & Becker, R. E. (2002). *Cognitive-behavioral group therapy for social phobia: Basic mechanisms and clinical strategies*. New York: Guilford.

Hoppes, K. (2006). The application of mindfulness-based cognitive interventions in the treatment of co-occurring addictive and mood disorders. *CNS Spectrum, 11,* 829-851.

Jain, S., Shapiro, S. L., Swanick, S., Roesch, S. C., Mills, P. J., Bell, I. et al. (2007). A randomized controlled trial of mindfulness meditation versus relaxation training: Effects on distress, positive states of mind, rumination, and distraction. *Annals of Behavioral Medicine, 33,* 11-21.

Jha, A. P., Krompinger, J., & Baime, M. J. (2007). Mindfulness training modifies subsystems of attention. *Cognitive, Affective, and Behavioural Neuroscience, 7,* 109-119.

Kabat-Zinn, J. (1982). An outpatient program in behavioral medicine for chronic pain patients based on the practice of mindfulness meditation: Theoretical considerations and preliminary results. *General Hospital Psychiatry, 4*, 33–47.

Kabat-Zinn, J. (1990). *Full catastrophe living: Using the wisdom of your body and mind to face stress, pain and illness.* New York: Dell.

Kenny, M. A., & Williams, J. M. G. (2007). Treatment-resistant depressed patients show a good response to mindfulness-based cognitive therapy. *Behaviour Research and Therapy, 45*, 617–625.

Kocovski, N. L., Fleming, J., & Rector, N. A. (2007). Mindfulness and acceptance-based group therapy for social anxiety disorder: Preliminary evidence from four pilot groups. Poster accepted for presentation at the 41st Annual Convention of the Association for Behavioral and Cognitive Therapies (ABCT), Philadelphia, November 15–18, 2007.

Kocovski, N. L., & Rector, N. A. (2007). Predictors of post-event rumination related to social anxiety. *Cognitive Behaviour Therapy, 36*, 112–122.

Kocovski, N. L., Vorstenbosch, V., & Rogojanski, J. (2007). Mindfulness and social anxiety: An examination of mediating variables. Poster presented at the 68th Annual Convention of the Canadian Psychological Association, Ottawa, June 7–9, 2007.

Koszycki, D., Benger, M., Shlik, J., & Bradwejn, J. (2007). Randomized trial of a meditation-based stress reduction program and cognitive behavior therapy in generalized social anxiety disorder. *Behaviour Research and Therapy, 45*, 2518–2526.

Kraemer, H. C., Stice, E., Kazdin, A., Offord, D., & Kupfer, D. (2001). How do risk factors work together? Mediators, moderators, and independent, overlapping, and proxy risk factors. *American Journal of Psychiatry, 158*, 848–856.

Lau, M. A., & McMain, S. F. (2005). Integrating mindfulness meditation with cognitive and behavioural therapies: The challenge of combining acceptance- and change-based strategies. *Canadian Journal of Psychiatry, 50*, 863–869.

Levitt, J. T., Brown, T. A., Orsillo, S. M., & Barlow, D. H. (2004). The effects of acceptance versus suppression of emotion on subjective and psychophysiological response to carbon dioxide challenge in patients with panic disorder. *Behavior Therapy, 35*, 747–766.

Linehan, M. M. (1993). *Cognitive-behavioral treatment of borderline personality disorder.* New York: Guilford.

Ma, S. H., & Teasdale, J. D. (2004). Mindfulness-based cognitive therapy for depression: Replication and exploration of differential relapse prevention effects. *Journal of Consulting and Clinical Psychology, 72*, 31–40.

Mason, M. F., Norton, M. I., Van Horn, J. D., Wegner, D. M., Grafton, S. T., & Macrae, N. (2007). Wandering minds: The default network and stimulus-independent thought. *Science, 315*, 393–395.

Melbourne Academic Mindfulness Interest Group. (2006). Mindfulness-based psychotherapies: A review of conceptual foundations, empirical evidence and practical considerations. *Australian and New Zealand Journal of Psychiatry, 40*, 285–294.

Newberg, A. B., & Iversen, J. (2003). The neural basis of the complex mental task of meditation: Neurotransmitter and neurochemical considerations. *Medical Hypotheses, 61*, 282–291.

Nolen-Hoeksema, S. (1991). Responses to depression and their effects on the duration of depressive episodes. *Journal of Abnormal Psychology, 100*, 569–582.

Orme-Johnson, D. W., & Haynes, C. T. (1981). EEG phase coherence, pure consciousness, creativity, and TM-Sidhi experiences. *The International Journal of Neuroscience, 13*, 23–29.

Orme-Johnson, D. W., Schneider, R. H., Son, Y. D., Nidich, S., & Cho, Z. (2006). Neuroimaging of meditation's effect on brain reactivity to pain. *Cognitive Neuroscience and Neuropsychology, 17*, 1359–1363.

Orme-Johnson, D. W., & Walton, K. (1998). All approaches to preventing or reversing effects of stress are not the same. *American Journal of Health Promotion, 12,* 297–299.

Ramel, W., Goldin, P. R., Carmona, P. E., & McQuaid, J. R. (2004). The effects of mindfulness meditation on cognitive processes and affect in patients with past depression. *Cognitive Therapy and Research, 28,* 433–455.

Roemer, L., & Orsillo, S. M. (2007). An open trial of an acceptance-based behavior therapy for generalized anxiety disorder. *Behavior Therapy, 38,* 72–85.

Segal, Z. V., Williams, J. M. G., & Teasdale, J. D. (2002). Mindfulness-based cognitive therapy for depression: A new approach to preventing relapse. New York: Guilford.

Shapiro, S. L., Carlson, L. E., Astin, J. A., & Freedman, B. (2006). Mechanisms of mindfulness. *Journal of Clinical Psychology, 62,* 373–386.

Teasdale, J. D., Moore, R. G., Hyhurst, H., Pope, M., Williams, S., & Segal, Z. V. (2002). Metacognitive awareness and prevention of relapse in depression: Empirical evidence. *Journal of Consulting and Clinical Psychology, 70,* 275–287.

Teasdale, J. D., Segal, Z. V., & Williams, J. M. G. (2003). Mindfulness training and problem formulation. *Clinical Psychology: Science and Practice, 10,* 157–160.

Teasdale, J. D., Segal, Z. V., Williams, J. M., Ridgeway, V. A., Soulsby, J. M., & Lau, M. A. (2000). Prevention of relapse/recurrence in major depression by mindfulness-based cognitive therapy. *Journal of Consulting and Clinical Psychology, 68,* 615–623.

Travis, F., & Arenander, A. (2006). Cross-sectional and longitudinal study of effects of transcendental meditation practice on interhemispheric frontal asymmetry and frontal coherence. *International Journal of Neuroscience, 116,* 1519–1538.

Wallace, R. K., Dillbeck, M., Jacobe, E., & Harrington, B. (1982). The effects of transcendental meditation and TM-Sidhi program on the aging process. *International Journal of Neuroscience, 16,* 53–58.

Walsh, R., & Roche, L. (1979). Precipitation of acute psychotic episodes by intensive meditation in individuals with a history of schizophrenia. *American Journal of Psychiatry, 136,* 1085–1086.

6

Emotional Memory, Mindfulness and Compassion

Paul Gilbert and Dennis Tirch

But when the universe becomes your self, when you love the world as yourself, all reality becomes your haven, reinventing you as your own heaven.

Lao Tzu, Translated by Ralph Alan Dale Tao Te Ching

Emotional Memory, Mindfulness and Compassion

This chapter considers the role that mindfulness and compassion can play in helping people who come from difficult and traumatic backgrounds. These individuals often have a highly elevated sense of threat – both from the outside (what others might do to them) and from the inside (feeling overwhelmed by aversive feelings or memories; or their own self-dislike/contempt for themselves). The basic view is that traumatic backgrounds sensitise people to become overly reliant on processing from their threat systems.

To explore this further we need to outline briefly the idea that the brain has evolved different types of affect-behaviour regulation systems (Panskepp, 1998). These systems coordinate attention, thoughts, emotions and actions. One way to conceptualise these affect regulations is as basic systems (Depue & Morrone-Strupinsky, 2005). These are as follows: (1) threat-protection system, (2) drive, seeking, and reward system and (3) a contentment-soothing system. These systems are in constant states of co-regulation and are shown in Figure 6.1

Various other sub-divisions have been suggested and described (Panskepp, 1998), but the three-systems approach offers a useful heuristic for compassion-focused therapy (Gilbert, 2005, 2007a,b). Looked at this way, our threat system can be seen as having certain defensive emotions (e.g. anger, anxiety, and disgust), a range of behaviour options (e.g. fight, flight, freeze, and submission; Marks, 1987), and various 'better safe than sorry' attentional and processing biases (Gilbert, 1998). There are also clear physiological systems that underpin the threat system (LeDoux, 1998). Once activated, it creates various physiological patterns in the body underpinning felt experiences, directs thinking and actions tendencies. The drive system on the other hand orientates us to things that are rewarding (e.g. food, sex, money, and status). It is associated with the activated affects of excitement-linked positive affects. In contrast, the 'contentment system' enables animals

Types of Affect Regulation Systems

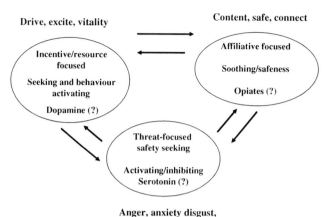

Figure. 6.1. Types of affect regulation systems.

to be quiescent when they no longer need to acquire resources and are not under any threat. This system appears to be associated with a sense of (soothing) peaceful well-being. During evolution the contentment system has evolved into a soothing system that can be triggered by social stimuli of affection, love and care (Carter, 1998; Depue & Morrone-Strupinsky, 2005).

The development, coordination and co-regulation of these three basic systems are dependent on gene-learning interactions. Indeed, biological organisms are designed to be changed and moulded by life experiences. Different experiences encourage and strengthen some neuronal connections and weaken others (LeDoux, 2002). For example, it is now known that harsh, neglectful and/or abusive backgrounds have major impacts on the maturing brain of young children, especially on those areas that regulate emotions such as connections between the prefrontal cortex (PFC) and amygdala (Cozolino, 2007; Schore, 1994; Siegel, 2001). Life experiences are coded as *emotional memories*, linked to synaptic sensitisation at one level–through to the complex brain systems dedicated to different types and forms of memory – such as episodic, semantic, and short- and long-term memory (LeDoux, 2002).

Understanding the way life experiences shape the brain's various sensitivities in threat and positive affect systems, and emotional memories, is important because we know that emotional disorders are linked to early affect sensitisation and emotional memories. Indeed, some therapists place the activation of emotional memories, at both implicit and explicit levels, centre stage to psychopathology (Brewin, 2006). Psychodynamic (Greenberg & Mitchell, 1983) and behavioural theorists (Ferster, 1973) have long argued that emotional memories, associations and conditioning need not be conscious but still highly influential on how people process and respond to life events and situations.

Most people who experience psychological problems, that require some kind of intervention, feel under threat from various aspects of their lives (e.g. in social relationships) or their inner experiences (e.g. being overwhelmed by emotions or memories or negative, ruminative thoughts). Thus, depression, anxiety, paranoia, eating disorder, phobias, PTSD and OCD are all related to threat-focused processing and efforts to regulate threat and get safe. Hence, most psychological therapies aim to help people recognise the early and current sources of heightened threat and loss sensitivities, various thoughts and feelings that automatically 'jump into mind', their ways of processing threats/losses from memory (Brewin, 2006), schematic representations of self and others (Beck, Freeman, Davis et al., 2003) and coping strategies (e.g. vigilance and avoidance). Through various interventions that may involve the therapeutic relationship, exposure, cognitive and emotional change, and new behaviour strategies, therapies try to reduce threat/loss sensitivities and threat/loss processing. In this way the external and internal stimuli that have activated threat/loss processing systems lose their power to do so.

One aspect that increases threat sensitivity and focuses threat processing is our human *meta-cognitive* abilities (Wells, 2000). These have given us huge advantages in being able to plan, anticipate and cooperate and are the source of culture, civilisation and science – but these abilities come with a cost. Chimpanzees probably do not worry that the pain in the chest could be a heart attack, or if they eat too much they will get fat and, in some social groups, might be rejected; they do not worry about their future prospects in family or work. Humans, however, live in both a world of 'is' (linked to direct sensory experiences) and one of 'imagination and meta-cognitions' where we can focus on the past and future, the feared, the lost and the hoped for (Gilbert, 2007a; Singer, 2006). We can construct plans and scenarios in our minds and then respond to them like real stimuli (Wells, 2000). Our imaginations are not physiologically neutral; rather fantasies (e.g. sexual) can stimulate physiological systems and produce arousal (e.g. sexual fantasies). When our attention is absorbed in this inner world of thinking, imagining or being overwhelmed by emotional memories, we are no longer open to live 'in' the present moment. We are dragged away from 'the present moment' because other systems in our brains are pulling on the field of consciousness demanding attention. For example, different emotional memories and conditioning means that we react quickly to things – our bodies might start reacting to a situation before we are consciously aware of it, and then our emotions rush us along, focusing our thoughts and behaviours.

Mindfulness

Mindfulness addresses both these problems. We can learn to be attentive to emotions and thoughts as they are triggered, to see them as linked to emotional memories and conditioning. We switch to an 'observer' mode – being able to notice and describe what happens inside us rather than be captured by it. Many therapies help people switch to this observing-describing mode of attention. Mindfulness also helps us to become more aware of the way our minds wander from the present moment into daydreams, the past and future, and with regret, anticipation or apprehension. By noticing the way consciousness is 'grabbed by these inner concerns' and our emotions affected, we are enabled to pull the attention back and thus reduce and calm the feedback loops between threat arousal and the maintaining effects of certain meta-cognitions and ruminations.

For over two and half thousand years Buddhist psychology has seen human psychology as dominated by the efforts of our minds to cope with the inevitability of threats, losses and harms that give rise to suffering; none of us are immune to life's frustrations, adversities and final decay and death of ourselves and of those we love. At the heart of the Buddhist approach is to train our minds in ways that enable us to 'face' but also 'flow with' the harsh realties of life. The two most important tasks in this mind training are those of mindfulness and compassion.

In the last 20 years mindfulness has attracted considerable attention as both a way to promote well-being and also a therapeutic process for specific difficulties (e.g. recurrent depression). For the most part these approaches focus on how to train one's attention so that we learn to pay attention to the present moment without judgement. Hence mindfulness is a mode of experiencing and is suggested to be a fundamental psychological state involved in the alleviation of suffering (Corrigan, 2004; Martin, 1997; Fulton & Seigel, 2005). The contemporary protégé Tibetan meditation master Yongyey Mingyur Rinpoche (2007) described mindfulness as 'the key, the *how* of Buddhist practice [that] lies in learning to simply rest in a bare awareness of thoughts, feelings and perceptions as they occur.'

Humans depend on verbal-linguistic and logico-mathematical processing in a great deal of their interactions with the environment. However, as noted above, the dominance of these processing mechanisms in human conscious experience can result in a disconnection from moment-to-moment experience and a reification and concretisation of internal emotional experiences (Hayes, Barnes-Holmes, & Roche, 2001; Hayes, Stroshal, Wilson, 1999). Because humans have meta-cognitive abilities, we can plan (what will happen if I do X; how can I get Y) and be fearful (what will happen if X happens) – all purely on the basis of our thoughts, attributions, exceptions and anticipations. As a result, humans may often spend their time responding to internal thoughts, predictions and intrusive memories as though they are real events. This 'literalisation' of mental representations has been referred to as 'cognitive fusion' (Hayes et al., 1999).

The distress that may arise in the presence of painful, literalised cognitions and emotional memories is clear and obvious. However, the way people try to cope with emotional sensitivities, intrusions, ruminations and memories – that pull on their thought processes – may be even more significant. For example, research has demonstrated that attempts at thought suppression or avoidance (both common coping strategies) often serve only to increase the frequency, pull and intrusiveness of painful thoughts, feelings and predictions (Hayes, Wilson, Gifford, Follette, & Strosahl, 1996; Wegner, Schneider, Knutson, & McMahon, 1991). Under such conditions, our emotional memories, associational learning patterns, and the nature of human relational responding create a paradoxical prison, wherein our attempts to reject and ignore painful experiences only serve to drag our attention back to the internal constructs which drive our suffering. Buddhist psychology describes such a phenomenon as *Samsara* (cyclic existence), a cycle of persistently re-experiencing (i.e. re-incarnating) our suffering through grasping at what we cannot have and rejecting that which we do not wish to experience. Historically, this re-experiencing was construed as a returning to lives of suffering after death. However, a post-modern, 21st-century, Western perspective may interpret this *Samsara* as a remarkably apt and concise description of a life spent experientially fused with emotional memories and dysfunctional cognitions. Mindfulness is a way of recognising the eruptions in thoughts and feelings, the pull and flow in our thinking that link to our personal sensitivities. It also trains the mind to be with them but not 'in' them.

We noted above that many of our personal threat sensitivities and the links between thoughts and emotions can be understood as emergent for the interplay of various neurophysiological systems. Mindfulness research has focused on its neurophysiological effects. In fact, research across a range of levels of analysis, from neuroimaging to clinical outcome studies, has demonstrated the effectiveness of mindfulness-based practice in helping people change their relationship to their emotions. Recent experimental research has found that a 15-minute focused breathing induction, which parallels aspects of mindfulness training, resulted in greater capacity for emotion regulation and a greater willingness to remain in the presence of emotionally aversive stimuli (Arch & Craske, 2006). Similarly, research has demonstrated that individuals who completed an eight-week mindfulness training intervention reported less-frequent negative automatic thoughts and believed that they were better able to 'let go' of these thoughts when they encountered them. This finding was supported by research on dispositional mindfulness, which indicated that individuals exhibiting a higher level of dispositional mindfulness reported fewer negative automatic thoughts and believed themselves capable of 'letting go' of such thoughts (Frewen, Evans, Maraj, Dozois, & Partridge, 2006).

Neuroimaging research has demonstrated that adept meditators practicing a mindfulness of breathing exercise exhibit stronger activation in the anterior cingulate cortex (ACC) during mindfulness of breathing, when compared to controls (Holzel, et al. 2007). It has been hypothesised that this group difference may be attributed to a more effective processing of distracting events and may involve more effective processing of emotional memories. The ACC is theorised to be involved in the resolution of conflict, emotional self-control and adaptive responses to changing conditions (Allman, Hakeem, Erwin, Nimchinsky, & Hof, 2001). It has been postulated that the ACC may be involved in a neural homeostatic mechanism that regulates an individual's response to distress (Corrigan, 2004).

People present with varying degrees of innate or dispositional mindfulness, reflecting their capacity to employ a mindful state of awareness to better address difficult emotional experiences and adapt to the presence of their emotional memories. fMRI data suggests that dispositional mindfulness is correlated with stronger widespread prefrontal cortical activity and reduced bilateral amygdala activity during the act of labelling emotions (Creswell, Way, Eisenberger, & Lieberman, 2007). Mindfulness training frequently employs the labelling of phenomenal emotional experiences (e.g. upon noticing a sad feeling, the meditator may label the experience 'sadness'). These findings suggest a possible component of mindfulness, this being enhanced prefrontal regulation of affect brought about through the act of noting and then labelling of affect – which requires cognitive work.

Recent neuroimaging data also suggests that the effectiveness of mindfulness may involve a shift in the perceived sense of self that is experienced during meditation. fMRI studies have contrasted the neural correlates involved in a 'narrative' mode of self-reference and an 'experiential' mode of self-reference (Farb et. al., 2007). A 'narrative' sense of self roughly corresponds to a conventional Western view of the self as a pervasive and ongoing separate individual identity enduring across time and situations. The narrative mode of self-reference has been found to be correlated with the medial prefrontal cortex (mPFC), which is involved in maintaining a sense of self across time, comparing one's traits to those of others, and the maintenance of self-knowledge (Farb et. al., 2007). The 'experiential mode' of self-reference corresponds to the present moment-focused awareness found in mindfulness meditation and represents the mode of being that has been described as an 'Observing Self' (Deikman, 1982).

Farb et al. (2007) research examined the neurological activity involved in these modes of self-reference among both experienced meditators and novice participants in an 8 week mindfulness training. Novice meditators exhibited a reduction in the activity of the mPFC while maintaining an experiential focus, which may reflect a reduction in a narrative sense of self-reference. More experienced mindfulness practitioners exhibited stronger reductions in this mPFC activity. Further, the trained participants also exhibited a more right lateralised network of cortical activity including the lateral PFC, viscerosomatic areas, and the inferior parietal lobule. This network of activity appeared to correlate with a phenomenology of an 'observing self' and may indicate a more effective mode of processing emotional memories from a mindful stance. Additionally, novice meditators evidenced a stronger coupling between areas of the PFC involved in narrative self-reference (mPFC) and areas which may be involved in the translation of visceral emotional states into conscious feelings (i.e. right insula) (Damasio, 1999).

More experienced meditators exhibited weaker coupling between these areas, which may reflect a cultivated capacity to disengage the habitual connection between an identified sense of self across time and the processing of emotional memories, yielding the previously described beneficial aspects of the experience of mindfulness.

The above outlines a variety of avenues by which mindfulness may help people recruit and train their brains to better ride the waves of emotions and thoughts that are in constant flow. Also it offer ways that people can better choreograph their affect regulation systems.

Compassion

Some practitioners of mindfulness suggest that compassion is an emergent quality of mind that comes with 'mindful practice'. This is in part because mindfulness helps us experience the illusions of the grasping, bounded ego-self, and instead experience insights/feelings of all being part and parcel of a unifying consciousness that pervades the universe. However, other schools of Buddhism (e.g. Mahayana) suggest it is important to specifically focus and practice developing a 'compassionate mind.' To do this they have developed a range of concepts on the nature and benefits of compassion and ways of thinking and behaving to practice and enhance compassion, including a range of compassion-focused mediations and imagery exercises (Leighton, 2003). Interestingly, many of the writings of the Dalai Lama (e.g. 1995, 2001) have focused less on the processes of mindfulness and far more on the nature and value of developing compassion.

There have been important explorations of Western and Eastern views of compassion and how to enhance compassion in all walks of life as well as personally (Davidson & Harrington 2002; Neff, 2003a,b). In some forms of mindfulness training, loving-kindness (compassion) mediations are added to standard procedures and may be one of the key ingredients of change (e.g. Shapiro, Astin, Bishop, & Cordova, 2005). Compassion-focused therapies are also emerging that specifically focus on developing compassion for self and others as a therapeutic process (Gilbert, 2000; Gilbert & Procter, 2006; Leary, Tate, Adams, Allen, & Hancock, 2007). While some of these are directly linked to Buddhist traditions (e.g. Neff, 2003a; Leary et al., 2007), others are focused on evolutionary psychology (e.g. attachment theory), social neuroscience and affect regulation (Gilbert, 2005, 2007).

Most theorists see compassion as a multifarious process. For example, McKay and Fanning (1992) view compassion as involving developing understanding, acceptance and forgiveness. Neff (2003a,b), from a social psychology and Buddhist tradition, has developed a self-compassion scale that sees compassion as consisting of bipolar constructs related to kindness, common humanity and mindfulness. *Kindness* involves understanding one's difficulties and being kind and warm in the face of failure or setbacks rather than harshly judgemental and self-critical. *Common humanity* involves seeing one's experiences as part of the human condition rather than as personal, isolating and shaming; *mindful acceptance* involves mindful awareness and acceptance of painful thoughts and feelings rather than over-identifying with them. Neff, Kirkpatrick & Rude (2007) have shown that self-compassion is different to self-esteem and is conducive to many indicators of well-being.

Gilbert's (1989, 2005, 2007a,b) evolutionary model suggests that the potential for compassion evolved with the caring-giving side of the attachment system. Hence, receiving compassion has the same effects as being cared for – that is it stimulates the soothing systems (see Figure 6.1) in the recipients of compassion, helping people feel safe and calmed. In this model human compassion-giving arises from specific motivational, emotional and cognitive competencies that can be enhanced through training. The six main components of compassion are as follows:

(1) Developing a motivation to care for one's well-being and the well-being of others. This motivational aspect also extends into a self-identity – that is to develop and become more compassionate. With this motivation people can then engage in seeking 'knowledge' and developing compassion skills, that will include the following:

(2) Developing one's sensitivity to one's own distress and needs and those of others; recognising how one's own threat emotions (e.g., anger, anxiety) can block such sensitivity

(3) Developing one's capacity for sympathy, which involves the ability to be emotionally open and moved by the feelings, distress and needs of others

(4) Developing one's capacity for distress and emotional tolerance, which is linked to the ability to 'be with' painful or aversive emotions within self or others without avoiding them or trying to subdue them. Thus, this is also linked to competencies for acceptance

(5) Developing empathy, which involves more cognitive and imaginal competencies of putting 'oneself in the shoes of the other' and developing insights into understanding why they may feel or act as they do. This is also linked to what is sometimes called mentalising, or theory of mind

(6) Developing non-judgement is a way of refraining from condemning and accusing. It evolved for empathy and deepening one's understanding of the human condition rather than being adopted as 'an instruction'. It does not mean non-preference. For example, the Dalai Lama (2001) would dearly love the world to be more compassionate.

When developing these qualities and competencies, they are all cultivated in the emotional atmosphere of warmth and kindness. Hence in this system, warmth and also mindfulness are ways of developing the compassion qualities and competencies. These are viewed as being interconnected and interdependent qualities – as shown in Figure 6.2.

Compassion training involves developing these qualities 'for the self'. They can then be utilised when individuals feel stressed but also to promote a sense of well-being and contentment. This occurs because training our minds for compassion can help us to stimulate these emotion systems and go some way to facilitating a sense of well-being.

Hence, unlike mindfulness, which is not designed to stimulate any particular affect system (but rather to develop the observing self), compassion work is design to stimulate the soothing system that evolved with attachment. This is because, as noted above, it is the system that is a natural regulator of the threat and drive systems, and underpins feelings of contentedness, connectedness and well-being.

There are many exercises and processes that can be used therapeutically to stimulate compassion for others and self. These involve the therapeutic relationship (Gilbert 2007b) and helping people develop compassionate attention, compassionate thinking, compassionate behaviour and compassionate

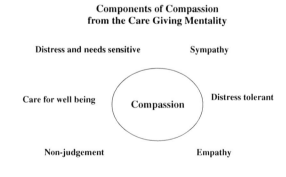

Figure. 6.2. Compassion circle.

feelings. Breathing and body focus, method-acting techniques, imagery, reframing and compassionate letter writing can all be used to advance these abilities (Gilbert 2007a in press; Gilbert & Irons 2005). Compassion-focused therapy utilises mindfulness but is also very focused and active, and therefore different to mindfulness both in formulation and in process. The major focus in compassion training is that whatever one undertakes and tries to do to facilitate change, one does it via creating feelings of warmth and support within the self. Although research is limited, there is some evidence for compassion development to be helpful (Gilbert & Procter, 2006; Mayhew & Gilbert, 2008). It should be noted, however, that much of the therapeutic work is often focused on the fear of, resistance to, or inability to, feel compassion for the self.

Conclusion

This chapter looked at a neurophysiological model of psychological sensitivities and explored ways in which mindfulness and compassion-focused therapies may impact on neurophysiological systems. Mindfulness operates through attentional training which facilitates different brain states and enables people to gain new insights and management over distressing thoughts, feelings and memories. Compassion-focused therapies utilise mindfulness but in the service of creating compassionate feelings and thoughts within oneself. One of the reasons for doing this is because trying to generate compassionate feelings within oneself will stimulate a particular kind of affect system which has soothing qualities. It was suggested that such a system evolved with attachment and gives rise to attachment-type feelings of calming, sense of connectedness and empathy for others.

Mindfulness teaches a non-judgemental observing of the arising and emergence of thoughts and feelings onto the screen of our consciousness. Compassionate mind training utilises this but also focuses on (re)directing attention, with a focus on trying to generate feelings of warmth, gentleness and kindness (Gilbert, 2000; Gilbert & Irons, 2005). When people feel threatened and traumatised and have few emotional memories or schema of being helped, loved or wanted, they may not be able to access their soothing and reassurance affect system. Through processes that involve learning to nurture compassionate attention, thinking, imagery, behaviour and feeling, people can be trained to develop a self-compassion orientation to themselves and difficulties. This orientation aims to shift focus from the threat system to the soothing system and may be especially helpful in the face of high affect and when engaging with painful emotional memories.

References

Allman, J. M., Hakeem, A., Erwin, J. M., Nimchinsky, E., & Hof, P. (2001). The Anterior cingulate cortex: The evolution of an interface between emotion and cognition. *Annals of The New York Academy of Science, 935*, 107–117

Arch, J. J., & M. G. Craske (2006). Mechanisms of mindfulness: Emotion regulation following a focused breathing induction. *Behaviour Research and Therapy, 44*, 1849–1858.

Beck, A.T., Freeman, A., Davis, D. D., & associates. (2003). *Cognitive therapy of personality disorders (Second Edition)*. New York: Guilford Press

Bifulco, A., & Moran, P. (1998). *Wednesday's child: Research into women's experiences of neglect and abuse in childhood, and adult depression*. London: Routledge.

Brewin, C. R (2006). Understanding cognitive behaviour therapy: A retrieval competition account. *Behaviour Research and Therapy, 44*, 765-784.

Carter, C. S. (1998). Neuroendocrine perspectives on social attachment and love. *Psychoneuroendocrinlogy, 23*, 779-818.

Corrigan, F. M. (2004). Psychotherapy as assisted homeostasis: Activation of emotional processing mediated by the anterior cingulate cortex. *Medical Hypotheses, 63*, 968-973.

Cozolino, L. (2007). The neuroscience of human relationships: Attachment and the developing social brain. New York: Norton.

Creswell, J. D., Way, B. M., Eisenberger, N. I., & Lieberman, M. D. (2007). Neural correlates of dispositional mindfulness during affect labeling. *Psychosomatic Medicine, 69*, 560-5.

Dalai Lama. (1995). *The power of compassion*. India: HarperCollins.

Dalai Lama. (2001). In N. Vreeland (Ed.), *An open heart: Practising compassion in everyday life*. London: Hodder & Stoughton.

Damasio, A. R. (1999). *The feeling of what happens: Body and emotion in the making of consciousness*. USA: Harcourt Trade Publishers.

Davidson, R. J., & Harrington, A. (2002, Eds). *Visions of compassion: Western scientists and tibetan buddhists examine human nature*. New York: Oxford University Press.

Deikman, A. (1982). *The observing self: Mysticism and psychotherapy*. Boston: Beacon Press.

Depue, R. A., & Morrone-Strupinsky, J. V. (2005). A neurobehavioral model of affiliative bonding. *Behavioral and Brain Sciences, 28*, 313-395.

Farb, N. A. S., Segal, Z. V., Mayberg, H., Bean, J., McKeon, D., Fatima, Z., & Anderson, A. K. (2007). Attending to the present: Mindfulness meditation reveals distinct neural modes of self-reference. *Social Cognitive Affective Neuroscience Advance Access*. 1-10.

Ferster, C. B. (1973). A functional analysis of depression. *American Psychologist, 28*, 857-870.

Frewen, A. P., Evans, E. M., Maraj, N., Dozois, D. J. A., & Partridge, K. (2006). Letting go: Mindfulness and negative automatic thinking. *Cognitive Therapy and Research. In press*.

Fulton, P. R., & Seigel, R. D. (2005). Buddhist and Western psychology: Seeking common ground. In C. K. Germer, R. D. Seigel, & P. R. Fulton (Eds.) *Mindfulness and Psychotherapy* (pp.55-72) New York: Guilford Press.

Gerhardt, S. (2004). *Why love matters. How affection shapes a baby's brain*. London: Routledge.

Gilbert, P. (1989). *Human nature and suffering*. London: Lawrence Erlbaum Associates.

Gilbert, P. (1998) The evolved basis and adaptive functions of cognitive distortions. *British Journal of Medical Psychology, 71*, 447-463

Gilbert, P. (2000). Social Mentalities: Internal 'social' conflicts and the role of inner warmth and compassion in cognitive therapy. In P. Gilbert, & K. G. Bailey (Eds.) *Genes on the couch: Explorations in evolutionary psychotherapy* (p.118-150). Hove: Psychology Press.

Gilbert, P. (2005). Compassion and cruelty: A biopsychosocial approach. In P. Gilbert (Ed.), *Compassion: Conceptualisations, research and use in psychotherapy* (pp. 9-74). London: Routledge.

Gilbert, P. (2007a). *Psychotherapy and counselling for depression*: 3rd edition. London: Sage.

Gilbert, P. (2007b). Evolved minds and compassion in the therapeutic relationship In P. Gilbert, & R. Leahy (Eds.). *The therapeutic relationship in the cognitive behavioural psychotherapies* (pp.106–142). London: Routledge.

Gilbert, P., & Irons, C. (2005). Focused therapies and compassionate mind training for shame and self attacking. In P. Gilbert (Ed.), *Compassion: Conceptualisations, research and use in psychotherapy* (pp. 263–325). London: Routledge.

Gilbert, P., & Procter, S. (2006). Compassionate mind training for people with high shame and self-criticism: A pilot study of a group therapy approach. *Clinical Psychology and Psychotherapy, 13*, 353–379.

Gilbert, P. (in press). *The Compassionate Mind. A New Approach to life's Challenges*. London Constable-Robin.

Greenberg, J. R., & Mitchell, S. A. (1983). Object Relations in Psychoanalytic Theory. Cambridge, Mass.: Harvard University press.

Hayes, S. C., Barnes-Holmes, D., & Roche, B. (2001) *Relational frame theory: A post-Skinnerian account of human language and cognition*. New York: Kluwer Academic/Plenum Press.

Hayes, S. C., Stroshal, K. D., & Wilson, K. G. (1999). *Acceptance and commitment therapy: An experiential approach to behavior change*. New York: Guilford Press.

Hayes, S. C., Wilson, K. G., Gifford, E. V., Follette, V. M., & Strosahl, K. (1996). Experiential avoidance and behavioral disorders: A functional dimensional approach to diagnosis and treatment. *Journal of Consulting and Clinical Psychology, 64*, 1152–1168

Holzel, B. K., Ott, U., Hempel, H., Hackl, A., Wolf, K., Stark, R., & Vaitl, D. (2007). Differential engagement of anterior cingulate and adjacent medial frontal cortex in adept meditators and non-meditators, *Neuroscience Letters, 421*(1), 16–21.

Leary, M. R., Tate, E. B., Adams, C. E., Allen, A. B., & Hancock, J. (2007). Self-compassion and reactions to unpleasant self-relevant events: The implications of treating oneself kindly. *Journal of Personality and Social Psychology, 92*,887–904.

LeDoux, J. (1998). *The emotional brain*. London: Weidenfeld and Nicolson.

LeDoux, J (2002). *Synaptic Self: How Our Brains Become Who We Are*. New York: Penguin.

Leighton T. D. (2003). *Faces of compassion: Classic bodhisattva archetypes and their modern expression*. Boston: Wisdom Publications.

Martin, J. R. (1997). Mindfulness: A proposed common factor. *Journal of Psychotherapy Integration, 7*, 291–312.

Marks, I. M. (1987). *Fears, phobias, and rituals: Panic, anxiety and their disorders*. Oxford: Oxford University Press.

Mayhew, S., & Gilbert, P. (2008). Compassionate Mind Training with people who hear malevolent voices: A case series report. *Clinical Psychology and Psychotherapy*.

McKay, M., & Fanning, P. (1992). *Self-esteem: A proven program of cognitive techniques for assessing, improving, and maintaining your self-esteem. Second Edition*. Oakland, C.A: New Harbinger Publishers.

Mingyur, Y. (2007). *The joy of living: Unlocking the secret and science of happiness*. New York: Harmony Books.

Neff, K. D. (2003a). Self-compassion: An alternative conceptualization of a healthy attitude toward oneself. *Self and Identity, 2*, 85–102.

Neff, K. D. (2003b). The development and validation of a scale to measure self-compassion. *Self and Identity, 2*, 223–250.

Neff, K. D., Kirkpatrick, K., & Rude, S. S. (2007). Self-compassion and its link to adaptive psychological functioning. *Journal of Research in Personality, 41*, 139–154.

Panskepp, J. (1998). *Affective neuroscience*. New York: Oxford University Press.

Schore, A. N. (1994). *Affect regulation and the origin of the self: The neurobiology of emotional development*. Hillsdale: N.J. Lawrence Erlbaum.

Shapiro, S. L., Astin J. A., Bishop, S. R., & Cordova, M. (2005). Mindfulness-based stress reduction for health care professionals: Results from a randomised control trail. *International Journal of Stress Management, 12*, 164-176.

Siegel, D. J. (2001). Toward an interpersonal neurobiology of the developing mind: Attachment relationships, "mindsight" and neural integration: *Infant Mental Health Journal, 22*, 67-94.

Singer, J. L. (2006). *Imagery in psychotherapy*. Washington DC: American Psychological Press.

Wegner, D. M., Schneider, D. J., Knutson, B., & McMahon, S. R. (1991). Polluting the stream of consciousness: The effect of thought suppression of the mind's environment. *Cognitive Therapy and Research, 15*, 141-151.

Wells, A. (2000). *Emotional disorders and metacognition: Innovative cognitive therapy*. Chichester: Wiley.

7

The Use of Metaphor to Establish Acceptance and Mindfulness

Alethea A. Varra, Claudia Drossel, and Steven C. Hayes

All instruction is but a finger pointing to the moon. He whose gaze is fixed upon the pointer will never see beyond.

Buddhist Allegory

Figurative speech plays two distinct roles in clinical psychology: It serves as a useful clinical tool and guides clinicians' conceptualizations of presenting problems and subsequent interventions (see Leary, 1990, for a discussion of metaphor in the history of psychology). Given its utility it is not surprising that metaphors, allegories, similes, analogies, adages, and maxims are found across therapeutic interventions (Blenkiron, 2005; Eynon, 2002; Lyddon, Clay, & Sparks, 2001; Otto, 2000). The current chapter focuses on the functions of figurative speech that are especially related to acceptance- and mindfulness-based approaches. We are emphasizing on acceptance and commitment therapy (ACT, said as one word, not initials; Hayes, Strosahl, & Wilson, 1999) both because we know it well and because it seems to raise the key issues in this area that apply to mindfulness approaches more generally.

ACT is a therapeutic approach that focuses on the creation of psychological flexibility by undermining the overextended impact of literal, temporal, and evaluative human language and cognition. The basic theory underlying ACT views human verbal abilities as a two-edged sword, allowing us to solve everyday problems and create a comfortable world, while simultaneously permitting us to bring our painful past to the present, to view the emotional echoes of our history as a problem to be solved, to compare ourselves to an unrealistic ideal, and to project fearful futures.

Metaphor as the Scientist-Practitioner's Conceptual Framework

While it is important to understand specific metaphors useful in therapy, it is also important to acknowledge the root metaphors underlying a given practitioner's conceptual framework. This is especially important in acceptance- and mindfulness-based practice because the fundamental assumptions are often different than those that predominate a great deal of medical and psychiatric practice.

Pepper (1970) identifies four "root metaphors" describing prevalent views of human affect, behavior, and cognition and their relation to other events. All scientific questions, subsequent research programs, and interventions mirror can be characterized according to these metaphors (Rosnow & Georgoudi, 1986; Hayes, Hayes, Reese, & Sarbin, 1993). Two of these metaphors are of special interest for clinical psychology. The metaphor of the *machine* views human beings and their problems as one would a complex clock. It prompts an examination of how components and forces work together to culminate in a perceived explanatory chain of events. This metaphor is the basis for the medical model and provides guidance to intervention as finding the broken part and fixing it.

A contextualistic metaphor, conversely, views all human events as one would a historically situated, purposive action, like going to the store or making love. This metaphor emphasizes the *nested, historical, and ongoing* nature of human action and introduces a focus on context and workability within that context. In a contextualistic metaphor, there is not something that is necessarily broken that needs to be fixed, but rather an interest in how a particular action functions, given the person's history and current situation. In contrast to other metaphors, the metaphor of ongoing purposive, historical actions assumes neither a final or complete analysis nor a "right way" to go about such an analysis. Instead, as illuminated by the root metaphor itself, analysis itself is just another ongoing action, embedded in uncountable layers of context and history:

> [The analysis itself] is categorically an event [....] In the extended analysis of any event we presently find ourselves in the context of that event, and so on, from event to event as long as we wish to go, which would be forever or until we got tired [...] there are many equally revealing ways to analyze an event (Pepper, 1942, p. 249-250).

ACT specifically and contextual psychology more broadly have explicitly adopted this latter metaphor (Hayes, Hayes, & Reese, 1988). They represent an approach to human behavior within its context, as interconnected, nested, historical, and ongoing events. We are writing this chapter largely from within the assumptions of a contextual approach.

The concept of mindfulness tends readily toward contextualistic perspective, for its focus at each moment is on the fundamentally interrelated nature of human experience. This contextual understanding resembles the teachings of many eastern philosophical schools that cultivate an intuitive, almost nonverbal knowledge of the interrelated quality the person experiences in the world through meditation and mindfulness practice. Contextual psychology avoids overlaying mindfulness practices from eastern traditions onto an essentially mechanistic root metaphor. Instead, mindfulness is a nature extension of the tenets of contextual psychology that have emerged from the basic and applied study of human affect, cognition, and behavior (Drossel, Waltz, & Hayes, in press).

It seems important to explicitly acknowledge the influence of root metaphors on scientific and clinical activities, because otherwise these assumptions present themselves, falsely, as data on the success of an approach. Root metaphors are the ground of analysis, not the result of analysis, and they need to be owned and stated, not thrust forward as an intellectual weapon in the battle with other views. The use of figurative speech for clinical change is thus itself embedded in the even deeper metaphors of clinical and scientific work. When we consider the value of mindfulness in clinical work, we need to do so within the set of assumptions we adopt that allows value itself to be known and to be a useful guide to intellectual activity; these assumptions themselves need to be grasped. In creatures as cognitively limited as human beings, there seems to be no better way to do that than to embrace our assumptions as embedded in a root metaphor.

Understanding Figurative Speech in ACT

ACT attempts to alter the normal, culturally, and linguistically established relationships among affect, cognition, and behavior so as to weaken barriers to change. While the *machine* metaphor of human behavior assumes a causal chain leading from sensation to perception, then to emotion and cognition, and finally to behavior, contextualists hold that behavior change is possible without a prerequisite alteration of the form or frequency of thoughts, feelings, or memories (e.g., Harmon, Nelson, & Hayes, 1980; Jacobson et al., 1996). The form or frequency does not need to change because the impact of the experience is embedded in context. With a change in context, the impact of the experience can change even when the form of the thought of felling remains the same.

We understand this fully in everyday life, but its implications are usually missed. A person on a roller coaster may be terrified, but the terror is not harmful. A person having a panic attack may be terrified, but that terror as it is carried forward may be life restricting. The difference is not so much the terror itself as the psychological context in which it occurs.

From an ACT perspective, many of the most important functional contexts for thoughts, feelings, memories, and sensations are those that are built into human language itself. For example, language communities find it useful to establish the social and practical functions of language to treat words largely as if they are their referents. A person being told how to walk to a destination is usually not harmed by treating the description and the images it evokes almost as if it is the actual experience of walking to the destination. Words and their referents are poured together, or "fused" (a word drawn from an ancient root meaning "to pour"), without damage. But a person doing the same thing while thinking "I'm bad" can be drawn into a lifelong struggle with shame and self-blame, without even noticing the illusion of language that demanded that this fight be fought. The person is having the thought "I'm bad"—not experiencing being bad—but if that is missed the functions of that thought are radically altered. From an ACT perspective, cognitions and emotions function as barriers in life when we—therapists, clients, and people in general—take them literally and treat them as static objects that must be avoided or complied with, or that constitute "good reasons" for engaging in some actions and withdrawing from others, or that prove further judgments and evaluations of oneself or the world.

The avoidance, alteration, or termination of unwanted thoughts, feelings, or memories are often futile and even counterproductive (Hayes, Wilson,

Gifford, Follette, & Strosahl, 1996; Wenzlaff & Wegner, 2000), but because these effects are contextual, people often experience them as automatic, and not a matter of behavioral choice. Western culture encourages such experiential avoidance as a coping strategy, through the media and commercialism in particular. Disengaging from particular experiences certainly provides some short-term relief. However, in the long term, language processes assure the more frequent or more influential occurrence of exactly those experiences one seeks to avoid.

For example, the rule "I should not think x" contains a verbal event ("x") that will tend to evoke x, and thus following that rule is likely to work only temporarily. As soon as the person following it checks to see if it is working, it no longer will. A lack of flexibility and perceived vitality is the result of such processes, and people feel "stuck" (Chödrön, 1997).

The reason figurative language is so frequently used in ACT is that it is a challenge to alter the functions of normal verbal processes by engaging in verbal processes. The theory on which ACT is based, Relational Frame Theory (RFT; Hayes, Barnes-Holmes, & Roche, 2001), provides a way out. RFT divides language functions into those that establish the meaning of terms based on their relations to other things (cf., Sidman, 1994) and those that give terms behavioral impact. Most therapeutic approaches to cognition focus on the relational context, that is, on methods that instigate different relations among terms and between terms of other events. Said in another way, these methods try to change thinking patterns. ACT focuses instead on the functional context, that is, on methods that alter the degree to which verbal events evoke behavior. Said in another way, these methods try to change the impact of thinking.

Some of these methods, such as defusion techniques, directly target functional contexts. For example, saying a word repeatedly aloud quickly diminishes the believability and emotional arousal to the term (Masuda et al., 2004). But it is also possible to use the relational context in a way that alters a functional context. Figurative language is an example. From an RFT point of view, figurative language brings together two or more entire sets of verbal relations. The number of derived relations that result are staggering, and functions that are dominant in one relational network may now be available with regard to another but often not in a way it is easy for the person influenced by the metaphor to describe. For example, the metaphor "anxiety is like quicksand" may bring functions that exist with regard to quicksand (e.g., do not struggle with it; maximize your contact with it by laying out flat) to bear on anxiety.

Interventions based on the "machine metaphor" assume that clients' presenting problems are due to atypical errors in the machinery and will subside with error correction (Mojtabai, 2000). The processes targeted in ACT maintain the root metaphor of nested, historical, and ongoing events. Thus, figurative speech in ACT is not so much designed to change think as it is designed to change the context of thinking. Figurative speech is used to reframe thinking, evaluating, judging, remembering, and feeling as ongoing human activities, and to decouple the culturally established link between these experiences and overt behavior, so that life transformation becomes possible even if unwanted private experience persists.

Figurative Speech Versus Direct Instruction

ACT employs a variety of figurative speech component as is shown in Table 7.1. In contrast to other therapies that may employ figurative speech as rhetorical tools to convince or persuade, figurative speech in ACT eschews

Table 7.1. Types and examples of figurative language.

Figure of speech	Definition	Examples (from Kittay, 1987)	ACT examples
Similes	"Compare one thing with another" (Oxford English Dictionary [OED] online)	"A wolf is like a dog" (literal simile) versus "A man is like a wolf" (figurative simile) (p. 18)	Struggling with anxiety is like struggling in quicksand (Stewart & Barnes-Holmes, 2001)
Analogies	Point to "the fact that the relation borne to any object by some attribute or circumstance corresponds to the relation existing between another object and some attribute or circumstance pertaining to it" (OED online)	"Just as the right and left foot are equally strong because they must equally carry the burden of the rest of the body, [. . .] so the right hand and the left hand could be equally matched were they equally trained" (p. 276)	Just as "things" can be described, approached, manipulated, or "bought," so can thoughts and feelings
Metaphors	Transfer a name or a descriptive word or phrase to an object or action different from [. . .] that to which it is literally applicable (OED online)		
Conventional	Metaphorical origins go unnoticed (Kittay, 1987)	"Hold your tongue" (p. 51)	Pervasive in vernacular discourse; ACT stresses metaphorical or word origin (e.g., discussion of "responsibility")
Conceptual	Concepts are applied to a variety of expressions pertaining to the same topic (Lackoff & Johnson, 1980)	"Love is a physical force" (p. 90)	Human affect, behavior, and cognition are nested, historical, and ongoing events (Hayes, Wilson, & Strosahl, 1999, pp. 18–26)
Creative	Similarity is generated and not preexisting (Black, 1962)	"The garden was a slum of bloom." (p. 17)	Emotions, thoughts, and impulses are the cargo of trains running on parallel tracks in one's mind (Hayes & Smith, 2005, p. 66)
Allegories	"Extended metaphors" (OED online)	Plato's *Allegory of the Cave*	The story of the person in the hole (Hayes et al., 1999, pp. 101–102)
Maxims	Express "a general truth drawn from science or experience" (OED online)		If you aren't willing to have it, you got it (Hayes et al., 1999, pp. 121)

direct instruction or detailed rule giving. A body of research in the 1980s (e.g., Barrett, Deitz, Gaydos, & Quinn, 1987; Catania, Matthews, & Shimoff, 1982; Hayes, Brownstein, Zettle, Rosenfarb, & Korn, 1986) demonstrated that people are less likely to meet the changing demands of situations after having received explicit instructions. In essence, excessive rule-following may be repertoire narrowing, decreasing the flexibility necessary to master life's challenges. Conversely, more strategic or less-detailed verbal rules may preserve flexible coping. The Buddhist allegory of *the finger and the moon* (Watts, 2003) provides an example: Meticulous instruction following (i.e., attending to the other person's pointing finger) may prevent contact with the actually prevailing conditions (seeing what is there to be seen).

Experiential exercises combined with the figurative speech in ACT are explicitly designed to minimize the role of instruction and to maximize personal engagement with subtle and complex social situations. They downplay the therapist's expert (and potentially coercive) role, amplify the importance of individual experience, and create a space where the client may begin to experience events "freely and without defense" (Hayes et al., 1999, p. 77). Flexible approach, rather than rigid avoidance, characterizes the engagement in life that ACT aims to promote. In line with this understanding, regardless of ACT's evidence base and the demonstrated usefulness of the approach, therapists have to assess whether the use of figurative speech has the desired impact on the client.

Theories of Figurative Speech

Modern theorists characterize figurative speech as the "constitutive form" of language and its "omnipresent principle" (Richards, 1936, p. 93). While similes and analogies explicitly extend comparative relations and proportions to other subject matters and were rather uninteresting to linguists, metaphors have always received more scholarly attention because they seemed to arise out of a random, creative process that involved an intentional, "degenerative, incidental, or non-conforming" (Ritchie, 2006, p. 3) misuse of language. After Lakoff and his colleagues pointed to the ubiquity of conceptual metaphors in language process (Lakoff & Johnson, 1980, 1999), linguistic scholars began to distinguish "conventional metaphors"—firmly engrained in vernacular use, sharing nonverbal experience or a conceptual basis—from the "creative metaphors" of extraordinary rhetorical construction in speech, poetry, and literature (Knowles & Moon, 2006; Rozik, 2007).

RFT (Hayes et al., 2001) reconciles these seemingly divergent views (Stewart & Barnes-Holmes, 2001). RFT shows (1) how correlations between different types of nonverbal or verbal experiences may influence descriptions and (2) how novel references to nonexisting events may emerge out of purely verbally constructed relationships. To illustrate, a child commenting that carbonated water tastes like "my foot's asleep" would be an example of the first type of metaphorical extension (Skinner, 1957, p. 92), Shakespeare's "O, beware, my lord, of jealousy. It is the green-eyed monster which doth mock the meat it feeds on" (3.3, 189–192) is an example of the second. RFT integrates nonverbal events with verbal ones and provides an account of how never-before-experienced events (e.g., a green-eyed monster) come to exert cognitive meaning as well as emotional effects. Unlike the current compartmentalized and discontinuous theories of figurative speech, RFT renders a consistent and comprehensive account of language and cognition that systematically spans all types of literal and figurative speech, from descriptions over similes to creative metaphors.

The Application of Metaphor

ACT is a theory-driven and contextually based therapy in which the appropriate intervention differs greatly, given the individual client and the presenting problem. In discussing common ACT metaphors, we encourage therapists to identify the purpose of the metaphor and adapt the story or technique to their individual client's experience. This is congruent with research that suggests that clinical effectiveness of metaphors is increased when metaphors are produced in collaboration with client, are frequently repeated, and are apt to the situation (Martin, Cummings, & Hallberg, 1992). Thus, while each of the following metaphors is commonly used by ACT therapists, therapists are encouraged to create their own, similar metaphors in conjunction with their clients.

Undermine or Avoid Reason Giving

The ACT approach to understanding human suffering postulates that language is the basis for a great deal of emotional pain and inflexible behavior. One of the common impediments to behavioral change is reason giving. Individuals find it difficult to do something new because they have a well-developed story about why they are doing something old. A classic example is discussing why a person continues to use a particular coping strategy that is clearly not working. One approach would be to identify the strategy and identify reasons the person should do something else. From the ACT perspective, this simply strengthens reason giving as an appropriate coping strategy and leaves clients further entrenched in their original suffering. Consider the following metaphor:

The Person in the Hole Metaphor

The situation you are in seems a bit like this. Imagine that you're placed in a field, wearing a blindfold, and you're given a little bag of tools. You're told that your job is to run around this field, blindfolded. That is how you are supposed to live life. And so you do what you are told. Now unbeknownst to you, in this field there are a number of widely spaced, fairly deep holes. You don't know that at first—you're naive. So you start running around and sooner or later you fall into this large hole. You feel around and sure enough you can't climb out and there are no escape routes you can find. Probably what you would do in such a predicament is take the bag of tools you were given and see what is in there: Maybe there is something you can use to get out of the hole. Now suppose that there is a tool in that bag but what you've been given is a shovel. It's seemingly all you've got. So you dutifully start digging, but pretty soon you notice that you're not out of the hole. So you try digging faster, and faster. But you're still in the hole. So you try big shovelfuls, or little ones, or throwing the dirt far away or not. But still you are in the hole. All this effort and all this work and oddly enough the hole has just gotten bigger and bigger and bigger. Hasn't it? So you come in to see me thinking "maybe he has a really huge shovel—a gold-plated steam shovel." Well, I don't. And even if I did I wouldn't use it because digging is not a way out of the hole—digging is what makes holes. So maybe the whole agenda is hopeless—you can't dig your way out, that just digs you in.

(Hayes et al., 1999, pp. 101–102)

One function of this metaphor is to undermine reason giving. The metaphor acknowledges that the person may have reasons and that those reasons make quite logical sense. However, the metaphor puts at the forefront the question of whether or not what the person is doing is working. Reasons are undermined in that they are less important than the measure of workability. The therapist need not debate the individual's reasons nor convince their clients of the supremacy of other reasons.

Undermine or Avoid Pliance

As discussed above, while rule-following may decrease the flexibility necessary to master life's challenges, sufficiently vague rules may preserve flexible coping. Metaphors are particularly useful in undermining pliance in part for this reason. There is often no correct response or answer following a metaphor. In ACT, this is sometimes addressed directly in discussion of the therapeutic relationship. This is an example:

Two Mountains Metaphor

It's like you're in the process of climbing up a big mountain that has lots of dangerous places on it. My job is to watch out for you and shout out directions if I can see places you might slip or hurt yourself. The question is how do I best do that? If I am at the top of your mountain, then I can't really see you very well. If I am leading you up the mountain, then I have the same view as you and that isn't much help either. I see it like I am actually on my own mountain, just the one across the valley. From there I have a good view of your path. I don't have to know anything about exactly what it feels like to climb your mountain to see where you are about to step. You are the expert on your mountain and what it feels like to be there. I have the advantage of being able to see from a different perspective. Together we might be able to figure out a way to climb.

At other times, the metaphor is used to give a specific message, but the expected change in behavior is not articulated by the therapist

The Rubber Hammer Metaphor

It would be as if you were to go to the doctor and say that you have a terrible headache, and the doctor looks at you and you're hitting yourself in the head with a rubber hammer. You may not know that you're hitting yourself, or you might have a very good reason for doing so. However, the first thing the doctor is likely to tell you is "you are hitting yourself over the head with a hammer, and your head is likely to continue to hurt until that stops."

In this situation, the patient must decide what the hammer is and what it means to stop hitting oneself over the head with it. Pliance is reduced because the therapist does not explicitly define the rule. The resulting effect more closely resembles contingency shaping than a direct rule because a very wide variety of actions could be relevant to the metaphor.

Weaken Literal Functions of Language

Because of the emphasis on language in ACT, there are many metaphors that specifically target the literal functions of language. These metaphors are used to highlight the pitfalls of taking our thoughts and the associated language literally, and seek to establish contexts in which that is less likely. This is an example.

Two Computers Metaphor

Imagine two computers, sitting side by side, each with an operator in front of them. These are identical machines, and they have the same programs and the same data in them. Now, the way computers work is that if you give them a particular input, they give a particular output. So suppose we push a key on these two machines and some read-out shows up on both screens. Suppose what comes up is, "Deep down, there's something wrong with me." Now imagine two different situations. In situation #1, the operator is totally lost in the operation of the computer. It's like being lost in a movie; you're not watching, you are in that movie, so when someone jumps out from behind a door, you jump. It is like that. The operator is sitting right in front of the monitor, nose touching the screen, lost in the read out and unable to distinguish between the machine and the person operating the machine. The operator has forgotten that there's any distinction. So the screen shows "Deep down there's something wrong with me." Now, from that place—with the operator indistinct from the machine—the operator's only choice is to try to reprogram the machine. Who's going to accept that deep down inside there's something wrong with them? That's like saying it would be OK to be eaten by the tiger. Situation #2: Same computer, same programming, everything is the same. The same readout comes up, "Deep down there's something wrong with me." But this person is sitting back a little, and is real clear that there is a distinction between the machine and the person. He's the operator of the machine, he's working on the machine, but he is not the machine. The operator can still see the read out very clearly, but because there's a distinction between himself and the machine, the read-out doesn't necessarily have to change. He could call over his friends and say "Look at this thing. I type in x and looks what comes out on the screen. Interesting, huh." It's like that. Your mind has been programmed by all kinds of people. So at one point, Mom comes over and works on the keyboard for a while; a little later Dad comes over. At various times, your husband (or wife), your teachers, your kids, your friends, your coworkers—they all spend a little time at the computer. And in certain situations—given the right input—you'll get a certain read-out. You might even believe it to be true. For example, it says on the screen, "Boy, I really need to use heroin!" It may or may not be accurate. The issue isn't whether the readout is true or false. The issue is whether there is any distinction between the person and the mental machinery. Is there any distinction between you and the stuff that is in your life?

This metaphor is designed to weaken literal functions of language on multiple levels. First, it equates thought and the associated language as computer output rather than actual truth. Second, it introduces the idea that these thoughts and language may be highly influenced by the "input" of other people, rather than the clients own experience. Third, it emphasizes the distinction between the person and their verbal products, increasing a sense of choice even in the presence of particular verbal formulations.

Provide a Commonsense Model of Paradoxical Processes

Many ACT concepts do not make logical sense even though they make good psychological sense. It is not that ACT is illogical; it is that the usefulness of ACT concepts is dependent more on experience than analysis. Metaphors provide a commonsense model that can reassure and guide the client when dealing with paradoxical concepts. Consider the following example:

The Feedback Screech Metaphor

You know that horrible feedback screech that a public address system sometimes makes? It happens when a microphone is positioned too close to a speaker. Then, when a person on stage makes the least little noise, it goes into the microphone, the sound comes out of the speakers amplified and then back into the mic, a little bit louder than it was the first time it went in, and at the speed of sound and electricity, it gets louder and louder until, in split seconds, it's unbearably loud. Your struggles with your thoughts and emotions are like being caught in the middle of a feedback screech. So what do you do? You do what anyone would. You try to live your life [whispering] *very quietly*, always whispering, always tip-toeing around. You can't really live without making noise. But notice that in this metaphor, it isn't how much noise you make that is the problem. It's the amplifier that's the problem. Our job in here is not to help you live your life quietly, free of all emotional discomfort and disturbing thoughts. Our job is to find the amplifier and to take it out of the loop.

This metaphor is used to describe the complex implications of experiential avoidance while, at the same time, to introduce the idea of acceptance. The commonsense model of a feedback screech is more clear than an in-depth description of how rules can interact with direct experiences to produce self-amplifying loops of emotions and thoughts.

Providing Evidence Without Argument

This allows the client to experience a concept without having to convince the person. An example in ACT is discussing our limits at achieving internal, emotional control.

The Polygraph Metaphor

Suppose I had you hooked up to the best polygraph machine that's ever been built. This is a perfect machine, the most sensitive ever made. When you are all wired up to it, there is no way you can be aroused or anxious without the machine knowing it. So I tell you that you have a very simple task here: all you have to do is stay relaxed. If you get the least bit anxious, however, I will know it. I know you want to try hard, but I want to give you an extra incentive, so I also have a .44 Magnum which I'll hold to your head. If you just stay relaxed, I won't blow your brains out, but if you get nervous (and I'll know it because you're wired up to this perfect machine), I'm going to have to kill you. Your brains will be all over the walls. So, just relax! . . . What do you think would happen? Guess what you'd get? Bam! How could it work otherwise? The tiniest bit of anxiety would be terrifying. You'd be going "Oh, my God! I'm getting anxious! Here it comes!" BAM! You're dead meat. How could it work otherwise? (Hayes et al., 1999, pp. 123–124).

In this example, it is easy for the individual client to imagine being anxious, despite their best efforts to control their anxiety. The extreme nature of the metaphor allows the clinician to reliably demonstrate the concept without having to convince the client of the outcome logically or argue that it fits the client's actual situation.

Structure Experiential Processes

From an ACT perspective, mindfulness involves acceptance, defusion, a focus on the present moment, and a transcendent sense of self. Experiential mindfulness exercises are used regularly in ACT. Metaphors can be used to help guide the client to use these mindfulness exercises in a way that is focused on these four ACT processes. The following metaphor is designed to help the client observe their thoughts mindfully.

Leaves on a Stream Metaphor

Imagine yourself sitting on the bank of gurgling stream. You are sitting, enjoying the beautiful day, and relaxing under a large oak tree. It is fall and as you sit you notice many leaves falling from the tree into the stream, and floating by. As you imagine this, I want you to pay attention to any thoughts that you may be having in each moment. Notice the thoughts coming and going as the leaves come and go, and imagine your thoughts are written on the leaves as they float by. One leave may say, "Am I doing this right," and another might say, "I feel tired today." Whatever thought you having—just picture it on one of the leaves and watch it as it goes by, without pushing it or pulling it. At some point you may have the sense that you are no longer doing the exercise, that you are caught up in the thoughts rather than just watching them go by. When that happens, I want you to back up a few seconds and see if you can catch what you were doing right before the leaves stopped. Then go ahead and sit under that tree and start putting your thoughts on the leaves again. I'll be quiet now while you engage in this process [several minutes of silence follow] (Hayes et al., 1999, pp. 158–162).

In this exercise, all four ACT processes that are thought to define mindfulness are put into a figurative image. The "person under the tree" represents a transcendent sense of self; looking at a thought like one looks at a leaf encourages defusion; neither pushing nor pulling the leaf is a metaphor for acceptance; and watching for thoughts as they arise is a focus on the present moment. The silence that follows allows the actual exercise, but the metaphor structures it so that it is likely to be successful in ACT terms.

Summary

We have reviewed the importance of metaphor in ACT, from the model underlying its philosophy of science to the use of figurative language to encourage ACT processes. We have argued that metaphor is a useful clinical tool in acceptance- and mindfulness-based practice in general because it is uniquely suited to address the concerns that contextual therapies hope to address. Metaphor is heavily used in ACT therapy and addresses the impact of language on human suffering by undermining or at least avoiding reason giving and pliance, weakening the literal functions of language, providing commonsense models of paradoxical processes, experientially demonstrating concepts, and helping to properly structure and guide more experiential processes.

References

Barrett, D. M., Deitz, S. M., Gaydos, G. R., & Quinn, P. C. (1987). The effects of programmed contingencies and social conditions on response stereotypy with human subjects. *Psychological Record, 37,* 489-505.

Blenkiron, P. (2005). Stories and analogies in cognitive behaviour therapy: A clinical review. *Behavioural and Cognitive Psychotherapy, 33,* 45-59.

Catania, A. C., Matthews, B. A., & Shimoff, E. (1982). Instructed versus shaped human verbal behavior: Interactions with nonverbal responding. *Journal of the Experimental Analysis of Behavior, 38*(3), 233-248.

Chödrön, P. (1997). *When things fall apart: Heart advice for difficult times.* Boston: Shambala.

Drossel, C., Waltz, T., & Hayes, S. C. (in press). An introduction to principles of behavior. In D. Woods & J. Kanter (Eds.), *Understanding behavior disorders: A contemporary behavioral perspective.* Reno, NV: Context Press.

Eynon, T. (2002). Cognitive linguistics. *Advances in Psychiatric Treatment, 8,* 399-407.

Harmon, T. M., Nelson, R. O., & Hayes, S. C. (1980). Self-monitoring of mood versus activity by depressed clients. *Journal of Consulting and Clinical Psychology, 48*(1), 30-38.

Hayes, S. C., Barnes-Holmes, D., & Roche, B. (Eds.) (2001). *Relational Frame Theory: A post-Skinnerian account of human language and cognition.* NY: Kluwer Academic/Plenum Publishers.

Hayes, S. C., Brownstein, A. J., Zettle, R. D., Rosenfarb, I. & Korn, Z. (1986). Rule-governed behavior and sensitivity to changing consequences of responding. *Journal of Experimental Analysis of Behavior, 45,* 237-256.

Hayes, S. C., Hayes, L. J., & Reese, H. W. (1988). Finding the philosophical core: A review of Stephen C. Pepper's "World hypotheses: A study in evidence." *Journal of the Experimental Analysis of Behavior, 50*(1), 97-111.

Hayes, S. C., Hayes, L. J., Reese, H. W., & Sarbin, T. R. (Eds.). (1993). *Varieties of scientific contextualism.* Reno, NV: Context Press.

Hayes, S. C., Strosahl, K. D., & Wilson, K. G. (1999). *Acceptance and Commitment Therapy: An experiential approach to behavior change.* NY: The Guilford Press.

Hayes, S. C., Wilson, K. W., Gifford, E. V., Follette, V. M., & Strosahl, K. (1996). Experiential avoidance and behavioral disorders: A functional dimensional approach to diagnosis and treatment. *Journal of Consulting and Clinical Psychology, 64,* 1152-1168.

Jacobson, N. S., Dobson, K. S., Truax, P. A., Addis, M. E., Koerner, K., Gollan, J. K., Gortner, E., & Prince, S. E. (1996). A component analysis of cognitive-behavioral treatment for depression. *Journal of Consulting and Clinical Psychology, 64*(2), 295–304.

Knowles, M. & Moon, R. (2006). *Introducing metaphor.* New York: Routlege.

Lakoff, G., & Johnson, M. (1980). *Metaphors we live by.* Chicago: The University of Chicago Press.

Lakoff, G. & Johnson, M. (1999). *Philosophy in the Flesh: The embodied mind and its challenges to western thought.* New York: Perseus Books.

Leary, D. E. (1990). *Metaphors in the history of psychology.* Cambridge: Cambridge Studies in the History of Psychology.

Lyddon, W. J., Clay, A. L., & Sparks, C. L. (2001). Metaphor and change in counseling. *Journal of Counseling and Development, 79,* 269–274.

Martin, J. Cummings, A. L., & Hallberg, E. T. (1992). Therapists' intentional use of metaphor: Memorability, clinical impact, and possible epistemic/motivational functions. *Journal of Consulting and Clinical Psychology, 60,* 143–145.

Masuda, A., Hayes, S. C., Sackett, C. F., & Twohig, M. P. (2004). Cognitive defusion and self-relevant negative thoughts: Examining the impact of a ninety year old technique. *Behaviour Research and Therapy, 42,* 477–485.

Mojtabai, R. (2000). Delusion as error: The history of a metaphor. *History of Psychiatry, 11,* 3–14.

Otto, M. (2000). Stories and metaphors in cognitive-behavior therapy. *Cognitive and Behavioral Practice, 7,* 166–172.

Pepper, S. C. (1970). *World Hypotheses: Prolegomena to systematic philosophy and a complete survey of metaphysics.* Berkley: University of California Press.

Richards, I. A. (1936). *The philosophy of rhetoric.* London: Oxford University Press.

Ritchie, L. D. (2006). *Context and connection in metaphor.* NY: Palgrave Macmillan.

Rosnow, R. L., & Georgoudi, M. (Eds.). (1986). *Contextualism and understanding in behavioral science.* New York: Praeger.

Rozik, E. (2007). Cognitive theories of metaphor. *The European Legacy, 12*(6), 745–748.

Sidman, M. (1994). *Equivalence relations and behavior: A research story.* Boston: Authors Cooperative.

Skinner, B. F. (1957). *Verbal behavior.* Acton, MA: Copley Publishing Group.

Stewart, I., & Barnes-Holmes, D. (2001). Understanding metaphor: A relational frame perspective. *The Behavior Analyst, 24*(2), 191–200.

Watts, A. (2003). The finger and the moon. In M. Watts (Ed.), *Become what you are* (pp. 12–18). Boston: Shambala.

Wenzlaff, R. M. & Wegner, D. M. (2000). Thought suppression. *Annual Review of Psychology, 51,* 59–91.

8

Mindfulness and Feelings of Emptiness

Fabrizio Didonna and Yolanda Rosillo Gonzalez

"Nothing is as unbearable for man as to be completely at rest, without passion, without business, without distraction, without application to something."
In such a state of rest man becomes aware of "his nothingness, his foresakenness, his insufficiency, his dependence, his impotence, his emptiness."
Incontinently there springs from the depth of his soul "the ennui, the blackness, the tristesse, the chagrin, the spite, the despair."

Blaise Pascal

Introduction

The feeling of emptiness is a common symptom or phenomenological experience found in clinical practice with several kinds of disorders. What is, however, more difficult is finding two patients who describe this experience in the same way. Patients report different experiences: "I feel an emptiness inside," "everything seems empty," "I feel like I'm falling into a great emptiness," "nothing makes sense because of the emptiness," and many others. Though at first sight they may appear to be very similar, some specific and distinctive characteristics surface on closer observation. The diagnoses that comprise these manifestations can be multiple and are recurrent in relation to a series of disorders: from common depressive episodes to personality disorders, even in comorbidity with other pathologies.

This phenomenon seems to be a universal human experience and might not always seem directly linked to a pathology. All of us, at some moment in our lives, can experience a "feeling of emptiness," without suffering from a mental disorder. Like many other nonspecific symptoms, the feeling of emptiness is neither a necessary nor a sufficient reason for a frank diagnosis although it has become one of the inclusion/exclusion nosological criteria of borderline personality disorder (BPD) in the Diagnostic and Statistical Manual of Mental Disorders (DSM-IV, American Psychiatric Association, 2000).

The experience of emptiness has aroused the interest of well-known scholars and has become the main subject of their writings. Unfortunately, few thorough or rigorous studies have focused specifically on emptiness. This may be because of the many methodological problems involved in this type of study. For example, what do we mean by experience of emptiness? Does this feeling of emptiness always present itself in the same way? Does it vary according to the disorder diagnosed? Although we will try to answer these questions, at least in part, in this chapter, the main aim is to take the reader through a theoretical reflection on the possible clinical use of mindfulness, to alleviate, reduce, or eliminate the suffering caused by the experience of emptiness as a pathological symptom.

Psychology and Emptiness

He who has a why to live, can bear almost any how
Nietzsche

The experience of emptiness has not been studied only by psychologists. Various categories of scholars, including philosophers and theologians, have been and still are interested in this phenomenon of human experience. However, if we focus specifically on psychology, we can highlight some epistemological approaches that, more than others, have tried to explain this psychological experience. Cognitive-behavioral theory (Linehan, 1993; Young, 1987), existential psychology (Frankl, 1975, 1963; May, 1950, 1953), and psychoanalysis (Kernberg, 1975; Kohut, 1971, 1977) are some of the theoretical perspectives that have provided important contributions to the understanding of the experience of emptiness. These contributions will be discussed in detail below.

Cognitive-Behavioral Theory and Feelings of Emptiness

Several cognitive-behavioral authors have suggested that the experience of emptiness can be a sort of dysfunctional avoidance strategy in a situation of deep subjective suffering (Beck, Freeman et al., 1990; Linehan, 1993; Young, 1987). Linehan (1993) bases her therapeutic model on the idea that the inability to regulate and modulate painful emotions is an essential element in explaining the behavioral difficulties of patients with BPD. These patients present a sort of intolerance to negative emotions: "Many borderline patients try to control their emotions simply by forcing themselves *not to feel* what they are experiencing" (Linehan, 1993). Other researchers, such as Fiore and Semerari (2003), speak of a state of *emotional anesthesia* to avoid any suffering by which patients detach themselves from everything and everyone.

Young, Klosko, and Weishaar (2003) have identified various *modes*, meaning the specific emotions, cognitions, and behavior active in a person in the here and now. Among these, the *detached protector mode* aims at isolating the person from his needs and feelings, creating a sort of detachment with a protection purpose. The main symptoms of this mode include depersonalization, self-harm, boredom, and feelings of emptiness. These theories can be associated with Hayes, Wilson, Gifford, Follette, and Strosahl's (1996) assertions on *experiential avoidance*.

Experiential avoidance is a putative pathological process recognized by a wide number of theoretical orientations. Experiential avoidance is the phenomenon that occurs when a person is unwilling to remain in contact with particular private experiences (e.g., bodily sensations, emotions, thoughts, memories, and behavioral predispositions) and takes steps to alter the form or frequency of these events and the contexts that occasion them. We occasionally use terms such as *emotional avoidance* or *cognitive avoidance* rather than the more generic *experiential avoidance* when it is clear that these are the relevant aspects of experience that the person seeks to escape, avoid, or modify. We recognize that thoughts, memories, and emotions are richly intermingled and do not mean to imply any necessary rigid distinction among them (although distinctions might be drawn by some theoretical perspectives without threat to the underlying principle of experiential avoidance) (Hayes et al., 1996).

The question, then, is what can a patient do if, as has been hypothesized by the aforementioned authors, the feared stimulus is one's own emotions? How can a person avoid something that is not outside, but part of his or her natural and theoretically adaptive response to the outside world? Certainly, a possibility is to try *not to feel*, as was said above. Experiencing this "emptiness" creates a detachment leading to actions aimed at distancing the subject from the stimulus situation, that is, the negative emotions, replacing them with physical pain (self-harm), numbness (alcohol or substance abuse), euphoria (acting out dangerous behaviors), or physical gratification (sexual promiscuity, bulimic crises), all manageable situations from the subject's point of view.

Referring to the BPD, Linehan (1993) claims that exposure to an invalidating environment, where inadequate and unforeseeable answers follow the manifestation of a person's inner experiences, leads to the *non-recognition* or *inhibition* of negative emotions. This continuous inhibition of negative emotions leads to emotional avoidance. The paradigm, the author claims, is similar to learning flight behavior to avoid painful stimuli. In this case, the emotions, meaning the complex response of the body (activation of the central nervous system accompanied on a neurovegetative, behavioral, and cognitive level by specific modifications), seem to be conditioned. This conditioning may have been caused by a repeated process of adverse association stimuli such as those previously described by Linehan regarding an invalidating environment. If we add this to specific circumstances, increases in fear not caused by events experienced by the subject but rather by the simple repeated presentation of discriminative and conditioned stimuli, connected to such events (Sanavio, 1991), we find that even simple physical sensations, previously associated with a negative emotion, can produce a phenomenon known as *incubation of fear*. The sense of emptiness could be triggered by the simple arising of one of these discriminative stimuli, preceding the activation of the negative emotions, which the subject avoids and sometimes fails to recognize.

Existential Psychology

Viktor Frankl coined the term "existential vacuum" (1963; 1973), and aspects of the meaning of this term come close in meaning to the term "emptiness" as described in this chapter. Frankl posits that humans have a "will to meaning," which is as basic to them as the will to power or the will to pleasure. The frustration of the will to meaning results, in Frankl's estimation, in a "noogenic neurosis" – an abyss experience (Hazell, 2003). If meaning is what you desire, then meaninglessness is a hole, an emptiness, in our lives. Whenever you have a vacuum, of course, things rush in to fill it. Frankl (1963) suggests that one of the most conspicuous signs of existential vacuum in our society is boredom. He points out how often people, when they finally have the time to do what they want, don't seem to want to do anything, for example, people go into a tailspin when they retire, students get drunk every weekend, and people submerge themselves in passive entertainment every evening. He calls this the "Sunday neurosis" and defines it as "that kind of depression which afflicts those who become aware of the lack of content in their lives when the rush of the busy week is over and the void within themselves becomes manifest" (Frankl, 1963, p. 169). The result of this is an attempt to fill our existential vacuums with "stuff" that, because it provides some satisfaction, we hope will provide ultimate satisfaction as well; for example, we might try to fill our lives with pleasure, eating beyond all necessity, having promiscuous sex, living "the high life;" we might seek power, especially the power represented by monetary success; we might fill our lives with "busyness," conformity, and conventionality; or we might fill the vacuum with anger and hatred and spend our days attempting to destroy what we think is hurting us. We might also fill our lives with certain neurotic "vicious cycles," such as obsession with germs and cleanliness, or fear-driven obsession with a phobic object. The defining quality of these vicious cycles is that, whatever we do, it is never enough.

Frankl conducted many studies where he interviewed people on "existential emptiness" (1975). At the Policlinic Hospital in Vienna, he found that 55% of patients had experienced a loss in the meaning of life, and a statistical survey showed that 25% of European and 50% of American students had had this experience. In Frankl's thinking, the experience of emptiness is made up of two feelings: a feeling that life is meaningless and a feeling of inner emptiness. This bifactorial quality in the experience of existential vacuum is sometimes undifferentiated from other concepts such as boredom and depression: "The existential vacuum manifests itself mainly in a state of boredom" (Frankl, 1963, p. 169). Another important representative of existential psychology, Rollo May (1950, 1953), has illustrated some useful ideas on the concept of the experience of emptiness. In his earlier work, May (1950) connects the experience of anxiety with the threat of nonbeing, that is, anxiety is the experience of being affirming itself against nonbeing: "Emptiness and loneliness, are thus the two phases of the basic experience of anxiety". In 1953 (p. 14), he wrote: ". . . the chief problem of problem in the mid-decade of the twentieth century is emptiness. By that I mean that not only do people not know what they want; they often do not have any clear idea of what they feel . . . they have no definite experience of their desires or wants." May relates the experience of emptiness with turning to drug use or to the use of sex in a mechanical way: ". . . the most common problem now is not social taboos on sexual activity or guilt feelings about sex itself, but the fact that sex for most people is an empty, mechanical and vacuous experience" (May, 1953, p. 15). This behavior, which is found rather frequently in some types of disorders such as BPD, is often traced back by the same patients to their own experience of emptiness. Other interesting reflections by the author refer to the relationship between the experiences of emptiness, helplessness, and powerlessness (May, 1953). The experience of emptiness rather generally comes from people's feeling that they are powerless to do anything effective about their lives or the world they live in. Inner vacuousness is the long-term accumulated result of a person's particular conviction toward himself, namely, that he or she cannot act as an entity in directing his or her own life, and since what he or she wants and what he or she feels can make no real difference, he or she gives up wanting and feeling. Apathy and lack of feeling are also defenses against anxiety (May, 1953, p. 22).

Psychoanalysis and Emptiness

As far as psychoanalysis is concerned, let us take a look at Otto Kernberg's work (1975) on the experience of emptiness. Kernberg used psychodynamics and object-relations theory as a means of explaining the various forms the experience might take. For him, the experience of emptiness arises when there is a loss of what Jacobson (1964) calls "self feeling". Kernberg points out that although there are several forms of the experience of emptiness, there are two broad reactions to the experience: that of "acting out" in a forced attempt to regain a sense of internal aliveness and that of submitting to the experience and going through one's daily activities in a split-off, mechanical fashion (Hazell, 2003).

Kernberg (1975) also highlights the difference between the two concepts of emptiness and loneliness, which at times can be confused in a clinical context: "loneliness implies elements of longing and the sense that there are others that are needed, and whose love is needed and who seem unavailable now." If this longing were present, the individual would not feel empty. Emptiness is the lack of others without the realization of the lack or the longing to fill the lack (Hazell, 2003). In general, Kernberg (1975, p. 220) posits that: "The experience of emptiness represents a temporary or permanent loss of the normal relationship of self with the object relations, that is, with the world of inner objects that fixates intrapsychically the significant experiences with others and constitutes a basic ingredient of ego-identity . . . . Therefore, all patients with the syndrome of identity diffusion (but not with identity crises) present the potential for developing experiences of emptiness." The author hypothesizes that the experience of emptiness could be different depending on the personality experiencing it, and he describes the feeling of emptiness as it may occur in four personality types (depressive, schizoid, narcissistic, and borderline), arguing that its form, intensity, and etiology will differ for each type. While Kernberg interprets the experience largely in terms of object relations, Heinz Kohut (1977, p. 243) uses the framework of "self psychology" to explain this experience: "The psychology of the self is needed to explain the pathology of the fragmented self and of the depleted self (empty depression, i.e., the world of unmirrored ambitions, the world devoid of ideals)." He argues that the experience of emptiness is a symptom of narcissistic personality disorders (NPDs). The self-structure matures gradually in response to optimal failures in mirroring and idealized figures. If the failures are sub-optimal, the self-structure becomes friable and labile. One of the experiential outcroppings of this is the experience of emptiness, especially in the face of criticism or lack of warmth or acclaim from the environment. Kohut argues that very often, in response to early traumatic environmental failures, reactions develop, very often in the way of a soothing mechanism, to cope with, and alleviate the pain of the inner emptiness (Hazell, 2003). On occasion, a person will develop "a psychic surface that is out of contact with an active nuclear self" (Kohut, 1977, p. 49). This concept sounds extremely close to the concept of "false self system" proposed by Winnicott (1965a,b) and developed by Laing (1969). The false self is like a mask or set of clothes, donned to adapt to society but cut off from the individual's real self that lies hidden, even to the individuals themselves. This psychological state can lead to frequent experiences of emptiness: When the person attempts to discover his or her "true feelings," he or she is so alienated from them through habit that he or she draws a blank and feels empty (Hazell, 2003).

Among the symptomatic responses to the experience of emptiness, Kohut cites the following: an excessive interest in words, pseudovitality, compulsive sexuality, addictions, and delinquency. Each of these is a reaction to the inner experience of emptiness and is employed as a means of counteracting the experience in some way. Kohut also posits that young adulthood and middle age are the critical testing grounds for the cohesiveness of the sense of self, and there are thus times when the individual is especially prone to experiences of emptiness.

Subtle variants of these psychodynamic explanations for the experience of emptiness, basically growing out of "object relations theory," can be found in a number of other works. Bowlby (1980) follows the thought of Winnicott in that he connects feeling of emptiness with the experience of loss. "Numbness" and "emptiness" are, in Bowlby's model, the first phases of the human being's reaction to a loss. For Bowlby this loss is confined to a loss through death. He argues, however, that a small loss may act as a trigger for a prior, more serious loss. Bowlby also offers a hint at an explanation for the feeling of emptiness or numbness although he does not propose it as such. He cites the disruption of habitual responses that occur to the person who has recently experienced a loss. This, in turn, leads to a vague sense of disorientation, much akin to the disorientation Bowlby mentions in his earlier works on attachment and separation (Bowlby, 1980, p. 94).

Feelings of Emptiness and Essential Needs

Other valuable hypotheses have been suggested by Almaas (1987) and Trobe-Krishnananda (1999). Almaas (1987), in the chapter called "The Theory of Holes," describes how energetic holes develop inside when an essential need is not met as a child. A hole is a feeling of emptiness inside in relation to some aspect of our being that was not nourished and therefore not developed. According to Trobe-Krishnananda (1999), because it is frightening and uncomfortable to feel these holes, we spend much of our time and energy in our daily life unconsciously trying to fill them. Much of our behavior is directed at getting others to fill them. There may be many reasons that these holes exist; many of them can be difficult to explain, but they are probably directly related to basic needs that remain unfulfilled. Although there is really only one hole inside, the author makes distinctions to help with clarity. Those of us who did not receive the support we needed to find out who we were may develop a *support hole*. When we did not get the recognition we needed, we have a *recognition hole*. We can have a *worthiness hole* when we feel that we are not good enough as a person or when we don't feel special or respected. In this latter case, we then hunger for someone to validate us with the hope that the hole can be filled. We may develop holes related to being perfectionists and self-critical or to having deep fears of survival; we may have holes connected to feeling unwanted and abandoned or to getting warmth, touch, and closeness; in this case, we become dependent on someone to provide that for us. We may also have a hole related to trust when we feel that opening up and being vulnerable exposes us to mistreatment, control, or manipulation by another.

The intensity and effects of these holes and the degree to which they can affect the development and life of an individual may depend on the particular way in which he or she is able to deal with this experience. In some cases, these holes create a *co-dependency* in which individuals continually push other people away while longing for closeness at the same time. Our holes create deep anxiety and our life becomes a constant unconscious compulsion to fill them. Every hole creates a dependency on the outside in some way, either by desiring another or a situation to fill it or by avoiding a person or situation because of the hole. Our holes have a powerful effect on the type of people and situations we attract. We have a compulsion to create situations that provoke our holes because that is often the only way we become aware that they are there. This is the way that we can learn about and develop what is missing inside. We need the challenge to grow (Trobe-Krishnananda, 1999).

When we don't have awareness or understanding of our holes and the way they are affecting our lives, we naturally feel that something on the outside has to change for us to be happy. This is one of the cardinal beliefs of what the Trobe-Krishnananda has called "emotional child" – an inner experience of self, derived from the childhood wounds and negative experiences full of fear, shame, and mistrust and covered with compulsive behavior. For example, people can find themselves repeating the same painful patterns in their relationships without understanding why; they can become lost in addictive behavior, or they may have repetitive accidents or illnesses or sabotage their life repeatedly (Trobe-Krishnananda, 1999). Because of the emptiness inside, when individuals are identified with the *emotional child*, they experience themselves as needy. It is not real, but it leads to their believing that life or others have to fill the hole. People have to start treating us better or give us more recognition, love, space, attention, and so on. Another reaction is that individuals try to fill the holes with things that make them feel better such as drugs, objects, or entertainment. It can be very difficult to find other ways to end the discomfort, pain, anxiety, and fear that holes cause, without filling them from the outside. People can realize that the efforts to fill the holes from the outside never work – it only creates deeper frustration. What does work is beginning to understand our holes – what they are, where they come from, and how we can fill them. To do this, it could be helpful to have a look at what the author calls "the essential needs".

As a child, we each have essential needs (see also Bowlby, 1980). When these needs are not met, we could live in a constant state of deprivation. That deprivation is the hole inside, longing to be filled. While the degree and types of deprivation vary, we all share a common experience of deprivation in some form. From our deprivation, we unconsciously project our unmet needs onto our lovers, children, close friends, and those we work with – in fact, on anyone with whom we relate. The closer the connection, the deeper the projection. The experience of being deprived is universal, and it is an important rite of passage. People usually start out in a state of denial, in which they are not even aware that they were deprived of certain essential needs or how. Trobe-Krishnananda (1999) highlighted some of individuals' *essential needs*: the need to feel wanted and to feel special and respected; the need to have our emotions, thoughts, and perceptions validated (see also Chapter 11 in this volume); the need to be encouraged to discover and explore our unique aptitudes and turns, sexuality, resourcefulness, creativity, joy, silence, and solitude; the need to feel secure, protected, and supported; the need to be physically touched with loving presence; the need to be inspired and motivated to learn; the need to know that it is right to make mistakes and to learn from them; the need to witness love and intimacy; the need to be encouraged and supported to separate; and the need to be given firm and loving limits and boundaries. This list is where an individual's deprivation comes from, and it is ever present. It is interesting to notice that when one starts a relationship with another person, very often he or she is unconsciously experiencing these unmet needs. When there is no awareness, the individual automatically moves into one of five behavioral patterns of the emotional child: reaction and control, expectation and entitlement, compromise, addictiveness, or magical thinking (Trobe-Krishnananda, 1999). For this author, the starting point for overcoming these holes, and feelings of emptiness, is recognizing how automatically people try to fill them from the outside. This process of watching and understanding releases energy to break the automatic behavior and just be with the experience of emptiness when it is provoked. This means feeling it and letting it be there without trying to fix or change anything. Mindfulness, as we will see in the last part of this chapter, can be the core strategy to developing this non-reactive attitude.

Mindfulness and Emptiness: The "Paradox" of Meditation

> If you say you are somebody, you are attached to name and form,
> so I will hit you thirty times.
> If you say you are nobody, you are attached to emptiness,
> so I will hit you thirty times.
> What can you do?
>   Soen Sa Nim (Cited in J. Kabat-Zinn, *Coming to Our Senses*)

As we mentioned in the introductory paragraph, the aim of this chapter is to theorize a possible clinical use of mindfulness to treat the pathological feeling of emptiness. To be able to speak about the relationship between mindfulness and emptiness, it is essential to know how it is conceived within the psychological and philosophical approaches and traditions that have given origin to meditative practice.

The concept of emptiness in Eastern psychology and culture is totally unrelated to that of the West, especially considering the negative value that is commonly ascribed to it in the West. An analysis of the classical texts of Taoism or Chinese Buddhism is enough to conclude that the Christian-Western concepts are basically opposite of those illustrated in Eastern thought.

The majority of Buddhist schools share a series of basic common principles. What interests us is called *Sunyata* (Sanskrit), generally translated into English as "emptiness" or "voidness." This is a concept of central importance in the teaching of Buddha since a direct realization of Sunyata is a requirement for achieving liberation from the cycle of existence (*samsara*) and full enlightenment. Widely misconceived as a doctrine of nihilism, the teaching on the emptiness of people and phenomena is unique to Buddhism, constituting an important metaphysical critique of theism with profound implications for epistemology and phenomenology.

Sunyata means that everything one encounters in life is empty of absolute identity, permanence, or "self." This is because everything is interrelated and mutually dependent – never wholly self-sufficient or independent. All things are in a state of constant flux where energy and information are forever flowing throughout the natural world giving rise to themselves undergoing major transformations with the passage of time. This teaching never connotes nihilism – nihilism is, in fact, a belief or point of view that Buddha explicitly taught was incorrect – a delusion, just as the view of materialism, is a delusion. In the English language, the word emptiness suggests the absence of spiritual meaning or a personal feeling of alienation, but in Buddhism the emptiness of phenomena enables liberation from the limitations of form in the cycle of uncontrolled rebirth. Kabat-Zinn (2005, p. 180) explains the concept:

> People can get scared even hearing such a thing, and may think that it is nihilistic. But it is not nihilistic at all; emptiness means empty of inherent self-existence, in other words that nothing, no person, no business, no nation or atom exists in and of itself as an enduring entity, isolated, absolute, independent of everything else. Nothing! Everything emerges out of the complex play of particular causes and conditions that are themselves always changing. This is a tremendous insight into the nature of reality."

Further he posits that "Emptiness is intimately related to fullness. Emptiness doesn't mean a meaningless void [...] emptiness is fullness, [...] is the invisible, intangible "space" within which discrete events can emerge and unfold. No emptiness, no fullness."

Rawson (1991) states that "One potent metaphor for the Void, often used in Tibetan art, is the sky. As the sky is the emptiness that offers clouds to our perception, so the Void is the 'space' in which objects appear to us in response to our attachments and longings." The Japanese use of the Chinese character signifying Sunyata is also used to connote sky or air.

Sunyata is a key theme of the *heart sutra* (one of the Mahayana Perfection of Wisdom Sutras), which is commonly chanted by Mahayana Buddhists worldwide. The *heart sutra* declares that the skandhas, which constitute our mental and physical existence, are empty of any such nature or essence. However, it also states that this emptiness is the same as form (which connotes fullness), that this is an emptiness which is at the same time not different from the kind of reality which we normally ascribe to events, and that it is not a nihilistic emptiness that undermines our world, but a "positive" emptiness that defines it.

The inability to experience emptiness (Sunyata), considered as the true nature of reality, would represent a sort of primordial ignorance of the human being (avidya). When this happens, it is called *nirvana* (the awakening) in Buddhism. This concept is a central part of all the Buddhist psychology, so much so that the teachings of Buddhism on the nature of reality develop in order to help understand this vacuity. Mark Medweth (2007) explains this notion of emptiness in Buddhism: "Emptiness has been a term used to describe many psychological states in the West, including the confusing numbness of the psychotic, incomplete feelings of the personality disorders, identity diffusion and existential meaninglessness (Epstein, 1989). Buddhists, however, refer to emptiness as the ultimate reality. Emptiness assumes a defining role in the notion of 'self'; it is the experience of emptiness that destroys the idea of a continuous, independent individual nature. Unlike many Western misconceptions, emptiness is not an end in itself nor is emptiness considered real in a concrete sense but merely a specific negative of inherent existence (Epstein, 1988). While the ordinary consciousness perceives things as permanent and independent, Buddhists would counter that perceived phenomena are interdependent and thus empty of permanence and without an identity based on their own assumed nature (Komito, 1984). In relation to the sense-of-self, in Buddhism, emptiness does not imply (as Westerners have often interpreted) the abandonment or annihilation of the ego, 'self,' or 'I' but simply a recognition that this 'self' actually never existed at all (Epstein, 1989). Buddhism is not an escape from the world but simply a refusal to extend or exaggerate the importance of conventional reality. In so doing, the mind becomes empty of struggle, allowing us to see things as they are in an ultimate sense. Thus, in Buddhist psychology, the empty quality of the mind is regarded as the true nature of a person." Therefore, a translation of this mental and experiential state in Western terms is what we called "*mindemptiness*".

The Feeling of Emptiness as an Indicator of Psychopathology

There are many psychological disorders in which the feeling of emptiness generally presents itself as a transitory symptom (e.g., eating disorders, obsessive compulsive disorders, PTSD, schizophrenia) or as a rather stable phenomenological condition (personality disorders). Describing all these disorders is beyond the scope of this chapter, so we will limit the following discussion to pathologies where the feeling of emptiness often appears to be a central and recurrent experience of the pathology.

Personality Disorders and Emptiness

All clinicians who have worked with personality disorders are familiar with the relationship between this type of disorder and the experience, often reported by patients during sessions, of the feeling of emptiness. The descriptions, the hypothesized causes, and the consequences of experiencing these sensations vary greatly even within the different disorders in Axis II (DSM-IV, 1994). We will now try to discuss what "emptiness" means when we come across a patient with a specific personality disorder.

Borderline Personality Disorder
The main characteristics of BPD, as reported in the DSM-IV (APA, 2000), are a pervasive instability condition of interpersonal relations, self-esteem, and mood and a marked impulsiveness, with onset in early adult age and occurring in several contexts. Among all the diagnostic criteria of the disorder,

criterion 7 specifies, "These individuals can be affected by chronic feelings of emptiness. They are easily bored, they are continuously searching for something to do." This state, as well as anger, has been a specific characteristic of this disorder since its first formalized empirical descriptions (Fiore & Semerari, 2003). Kernberg (1975), in his descriptive analysis, considers it a minor criterion. Other important authors like Gunderson and Singer (1975) or Spitzer (1975) consider this diagnostic criterion a discriminating feature of this disorder.

As previously pointed out, several authors in the field of cognitive-behavioral therapy think that the experience of emptiness in BPD can be a sort of dysfunctional avoidance strategy in situations of clear subjective suffering and associated with a major risk of abuse or injuries to self and others (Beck, Freeman et al., 1990; Linehan, 1993; Young, 1987). According to Fiore and Semerari (2003), the perception, in this type of patient, of the "unworthy self" and the "vulnerable self" can expose them to intolerable pressure. At times, patients succeed in escaping this pressure, detaching themselves from everybody and everything and entering into a state of numbness. This is the condition where frequent suicide attempts and self-injuries occur more frequently, representing a state of complete detachment from the world or a way to evoke such detachment. Other times, according to these authors, the emptiness can be perceived as "a painful sense of lack of purpose." In these cases, patients tend to react by raising their level of arousal, for example, seeking promiscuous sexual relationships, dangerous acting out, and alcohol or substance abuse to the point of no return or bulimic crises.

From a psychodynamic perspective, Pazzagli and Monti (2000) for research purposes consider that two of the criteria listed in the DSM-IV for BPD diagnosis, chronic feelings of emptiness and efforts to avoid abandonment, can be appropriately grouped together in the concepts of "solitude and emptiness." According to the authors, the borderline person functions via osmosis: He is empty but, at the same time, intolerant of a solitude in which he keeps looking for objects to fill this inner sense of emptiness. The solitude of the BPD patient is actually an intolerance of true solitude, the solitude of being able to be alone. It is a solitude dominated by emptiness: a void in the outside world, made up of inadequate objects, sporadic, stormy, and superficial relationships prone to sudden break-ups, and a void in the inner world, always subject to the threat of rupturing and the loss of limits.

In a research study conducted by Rogers, Widiger, and Krupp (1995) aimed at identifying the qualitative differences of depression diagnosed in patients with BPD and others, the most frequent aspects associated with depression were found to be self-condemnation, emptiness, abandonment fears, self-destructiveness, and hopelessness. The authors conclude that the depression associated with borderline pathology is unique in certain aspects. The implications of the study outline the importance of considering the phenomenological aspects of depression, among which is the experience of emptiness, in the BPD. Leichsenring (2004) reports the following in another study: "Clinical observations suggest that depressive experiences in patients with borderline personality disorder have a specific quality. These experiences are characterized by emptiness and anger ('angry depression')." In this study, this observation was tested empirically. Westen et al. (1992) found an interpersonally focused "borderline depression" that was phenomenologically characterized by emptiness, loneliness, despair, and an unstable negative affectivity. The quality of the depression may also have consequences for pharmacotherapy (Westen et al., 1992, p. 391). The qualitative experience of depression (e.g., emptiness or anger) may influence a patient's reaction to drugs more strongly than the diagnosis (depression).

Narcissistic Personality Disorder

The essential characteristic of NPD is a pervasive picture of grandiosity, necessity of admiration, and lack of empathy, with onset in early adult age and present in a variety of contexts (DSM-IV, APA, 2000). On the whole, we can say that the authors studying the disorder can be divided into those who describe some subtypes (Gabbard, 1989; Millon, 1999) and those who lean more to a Horowitz-type interpretation assuming that a subject experiences a set of multiple distinct mental states. These authors observe how the narcissists oscillate between states of grandiosity, emptiness, shame, anguished depression, and dysregulated affect with acting-out tendencies (Horowitz, 1989; Young & Flanagan, 1998; Dimaggio et al., 2002). A substantial agreement exists between the various authors: It is most probable that the narcissist experiences on the whole mental states described in the literature and that the diagnosed subtype is characterized by the most important and manifest of mental states. Dimaggio et al. (2002) have identified in their work four mental states: grandiosity, transition, frightening depression, and devitalized emptiness. In this state of devitalized emptiness, the emotional experience is completely shut down; not only are feelings of weakness and fragility "scotomized" (obscured, clouded), but also feelings overall are. Subjects feel cold, detached, distanced from others and from their own inner experience, and they perceive an almost unreal world; their body is annoyingly far away and they are anhedonic. The experience is not at all intensely unpleasant; for a long time narcissists dwell in this state where they are untouchable, not subject to self-esteem fluctuations and to the complex, annoying, and incomprehensible demands of others.

The fantasy of success and almightiness can fill up mental life even though these subjects lack the triumphant echoes overwhelming the state of grandiosity. The aims are mostly inactive. This state largely coincides with the clinical descriptions of Modell (1984), which describes patients as being closed up as if in a "cocoon." In the long run, this state becomes ego-dystonic: The subject perceives life as empty and boring, the emotional coldness touches him, and his need for relationships surfaces unconfessed (Dimaggio, Petrilli, Fiore, & Mancioppi, 2003).

The sense of emptiness as an important and distinctive experience in NPD has been indicated by a large number of authors. Forman (1975) made a summary of the characteristics that emerge from the descriptions of Kohut (1971). The most important are low self-esteem, a tendency to have hypochondriac episodes, and a feeling of emptiness or a deficiency of vital force. Millon (1996) gives us the following description of the narcissistic prototype at a biopsychological level in clinical settings: "the narcissistic personality presents a general indifference, unflappability, and fake tranquility...except when his narcissistic confidence is threatened, where brief demonstrations of anger, shame or feelings of emptiness appear." Millon identifies rationalization as a mechanism of defense in NPD; if the rationalization fails, these individuals often feel rejected and embarrassed, and experience feelings of emptiness. Kernberg (1975) explains how the experience of emptiness in narcissists is characterized by the addition of strong feelings of boredom and restlessness: "Patients with depressive personality and even schizoid patients, are able to empathize deeply with human feelings and experiences involving other people, and may feel painfully excluded from and yet able to empathize with love and emotion involving others. . .patients with narcissistic personalities, on the other hand, do not have that capacity for empathizing with human experience in depth. Their social life, which gives them opportunities to obtain confirmation in reality or fantasy of their needs to be admired, and offers them direct instinctual gratifications, may provide them with an immediate sense of meaningfulness, but this is temporary. When such gratifications are not forthcoming, their sense of emptiness, restlessness and boredom take over. Now their world becomes a prison from which only new excitement, admiration, or experiences implying control, triumph or incorporation of supplies, are an escape. Deep emotional reactions to art, the investment in value systems or in creativity beyond gratification of their narcissistic aims, is often unavailable and indeed strange to them" (1975, p. 218)

Schizoid Personality Disorder

The essential characteristics of schizoid personality disorder are a pervasive condition of detachment from social relations and a restricted range of emotional experiences and expressions in interpersonal contexts. The onset of this condition is in early adult age, and it is present in a variety of contexts (DSM-IV, APA, 2000).

Kernberg (1975), as previously indicated, thinks that the experience of emptiness varies in form, intensity, and etiology in relation to the type of personality disorder affecting the patient. Even in schizoid disorders, specific characteristics of emptiness are obviously present. According to the author, these individuals can experience the emptiness as an inborn quality that makes them different from others: "in contrast to others, they cannot feel anything and they may feel guilty because they do not have feelings of love, hatred, tenderness, longing or mourning which they observe and understand in other people, but feel they cannot count on to experience themselves" (1975, p. 215). For these schizoid patients, the experience of emptiness can be less painful than for the depressed because the contrast between the periods when they feel empty and those when they would like to have emotional relations with others is less violent. A feeling of inner fluctuation, of subjective unreality, and the appeasement derived from this same unreality make the vacuous experience more acceptable to schizoids, allowing them to fill in time with the awareness of external reality opposed to their subjective experience.

Depression and Emptiness

Many people who come to therapy complain about having a senseless life. Their words express the idea of deep and anguishing "emptiness" leading them to wish for death as a liberation from this state. These patients often suffer from depression, and what has been described is only the manifestation of one of the many emotional, cognitive, and physical symptoms marking the disease.

Maureta Reyes (2007) defines this existential emptiness as:

> the feeling of a lack of a sense in life, of tediousness, of not knowing the reason for living, leading to isolation and impoverishment of the relation with family and society [...] patients with this problem, usually experience moments of strong tension and anxiety attacks without a valid reason, they worry about everything, but nothing seriously, they have lost the motivation and interest for everything and this makes them think that living is the worst thing that can happen to them. When this situation is prolonged, becoming more intense, it can lead to suicide.

This type of experience, described as such, appears more frequently in certain periods of life, for example, during old age, retirement, or the course of a terminal illness, or in the so-called empty-nest syndrome when adult children abandon the family home. In the latter case, women, seeing their role as mothers ending – their children having little need for them and their husbands busy at work, spending little time with them – are more prone to feeling depressive symptoms and a sense of emptiness. Old age, though, is surely a period where this type of feeling of emptiness becomes more present. Faced with fears associated with becoming old, such as isolation, solitude, physical decline, no longer being desired, uselessness, the loss of every role in society or in the family, and illness, it is easy to imagine how the lack of one's own sense of life leads to experiencing emptiness.

The feeling of emptiness in depression is often associated with significant experiences of loss (see also Bowlby, 1980), above all in conjunction with a first depressive episode (see also Chapter 12). In some cases, the feeling of emptiness is connected not only to what is no longer there, but also to what will no longer be there in the future.

In the following case example, a 41-year-old depressed patient describes her deep sense of emptiness derived from the loss of her 15-year-old son who died tragically in a car accident:

I would never have thought that, from one day to another, life could change so violently and destructively. With N's death, I find myself having to reinvent everything, fighting against this harsh reality, with all its emotions and feelings. It is unthinkable that he is no longer here with me and that he has left this immense emptiness just in this moment: a life yet to start, come to a sudden end by such an unfair destiny.

The pain is so great that with its presence, it is actually physical every time I think of the things N. liked and loved to spend his time on, his determination and will to live. It's like suddenly opening a door without expecting to find someone there: an icy wave, a shock which rises up from my feet and leaves me momentarily incredulous that all this belongs to me. A great weakness is left behind and a loss of feeling pervades my arms and hands. I get a tingling which becomes all one with a pain in my stomach as if it were knotted. These are very hard moments that make me realize that I'll never have him near me again. This great emptiness that I perceive projects itself not so much in my past memories which are alive, but based on the fact that I will never experience some situations or share them with him. There is only emptiness when I think I'll never be able to listen to his secrets, there won't be any requests of advice, I won't be able to see him growing up, becoming a man. I won't be able to get excited about his first love, a disappointment, a defeat or a victory. There will only be the lack of a relationship based on participation, bonding, joining of forces that was just starting and I was really waiting for. Why has all this been denied me? Everything has become null and void when I think of all that has been left suspended: it's like an abnormal condition in my life that I don't know how long will last. It's as if, while I'm watching a TV programme, this suddenly changes and I'm left here waiting in vain for everything to go back to normal, to the previous programme.

In this patient, like in other individuals suffering from major depression, the deep and overwhelming feeling of emptiness was determined on the one hand by what was no longer in her life, but on the other hand by the loss of what there would not be in the future and that never more will be, that is, the ineluctable interruption of a plan, a *loss in the future*.

How Mindfulness Can Help to Deal with and Overcome the Feeling of Emptiness

There is nothing greater than anything else

Plutarco, Adversus Colotem

Mindfulness as an Anti-avoidance Strategy

If we hypothesize the feeling of emptiness as a sort of emotional avoidance of a phobic stimulus situation (negative emotion), it is then right to think that the treatment should include the exposure to the stimulus provoking fear in the absence of the feared consequences. During this exposure, the patient is asked to pay attention to the stimuli that he or she usually systematically avoids in a controlled way, showing him or her with the same stimuli (imaginatively or in vivo), thereby hampering avoidance so that the patient can experience the harmlessness of the stimulus.

It is assumed that exposure causes habituation to the stimulus or a process of extinction of the avoided reactions, favoring the emotional coping, that is, preparing the subject to face the emotions resulting from feared situations. Baer (2003) affirms that among the mechanisms explaining the clinical effectiveness of mindfulness, one of the most important is experimenting through exercises a form of "exposure" to various types of information (extereoceptive and interoceptive) that are usually avoided and/or suppressed. Kabat-Zinn (1982) used mindfulness on patients affected by chronic pain. The author has stated that guiding patients to develop a non-judgmental attitude with respect to their own feelings of pain, and helping them to curiously observe them without reacting impatiently or intolerantly, resulted in a significant reduction in suffering, not related to the sensory perception of pain but to their own emotional reactivity (aversion) toward the perceived feelings. This can be considered an extended exposure associated with an attitude of acceptance of physical pain. The result would be an increase in tolerance toward the suffering and a reduction in the reactive emotionality.

Linehan (1993) starts from the theoretical assumption that BPD emotional distress is mainly derived from secondary responses (e.g., deep shame, anxiety, anger, or guilt) to the primary emotions that often, instead, would be adaptive and context appropriate. A reduction in this secondary stress requires exposure to primary emotions in non-judgmental circumstances. In a similar context, awareness and non-judgmental attention toward one's own emotional responses can be considered a technical exposure. The basic concept is that exposure to intense or painful emotions, without associating negative consequences, will extinguish their ability to stimulate negative secondary affects. If a patient judges negative emotions as "bad" or "wrong," it is obvious that every time he or she experiences them, he or she will have feelings of guilt, anger, and/or anxiety. Adding these feelings to an already negative situation will only increase the patient's distress and will only make it more difficult to put up with the anguish. Mindfulness is the ability to ensure or the set of skills capable of ensuring that the patient enacts this form of perception, taking advantage of all the assumptions needed for it to be effective. During the practice of mindfulness, we can keep frequency and duration of the exposure under control. The exercises can be guided so that they will be clearly specified and last long enough. Intensity can also be managed by leading patients to set their non-judgmental attention and awareness on elements outside themselves and far from anxiety-producing stimuli: As they progress in the process, they bring themselves closer to their physical sensations, thoughts and, lastly, to their negative emotions. The validating environment, during mindfulness training, accepts any experience originating from practice, informing patients that accepting reality does not necessarily mean approving it.

Exposure is probably not the only active factor in the process of mindfulness clinical effectiveness that could refer to the experience of emptiness. The mechanisms implementing these effects are in our opinion closely related to the development and initiation of meta-cognitive processes regarding the aforementioned experience.

Detachment and Decentering

One of the more important processes in the state of mindfulness is detachment (*detached mindfulness*; Wells, 1997, 2000, 2006; see also Chapters 5 and 11). According to the author, this attitude would be characterized by meta-awareness (a form of objective conscience of thoughts), cognitive decentering (acquired consciousness that thoughts are just thoughts, not facts), attentive flexibility (self-regulation of attention including both *sustained attention* and *skills in switching*, and meta-attention; see also next paragraph and Chapter 11 of this volume), low levels of conceptual processing (low levels of inner dialogue), and a low level of coping behaviors aimed at the avoidance or reduction of the threat. This is the equivalent of affirming that the patient becomes aware of his or her feelings mainly due to the ability to observe them, implementing a decentering from them, and developing a better understanding of his or her own cognitive functioning.

Self-Regulation of Attention

Bishop et al. (2004) consider self-regulation of attention to be central among the main cognitive processes that lead to mindfulness (see also Chapters 5 and 11 of this volume). Wallance and Shapiro (2006) also say that there are two types of attentive ability: One deals with the ability to continuously support voluntary attention on a familiar object without forgetfulnesses or distractions; the other, called "meta-attention," refers to the ability to monitor the quality of the attention, quickly recognizing if he or she has yielded to sluggishness or excitement. The concept of self-regulation of attention would then include three sub-functions: the ability to shift attention from one content to another, the ability to stay focused on a single object, and the meta-attentive ability leading to recognizing the moments where the attention has shifted toward other mental objects. In the process of dynamics, the self-regulation of attention constantly interacts with two other factors: the unconditioned openness of behavior toward the tried experience (acceptance equanimity) and the continual consideration given to the functional objectives of the momentary task (intention). The self-regulation of attention becomes extremely useful in helping subjects to focus on the components of the experience of emptiness, overcoming the difficulties that are often present in deciphering their own emotional and cognitive state.

Acceptance

Acceptance, another basic component of the state of mindfulness, has an essential role in allowing the patient to stay in touch with his or her own experience of emptiness, thus allowing the exposure to painful stimuli, whichever they are. Acceptance allows the patient, in a state of psychological openness and willingness, and through a gentle curiosity to approach various sources of aversive stimulation that has till that moment caused the person behavioral patterns of escape, refusal, or avoidance. For Hayes (1994), acceptance is a position relative to which previously intrinsically problematic or painful events become an opportunity of personal growth and development. Donaldson (2003) and Wells (2002) consider it a meta-cognitive process operating at a higher level than that of immediate experience, a "meta" level implying the direct perception of thoughts, feelings, or intentions of purpose.

Accepting is receiving, welcoming the experience of the moment, staying fully in touch with one's own thoughts, emotions and physical feelings, without reacting to and developing a decentered ability to observe them. Acceptance gives us the possibility to see our experience in the moment as it really is. However, accepting does not actually mean appreciating what we accept. The experience of emptiness could for a certain period of time be admitted and accepted. This would give the patient the opportunity to observe the consequences of this contact without negatively labeling it through judgment.

In a state of acceptance, the person recognizes that some aspects of the experience cannot be changed while he succeeds in realizing the elements that can. The patient will, therefore, channel his or her energies toward these latter ones, trying to *respond*, where possible, through a thoughtful action, rather than *reacting* (with automatic and impulsive actions) to the distressing experience in order to reduce, and often cancel out, the aversive psychological component of the experience. All the signs that accompany the experience of emptiness are usually submitted to meta-evaluation (a meta-cognitive process) by the subject; that is, they are affected by a negative meaning considered highly disagreeable or unbearable, leading the individual to various attempts of suppression or avoidance. Unconditioned acceptance would be a different way to relate to the experience that would reduce cognitive avoidance, thereby eliminating one of the factors responsible for the suffering (Didonna, 2007).

Letting Go

Letting go is the ability directly connected to acceptance that can fail to be immediately experienced when the patient comes into contact with certain disagreeable thoughts or feelings. Kabat-Zinn (1990) states that in the practice of meditation, we deliberately put aside that part of the mind clinging to certain aspects of our experience and reject others. The non-attachment, the letting go, is a form of acceptance of the things as they are. This ability allows patients to give the same attention to all stimuli, regardless of his or her need to hold on to or distance him/herself from those aspects of the experience of emptiness that cause suffering, or "entrapping" them in a certain mental state.

Not Striving

Not striving is the attitude where the patient does not pursue any precise aim during the practice of mindfulness. There is nothing that he or she should or should not do. Nothing has to be reached. It is enough "to be" and to remain in the present, bringing his or her own attention to himself/herself. We need to ask patients not to want to attain any changes or expect to modify their own experience of emptiness. The only thing they are to do is to remain there and observe. The change, if it happens, will paradoxically be the result of not having sought it out.

Identifying the Precocious Signs of Emptiness

Another important mechanism of change of mindfulness for the experience of emptiness could be the precious aid given to the ability to identify the feelings, thoughts, or situations leading to the feeling of emptiness early. Mindfulness allows patients to gather these signs, which differ depending on each patient's own experience, from the onset, helping to identify the suitable moment in order to use appropriate coping strategies and not to remain "entrapped" in the emptiness that leads to having to resort to dysfunctional solutions. Baer (2003) suggests that mindfulness training may promote recognition of early signs of a problem, at a time when application of previously learned skills will be most likely to be effective in preventing the problem.

Clinical Application of Mindfulness to the Experience of Emptiness

Practical Issues

A mindfulness-based intervention with patients affected from a pathological "feeling of emptiness" should be carried out by an expert therapist in the practice of meditation. In addition, the therapist should have good clinical competence with respect to all the psychological problems of the patient toward which the intervention is directed. The therapist should be ready to effectively deal with the eventual intense reactions that could be activated during the sessions, including dissociative crises and intense states of anxiety or escape.

Many patients who feel emptiness have a long history in invalidating environments where their emotions, feelings, and needs have been denied recurrently, and the only remaining inner criteria is the one labeling their own inner experience of the moment as unreliable or dangerous. It is therefore useful and important to help the patient trust and believe what he or she is feeling, in his or her own cognitive, emotional, and sensory experience, learning to listen to herself/himself. Furthermore, a regular practice of mindfulness by the patient outside of the therapeutic setting is necessary. It is vital that he/she has the possibility to find a small amount of time to dedicate to meditative practice every day (even 10–15 minutes). This intervention could be integrated in a structured mindfulness-based program (e.g., MBSR, MBCT) or form a specific independent intervention that could be implemented in an individual or group setting.

The final goal of this training is to lead the patient to explore and confront his or her own emotions, mainly anxiety, which, as we have hypothesized above, appears to be strictly related to the emptiness experienced in certain types of disorders. As suggested by Trobe-Krishnananda (1996), the objective is to penetrate the fear in depth, but with awareness, compassion, and understanding, giving value to these feelings and creating an inner space to allow patients to feel, observe, and accept.

Venturing into this layer of vulnerability is not an easy task for the patient affected by feelings of pathological emptiness. As we have previously explained, these people are used to activating a set of avoidance strategies and mechanisms in order not to feel the suffering. This "shell" keeps psychological fear and pain away, even at the cost of developing alexithymia or turning psychological suffering into a physical one, sometimes putting the patient's life at risk.

In our opinion, approaching the emotional sphere should take place in a gradual way, with the utmost caution. The activation of emotions at a neurovegetative level is often undifferentiated and can be the same for different emotions. Any element of this activation can lead the patient back to a state of emptiness, given the strong evocative potential for emotions associated thereto. Every session, in such a structured intervention, should include a gradual increase in the level of difficulty, that is, taking the patient a little closer to the stimuli, situations, and feelings connected to emptiness. Everything has to take place in a completely acceptable and non-judgmental framework. In order to do this, we suggest starting the intervention by teaching patients to initially focus attention on exteroceptive stimuli, which are usually less anxiety inducing, doing exercises like mindful seeing or hearing, or mindful walking (see Appendix A). Only at a later stage, during the course of the program, are they conscientiously drawn closer to their inner feelings and, therefore, to the enteroceptive experiences; some exercises such as body scan or sitting meditation (see Appendix A) would be suitable for this purpose (Didonna, 2007, paper submitted for publication).

Once these abilities have been consolidated, for example, "letting go," not passing judgment on their own experience, or "trusting" their own perceptions (see also Chapter 11), patients should be in a position to be in contact with thoughts, feelings, and negative mindsets without enacting avoidance behaviors. Moreover, during the course of the treatment, patients have the opportunity to observe their own state of emptiness, to become aware of its components, and above all, to perceive how secondary emotions and the increase in emotional reactivity in those situations have decreased, reducing the level of suffering of this experience. The patient should no longer judge or blame himself/herself for feeling what he or she feels.

Staying in Touch with the Feeling of Emptiness

At a certain point in the therapeutic program, the patient should directly face the experience of emptiness. Specific exercises can be developed to help the patient to voluntarily enter into such a state. The fear of feeling pain can keep patients distanced from their own feelings. A particular atmosphere of acceptance, presenting them with a gentle invitation to get in touch with what they fear, is required. There must be no pressure or judgment. In order to recreate this state, it might be sufficient to ask patients to remember the last time they felt this way, or the time when the feeling was so strong that they did something particular in order not to feel it. Being "with themselves" in those moments was not a pleasant feeling.

These experiences can be explored with the guidance of the therapist, helping patients to focus their attention on certain aspects in order not to let themselves go, thereby avoiding passing judgment on themselves. The most important thing is to learn to recognize what is happening, intimately bonding with what was previously avoided. The instructions could invite the patient to focus their own attention on those aspects, for example, allowing them to remain inside their experience, preventing the activation of the escape behavior, or observing how the sense of threat is perceived, or simply examining when and which type of impulses occur during the session. This could help, in some cases, to identify even the nature of their own fear connected with the feeling of emptiness (abandonment, failure, violence, judgment, and the thought that the fear will never end) more easily recognized observing the contents of thoughts in this state.

It is natural for these patients to fear being overwhelmed by the feeling of emptiness they encounter. The idea of being in contact and remaining with the feeling is terrifying. For this reason, the method used needs to be well consolidated, offering a "safe base" made up of previously acquired experiences and abilities, which are needed to deal with stimuli with greater aversive potential. The approach has to happen gradually, with the maximum sensitivity and without haste, but with the knowledge that with mindfulness meditation, the individual needs to go through the feeling of emptiness if he or she wants to be free.

Some possible instructions that can be used in order to allow patients to better understand and stay in touch with the feeling of emptiness, in a mindful way, are the following (adapted from Trobe-Krishnananda, 1999):

1. Look over your childhood essential needs. Ask yourself: "Do I have a hole related to this need?"
2. Then focusing on this particular hole, ask yourself: "How does this hole affect the way I relate to myself?" and "How does this hole affect the way I relate to people and life?"
3. Staying with this hole, ask yourself: "How do I feel this hole inside?" and "Which sensations do I feel right now and where in the body?" Allow yourself to notice your feelings in this moment and realize how they are, however, different from you, they aren't you...breathe with them. Try to observe them, without judging them, carrying a sense of gentle curiosity toward that experience. You can approach or recede from these feelings, and finally try to let them go.
4. Explore your needs: "What thoughts and feelings arise when you consider your needs?" (e.g., "I am weak or needy if I want this" or "I don' t feel I have the right to want or need this"). Let's grant them the possibility and the necessary time to cross our mind ...; "We accept and are compassionate toward these thoughts, realizing that when they were formed, they certainly made sense and had a function even though we have now lost them...let's try to think how much they need us to exist, without us they don't have strength or meaning...let's allow ourselves to observe and understand them without judging ..."; "Let's give ourselves permission to immerse ourselves in our inner experience even though it hurts and causes pain, breathing together, crossing it and letting it envelop us in order to reemerge at a certain point...let's try to observe what happens, what changes...trusting our experience."

- We may also ask the patient to write down, if possible, what beliefs he or she holds inside about having or expressing these needs.
- And eventually may ask: "What were you taught as a child about having and expressing your needs?" (e.g., "It is selfish to have needs and wants" and "Men should not have needs and wants"). "Be kind and do not judge yourself and your own thoughts. There is nothing that you need to do or not do in this moment. Just stay with yourself and your breath now, moment by moment ...".

What Can the Instructor Do

- **Consider that sense of pathological emptiness is only the manifestation of a wider range of psychological difficulties of the patient**. According to Teasdale (2004), it is necessary to keep in mind the specificity of emotional disorders examined as well as some specific interventions likely to help the patient in the effort to modify the processes (apart from the contents) of his or her own modes of mind. Mindfulness must be used in an overall therapeutic strategy within a framework of clear understanding of the emotional problems of the patient.

- **Share with the patient a new conceptualization/formulation of his problem**, helping him or her to formulate an alternative vision of the feeling of emptiness through a cognitive-behavioral model of understanding the functioning of his or her problem. Some mindfulness-based training, like MBSR, MBCT, or ACT, use homework (ABC, self-monitoring form, diary, etc.) as a vehicle for explaining the various cognitive processes at the basis of the disorder and of their functioning modes when they occur.
- **Welcome the difficulties of the method reported by patients from the onset.** We need to use the difficulties from the beginning as an opportunity to teach new attitudes for facing the problems. Relating to the difficulties with curiosity and interest, trying to accept them rather than reject them, defines the bases for a mindfulness approach to thoughts and negative emotions, especially those deriving from experiences of emptiness.
- **Share one's own experience during the meditative practice, inviting patients to do the same.** Segal, Willians, and Teasdale (2002, p. 55) talk about the approach and attitude of the instructors observed in the MBSR mindfulness program: "the stance of the instructor was itself 'invitational'. In addition, there was always the assumption of 'continuity' between the experience of instructor and the participants (...)". The assumption was simple: Different minds work in a similar way, and there is no reason to discriminate between the mind of the person asking for help and of the person offering it.

    Conti and Semerari (2003) describe *sharing* in a therapeutic context as a set of explicit interventions where it is stressed that some aspects of the patient's experience are shared or shareable by the therapist himself/herself. Sharing interventions include elements of both validation and self-disclosure. With this technique, in fact, the therapist implicitly validates the patients' experience through the acceptance and recognition of the shared dimension and, in so doing, reveals one's own mental state. However, this does in no way imply that the patients should feel forced to report their own experience. It must be clear that it is a free choice that does not affect the practice. It is enough to be present and to listen in order to take part in this intervention.
- **Eliminate any type of judgment during the practice or the sharing, and invite patients to do the same.** Often, especially at the beginning, patients tend to judge the "success" of the practice sessions, the positive or negative changes, their own feelings at the time, or their mental contents. Following the examples and instructions of the leader, they initially learn not to pass judgment on the experience of others; as the practice slowly goes ahead, they will acquire the ability not to judge themselves and their own experience, which is much more complex.
- **Communicate clearly that meditating implies the unconditioned acceptance of anything arising moment by moment.** The first thing that we can suggest to a patient is to note and record (without judging himself/herself) during the early experiences with the practice of mindfulness the moments when he or she would tend to react (or actually reacts) to the disturbing experience, noticing the type of evaluations that lead to the non-acceptance and to the dysfunctional reactions as well.

- **Refrain from offering solutions or answers**. At any time during the individual or group intervention, patients are simply asked to become aware of their difficulties and remain in contact with them. The aim is to promote acceptance, "being" and not "doing", suggesting the detachment from a reactive way, aiming at getting results and answers to any problem.

- **Validate the patient's emptiness experience together with all the elements connected thereto**: Validation, according to Linehan (1993), is a therapeutic strategy consisting in giving value to the subjective experience of a patient. In particular, it is needed when the individual finds himself/herself in a *self-invalidating state*, a mental state where he or she negatively judges or tries to suppress any aspect of his or her own experience, considering it dishonorable, wrong, horrible, or unacceptable by others. In this condition, totally aimed at judging or denying, rather than at understanding one's own mental states, the patient is not in a position to reflect on it in a constructive way. The simple fact of succeeding in sharing one's own perceptions of the feelings of emptiness, being able to feel that they are accepted, not receiving any type of judgment while they are reported, and not feeling pressured to modify or find a solution to them validates the experience as of itself.

Possible Usefulness and Effects of the Intervention

Clinical observation suggests that a mindfulness-based intervention may help a patient deal with his/her experience of emptiness in many ways. This approach might make it possible to

- identify the prodromes or the early signs of emptiness before it starts, as well as at-risk situations;
- succeed in identifying the components of one's own "emptiness": thoughts, physical feelings, emotional states and impulses, acquiring awareness;
- neutralize the tendency to self-invalidate one's own experience, developing the ability to cross one's own inner state;
- become able to remain in that state without exasperating it by activating *secondary emotions* (guilt, shame, anger) or with an escalation of anxiety;
- accept being in contact with the experience of emptiness without enacting dysfunctional behavior in order to escape it, also thanks to the awareness of its transience;
- lower the intensity of suffering experienced in the feeling of emptiness and its frequency;
- succeed in sharing what patient feels with others and accept their support.

Summary and Future Directions

The feeling of emptiness may be one of the most difficult psychological phenomena to explain and describe, but it is also not an unusual symptom to find in both normal and pathological human experience. In this chapter, the authors have tried to illustrate the state of the art present in the literature with respect to the clinical problem of emptiness and show how the concept of emptiness is utilized in radically antithetical ways in Western psychology compared to its meaning in Eastern psychology.

The authors have proposed some hypotheses to explain the possible mechanisms of actions of mindfulness with regard to the clinical experience of emptiness. The potential clinical effectiveness of mindfulness with respect to feelings of emptiness should mostly be due to exposure to the different stimuli configuring the aversive experience, usually avoided or suppressed, most often dysfunctionally. Surely there are also other possible mechanisms of change in the potential clinical relevance of mindfulness on the feeling of emptiness. Different meta-cognitive processes are developed and strengthened during its use of mindfulness such as detachment or the self-regulation of attention. Becoming aware of what one really feels inside an experience of emptiness; identifying emotions, thoughts, and feelings related thereto; managing to observe everything by decentering; and reflecting on one's own cognitive functioning and on the consequences of the dysfunctional behavior actually mean improving the meta-cognitive functions implying controlling and regulating of one's own mental states.

Some treatment guidelines have been proposed on pathological emptiness, but it is important to stress that these interventions are never a substitute for an overall psychological therapy for the pathology that is at the root of the feeling of emptiness. Furthermore, we believe that this type of intervention must be carried out by therapists expert in the disorder presenting emptiness as a symptom and with a long and regular mindfulness practice. At the moment there are few studies that have investigated the phenomenological experience of emptiness and there are even fewer that have certified the effectiveness of the treatments carried out thereon.

Future research is needed to more thoroughly study this clinical phenomenon since it is common to numerous nosographic frames that are extremely different from one another. The importance of methodologically sound research in this area cannot be overstated as this could lead to a better understanding of the activating and maintenance mechanisms of the phenomenon, as well as how therapeutic intervention like mindfulness-based training, used for the pathology presenting these symptoms, modify and improve this challenging and disabling experience.

I am tired of being bedridden with the feeling that something must happen.

I don't understand what is happening to me. I have never been afraid of the dark: but maybe mine is not fear of the dark. I have exchanged day for night. At night I open the shutters and I always keep the light on...during the day I close everything in order to isolate myself from the thought that everyone is working or doing something. Lately I have started to go to bed dressed and putting the pillow on top of the blankets for thickness.

Maybe it is just a habit, I cannot look for a meaning in everything I do. In so doing, I miss out on so many things that could make me feel alive...Well, all these thoughts are partly a defense against those feelings of emptiness that otherwise I would experience. In other words, the truth is that inventing all these small manias and fears or choosing to live the depression is a more acceptable way of saying that you do not know what to do with yourself and your life.

Angela, a 21-year-old depressed patient

References

Aalmas, A. H. (1987). *The diamond heart series book 1*. Boston: Shambala Publications.

American Psychiatric Association (APA). (2000). *Diagnostic and statistical manual of mental disorders* (4th ed., Text Rev.). Washington, DC: Author.

Baer, R. A., (2003). Mindfulness training as a clinical intervention: a conceptual and empirical review. *Clinical Psychology: Science and Practice, 10*, 125-143.

Beck, A. T., Freeman, A. et al., (1990). *Cognitive therapy of personality disorder*. New York: Guilford.

Bishop, S. R., Lau, M., Shapiro, S., Carlson, L., Anderson, N. D., Carmody, J., et al., (2004). Mindfulness: A proposed operational definition. *Clinical Psychology: Science and Practice, 11*, 230-241.

Bowlby, J., (1980). *Loss*. New York: Basic Books

Conti, L., & e Semerari, A., (2003). *Linee generali di trattamento dei disturbi della personalità*, In G. Dimaggio & A. e Semerari (Eds.), *I disturbi di personalità. Modelli e trattamento*. Roma: Editori Laterza (GLF).

Didonna, F. (paper submitted). Mindfulness and its clinical applications for severe psychological problems: Conceptualization, rationale and hypothesized cognitive mechanisms of change. Paper submitted to: *International Journal of Cognitive Therapy*.

Dimaggio, G., Semerari, A., Falcone, M., Nicolò, G., Carcione, A., & Procacci, M. (2002). Metacognition, states of mind, cognitive biases and interpersonal cycles. Proposal for an integrated narcissism model. *Journal of Psychotherapy Integration, 12*(4), 421-451.

Dimaggio, G., Petrilli, D., Fiore, D., & e Mancioppi, S., (2003). *Il disturbo narcisistico di personalità: la malattia della grande vita*, In G. Dimaggio & A. e Semerari (Eds.), *I disturbi di personalità. Modelli e trattamento*. Roma: Editori Laterza (GLF).

Donaldson, E., (2003). Psychological Acceptance: Why every OH/HR practioner should know about it. *Occupational Health Review, 101*, 31-33.

DSM-IV, (1994). *Diagnostic and statistical manual of mental disorders*, (4th ed.). Washington, D.C: American Psychiatric Association.

Epstein, M., (1988). The deconstruction of the self: Ego and "egolessness" in Buddhist insight meditation. *The Journal of Transpersonal Psychology, 20*(1), 61-69.

Epstein, M., (1989). Forms of emptiness: Psychodynamic, meditative and clinical perspectives. *The Journal of Transpersonal Psychology, 21*(1), 61-71

Fiore, D., & e Semerari, A., (2003). *Il disturbo borderline di personalità: il modello*, In G. Dimaggio & A. e Semerari (Eds.), *I disturbi di personalità. Modelli e trattamento*. Roma: Editori Laterza (GLF)

Forman, M., (1975). *Narcissistic personality disorders and the oedipal fixations*. Annual of Psychoanalysis, 3, 65-92. New York: International Universities Press.

Frankl, V. E. (1963). (I. Lasch, Trans.) *Man's search for meaning: An introduction to logotherapy*. New York: Washington Square Press. (Earlier title, 1959: From Death-Camp to Existentialism. Originally published in 1946 as Ein Psycholog erlebt das Konzentrationslager).

Frankl, V. E. (1973). (R. and C. Winston, Trans.) *The doctor and the soul: From psychotherapy to logotherapy*. New York: Vintage Books. (Originally published in 1946 as Ärztliche Seelsorge.)

Frankl, V. E. (1975). *The unconscious god: Psychotherapy and theology*. New York: Simon and Schuster. (Originally published in 1948 as Der unbewusste Gott. Republished in 1997 as Man's Search for Ultimate Meaning.)

Gabbard, G. O. (1989). Two subtypes of narcissistic personality disorder. *Bulletin of Meninger clinic, 53*, 527-532

Gunderson, J. G., & e Singer, M. T., (1975). Defining borderline patients: an overview. *American Journal of Psychiatry, 132*, 1-9.

Hayes, S. C., (1994). *Content, context and the types of psychological acceptance.* In S. C. Hayes, N. S. Jacobson, V. M. Follette, & M. J. Dougher (Eds.), *Acceptance and change: Content and context in psychotherapy* (pp. 13-32), Reno NV: Context Press.

Hayes, S. C., Wilson, K. G., Gifford, E. V., Follette, V. M., & Strosahl, K., (1996). Experiential avoidance and behaviour disorder: A functional dimensional approach to diagnosis and treatment. *Journal of Consulting and Clinical Psychology, 64*, 1152-1168.

Hazell, C., (2003). *The experience of emptiness.* Bloomington, IN: 1stBooks.

Horowitz, M. J., (1989). Clinical phenomenology of narcissistic pathology. *Psychiatric Clinic of North America, 12*, 531-539.

Jacobson, E., (1964). *The self and the object world.* New York: International Universities Press.

Kabat-Zinn, J., (1982). An autpatient program in behavioural medicine for chronic patients based on the practice of mindfulness meditation: Theoretical considerations and preliminary results. *General Hospital Psychiatry, 4*, 33-47.

Kabat-Zinn, J., (1990). *Full catastrophe living: Using the wisdom of your body and mind to face stress, pain and illness.* New York: Dell publishing.

Kabat-Zinn, J. (2005). *Coming to our senses.* London: Piatkus Books Ltd.

Kernberg, O., (1975). *Borderline conditions and phatological narcissism.* New York: Jason Aronson.

Kohut, H., (1971). *The analysis of self.* New York: International Universities Press.

Kohut, H., (1977). *The restoration of the self.* New York: International Universities Press.

Komito, D. R., (1984). Tibetan Buddhism and psychotherapy: Further conversations with the Dalai Lama. *The Journal of Transpersonal Psychology, 16*(1), 1-24.

Laing, R. (1969). *The divided self.* New York: Pantheon.

Leichsenring, F. (2004). Quality of depressive experiences in borderline personality disorders: Differences between patients with borderline personality disorder and patients with higher levels of personality organization. *Bulletin of the Menninger Clinic, 68*(1), 9-22.

Linehan, M., (1993). *Cognitive-behavioral treatment of borderline personality disorder.* New York: The Guilford Press.

Maureta Reyes, M. (2007). In Vacio esistencial, un mal contemporaneo. Mejia, R. www.amapsi.org

May, R. (1950). *The meaning of anxiety.* New York: Simon and Schuster.

May, R. (1953). *Man's search for himself.* New York: Signet Norton.

Medweth, M. HYPERLINK "http://www.jefallbright.net/node/2901" *Becoming Nobody.* Department of Psychology. Simon Fraser University. Web site: http://www.purifymind.com/BecomingNobody.htm

Millon, T. (1996). *Disorders of personality. DSM-IV and beyond.*, New York: John Wiley & Sons.

Millon, T. (1999). *Personality-Guided therapy.* New York: John Wiley & Sons.

Modell, A. H., (1984). *Psychoanalysis in a new context.* New York: International University Press.

Pascal, B. (1965). *Pensees,* Paris: Armand Colin.

Pazzagli, A., & e Monti, M. R., (2000). Dysphoria and aloneness in borderline personality disorder. *Psychopathology, 33*(4), 220-226 July–August.

Rawson, P., (1991). *Sacred tibet.* London: Thames and Hudson.

Rogers, J. H., Widiger, T. A., & Krupp, A., (1995). Aspects of depression associated with borderline personality disorder. *American Journal of Psychiatry, 152*(2), 268-270 February.

Sanavio, E., (1991). *Psicoterapia Cognitiva e Comportamentale.* Roma: La Nuova Italia Scientifica.

Segal, Z. V., Williams, J. M., & y Teasdale, J. D., (2002). *Mindfulness-based cognitive therapy for depression. A new approach to preventing relapse.* New York: Guilford.

Spitzer, R. L., (1975). Crossing the border into borderline personality and borderline schizophrenia. The development criteria. *Archives of General Psychiatry, 36,* 17-24

Sunyata (2007). http://en.wikipedia.org/wiki/Shunyata

Teasdale, J. D., (2004) *Minfulness and the third wave of cognitive-behavioural therapies.* Keynote address presented at the 34th Annual Conference of the EABCT, Manchester, England.

Trobe-Krishnananda, T. (1996). *Face to face with fear.* Verlag: Koregaon Publications

Trobe-Krishnananda, T. (1999). *Stepping out of fear.* Verlag: Koregaon Publications.

Wallance, A. B., & e Shapiro, S. L., (2006) Mental balance and well-being: Building bridges between Buddhism and western psychology. *American Psychologist, 61,* 690-701.

Wells, A., (1997). *Cognitive therapy of anxiety disorders.* Chicester: Wiley.

Wells, A., (2000). *Emotional disorders and metacognition: Innovative cognitive therapy.* Chicester: Wiley.

Wells, A., (2002). Gad, metacognition and mindfulness: An information processing analysis. *Clinical Psychology: Science and Practice, 9,* 95-100.

Wells, A., (2006). Detached mindfulness in cognitive therapy: a metacognitive analysis and ten techniques. *Journal of Rational-Emotive and Cognitive-Behavior Therapy, 3,* 337-335.

Westen, D., Moses, M. J., Silk, K. R., Lohr, N. E., Cohen, R., & Segal, H. (1992). Quality of depressive experiences in borderline personality disorder and major depression: When depression is not just depression. *Journal of Personality Disorders, 6,* 382-393.

Winnicott, D. W., (1965a). *The maturaional processes and the facilitating environment.* New York: IUP.

Winnicott, D. W., (1965b). *The family and individual development.,* London: Tavistock Publications.

Young, J. E., (1987). Schema-focused cognitive therapy for personality disorders. *International cognitive therapy newsletter, 4, 5,* 13-14

Young, J. E., & Flanagan, C. (1998). Schema-focused therapy for Narcissistic Patients, In E. F. Ronninggstam (Ed.), *Disorders of narcissism: Diagnostic, clinical, and empirical implications.* New York: American Psychiatric Press.

Young, J. E., Klosko, J. S., & Weishaar, M., (2003). *Schema therapy: A practitioner's guide.* New York: Guilford Publications.

9

Assessment of Mindfulness

Ruth A. Baer, Erin Walsh, and Emily L. B. Lykins

Mindfulness can be cultivated by paying attention in a specific way, that is, in the present moment, and as non-reactively, non-judgmentally and openheartedly as possible.

Kabat-Zinn (2005, p. 108)

Mindfulness-based interventions have been developed for a wide range of problems, disorders, and populations and are increasingly available in a variety of settings. Empirically supported interventions that are based on or incorporate mindfulness training include acceptance and commitment therapy (ACT; Hayes, Strosahl, & Wilson, 1999), dialectical behavior therapy (DBT; Linehan, 1993), mindfulness-based cognitive therapy (MBCT; Segal, Williams, & Teasdale, 2002), and mindfulness-based stress reduction (MBSR; Kabat-Zinn, 1982, 1990). Variations on these approaches, including integration of mindfulness training into individual psychotherapy from diverse perspectives, also have been described (Germer, Siegel, & Fulton, 2005). As the empirical evidence for the efficacy of these interventions continues to grow, the importance of investigating the mechanisms or processes by which they lead to beneficial outcomes is increasingly recognized (Bishop et al., 2004; Shapiro, Carlson, Astin, & Freedman, 2006). Addressing this question requires psychometrically sound measures of mindfulness (Baer, Smith, & Allen, 2004; Brown & Ryan, 2004; Dimidjian & Linehan, 2003). Without such measures it is impossible to determine whether the practice of mindfulness leads to increased levels of mindfulness and whether these changes are responsible for the improvements in psychological functioning that are often observed.

The development of tools for assessing mindfulness requires clarity about its definition. According to Clark and Watson (1995), a sound measure must be based on "a precise and detailed conception of the target construct" (p. 310). Although the current literature includes many descriptions of mindfulness, several authors have noted that mindfulness is a subtle and somewhat elusive construct and that defining it in concrete terms is difficult (Block-Lerner, Salters-Pednault, & Tull, 2005; Brown & Ryan, 2004). Compounding the difficulty is the necessity of understanding closely related constructs such as acceptance and decentering. These are sometimes described as components or elements of mindfulness (Block-Lerner et al., 2005; Dimidjian & Linehan, 2003), whereas others argue that they are better understood as outcomes of practicing mindfulness (Bishop et al., 2004) or as skills that aid in fostering mindfulness (Brown, Ryan, & Creswell, in press). This chapter will provide an overview of current definitions and descriptions of mindfulness, instruments that have been developed to measure it, and findings based on the use of these instruments. Assessment of acceptance and decentering will be addressed, and future directions for research on the assessment of mindfulness will be discussed.

Definitions and Descriptions of Mindfulness

Perhaps the most commonly cited definition is provided by Kabat-Zinn (1994), who describes mindfulness as "paying attention in a particular way: on purpose, in the present moment, and nonjudgmentally." Several other definitions are similar. For example, Marlatt and Kristeller (1999) describe mindfulness as "bringing one's complete attention to the present experience on a moment-to-moment basis" (p. 68), and Brown and Ryan (2003) define it as "the state of being attentive to and aware of what is taking place in the present" (p. 822). Other descriptions are somewhat more detailed. According to Bishop et al. (2004), mindfulness is "a process of regulating attention in order to bring a quality of non-elaborative awareness to current experience and a quality of relating to one's experience within an orientation of curiosity, experiential openness, and acceptance" (p. 234). Segal et al. (2002) note that "...in mindfulness practice, the focus of a person's attention is opened to admit whatever enters experience, while at the same time, a stance of kindly curiosity allows the person to investigate whatever appears, without falling prey to automatic judgments or reactivity" (p. 322–323). These authors also note that mindfulness can be contrasted with behaving mechanically, without awareness of one's actions, in a manner often called *automatic pilot*. Kabat-Zinn (2003) states that "mindfulness includes an affectionate, compassionate quality within the attending, a sense of openhearted friendly presence and interest" (p. 145). Similarly, Marlatt & Kristeller (1999) suggest that mindfulness involves observing one's experiences "with an attitude of acceptance and loving kindness" (p. 70).

Commonly used instructions for teaching mindfulness are consistent with these definitions and descriptions. Participants in mindfulness training are often encouraged to focus their attention on particular types of stimuli that are observable in the present moment, such as sounds that can be heard in the environment or the movements and sensations of breathing. If thoughts, emotional states, urges, or other experiences arise, participants are encouraged to observe them closely. Brief, covert labeling of observed experiences, using short words or phrases, is often encouraged. For example, participants might silently say "sadness," "thinking," "aching," "urge," or "sound" as they observe internal or external phenomena. Participants are typically asked to bring a stance of acceptance, willingness, allowing, openness, curiosity, kindness, and friendliness to all observed experiences, and to refrain from efforts to evaluate, judge, change, or terminate them, even if they are unpleasant. In DBT (Linehan, 1993), mindfulness has been operationalized as a set of interrelated skills; three related to what one does while practicing mindfulness, and three related to how one does it. The "what" skills include *observing* (noticing or attending to) current experience, *describing* (noting or labeling observed experiences with words), and *participating* (focusing full attention on the current activity). The "how" skills include being *nonjudgmental* (accepting, allowing, or refraining from evaluation), being *one-mindful* (with undivided attention), and being *effective* (using skillful means).

This collection of definitions, descriptions, and instructions for teaching mindfulness suggests that mindfulness may be usefully conceptualized as a multifaceted construct that includes attending to (observing or noticing) present moment experiences, labeling them with words, and acting with awareness or avoiding automatic pilot. Particular qualities of attention also appear to be important. Terms used to capture these qualities include acceptance, openness, allowing, nonjudging, willingness, kindness, and curiosity.

Instruments for Measuring Mindfulness

Several measures of mindfulness have been developed in recent years. Most use self-report methods to assess a general tendency to be mindful in daily life and are based on one or more of the descriptions of mindfulness just summarized. These instruments have shown promising psychometric characteristics and have contributed to increased understanding of the nature of mindfulness, its relationships with other psychological constructs, and the changes that occur as individuals practice mindfulness meditation. Recently developed mindfulness questionnaires are described in the following paragraphs.

Freiburg Mindfulness Inventory

The Freiburg mindfulness inventory (FMI; Buchheld, Grossman, & Walach, 2001) is a 30-item instrument designed to assess nonjudgmental present-moment observation and openness to negative experience in experienced meditators. Items include, "I watch my feelings without becoming lost in them" and "I am open to experience in the present moment." The FMI was developed with participants in intensive mindfulness meditation retreats and has high internal consistency in this sample (alpha = 0.93). From pre- to post-retreat, mean scores increased by approximately one standard deviation. Although factor analyses revealed that the FMI captures several components of mindfulness, factor structure was not stable across administrations, and the authors recommend a unidimensional interpretation.

In a subsequent study, Walach, Buchheld, Buttenmüller, Kleinknecht, and Schmidt (2006) developed a 14-item form of the FMI for use in nonmeditating samples. This version demonstrated adequate to good internal consistency in several samples and showed differences in the expected direction between meditators, nonmeditators, and clinical groups. Higher scores on both versions of the FMI were related to increased private self-awareness and self-knowledge, decreased dissociation, and lower psychological distress in meditating and general adult samples. The authors recommend using the longer form in samples familiar with mindfulness or Buddhist concepts and the short form in populations without such experience.

In a sample of undergraduate students, Leigh, Bowen, and Marlatt (2005) found that the FMI was internally consistent and modestly related to measures of spirituality. Surprisingly, they also found that higher scores on the FMI were associated with increased alcohol and tobacco use, possibly because of an increased tendency to notice bodily sensations in those who use these substances.

Mindful Attention Awareness Scale

The mindful attention awareness scale (MAAS; Brown & Ryan, 2003) is a 15-item measure assessing the general tendency to be attentive to and aware of present-moment experiences in everyday life. Items describe being on automatic pilot, preoccupied, and inattentive and are reverse scored, so that higher scores represent higher levels of mindfulness. Factor analyses revealed a single-factor structure. Example items include, "I find it difficult to stay focused on what's happening in the present" and "I break or spill things because of carelessness, not paying attention, or thinking of something else." In undergraduate and general adult samples the MAAS has demonstrated good internal consistencies (alphas = 0.82 and 0.87, respectively). Evidence for convergent and discriminant validity includes positive correlations with openness to experience, emotional intelligence, and well-being; negative correlations with rumination and social anxiety; and a nonsignificant relationship to self-monitoring. Additionally, Zen Buddhist practitioners scored significantly higher on the MAAS than matched community controls.

In recent investigations, the single-factor structure has been further validated in a population of cancer outpatients (Carlson & Brown, 2005), as well as in a large undergraduate student sample (MacKillop & Anderson, 2007). However, MacKillop and Anderson (2007) reported that the MAAS did not discriminate between novice meditators and individuals with no prior meditation experience. Higher scores on the MAAS have been associated with increases in psychological mindedness (Beitel, Ferrer, & Cecero, 2005), decreases in mood disturbance and symptoms of stress in cancer outpatients (Carlson & Brown, 2005), and decreases in the tendency to experience lapses of attention (Cheyne, Carriere, & Smilek, 2006).

Kentucky Inventory of Mindfulness Skills

The Kentucky inventory of mindfulness skills (KIMS; Baer et al., 2004) is based largely on the DBT conceptualization of mindfulness skills and includes 39 items measuring four facets of mindfulness: observing, describing, acting with awareness, and nonjudgmental acceptance. The KIMS assesses the general tendency to be mindful in daily life and does not require experience with mediation. Items include, "I notice when my moods begin to change" (observe); "I'm good at finding words to describe my feelings" (describe); "When I do things, my mind wanders and I am easily distracted" (act with awareness); and "I tell myself I shouldn't be feeling the way I'm feeling" (acceptance). The authors reported internal consistencies ranging from 0.76 to 0.91 for the four subscales. The four-factor structure was supported by exploratory and confirmatory factory analyses. Evidence for convergent and discriminant validity was provided by correlations in the expected directions with constructs including openness to experience, emotional intelligence, alexithymia, and experiential avoidance.

Cognitive and Affective Mindfulness Scale

The cognitive and affective mindfulness scale-Revised (CAMS-R; Feldman, Hayes, Kumar, Greeson, & Laurenceau, 2007) is a 12-item measure of attention, present focus, awareness, and acceptance of thoughts and feelings in general daily experience. These components are not measured separately but are combined to provide a total mindfulness score. Items include, "I try to notice my thoughts without judging them," "It is easy for me to concentrate on what I am doing," and "I am able to accept the thoughts and feelings I have." Internal consistency for the 12-item scale ranged from 0.74 to 0.77, and confirmatory factor analyses supported the proposed model. The CAMS-R was positively correlated with the FMI and MAAS, well-being, adaptive emotion regulation, cognitive flexibility, problem analysis, and plan rehearsal and negatively correlated with symptoms of distress, worry, rumination, brooding, thought suppression, experiential avoidance, and stagnant deliberation.

Southampton Mindfulness Questionnaire

The Southampton mindfulness questionnaire (SMQ; Chadwick, Hember, Mead, Lilley, & Dagnan, 2005) is a 16-item inventory assessing the degree to which individuals mindfully respond to distressing thoughts and images. Although the SMQ is designed to capture four aspects of mindfulness (mindful observation, non-aversion, nonjudgment, and letting go), the authors recommend use of a single total score. Each item begins with, "Usually when I have distressing thoughts or images" and is followed by a statement, such as, "I am able to just notice them without reacting" and "they take over my mind for quite a while afterwards". The SMQ demonstrated good internal consistency (alpha = 0.89), was significantly correlated with the MAAS ($r = 0.57$), and differentiated between meditating and non-meditating individuals in expected directions. Scores on this instrument were positively correlated with pleasant mood ratings and significantly increased following participation in an MBSR course.

Philadelphia Mindfulness Scale

This 20-item measure (Cardaciotto, Herbert, Forman, Moitra, & Farrow, 2007) includes two factors that are scored separately: awareness and acceptance. Awareness refers to the ongoing monitoring of internal and external experience (e.g., "I'm aware of thoughts I'm having when my mood changes"). Acceptance refers to an attitude of nonjudging or openness about experience, and refraining from attempts to avoid or escape it (e.g., "I try to distract myself when I feel unpleasant emotions"). In several clinical and nonclinical samples, good internal consistency was demonstrated, most correlations with other constructs were significant in the expected directions, and clinical samples generally had lower scores than nonclinical samples.

Five-Facet Mindfulness Questionnaire

Using large student samples, Baer, Smith, Hopkins, Krietemeyer, and Toney (2006) studied five of the mindfulness questionnaires described earlier (all but the Philadelphia Mindfulness Scale [PHLMS], which was not available) and found them to be internally consistent, significantly correlated with each other, and correlated in expected directions with several other variables predicted to be related to mindfulness, including openness to experience, emotional intelligence, thought suppression, alexithymia, and experiential avoidance. However, differences in their content and relationships with other constructs suggested that these questionnaires might be measuring somewhat different elements or facets of mindfulness. The MAAS appeared to emphasize an aspect of mindfulness that is inversely associated with dissociation and absent mindedness, whereas the SMQ was most strongly associated (negatively) with experiential avoidance and difficulties in emotion regulation. To examine facets of mindfulness systematically, Baer et al. (2006) combined responses to all five of these questionnaires into a single data set and conducted exploratory factor analysis to examine underlying dimensions. This analysis allowed items from different instruments to combine to form factors, yielding an empirical integration of these independent attempts to operationalize mindfulness. Findings suggested a five-factor solution. *Observing* includes noticing or attending to internal and external stimuli, such as sensations, emotions, cognitions, smells, sounds, and sights. *Describing* refers to labeling observed experiences with words. *Acting with awareness* includes attending to the activities of the moment and can be contrasted with automatic pilot, or behaving mechanically, without awareness of one's actions. *Nonjudging of inner experience* refers to taking a nonevaluative stance toward cognitions and emotions. *Nonreactivity to inner experience* is the tendency to allow thoughts and feelings to come and go, without getting carried away by them or caught up in them. The five-facet mindfulness questionnaire (FFMQ), which contains 39 items, was created by selecting the seven or eight items with the highest loadings on their respective factors and low loadings on all other factors. The five-facet scales demonstrated adequate to excellent internal consistency (alphas ranging from 0.75 to 0.91), and relationships between the facet scales and other variables were consistent with predictions in most cases (Baer et al., 2006).

Recent findings with the FFMQ support the utility of measuring facets of mindfulness separately and help to clarify the skills that are cultivated by the practice of mindfulness meditation. Baer et al. (2007) administered the FFMQ in a sample of experienced meditators and several nonmeditating comparison samples. Scores on four of the facets (all but *acting with awareness*) were significantly correlated with extent of meditation experience and meditators scored higher than nonmeditators. In the group of experienced meditators, all facets were significantly negatively correlated with psychological symptoms and positively correlated with psychological well-being. Several of the facets demonstrated incremental validity over the others in predicting well-being and contributed to the significant mediation of the relationship between meditation experience and well-being. These results support the common assumption that meditation cultivates mindfulness skills, which in turn facilitate psychological health. Findings also suggest that consideration of multiple facets of mindfulness is helpful in understanding the relationship between mindfulness and psychological adjustment.

In samples of experienced meditators and demographically similar nonmeditators, Lykins and Baer (in press) examined relationships between meditation experience and several proposed mechanisms by which mindfulness training may exert beneficial outcomes. These mechanisms include reduced rumination (Segal et al., 2002), desensitization through exposure to negative emotion (Linehan, 1993), and improved ability to behave constructively when experiencing unpleasant emotions or sensations (Kabat-Zinn, 1982).

Lykins and Baer (in press) showed that the acting with awareness, *nonjudging* and *nonreactivity* facets of mindfulness completely mediated the relationships between meditation experience and rumination, fear of emotion, and ability to engage in goal-directed behavior when upset. Two of these variables also were shown to partially mediate relationships between mindfulness and psychological well-being. Overall, results support the idea that increased mindfulness improves psychological functioning by reducing rumination and fear of emotion.

In another recent study, Carmody and Baer (2008) administered the FFMQ to 174 individuals with stress, anxiety, and illness-related complaints who completed MBSR, an 8-week group program based on the intensive practice of several forms of mindfulness meditation (see other chapters in this volume for more detail). Scores on all five facets of mindfulness increased significantly from pre- to post-treatment. For four of the facets (all but *describing*) increases were related to the amount of home practice of meditation exercises that participants completed during the program. Increases in mindfulness also were shown to mediate the relationship between extent of home practice and improvement in psychological symptoms and stress levels. Weaker findings for the *describing* facet may not be surprising in this case, as MBSR places very little emphasis on verbal labeling of experiences. In contrast, DBT and ACT include exercises for the labeling of emotions, cognitions, and sensations. Study of the *describing* facet with these interventions is warranted.

Overall, preliminary evidence from studies of the FFMQ supports two general conclusions. First, the five subscales of the FFMQ appear to measure skills that are cultivated by the practice of mindfulness, both in long-term meditators and in relative novices. Second, increases in levels of mindfulness appear to be related to changes in other aspects of psychological functioning that promote well-being.

Assessment of Mindfulness as a State

The instruments discussed in previous sections measure a trait-like general tendency to be mindful in daily life. In contrast, Bishop et al. (2004) view mindfulness as a state-like quality that occurs when attention is intentionally directed to sensations, thoughts, and emotions, with an attitude of curiosity, openness, and acceptance. The Toronto Mindfulness Scale (TMS; Lau et al., 2006) assesses attainment of a mindful state during an immediately preceding meditation session. Participants first practice a meditation exercise for about 15 minutes and then rate the extent to which they were aware and accepting of their experiences during the exercise. This instrument has two factors. The *curiosity* factor reflects interest and curiosity about inner experiences and includes items such as "I was curious to see what my mind was up to from moment to moment." The *decentering* factor emphasizes awareness of experiences without identifying with them or being carried away by them, and includes items such as "I experienced myself as separate from my changing thoughts and feelings." Findings showed good internal consistency for each factor and significant correlations with other measures of self-awareness. Scores increased with participation in MBSR, and decentering scores predicted reductions in psychological symptoms and stress levels. This measure has good psychometric properties and is likely to be useful in the study of mindfulness meditation. However, as the authors note, scores reflect the experience of mindfulness during a specific meditation session and may not be related to the tendency to be mindful in ordinary daily life. The authors also recommend multiple assessments, because the extent to which a mindful state was attained during a single meditation session may not reflect participants' general tendency to be mindful while meditating, due to factors such as fatigue or stress on a particular occasion.

Mindfulness as a state has also been assessed using experience sampling in participants asked to carry pagers for a few weeks (Brown & Ryan, 2003). When paged at quasi-random intervals during each day, participants immediately responded to a subset of MAAS items asking about the extent to which they were attending to their activity of the moment or were behaving automatically. Results showed that momentary-state mindfulness was significantly correlated with baseline levels of trait mindfulness as assessed by the original form of the MAAS. State mindfulness also predicted higher levels of positive emotion and autonomy and lower levels of negative emotion while engaged in the activity of the moment.

Assessment of Closely Related Constructs

Acceptance

Acceptance has been most comprehensively described in writings on ACT (Hayes et al., 1999; Hayes & Strosahl, 2004) and usually refers to willingness to experience a wide range of internal experiences (such as bodily sensations, cognitions, and emotional states) without attempting to avoid, escape, or terminate them, even if they are unpleasant or unwanted. Acceptance is generally an issue when attempts to avoid or escape these experiences are harmful or counterproductive. This is often true in situations that involve competing contingencies or approach-avoidance conflicts (Dougher, 1994). For example, initiating conversation with a stranger may offer both reinforcing and punishing consequences (social interaction and development of a relationship versus shame or humiliation if rejected) and may therefore elicit anxiety. Avoiding the anxiety by refraining from conversation will be counterproductive if it perpetuates loneliness. Attempts to eliminate the anxiety with alcohol or drugs may be harmful if these substances contribute to socially inappropriate or ineffective behavior or maladaptive health consequences. Thus, acceptance of feelings of anxiety (allowing them to be present while continuing with goal-consistent behavior) may be more adaptive.

The Acceptance and Action Questionnaire (AAQ; Hayes, Strosahl, et al., 2004) is a nine-item self-report instrument whose items describe elements of experiential avoidance, including negative evaluation of and attempts to control or avoid unpleasant internal stimuli, and inability to take constructive action while experiencing these stimuli. If reverse scored, it serves as a measure of acceptance. Its internal consistency is adequate (alpha = 0.70), and it is correlated with many forms of psychopathology. A revised version by Bond and Bunce (2003) includes 16 items and has two subscales: Willingness and

Action. The first measures willingness to experience negative thoughts and feelings and includes items such as "I try hard to avoid feeling depressed or anxious." The Action subscale measures ability to behave consistently with goals and values even while having unpleasant thoughts and feelings and includes items such as "When I feel depressed or anxious, I am unable to take care of my responsibilities." A revised version of the AAQ is currently in development.

Measures based on the AAQ but modified for specific populations have also been developed. For example, the Chronic Pain Acceptance Questionnaire (CPAQ; McCracken, 1998; McCracken & Eccleston, 2003; McCracken, Vowles & Eccleston, 2004) measures recognition that pain may not change, ability to refrain from fruitless efforts to avoid or control pain, and engaging in valued life activities despite the presence of pain. Items include, "I am getting on with the business of living no matter what my pain level is." Internal consistency is good (alpha = 0.85). Scores are correlated positively with daily activity level and improved work status and negatively with depression, anxiety, and disability, even when pain intensity is controlled. Also derived from the AAQ, the Acceptance and Action Diabetes Questionnaire (AADQ; Gregg, Callaghan, Hayes, & Glenn-Lawson, 2007) assesses acceptance of diabetes-related thoughts and feelings and ability to engage in valued actions while having these experiences (e.g., "I do not take care of my diabetes because it reminds me that I have diabetes"). Internal consistency is high (alpha = 0.94), and scores improved significantly in a group of diabetics who participated in an ACT workshop, but not for those in a control condition. Other measures currently in development include the AAQ-Weight (Lillis & Hayes, 2008) for weight loss and weight maintenance contexts, and the Avoidance and Fusion Questionnaire for Youth (AFQ-Y; Greco, Ball, Dew, Lambert, & Baer, 2008), a measure for children and adolescents.

Decentering

Decentering is defined as the ability to observe one's thoughts and feelings as temporary events in the mind, rather than reflections of the self that are necessarily true (Fresco, Moore, et al., 2007). It includes taking a present-focused, nonjudgmental stance toward thoughts and feelings and accepting them as they are (Fresco, Segal, Buis, & Kennedy, 2007). Decentering (also called distancing) has long been recognized as an important process in cognitive therapy for depression (Beck, Rush, Shaw, & Emery, 1979), but is often viewed as a step in the process of changing thought content rather than as an end in itself. Patients in cognitive therapy learn to adopt a decentered perspective on thoughts by viewing them as ideas to be tested, rather than truths (Hollon & Beck, 1979). However, they then go on to dispute distorted thoughts and generate more rational ones. Several authors have suggested that decentering alone may be the central ingredient in the effectiveness of cognitive therapy in preventing relapse of depression (Ingram & Hollon, 1986; Segal et al., 2002). It is a central ingredient in MBCT, which uses the intensive practice of mindfulness meditation to teach decentering, which in turn reduces rumination and lowers the likelihood of relapse.

Decentering can be measured with two recently developed tools. The Measure of Awareness and Coping in Autobiographical Memory (MACAM; Moore, Hayhurst, & Teasdale, 1996) is a vignette-based, semistructured clinical interview in which participants are asked to imagine themselves in several mildly depressing situations and to feel the feelings that would be elicited. They are then asked to recall specific occasions from their own lives that the vignettes bring to mind and to describe these occasions in detail, including their feelings and how they responded to them. Responses are tape recorded, and trained raters then code the responses for the presence of decentering or awareness of thoughts and feelings as separate from the self. Teasdale et al. (2002) found that decentering scores were higher for a group of never-depressed adults than for a previously depressed group. Previously depressed patients who completed MBCT showed larger increases in decentering than a control group who received treatment as usual. Finally, lower baseline levels of decentering predicted earlier relapse following treatment for depression with either cognitive therapy or medication. Overall, these findings support the idea that the ability to adopt a decentered perspective on thoughts and feelings is centrally related to recovery from depression and prevention of relapse.

Although the MACAM appears to have good psychometric properties, it is time consuming and difficult to use. For this reason, Fresco, Moore, et al. (2007) conducted a psychometric evaluation of the experiences questionnaire (EQ), a rationally derived self-report instrument designed by Teasdale to assess decentering and rumination. Analyses by Fresco et al. (in press) yielded an 11-item decentering factor, which includes items such as "I can observe unpleasant feelings without being drawn into them" and "I can separate myself from my thoughts and feelings." The EQ showed good internal consistency and was correlated in expected directions with measures of depressive rumination, experiential avoidance, emotion regulation, and depression. Depressed patients showed lower levels of decentering than healthy controls (Fresco et al., in press). In a second study, Fresco, Segal, et al. (2007) showed that depressed patients who responded to CBT showed greater gains in decentering than those successfully treated with medication. In addition, high levels of decentering post-treatment were associated with lower rates of relapse during an 18-month follow-up period.

Fresco, Moore, et al. (2007) note that the EQ was not designed to be a measure of mindfulness. However, definitions of decentering are very similar to descriptions of mindfulness summarized earlier. Empirical investigations of relations between the EQ and measures of mindfulness have not yet been conducted.

Performance-Based Tasks

Self-report methods can be subject to demand characteristics or response biases, and some aspects of mindfulness may be difficult for individuals to report on, especially if they have no meditation experience. Thus, it is important to develop additional tools for assessing mindfulness that do not rely on self-report methods. Unfortunately, very little research has examined the assessment of mindfulness by non-self-report methods. Bishop et al. (2004)

suggested several laboratory- or computer-based tasks for which performance may reflect aspects of the tendency or ability to be mindful. For example, as the practice of mindfulness should cultivate both sustained attention and flexibility of attention, more mindful individuals should score higher on established tests of vigilance and attention switching. In addition, mindfulness encourages observation of stimuli without secondary elaborative processing. Therefore, more mindful individuals should perform better on tasks that require inhibition of semantic processing, such as the emotional Stroop task (Williams, Mathews, & MacLeod, 1996). The Implicit Associations Test (Greenwald, McGhee, & Schwartz, 1998) could provide a method for assessing the tendency to associate negative emotions with avoidance rather than approach. Because the practice of mindfulness encourages acceptance and allowing of negative emotion, this tendency should be lower in more mindful individuals.

Some authors have suggested that responses to stressful or unpleasant experiences in a laboratory setting might reflect levels of mindfulness or acceptance. Several studies have shown that participants who are instructed to adopt a mindful perspective while experiencing short-term, laboratory-induced pain, negative mood, or panic-like symptoms show quicker recovery or greater willingness to repeat the experience than those given suppression, distraction, or rumination instructions (e.g., Broderick, 2005; Levitt, Brown, Orsillo, & Barlow, 2004). Zettle and colleagues found that participants who scored higher on experiential avoidance (as measured by the AAQ) also showed lower pain tolerance (Zettle et al., 2005) and were more distressed by unpleasant sensations (Zettle, Peterson, Hocker, & Provines, 2007). However, whether such tasks provide adequate indices of individuals' levels of mindfulness or acceptance requires more investigation.

Conclusion

No single method of psychological assessment can provide a complete picture of the characteristic it is designed to measure. Self-report questionnaires, structured interviews, performance-based measures, and other methods all have strengths and weaknesses, and each may yield useful data not provided by the others (Meyer et al., 2001). Mindfulness, as noted earlier, appears to be unusually difficult to define and conceptualize, perhaps because it is associated with the "mysterious territory" of consciousness (Brown & Ryan, 2004, p. 242, see also Chapter 4 of this volume) or because mindful acceptance is an atypical way of meeting adversity in our culture (Santorelli, 1999). Mindfulness-based interventions address these difficulties through extensive use of experiential methods and by placing less emphasis on intellectual learning (Hayes et al., 1999; Segal et al., 2002). Given the difficulty of translating mindfulness and acceptance into the concrete operational definitions required by scientific methods of assessment and the importance of understanding of how mindfulness-based treatments work, it is essential that we continue to strive for the most productive combination of critical thinking and open mindedness about how to assess these constructs.

Appendix: Five-Facet Mindfulness Questionnaire

Please rate each of the following statements using the scale provided. Write the number in the blank that best describes your own opinion of what is generally true for you.

1	2	3	4	5
never or very rarely true	rarely true	sometimes true	often true	very often or always true

_____1. When I'm walking, I deliberately notice the sensations of my body moving.

_____2. I'm good at finding words to describe my feelings.

_____3. I criticize myself for having irrational or inappropriate emotions.

_____4. I perceive my feelings and emotions without having to react to them.

_____5. When I do things, my mind wanders off and I'm easily distracted.

_____6. When I take a shower or bath, I stay alert to the sensations of water on my body.

_____7. I can easily put my beliefs, opinions, and expectations into words.

_____8. I don't pay attention to what I'm doing because I'm daydreaming, worrying, or otherwise distracted.

_____9. I watch my feelings without getting lost in them.

_____10. I tell myself I shouldn't be feeling the way I'm feeling.

_____11. I notice how foods and drinks affect my thoughts, bodily sensations, and emotions.

_____12. It's hard for me to find the words to describe what I'm thinking.

_____13. I am easily distracted.

_____14. I believe some of my thoughts are abnormal or bad and I shouldn't think that way.

_____15. I pay attention to sensations, such as the wind in my hair or sun on my face.

_____16. I have trouble thinking of the right words to express how I feel about things

_____17. I make judgments about whether my thoughts are good or bad.

_____18. I find it difficult to stay focused on what's happening in the present.

_____19. When I have distressing thoughts or images, I "step back" and am aware of the thought or image without getting taken over by it.

_____20. I pay attention to sounds, such as clocks ticking, birds chirping, or cars passing.

_____21. In difficult situations, I can pause without immediately reacting.

_____22. When I have a sensation in my body, it's difficult for me to describe it because I can't find the right words.

_____23. It seems I am "running on automatic" without much awareness of what I'm doing.

_____24. When I have distressing thoughts or images, I feel calm soon after.

_____25. I tell myself that I shouldn't be thinking the way I'm thinking.

_____26. I notice the smells and aromas of things.

____27. Even when I'm feeling terribly upset, I can find a way to put it into words.

____28. I rush through activities without being really attentive to them.

____29. When I have distressing thoughts or images I am able just to notice them without reacting.

____30. I think some of my emotions are bad or inappropriate and I shouldn't feel them.

____31. I notice visual elements in art or nature, such as colors, shapes, textures, or patterns of light and shadow.

____32. My natural tendency is to put my experiences into words.

____33. When I have distressing thoughts or images, I just notice them and let them go.

____34. I do jobs or tasks automatically without being aware of what I'm doing.

____35. When I have distressing thoughts or images, I judge myself as good or bad, depending on what the thought/image is about.

____36. I pay attention to how my emotions affect my thoughts and behavior.

____37. I can usually describe how I feel at the moment in considerable detail.

____38. I find myself doing things without paying attention.

____39. I disapprove of myself when I have irrational ideas.

References

Baer, R. A., Smith, G. T., Lykins, E., Button, D., Krietemeyer, J., Sauer, S., Walsh, E., Duggan, D., & Williams, J. M. G. (2007). Construct validity of the Five Facet Mindfulness Questionnaire in meditating and nonmeditating samples. *Assessment, 15,* 329–342.

Baer, R. A., Smith, G. T., & Allen, K. B. (2004). Assessment of mindfulness by self-report: The Kentucky Inventory of Mindfulness Skills. *Assessment, 11,* 191–206.

Baer, R. A., Smith, G. T., Hopkins, J., Krietemeyer, J., & Toney, L. (2006). Using self-report assessment methods to explore facets of mindfulness. *Assessment, 13,* 27–45.

Beck, A. T., Rush, A. J., Shaw, B. F., & Emery, G. (1979). *Cognitive therapy of depression.* New York: Guilford Press.

Beitel, M., Ferrer, E., & Cecero, J. J. (2005). Psychological mindedness and awareness of self and others. *Journal of Clinical Psychology, 61,* 739–750.

Bishop, S. R., Lau, M., Shapiro, S., Carlson, L., Anderson, N. C., Carmody, J., et al. (2004). Mindfulness: A proposed operational definition. *Clinical Psychology: Science and Practice, 11,* 230–241.

Block-Lerner, J., Salters-Pednault, K., & Tull, M. T. (2005). Assessing mindfulness and experiential acceptance: Attempts to capture inherently elusive phenomena. In S. M. Orsillo & L. Roemer (Eds.), *Acceptance and mindfulness-based approaches to anxiety: Conceptualization and treatment* (pp. 71–100). NY: Springer.

Bond, F. W. & Bunce, D. (2003). The role of acceptance and job control in mental health, job satisfaction, and work performance. *Journal of Applied Psychology, 88,* 1057–1067.

Broderick, P. C. (2005). Mindfulness and coping with dysphoric mood: Contrasts with rumination and distraction. *Cognitive Therapy and Research, 29,* 501–510.

Brown, K. W. & Ryan, R. M. (2003). The benefits of being present: Mindfulness and its role in psychological well-being. *Journal of Personality and Social Psychology, 84,* 822–848.

Brown, K. W. & Ryan, R. M. (2004). Perils and promise in defining and measuring mindfulness: Observations from experience. *Clinical Psychology: Science and Practice, 11*, 242–248.

Brown, K. W., Ryan, R. M., & Creswell, J.D. (2007). Mindfulness: Theoretical foundations and evidence for its salutary effects. *Psychological Inquiry, 18*, 211–237.

Buchheld, N., Grossman, P., & Walach, H. (2001). Measuring mindfulness in insight meditation and meditation-based psychotherapy: The development of the Freiburg Mindfulness Inventory (FMI). *Journal for Meditation and Meditation Research, 1*, 11–34.

Cardaciotto, L., Herbert, J. D., Forman, E. M., Moitra, E., & Farrow, V. (2007). The assessment of present-moment awareness and acceptance: The Philadelphia Mindfulness Scale. *Assessment, 15*, 204–223.

Carlson, L. E., & Brown, K. W. (2005). Validation of the Mindful Attention Awareness Scale in a cancer population. *Journal of Psychosomatic Research, 58*, 29–33.

Carmody, J., & Baer, R. A. (2008). Relationships between mindfulness practice and levels of mindfulness, medical and psychological symptoms and well-being in a mindfulness-based stress reduction program. *Journal of Behavioral Medicine, 31*, 23–33.

Chadwick, P., Hember, M., Mead, S., Lilley, B., & Dagnan, D. (2005). Responding mindfully to unpleasant thoughts and images: Reliability and validity of the Mindfulness Questionnaire. Manuscript under review.

Cheyne, J. A., Carriere, J. S. A., & Smilek, D. (2006). Absent-mindedness: Lapses of conscious awareness and everyday cognitions. *Consciousness and Cognition, 15*, 578–592.

Clark, L. A. & Watson, D. (1995). Constructing validity: Basic issues in objective scale development. *Psychological Assessment, 7*, 309–319.

Dimidjian, S., & Linehan, M. M. (2003). Defining an agenda for future research on the clinical application of mindfulness practice. *Clinical Psychology: Science and Practice, 10*, 166–171.

Dougher, M. J., (1994). The act of acceptance. In S. C. Hayes, N. S. Joacobson, V. M. Follette, & M. J. Dougher (Eds.), *Acceptance and change: Content and context in psychotherapy* (pp. 37–45). Reno, NV: Context Press.

Feldman, G. C., Hayes, A. M., Kumar, S. M., & Greeson, J. G, and Laurenceau, J. P. (2007). Mindfulness and emotion regulation: The development and initial validation of the Cognitive and Affective Mindfulness Scale-Revised (CAMS-R). *Journal of Psychopathology and Behavioral Assessment, 29*, 177–190.

Fresco, D. M., Moore, M. T., van Dulmen, M., Segal, Z. V., Teasdale, J. D., Ma, H., & Williams, J. M. G. (2007). Initial psychometric properties of the experiences questionnaire: A self-report survey of decentering. *Behavior Therapy, 38*, 234–246.

Fresco, D. M., Segal, Z. V., Buis, T., & Kennedy, S. (2007). Relationship of posttreatment decentering and cognitive reactivity to relapse in major depression. *Journal of Consulting and Clinical Psychology, 75*, 447–455.

Germer, C. K., Siegel, R. D., & Fulton, P. R. (2005). *Mindfulness and psychotherapy*. NY: Guilford Press.

Greco, L. A., Lambert, W., & Baer, R. A. (2008). Psychological inflexibility in childhood and adolescence: Development and evaluation of the Avoidance and Fusion Questionnaire for Youth. *Psychological Assessment, 20*, 93–102.

Gregg, J. A., Callaghan, G. M., Hayes, S. C., & Glenn-Lawson, J. L. (2007). Improving diabetes self-management through acceptance, mindfulness, and values: A randomized controlled trial. *Journal of Consulting and Clinical Psychology, 75*, 336–343.

Greenwald, A. G., McGhee, D. E., & Schwartz, J. L. K. (1998). Measuring individual differences in implicit cognition: The Implicit Association Test. *Journal of Personality and Social Psychology, 74*, 1464–1480.

Hayes, S. C. & Strosahl, K. D. (2004). *A practical guide to Acceptance and Commitment Therapy*. New York: Springer.

Hayes, S. C., Strosahl, K., & Wilson, K. G. (1999). *Acceptance and commitment therapy: An experiential approach to behavior change*. New York: Guilford.

Hayes, S. C., Strosahl, K., Wilson, K. G., Bissett, R. T., Pistorello, J., Toarmino, D., et al. (2004). Measuring experiential avoidance: A preliminary test of a working model. *The Psychological Record, 54*, 553-578.

Hollon, S. D., & Beck, A. T. (1979). Cognitive therapy of depression. In P. C. Kendall & S. D. Hollon (Eds.), *Cognitive-behavioral interventions: Theory, research, and procedures* (pp. 153-203). New York: Academic Press.

Ingram, R. E., & Hollon, S. D. (1986). Cognitive therapy for depression from an information processing perspective. In R. E. Ingram, (Ed.), *Information processing approaches to clinical psychology* (pp. 259-281). San Diego, CA: Academic Press.

Kabat-Zinn, J. (1982). An outpatient program in behavioral medicine for chronic pain patients based on the practice of mindfulness meditation: Theoretical considerations and preliminary results. *General Hospital Psychiatry, 4*, 33-47.

Kabat-Zinn, J. (1990). *Full catastrophe living: Using the wisdom of your mind and body to face stress, pain, and illness*. New York: Delacorte.

Kabat-Zinn, J. (1994). *Wherever you go, there you are: Mindfulness meditation in everyday life*. New York: Hyperion.

Kabat-Zinn, J. (2003). Mindfulness-based interventions in context: Past, present and future. *Clinical Psychology: Science and Practice, 10*, 144-156.

Lau, M. A., Bishop, S. R., Segal, Z. V., Buis, T., Anderson, N. D., Carlson, L., et al. (2006). The Toronto mindfulness scale: Development and validation. *Journal of Clinical Psychology, 62*, 1445-1467.

Leigh, J., Bowen, S., & Marlatt, G. A. (2005). Spirituality, mindfulness and substance abuse. *Addictive Behaviors, 30*, 1335-1341.

Levitt, J. T., Brown, T. A., Orsillo, S. M. & Barlow, D. H. (2004). The effects of acceptance versus suppression of emotion on subjective and psychophysiological response to carbon dioxide challenge in patients with panic disorder. *Behavior Therapy, 35*, 747-766.

Lillis, J. & Hayes, S. C. (2008). Measuring avoidance and inflexibility in weight related problems. Manuscript under review.

Linehan, M. M., (1993). *Cognitive-behavioral treatment of borderline personality disorder*. New York: Guilford.

Lykins, E. L. B., & Baer, R. A. (in press). Psychological functioning in a sample of long-term practitioners of mindfulness meditation. *Journal of Cognitive Psychotherapy*.

MacKillop, J., & Anderson, E. J. (2007). Further psychometric validation of the Mindful Attention Awareness Scale. *Journal of Psychopathology and Behavioral Assessment, 29*, 289-293.

Marlatt, G. A., & Kristeller, J. L. (1999). Mindfulness and meditation. In W. R. Miller (Ed.), *Integrating spirituality into treatment* (pp. 67-84). Washington, DC: APA.

McCracken, L. M. (1998). Learning to live with pain: Acceptance of pain predicts adjustment in persons with chronic pain. *Pain, 74*, 21-27.

McCracken, L. M., & Eccleston, C. (2003). Coping or acceptance: What to do about chronic pain? *Pain, 105*, 197-204.

McCracken, L. M., Vowles, K. E., & Eccleston, C. (2004). Acceptance of chronic pain: Component analysis and a revised assessment method. *Pain, 107*, 159-166.

Meyer, G. J., Finn, S. E., Eyde, L. D., Kay, G. G., Moreland, K. L., Dies, R. R., et al. (2001). Psychological testing and psychological assessment: A review of evidence and issues. *American Psychologist, 56*, 128-165.

Moore, R. G., Hayhurst, H., & Teasdale, J. D. (1996). *Measure of Awareness and Coping in Autobiographical Memory: Instructions for administering and coding.*

Unpublished manuscript, Department of Psychiatry, University of Cambridge, Cambridge, United Kingdom.

Santorelli, S. (1999). *Heal thyself: Lessons on mindfulness in medicine.* New York: Bell Tower.

Segal, Z. V., Williams, J. M. G., & Teasdale, J. D. (2002). *Mindfulness-based cognitive therapy for depression: A new approach to preventing relapse.* New York: Guilford.

Shapiro, S. L., Carlson, L. E., Astin, J. A., & Freedman, B. (2006). Mechanisms of mindfulness. *Journal of Clinical Psychology, 62,* 373-386.

Teasdale, J. D., Moore, R. G., Hayhurst, H., Pope, M., Williams, S., & Segal, Z. (2002). Metacognitive awareness and prevention of relapse in depression: Empirical evidence. *Journal of Consulting and Clinical Psychology, 70,* 275-287.

Walach, H., Buchheld, N., Buttenmuller, V., Kleinknecht, N., & Schmidt, S. (2006). Measuring mindfulness: The Freiburg Mindfulness Inventory (FMI), *Personality and Individual Differences, 40,* 1543-1555.

Williams, J. M. G., Mathews, A., & MacLeod, C. (1996). The emotional Stroop task and psychopathology. *Psychological Bulletin, 120,* 3-24.

Zettle, R. D., Hocker, T. L., Mick, K. A., Scofield, B. E., Peterson, C. L., Song, H., & Sudarijanto, R. P. (2005). Differential strategies in coping with pain as a function of level of experiential avoidance. *Psychological Record, 55,* 511-524.

Zettle, R. D., Peterson, C. L., Hocker, T. R., & Provines, J. L. (2007). Responding to a challenging perceptual-motor task as a function of level of experiential avoidance. *Psychological Record, 57,* 49-62.

Part 3

Mindfulness-Based Interventions for Specific Disorders

10

Mindfulness and Anxiety Disorders: Developing a Wise Relationship with the Inner Experience of Fear

Jeffrey Greeson, Jeffrey Brantley

> *... the term mental disorder unfortunately implies a distinction between "mental" disorders and "physical" disorders that is a reductionistic anachronism of mind/body dualism. A compelling literature documents that there is much "physical" in mental disorders and much "mental" in physical disorders.*
> – American Psychiatric Association (DSM-IV-TR, 2000)

Introduction

Perhaps no condition better illustrates the intimate relationship between brain and behavior – mind and body – as the inner experience of fear. In this chapter, we present an integrative scientific view of anxiety and clinical anxiety disorders, with an emphasis on awareness and acceptance as a foundation for mind/body health. Whereas anxiety-related psychopathology is characterized by a desire to avoid the inner experience of fear, we postulate that practicing mindfulness can promote a wise and accepting relationship with one's internal cognitive, emotional, and physical experience, even during times of intense fear or worry. Further, we suggest that the "wise relationship" that develops by turning toward fear, anxiety, and panic with stable attention, present focused awareness, acceptance, and self-compassion can promote psychological freedom from persistent anxiety and greater behavioral flexibility.

Mindfulness is a word that refers to a basic human capacity for non-conceptual, non-judging, and present-moment-centered awareness. This awareness arises from intentionally paying attention, from noticing on purpose what is occurring inside and outside of oneself, with an attitude of friendliness and acceptance toward what is happening while it is happening. Mindfulness has been cultivated by human beings using "inner technologies" of meditation in various spiritual contexts for literally thousands of years. In the past 25–30 years, Western medical science has turned increasing attention to the psychological and physical correlates of meditation and mindfulness practices (Walsh & Shapiro, 2006). Modern clinical investigators have joined meditation teachers in offering definitions of mindfulness (see Table 10.1).

Table 10.1. Definitions of mindfulness.

Definition	Reference
"the non-judgmental observation of the ongoing stream of internal and external stimuli as they arise."	Baer (2003)
"self-regulation of attention [and] adopting a particular orientation toward one's experience in the present moment, an orientation that is characterized by curiosity, openness, and acceptance."	Bishop et al. (2004)
"friendly, nonjudging, present-moment awareness."	Brantley (2003)
"awareness, of present experience, with acceptance."	Germer (2005)
"the awareness that emerges through paying attention on purpose, in the present moment, and nonjudgmentally to the unfolding of experience moment by moment."	Kabat-Zinn (2003)
"the state of being fully present, without habitual reactions."	Salzberg and Goldstein (2001)

Our central thesis in this chapter is that practicing mindfulness offers a healthier and more effective means for relating to one's inner experience of fear and anxiety, through self-regulation built on intentional, non-judging awareness.

In the sections that follow, we present current theoretical, scientific, and clinical evidence in support of our hypothesis that practicing mindfulness enables a "wise relationship" to develop toward one's own inner life, particularly the internal experience of anxiety and fear. By bringing inner processes of thinking, feeling, and physical sensations into consciousness using mindfulness practice, identification with and perpetuation of unconscious patterns in mind and body can be transformed into interactions that are "wise", that is, based in accurate perception and inclusive of all the domains of experience available to each human being in each moment. The healing benefits of mindfulness practice to the conditions of anxiety and fear follow from this more conscious, wise relationship.

Prevalence, Characteristics, and Current Treatment of Anxiety Disorders

Human anxiety occurs along a continuum, from normal fear reactions that help avert clear and present danger to uncontrollable panic and maladaptive avoidance of people, places, and things in an effort to feel safe from harm. The experience of acute fear and mild-to-moderate anxiety is ubiquitous in the human condition. When it occurs in the appropriate context, some fear and anxiety can increase attention to threatening circumstances or enhance effective performance in the face of a challenge. Thus, some degree of anxiety is good.

However, when anxiety is unwarranted, excessive, and persistent, and/or it interferes with everyday functioning, it can be categorized as a psychiatric disorder (American Psychiatric Association, 2000). The Diagnostic and Statistical Manual of Mental Disorders, 4th edition, Text Revision (DSM-IV-TR) includes six primary anxiety disorders (see Table 10.2). Each anxiety disorder shares characteristic symptoms of intrusive and disturbing thoughts,

Table 10.2. Primary anxiety disorders, clinical descriptions, and lifetime prevalence.

Diagnostic category	Clinical description	Lifetime prevalence[*]
Generalized anxiety disorder	Persistent, pervasive worry that is difficult to control	5%
Obsessive-compulsive Disorder	Obsessive thinking about possible threats to safety and compulsive ritualistic behaviors to allay fear	2.5%
Panic disorder	Sudden, overwhelming, intense fear of something going wrong	1.0–3.5%
Post-traumatic stress disorder	Intrusive thoughts, hyperarousal, and reexperience of past trauma	8%
Social anxiety disorder	Fear of negative social evaluation	Up to 13%
Specific phobia	Fear of a specific object or situation	7–11%

[*]Obtained from DSM-IV-TR, American Psychiatric Association (2000).

heightened psychophysiological arousal, and intensely unpleasant appraisals of one's internal emotional experience (Brantley, 2003). Taken together, anxiety disorders are the most prevalent category of mental health diagnoses, affecting an estimated 25–30 million Americans during their lifetime (Lepine, 2002; Narrow, Rae, Robins, & Regier, 2002).

Anxiety disorders are often conceptualized as a *fear of fear* that results in high levels of subjective distress, somatic symptom manifestation, and disruption of daily living (Barlow, 2002). Worry has been described as the persistent activation of one's cognitive representation of anxiety, including disturbing thoughts, stories, or images about a possible danger or threat (Borkovec, Ray, & Stober, 1998). Despite its useful function in helping one to cope, feel safe, and prepare for what may come, persistent worry and its associated affective distress and physiological arousal can produce defensive, self-protective, and avoidant behavior out of context, typical of psychiatric disorder (Barlow, 2002; Borkovec et al., 1998).

The Psychobiological Nature of Fear and Anxiety

The psychological experience of fear occurs concomitantly with a pattern of stress-related physiological activation designed to promote survival by avoiding danger through fight-flight-or-freeze behavior (Barlow, 2002). A startle response initiated by sensory detection of a potentially threatening stimulus, such as a sudden loud noise, a looming shadow, or an unexpected touch, immediately signals the subcortical structures in the brain (i.e., the limbic system) that perceive threat and mediate an alarm reaction. This alarm reaction descends from the limbic system through the brainstem, spinal cord, and peripheral nervous system, ultimately activating a broad-spectrum physiological response throughout the body. Integrated psychophysiological activation in response to a perceived threat enables one to cope through vigorous defensive action, such as fighting or fleeing (Schneiderman & McCabe, 1989). These adaptive responses are generated by activation of multiple body systems, including the central and peripheral nervous systems, cardiovascular system, endocrine system, metabolic system, neuromuscular system, and immune system (Selye, 1976). Conversely, select biological systems unessential for survival in the face of an immediate threat, including the digestive system and the reproductive system, are deactivated under conditions of fear or stress (Selye, 1976).

Psychophysiological activation and accompanying energy mobilization is certainly useful in supporting escape behavior when actual escape is possible. When a threat outweighs one's perceived ability to escape or otherwise cope, however, behavioral freezing and cognitive hypervigilance may occur in an attempt to passively avoid harm (Schneiderman & McCabe, 1989). Under conditions of passive avoidance rather than active coping or escape, the physiological effort and energy generated can go unused. While acute, time-limited onset and recovery of stress-related mental and physical activation clearly provides an adaptive advantage in the face of a true threat (i.e., when actual fighting, fleeing or freezing is needed to promote survival), chronic or unwarranted activation of fear-related psychophysiology can be detrimental to health. Indeed, a growing body of animal and human research indicates that repeated, exaggerated, or prolonged activation of stress physiology, as well as delayed recovery of biological responses to stress, can contribute to premature breakdown of organ systems that may increase susceptibility to disease (McEwen, 1998).

Mind/Body Connections and Processes Underlying Clinical Anxiety

Anxiety disorders can be characterized by a set of dysregulated cognitive, affective, physiological, and behavioral processes that manifest as maladaptive ways of responding to one's inner experience of fear. Dysregulated cognitive processes in anxiety disorders typically include the following:

- a narrow focus of attention on some disturbing aspect of internal experience, such as a distressing thought or physical sensation,
- misappraisal of threat in the absence of real danger, and
- distortion of the magnitude of a true threat or challenge through magnifying, catastrophizing, or fortune telling (Barlow, 2002).

In addition, from a cognitive standpoint, anxiety disorders can be characterized by a focus of attention on future-oriented concerns about possible misfortune (Barlow, 2002). The narrow focus of attention on disturbing thoughts or physical sensations, coupled with a future-oriented tendency to worry about *potential* threats of harm, can predispose an individual to a lack of awareness of what is actually happening in the present moment (Brantley, 2003).

When one is unaware of what is actually happening in the present moment, one's attentional focus is more susceptible to being hijacked by a train of cognitive interpretations about one's experience that may be inaccurate and distress provoking. For instance, in the case of depression, the "downward spiral" of automatic, negatively biased information processing, or "depressogenic thinking," can transform momentary emotional distress into longer-lasting mood disturbance, which in turn, can increase susceptibility to depressive relapse (Segal, Williams, & Teasdale, 2002). Similarly, in the case of anxiety, a cognitive style marked by a narrow focus of attention, orientation to future events as opposed to present moment experience, and a propensity to catastrophically appraise or misinterpret mental or physical phenomena can result in the arousal of anxiety and other emotional disturbances such as anger, sadness, and loneliness.

While the perception of fear and anxiety occurs in the brain, the response can be most noticeable in the body. The induction of fear and other forms of negative affect stimulates widespread sympathetic activation, which originates from pathways in the cerebral cortex and subcortical limbic structures (e.g., amygdala, hippocampus, hypothalamus), and descends through the brainstem, spinal cord, and peripheral sympathetic nerves to organ systems throughout the body (Thayer & Brosschot, 2005). Consequently, fearful cognitive interpretations and associated emotional and physiological arousal can manifest in an array of somatic symptoms, including painful muscle tension, racing pulse, elevated blood pressure, cardiac arrhythmia, labored respiration, and gastrointestinal disturbance. Moreover, given one's anxiety-prone cognitive style, somatic symptoms can be interpreted as evidence of harm, which may result in even narrower attention to the symptoms, catastrophic thinking, acute panic, emotional distress, and even a sense of impending doom. Because these internal experiences are unpleasant and aversive, they are typically avoided by actively attempting to distract attention away from the inner experience when it is present and attempting to prevent recurrent anxiety in the future by avoiding associated people, places, or things. Taken together, it has been noted that "reactions (both cognitive and emotional) to one's own internal experiences (thoughts, feelings, bodily sensations) may underlie the development and/or maintenance of anxiety disorders," which categorically manifest as psychological and behavioral inflexibility (Orsillo, Roemer, & Holowka, 2005).

Overview of Current Treatments for Anxiety

Given the integrated mind/body nature of fear and experiential anxiety, it is logical that effective treatment strategies for anxiety disorders address both mental and physical functioning. Standard treatment approaches for clinical anxiety include psychotherapy and medication, both of which are intended to modulate cognitive, affective, physiological, and/or behavioral reactions to perceived threat (American Psychiatric Association, 2005). Several different psychotherapies and medications are equally efficacious in the short-term amelioration of anxiety-related symptoms (American Psychiatric Association, 2005). Effective psychotherapies include behavior therapy in which an individual is systematically exposed to a feared condition without being permitted to engage in an automatic, avoidant behavioral response, and cognitive-behavioral therapy (CBT), in which distorted beliefs, misappraisals, contextually inappropriate emotional reactions, and inflexible behavior patterns are identified and corrected using self-monitoring, cognitive restructuring, and relaxation training (for detailed reviews see Barlow, 2002). CBT for anxiety has demonstrated to be superior to medication for long-term symptom reduction (Otto, Smits, & Reese, 2005). There are many "active ingredients" in psychotherapeutic approaches to anxiety disorders, and it remains unclear to what extent specific cognitive, affective, behavioral, or psychoeducational components account for therapeutic change, as opposed to non-specific factors such as therapist attention, empathy and positive regard, or perceived social support (Barlow, 2002). Effective medications for the treatment of clinical anxiety include benzodiazepines, tricyclic antidepressants, monoamine oxidase inhibitors, and selective serotonin reuptake inhibitors (Sheehan & Harnett Sheehan, 2007). In chronic and/or treatment refractory cases, psychotherapy may be effectively combined with pharmacotherapy (Sheehan & Harnett Sheehan, 2007).

In recent years, mindfulness- and acceptance-based approaches have been combined with traditional change-based approaches such as CBT in an attempt to enhance effective treatment of psychopathology, including anxiety and depressive disorders (for reviews see Feldman, 2007; Hayes, 2005; Lau & McMain, 2005; Orsillo & Roemer, 2005; Segal et al., 2002). Because individuals who experience clinically relevant anxiety typically have a strongly conditioned desire to avoid distressing internal experiences – despite the tendency of experiential avoidance to prolong or even exacerbate distressing sensations – mindfulness practice offers a fundamentally different orientation in which anxiety is deliberately noticed, allowed, and responded to with openness, curiosity, and acceptance. Therefore, practicing mindfulness may increase distress tolerance, interrupt habitual avoidance, and ultimately promote adaptive self-regulation and healthy mind/body functioning.

How Mindfulness May Target the Shared Roots of Anxiety-Related Suffering

Modern-day responses to psychological stress, fear, and uncertainty are often marked by rumination, worry, anticipatory anxiety, and stagnant deliberation. These habits of thinking continue to stimulate fear reactions in the body, which in turn, feed back to fuel worried thoughts, causing a cycle of unpleasant experience (Brosschot, Gerin, & Thayer, 2006; Feldman, Hayes, Kumar, Greeson, & Laurenceau, 2007). Consequently, one might say that human beings today are more likely to fight the *unpleasantness* of their own inner experience of threat rather than fight off the threat itself. In the short term, strategies for avoiding one's inner experience of anxiety, such as distraction, thought suppression, or the use of emotion-regulating substances including cigarettes, alcohol, illicit drugs or food, may be effective in reducing distress temporarily. This behavioral approach can certainly be reinforcing, and thus can become quite habitual, automatic, and rigid. However, attempts to avoid the inner experience of fear, anxiety, and panic not only fail to ameliorate the root cause of emotional upset, but also paradoxically exacerbate the inner experience of suffering by reinforcing maladaptive (i.e., avoidant) coping behaviors that permit an emotionally upsetting experience to recur indefinitely outside of an appropriate context.

Knowing Without Identifying or Reacting

From the perspective of mindfulness, thoughts, emotions, physical sensations, and impulses that arise in association with one's internal experience of fear, anxiety or panic are merely events in the broad field of one's present-moment awareness (Brantley, 2003). Mindfulness practice is believed to improve effective self-regulation of anxiety-related cognition, emotion, sensation and behavior, although the precise mechanisms are not yet clear (Baer, 2003; Bishop, 2002; Garland, 2007; Kabat-Zinn, 1990; Shapiro, Carlson, Astin, & Freedman, 2006; Shapiro, & Schwartz, 2000).

Central to the self-regulatory capacity of mindfulness is a fundamental shift in one's relationship with one's inner life and the outer world. In essence, mindfulness enables conscious awareness of inner life and physical sensations. This shift in awareness brought about by mindfulness has variably been termed "reperceiving," "decentering," "detachment," "metacognitive awareness," "bare attention," and "clear seeing" (Salzberg & Goldstein, 2001; Segal et al., 2002; Shapiro et al., 2006; Teasdale et al., 2002). Shapiro et al. (2006), for instance, have described reperceiving as "rather than being immersed in the drama of our personal narrative or life story, we are able to stand back and simply witness it."

The capacity for mindfulness – and its resultant perspective shift on the inner life – is traditionally cultivated by regular meditation practice (Hahn, 1976; Kabat-Zinn, 1990; Salzberg & Goldstein, 2001; Brantley, 2003). Meditation can be understood as an intentional training of attention, embedded with acceptance, and the resulting awareness and understanding that emerge (Brantley, 2003). As observed by Goleman (1980), "The first realization in 'meditation' is that the phenomena contemplated are distinct from the mind contemplating them."

Walsh and Shapiro (2006) have emphasized that meditation training typically differs from other self-regulatory strategies such as self-hypnosis, visualization, and psychotherapy in that meditation primarily aims to train attention and awareness, whereas other approaches primarily intend to change mental contents (i.e., thoughts, images, beliefs, emotions) and modify behavior. Although mindfulness has been described as the "heart of Buddhist meditation," being mindful is considered an innate human capacity that is universal, secular, and compatible with nearly every major world religion (Kabat-Zinn, 2005). Indeed, mindfulness and the ability to reperceive are conceptualized as part of a developmental process (Shapiro et al., 2006).

From a meditation teacher's perspective, practicing mindfulness may help in the following way. As one pays attention on purpose to one's actual direct experience of anxiety, as opposed to being identified with what one *thinks* about anxiety, one gains significantly greater understanding and insight about the experience of anxiety and about oneself in relation to one's world (Goldstein, 1976). Such understanding and insight can provide a foundation for more skillful responses in the face of fear, anxiety and panic, including equanimity rather than reactivity and wise self-regulation rather than aversion. By virtue of the psychological and behavioral flexibility mindfulness can afford in the present moment, one might be better able to consciously choose actions that are effective in meeting one's needs for safety, a sense of security, and calm.

"How Are You Treating Anxiety?" Establishing Wise Relationship

Put simply, distress seems to increase as we stray further from the present moment. As Mark Twain, a famous worrywart, once said, "There has been much tragedy in my life; at least half of it actually happened." The consequences for psychological suffering are clear when we live in the future. Moreover, reflexively and rigidly attempting to avoid one's inner experience of fear, anxiety, and panic not only fails to address the problem, but actually functions to exacerbate it and prolong suffering. But, what happens when one deliberately takes a different relationship to one's inner life experience? A more conscious and allowing relationship? Can such an act of intention, attention, and acceptance increase one's awareness of the mind/body connection, including implications for self-regulation, wise action, and optimal health?

When one changes their relationship to their internal experience from that of automatic judgment, rigid thinking, and disconnection to one of acceptance, openness, and intentional connection, an immediate impact occurs in the circuits and feedback loops of mind and body. Because mindfulness represents a completely different perspective than the prevailing Western cultural norm of narrowly focused attention, avoidance of unpleasantness, and behavioral reactivity contingent on environmental circumstances, it has been described as an "orthogonal rotation" in consciousness (Kabat-Zinn, 2005).

Many mindfulness teachers emphasize that practicing mindfulness is an invitation to relate to life differently. In more practical terms, mindfulness may be described as an intentional willingness to fully and completely engage with one's direct experience of living, on a moment-to-moment basis, with whatever pleasant, unpleasant, or neutral events that arise. The central goal of living mindfully is to open to the fullness and richness of each moment, and not to add, subtract, or modify any part of one's psychological or physical experience. At its core, mindfulness is intended to help one live a life of deep meaning, value, direction, and purpose even when emotional or physical pain is present (Kabat-Zinn, 2003). By awakening to the possibilities available in the present moment, one often becomes empowered to choose a wise response in the face of an upsetting internal experience or external event, as opposed to having an upsetting experience or event dictate how one responds.

Scientific Evidence to Support Mindfulness as a Model Self-Regulatory Mechanism

Mindfulness enables one to establish a radically different relationship to one's experience of internal sensations and outer events by cultivating present-moment awareness based on an attitude of allowance and a behavioral orientation based on wise responsivity rather than automatic reactivity. As shown in Figure 10.1, mindfulness offers an alternative response to the reactive elements of fear and anxiety in the mind and body. By purposefully engaging higher order mental functions, including attention, awareness, and attitudes of kindness, curiosity and compassion, mindfulness may effectively activate control over emotional reactions via cortical inhibition of the limbic system. Mindfulness practice, therefore, not only offers a new way of seeing, a new way of being, in relationship to one's interior life and external world, but also provides a possible means for effective self-regulation of the mind/body connection (Kabat-Zinn, 2005, 1994, 1990).

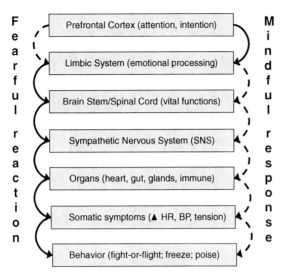

Figure. 10.1. An automatic reaction versus a mindful response to the inner experience of fear. In the case of a fearful reaction, higher-order thinking centers in the prefrontal cortex are taken "offline" (dashed line on left) so that one's mind/body experience is dictated by activation of the subcortical limbic system. Unencumbered by conscious thought, activation of fear circuitry in the limbic system stimulates sympathetic nerves that originate in the brain stem, descend through the spinal cord, and innervate internal organs to prepare the body for vigorous defensive behavior (e.g., "fight-or-flight"; solid lines on left). In the case of anxiety disorders, one's perception of threat may be greatly magnified or completely imagined. In this context, mindfulness, including paying attention on purpose to one's internal experience in the present moment, may activate prefrontal cortex areas to come "online" (solid line on right), which in turn, can inhibit reactive emotional circuitry, fear-related physiological arousal, and automatic behavior (dashed lines on right).

Considerable data support the rationale for a model of conscious, accepting attention to unfolding mind/body experiences as a skillful self-regulatory process. A brief review of several psychological and biological pathways through which mindful attention, awareness, and attitudes may influence brain and body functioning follows.

First, mindfulness practice may increase one's ability to maintain a stable focus of attention that is intentional and chosen, as opposed to automatically driven or hijacked by emotional reactivity (Jha, Krompinger, & Baime, 2007). Consequently, one may be more likely to avoid maladaptive, unconscious patterns of anxiety-producing thinking, including perseveration on upset, unpleasantness, or discomfort. Many forms of perseverative cognition, including worry, anticipatory anxiety, and rumination are associated with increased sympathetic arousal and dysregulated (persistently activated) cardiovascular, neuroendocrine, metabolic, neuromuscular, and immune processes (Brosschot et al., 2006; Brosschot, Pieper, & Thayer, 2005; Thayer & Brosschot, 2005). Notably, trait mindfulness has been associated with lower levels of worry, rumination, thought suppression, experiential avoidance, and stagnant deliberation (Baer, Smith, Hopkins, Krietemeyer, & Toney, 2006a; Feldman et al., 2007). In addition, formal training in mindfulness meditation has produced significant reductions in the tendency to ruminate and to problem-solve using an inflexible cognitive style (Feldman, Hayes,

& Greeson, 2006; Jain et al., 2007; Ramel, Goldin, Carmona, & McQuaid, 2004). Based on these shifts in attention, awareness, and cognitive processing, one might also expect mindfulness to correlate with decreased physiological arousal and somatic symptom manifestation.

A second line of scientific inquiry for the self-regulatory capacity of mindfulness practice involves the investigation of autonomic nervous system regulation. Preliminary evidence for such regulation was recently demonstrated by a study in which mindful body scan meditation produced greater parasympathetic activation than progressive-muscle relaxation (Ditto, Eclache, & Goldman, 2006). In a different study, practice of a mindful body scan meditation immediately prior to a standardized psychosocial stress task was associated with normal stress-related activation of the hypothalamic-pituitary-adrenal (HPA) axis among medical students trained in mindfulness-based stress reduction (Greeson, Rosenzweig, Vogel, & Brainard, 2001). In addition to possible attenuating effects on stress-related physiological activation, mindfulness and meditation may also induce a relaxation response, characterized by relaxed alertness, passive disregard for internal stimuli or external events, and low-level physiological arousal (Benson & Klipper, 1975).

A third line of scientific inquiry into the self-regulatory effects of mindfulness practice is the rapidly growing field of contemplative neuroscience. This burgeoning area of investigation is beginning to reveal some of the ways in which paying attention on purpose, cultivating inner attitudes of acceptance and non-judgment, and setting meaningful intentions such as to direct lovingkindness toward oneself or others can actually modify brain activity, including perception, higher order cognition, and emotion regulation (Cahn & Polich, 2006; Siegel, 2007; Wallace, 2006). One recent analysis based on a comprehensive review of the current scientific literature spanning neuroscience and meditation concluded that neural plasticity may indeed enable humans, including adults, to gradually transform mindful *states* into *traits* based on repeated exposure to experiential shifts in perspective, emotional processing, and behavioral responses (Begley, 2007). A landmark clinical intervention study by Davidson, Kabat-Zinn et al. (2003) demonstrated for the first time that systematic mindfulness training in a real-world setting can produce observable changes in the brain, namely greater left prefrontal activation, which has previously been associated with positive emotion. Of particular interest, the study by Davidson, Kabat-Zinn et al. (2003) further revealed a connection between change in the brain, and change in the body, as greater intervention-related shifts toward left prefrontal activation corresponded with more vigorous antibody responses to influenza vaccination. The connection between changes in central nervous system activity and peripheral immune function is well established (Ader, 2007). Two very recent examples of the power of the mind to change the brain include modification of attentional subsystems following eight weeks of group-based mindfulness meditation training (Jha et al., 2007), as well as enhanced prefrontal cortex regulation of affect through labeling negative emotions, a core mindfulness skill (Creswell, Way, Eisenberger, & Lieberman, 2007).

Finally, behavioral scientific evidence suggests that mindfulness practice can positively impact health-related behaviors through its effects on cognitive, affective, and physiological self-regulation. Specifically, mindfulness practice appears to increase behavioral flexibility in conditions previously associated with maladaptive rigidity, such as fear-related avoidance of normal everyday activities. A "third wave" of behavioral psychotherapies has recently emerged in which mindfulness- and acceptance-based approaches have been combined with traditional cognitive-behavioral treatment of anxiety and other emotionally dysregulated conditions, including depression, chronic pain, eating disorders, and borderline personality disorder (Baer, Fischer, & Huss, 2006b; Hayes, 2005; Lau & McMain, 2005). These new integrated psychotherapies include mindfulness-based cognitive therapy (MBCT) for active depression and anxiety as well as the prevention of depressive relapse (Finucane & Mercer, 2006; Segal et al., 2002); acceptance and commitment therapy (ACT) for anxiety disorders and chronic pain (Eifert & Forsyth, 2005; Dahl, Wilson, Luciano, & Hayes, 2005); dialectical behavior therapy (DBT) for borderline personality disorder (Linehan, 1993); and mindfulness-based eating awareness training (MB-EAT) for binge eating disorder (Kristeller, Baer, & Quillian-Wolever, 2006). The primary objective of integrating mindfulness meditation with traditional CBT is to increase treatment efficacy by exploring the relationship between acceptance of one's present moment experience as a catalyst of desired behavior change, including modification of self-destructive ways of thinking, feeling, and acting (Lau & McMain, 2005).

There is a burgeoning literature to support the integration of mindfulness- and acceptance-based strategies with traditional change-based strategies in the treatment of anxiety disorders in particular. This area of clinical investigation has recently been reviewed in special journal issues, professional handbooks, and practitioner's treatment guides (for detailed reviews see Borkovec, 2002; Craske & Hazlett-Stevens, 2002; Eifert & Forsyth, 2005; Germer, 2005; Orsillo & Roemer, 2005; Roemer, Salters-Pedneault, & Orsillo, 2006; Roemer & Orsillo, 2002; Wells, 2002). In addition, several literature reviews have concluded that mindfulness-based stress reduction programs in both controlled research and real-world community settings have produced clinically significant reductions in anxiety, mood disturbance, and stress-related physical symptoms (Baer, 2003; Brantley, 2005; Grossman, Niemann, Schmidt, & Walach, 2004; Lazar, 2005; Shigaki, Glass, & Schopp, 2006; Smith, Richardson, Hoffman, & Pilkington, 2005).

Whereas a number of different mindfulness-based clinical interventions have demonstrated effectiveness in ameliorating maladaptive cognition, negative affect, and somatic symptoms, one should note that the core intention of mindfulness practice centers around personal growth, transformation, and the pursuit of what is possible, meaningful, and truly valued in life despite any particular diagnosis, limitation, or pathology (Shapiro, Schwartz, & Santerre, 2002). By virtue of progressively awakening to one's senses, core values, intended life direction, and even spiritual purpose, mindfulness practice may be effectively coupled with other positively oriented behavior-change interventions like hypnosis to further increase contact with what is affirming, comforting, and fulfilling (Lynn, Das, Hallquist, & Williams, 2006).

Illustrative Case Report

Background: "John" is 25-year-old, single, Caucasian male graduate student with an 18-month history of treatment refractory hypertension, non-cardiac chest pain, and irregular heartbeat. He was referred for psychotherapeutic management of anxiety and recurrent panic attacks. Extensive biomedical workup prior to psychotherapy revealed no known medical cause for his physical or psychological symptoms, which were consistent with a diagnosis of panic disorder. Hypertension was reportedly non-responsive to combination treatment with a beta-blocker (Toprol XL) and diuretic (hydroxychlorothiazide; average blood pressure reading before and after medication = 145/95). The client reported that healing touch, breathwork with heartrate variability (HRV) biofeedback, and yoga instruction had been "somewhat beneficial" in reducing physical symptoms and anxiety, but not blood pressure. Several months of individual counseling for the treatment of anxiety and panic was reportedly "not helpful." Current self-care activities included yoga 5 days per week, running 1 day per week, avoiding foods with processed sugar and added sodium, eating more fruits and vegetables, and nightly deep breathing with sound therapy. The client denied illicit substance use and reported minimal alcohol use (1 drink per month). Family psychiatric history was significant for anxiety in mother and father.

Intervention: Nine individual therapy sessions, which included a combination of formal mindfulness training, anxiety-specific cognitive-behavioral skills training, and supportive psychotherapy to aid the client in clarifying his vision of optimal health, wholeness, and life direction. Treatment goals included the following: (1) ability to tolerate distressing physical symptoms without panic, (2) reduction in muscle tension, including chest pain, and (3) reduction in blood pressure. Each session emphasized formal mindfulness meditation practice (i.e., awareness of breath; body scan; mindfulness of thoughts, feelings, physical sensations, and sounds), cognitive-behavioral strategies to reduce anxiety and related physiological symptoms (e.g., cognitive restructuring, exposure therapy with response prevention), and self-help readings to reinforce learning and to provide structured mindfulness-based exercises (e.g., the book *Calming Your Anxious Mind*). In-session meditation practices were recorded for home use. During the course of treatment, "John" stated that he experienced a shift in his relationship to worrisome thoughts, noting that "[his] feelings are temporary." In addition, "John" stated that he was "not focusing on what *could* happen, but focusing on what *is* happening." The client further described a shift in his relationship to "strange pains" and other unpleasant physical sensations, noting that "[his] experience of chest tightness dissipated with allowance." Notably, "John" did not experience a panic attack during his 9 weeks of therapy, which he attributed to the shifts in perspective he experienced. Midway through therapy, he described feeling "a bit nervous, but okay" in situations that he typically feared and avoided, such as flying and being outdoors in remote areas. By the end of treatment, "John" had experienced a significant reduction in self-reported levels of anxiety and muscle tension, as well as a decrease in blood pressure readings following his regular yoga, breathwork, and mindfulness exercises. He insightfully reported discovering how to "be in control by letting go." Moreover, "John" was no longer avoiding formerly feared social situations. He reported actively engaging with co-workers, community members, and spiritual guides. And at the final session he enthusiastically shared that he had become engaged to his long-time girlfriend, because "[he] was no longer afraid." Taken together, the multimodal intervention approach with mindfulness as a core self-regulatory skill resulted in marked improvements the client's quality of life, including mental, physical, and social functioning.

Illustrative Mindfulness Practice: "Awareness of Breath"

Paying attention on purpose to your breath sensations is an effective way to reconnect with your inner experience as it is unfolding moment to moment.

(1) Notice and follow the full duration of an in breath...an out breath...and the spaces between them....

(2) Noticing the physical sensations of the breath with a sense of curiosity and kind attention...allowing the sensations to unfold moment to moment...breath by breath...observing as best you can....

(3) Noticing whether your attention is on the breath in this moment...and if it is not, where did the mind go...perhaps it began thinking, telling some sort of story about your experience, or analyzing...just noticing these thoughts or judgments as mere events in the field of your own spacious awareness....

(4) Noticing the transient nature of these mental events as you continue to surf the rising and falling waves of the in breath and the out breath...consciously choosing to acknowledge and let go of thoughts, feelings, body sensations, or impulses with the next exhale....

(5) Gently escorting your attention back to your focus on the present moment...using the sensations of the breath as your anchor for mindfulness...dropping back into your direct experience of what is here in the present moment whenever you choose....

(6) And whenever you are ready, reorienting to the room...noticing where your body makes contact with the furniture...perhaps stretching gently...and gradually opening your eyes.

Future Directions

A growing body of scientific literature demonstrates that mindfulness- and acceptance-based treatment approaches to anxiety work, in part by creating a fundamental shift in perspective toward one's inner life. Much work, however, remains to be done across conceptual, definitional, and research fronts applied to mindfulness-based interventions for fear and anxiety. In addition, there is theoretical and empirical support for the concept that paying attention on purpose to the inner experience of fear and anxiety with a sense of openness, curiosity, and acceptance can actually change one's experience by directly modifying habitual circuits and mind/body feedback loops in the brain. Additional research is needed to examine more deeply the aspects of consciousness, including awareness, attention and intention, which may be used to effectively self-regulate mind-brain-body-behavior systems implicated in anxiety and anxiety disorders. Questions that await further inquiry include: Who benefits most (and least) from mindfulness training in the context of clinical anxiety? How can mindfulness training be integrated most effectively with existing evidence-based treatment approaches, including CBT and/or medication? And finally, what is the role that institutions and communities may play in facilitating the development of greater mindfulness, individually, and collectively?

Conclusion

Human beings have the capacity for accurate, present-moment awareness of the flow of their inner life. Mindfulness is a name for this accepting and accurate awareness. Mindfulness arises from paying attention on purpose. Practicing mindfulness appears to complement and enhance established psychotherapeutic approaches to the treatment of anxiety and underlying mind/body dysregulation. Taken together, mindfulness practice appears to offer a healthy and effective means of relating to one's inner experience of fear and anxiety, in part through cultivating the ability to pay attention on purpose with an open, curious, and accepting attitude toward oneself and one's outer world. This "wise relationship" offered by mindfulness practice may help ease the suffering of excessive fear, anxiety or panic by encouraging an individual to "reperceive" the transient conditions of internal discomfort by maintaining equanimity as one's experience unfolds, moment by moment. Using the higher-order skill of "metacognitive awareness," one may more easily perceive unpleasant internal stimuli or external events simply as they are, without creating a story about one's present-moment experience that can fuel perseverative thinking, upsetting feelings, disconcerting physiological arousal, and reactive behavior in an attempt to avoid distress. With practice, as automatic reactions are deliberately acknowledged and let go and consciously chosen behavioral responses are selected, one begins to realize increasing wisdom, psychological freedom, and behavioral flexibility. These characteristics afforded by mindfulness practice define healthy, adaptive mental functioning, which includes acknowledging fear and anxiety, but does not allow fear to control or distort one's life.

References

Ader, R. (Ed.). (2007). *Psychoneuroimmunology* (4th ed.), Vol. 1. San Diego, CA: Academic Press.

American Psychiatric Association. (2000). *Diagnostic and statistical manual of mental disorders* (DSM-IV, 4th ed., text revision). Washington, DC: American Psychiatric Association.

American Psychiatric Association. (2005). *Let's talk facts about anxiety disorders.* Available at http://www.HealthyMinds.org

Baer, R. A. (2003). Mindfulness training as a clinical intervention: A conceptual and empirical review. *Clinical Psychology: Science and Practice, 10,* 125–143.

Baer, R. A., Fischer, S., & Huss, D. B. (2006b). Mindfulness and acceptance in the treatment of disordered eating. *Journal of Rational-Emotive & Cognitive-Behavior Therapy, 23,* 281–300.

Baer, R. A., Smith, G. T., Hopkins, J., Krietemeyer, J., & Toney, L. (2006a). Using self-report assessment methods to explore facets of mindfulness. *Assessment, 13,* 27–45.

Barlow, D. H. (Ed.). (2002). *Anxiety and its disorders: The nature and treatment of anxiety and panic* (2nd ed.). New York: Guilford.

Begley, S. (2007). *Train your mind, change your brain: How a new science reveals our extraordinary potential to transform ourselves.* New York: Ballantine.

Benson, H., & Klipper, M. Z. (1975). *The relaxation response.* New York: HarperCollins.

Bishop, S. D. (2002). What do we really know about mindfulness-based stress reduction? *Psychosomatic Medicine, 64*, 71-83.

Bishop, S. R., Lau, M., Shapiro, S., Carlson, L., Anderson, N. D., Carmody, J., et al. (2004). Mindfulness: A proposed operational definition. *Clinical Psychology: Science and Practice, 11*, 230-241.

Borkovec, T. D. (2002). Life in the future versus life in the present. *Clinical Psychology: Science and Practice, 9*, 76-80.

Borkovec, T. D., Ray, W. J., & Stöber, J. (1998). Worry: A cognitive phenomenon intimately lined to affective, physiological, and interpersonal behavioral processes. *Cognitive Therapy and Research, 22*, 561-576.

Brantley, J. (2003). *Calming your anxious mind: How mindfulness and compassion can free you from anxiety, fear, and panic.* Oakland, CA: New Harbinger.

Brantley, J. (2005). Mindfulness-based stress reduction. In S. M. Orsillo, & L. Roemer (Eds.), *Acceptance and mindfulness-based approaches to anxiety* (pp. 131-145). New York: Springer.

Brosschot, J. F., Gerin, W., & Thayer, J. F. (2006). The perseverative cognition hypothesis: A review of worry, prolonged stress-related physiological activation, and health. *Journal of Psychosomatic Research, 60*, 113-124.

Brosschot, J. F., Pieper, S., & Thayer, J. F. (2005). Expanding stress theory: Prolonged activation and perseverative cognition. *Psychoneuroendocrinology, 30*, 1043-1049.

Cahn, B. R., & Polich, J. (2006). Meditation states and traits: EEG, ERP, and neuroimaging studies. *Psychological Bulletin, 132*, 180-211.

Craske, M. G., & Hazlett-Stevens, H. (2002). Facilitating symptom reduction and behavior chance in GAD: The issue of control. *Clinical Psychology: Science and Practice, 9*, 69-75.

Creswell, J. D., Way, B. M., Eisenberger, N. I., & Lieberman, M. D. (2007). Neural correlates of dispositional mindfulness during affect labeling. *Psychosomatic Medicine, 69*, 560-565.

Dahl, J., Wilson, K. G., Luciano, C., & Hayes, S. C. (2005). *Acceptance and commitment therapy for chronic pain.* Reno, NV: Context Press.

Davidson, R. J., Kabat-Zinn, J., Schumacher, J., Rosenkranz, M., Muller, D., Santorelli, S. F., et al. (2003). Alterations in brain and immune function produced by mindfulness meditation. *Psychosomatic Medicine, 65*, 564-570.

Ditto, B., Eclache, M., & Goldman, N. (2006). Short-term autonomic and cardiovascular effects of mindfulness body scan meditation. *Annals of Behavioral Medicine, 32*, 227-234.

Eifert, G. H., & Forsyth, J. P. (2005). *Acceptance and commitment therapy for anxiety disorders.* Oakland, CA: New Harbinger.

Feldman, G. (2007). Cognitive and behavioral therapies for depression: Overview, new directions, and practical recommendations for dissemination. *Psychiatric Clinics of North America, 30*, 39-50.

Feldman, G., Hayes, A., Kumar, S., Greeson, J., & Laurenceau, J.-P. (2007). Mindfulness and emotion regulation: The development and initial validation of the Cognitive and Affective Mindfulness Scale-Revised (CAMS-R). *Journal of Psychopathology and Behavioral Assessment, 29*, 177-190.

Feldman, G. C., Hayes, A. M., & Greeson, J. M. (2006, November). *Reductions in stagnant deliberation during mindfulness training: A pilot study* [Abstract]. Proceedings of the 40th Annual Convention of the Association for Cognitive and Behavioral Therapies, Chicago, IL.

Finucane, A., & Mercer, S. W. (2006). An exploratory mixed methods study of the acceptability and effectiveness of mindfulness-based cognitive therapy for patients with active depression and anxiety in primary care. *BMC Psychiatry, 6*, 14.

Garland, E.L. (2007). The meaning of mindfulness: A second-order cybernetics of stress, metacognition, and coping. *Complementary Health Practice Review, 12*, 15–30.

Germer, C. K. (2005). Anxiety disorders: Befriending Fear. In C. K. Germer, R. D. Siegel, & P. R. Fulton (Eds.), *Mindfulness and psychotherapy* (pp. 152–172). New York: Guilford.

Goldstein, J. (1976). *The experience of insight: A natural unfolding.* Santa Cruz, CA: Unity Press.

Goleman, D. (1980). A map for inner space. In R. N. Walsh & F. Vaughan (Eds.), *Beyond ego* (pp. 141–150). Los Angeles: J.P. Tarcher.

Greeson, J. M., Rosenzweig, S., Vogel, W. H., & Brainard, G. C. (2001). Mindfulness meditation and stress physiology in medical students [Abstract]. *Psychosomatic Medicine, 63*, 158.

Grossman, P., Niemann, L., Schmidt, S., & Walach, H. (2004). Mindfulness-based reduction and health benefits: A meta-analysis. *Journal of Psychosomatic Research, 57*, 35–43.

Hahn, T. N. (1976). *The miracle of mindfulness: An introduction to the practice of meditation.* Boston: Beacon.

Hayes, S. C. (2005). Acceptance and commitment therapy, relational frame theory, and the third wave of behavioral and cognitive therapies. *Behavior Therapy, 35*, 639–665.

Jain, S., Shapiro, S. L., Swanick, S., Roesch, S. C., Mills, P. J., Bell, I. et al. (2007). A randomized controlled trial of mindfulness meditation versus relaxation training: effects on distress, positive states of mind, rumination, and distraction. *Annals of Behavioral Medicine, 33*, 11–21.

Jha, A. P., Krompinger, J., & Baime, M. J. (2007). Mindfulness training modifies subsystems of attention. *Cognitive, Affective, & Behavioral Neuroscience, 7*, 109–119.

Kabat-Zinn, J. (1990). *Full catastrophe living: using the wisdom of your body and mind to face stress, pain, and illness.* New York: Delacorte.

Kabat-Zinn, J. (1994). *Wherever you go, there you are: Mindfulness meditation in everyday life.* New York: Hyperion.

Kabat-Zinn, J. (2003). Mindfulness-based interventions in context: Past, present, and future. *Clinical Psychology: Science and Practice, 10*, 144–156.

Kabat-Zinn, J. (2005). *Coming to our senses: Healing ourselves and the world through mindfulness.* New York: Hyperion.

Kristeller, J. L., Baer, R. A., & Quillian-Wolever, R. (2006). Mindfulness-based approaches to eating disorders. In R. A. Baer (Ed.), *Mindfulness-based treatment approaches* (pp. 75–91). San Diego, CA: Academic Press.

Lau, M. A., & McMain, S. F. (2005). Integrating mindfulness meditation with cognitive and behavioural therapies: The challenge of combining acceptance- and change-based strategies. *Canadian Journal of Psychiatry, 50*, 863–869.

Lazar, S. W. (2005). Mindfulness research. In C. K. Germer, R. D. Siegel, & P. R. Fulton (Eds.), *Mindfulness and psychotherapy* (pp. 220–238). New York: Guilford.

Lepine, J. P. (2002). The epidemiology of anxiety disorders: Prevalence and societal costs. *Journal of Clinical Psychiatry, 63 suppl 14*, 4–8.

Linehan, M. M. (1993). *Cognitive behavioral therapy for borderline personality disorder.* New York: Guilford.

Lynn, S. J., Das, L. S., Hallquist, M. N., & Williams, J. C. (2006). Mindfulness, acceptance, and hypnosis: Cognitive and clinical perspectives. *International Journal of Clinical Hypnosis, 54*, 143–166.

McEwen, B. S. (1998). Protective and damaging effects of stress mediators. *New England Journal of Medicine, 338,* 171–179.

Narrow, W. E., Rae, D. S., Robins, L. N., & Regier, D. A. (2002). Revised prevalence based estimates of mental disorders in the United States: Using a clinical significance criterion to reconcile 2 surveys' estimates. *Archives of General Psychiatry, 59,* 115–123.

Orsillo, S. M., & Roemer, L. A. (Eds.). (2005). *Acceptance and mindfulness-based approaches to anxiety: Conceptualization and treatment.* New York: Springer.

Orsillo, S. M., Roemer, L., & Holowka, D. W. (2005). Acceptance-based behavioral therapies for anxiety. In: S.M. Orsillo & L. Roemer (Eds.), *Acceptance and mindfulness-based approaches to anxiety* (pp. 3–35). New York: Springer.

Otto, M. W., Smits, J. A. J., & Reese, H. E. (2005). Combined psychotherapy and pharmacotherapy for mood and anxiety disorders in adults: Review and analysis. *Clinical Psychology: Science and Practice, 12,* 72–86.

Ramel, W., Goldin, P. R., Carmona, P. E., & McQuaid, J. R. (2004). The effects of mindfulness meditation on cognitive processes and affect in patients with past depression. *Cognitive Therapy and Research, 28,* 433–455.

Roemer, L., & Orsillo, S. M. (2002). Expanding our conceptualization of and treatment for generalized anxiety disorder: Integrating mindfulness/acceptance-based approaches with existing cognitive-behavioral models. *Clinical Psychology: Science and Practice, 9,* 54–68.

Roemer, L., Salters-Pedneault, K., & Orsillo, S. M. (2006). Incorporating mindfulness- and acceptance-based strategies in the treatment of generalized anxiety disorder. In R. A. Baer (Ed.), *Mindfulness-based treatment approaches* (pp. 51–74). San Diego, CA: Academic Press.

Salzberg, S., & Goldstein, J. (2001). *Insight meditation.* Boulder, CO: Sounds True.

Schneiderman, N., & McCabe, P. M. (1989). Psychophysiologic strategies in laboratory research. In N. Schneiderman, S. M. Weiss, & P. G. Kaufmann (Eds.), *Handbook of research methods in cardiovascular behavioral medicine.* New York, Plenum.

Segal, Z. V., Williams, J. M., & Teasdale, J. D. (2002). *Mindfulness-based cognitive therapy for depression: A new approach to preventing depressive relapse.* New York: Guilford.

Selye, H. (1976). *The stress of life* (2nd ed.). New York: McGraw-Hill.

Shapiro, S. L., Carlson, L. E., Astin, J. A., & Freedman, B. (2006). Mechanisms of mindfulness. *Journal of Clinical Psychology, 62,* 373–386.

Shapiro, S. L., Schwartz, G. E. R., & Santerre, C. (2002). Meditation and positive psychology. In C. R. Snyder & S. J. Lopez (Eds.), *Handbook of Positive Psychology* (pp. 632–645), New York: Oxford University Press.

Shapiro, S. L., & Schwartz, G. E. R. (2000). Intentional systemic mindfulness: An integrative model for self-regulation and health. *Advanced in Mind/body Medicine, 16,* 128–134.

Sheehan, D. W., & Harnett Sheehan, K. (2007). Current approaches to the pharmacologic treatment of anxiety disorders. *Psychopharmacology Bulletin, 40,* 98–109.

Shigaki, C. L., Glass, B., & Schopp, L. H. (2006). Mindfulness-based stress reduction in medical settings. *Journal of Clinical Psychology in Medical Settings, 13,* 209–216.

Siegel, D. J. (2007). *The mindful brain: Reflection and Attunement in the Cultivation of well-being.* New York: W.W. Norton.

Smith, J. E., Richardson, J., Hoffman, C., & Pilkington, K. (2005). Mindfulness-based stress reduction as a supportive therapy in cancer care: A systematic review. *Journal of Advanced Nursing, 52,* 315–327.

Teasdale, J. D., Moore, R. G., Hayhurst, H., Pope, M., Williams, S., & Segal, Z. V. (2002). Metacognitive awareness and prevention of relapse in depression: Empirical evidence. *Journal of Consulting and Clinical Psychology, 70,* 275–287.

Thayer, J. F., & Brosschot, J. F. (2005). Psychosomatics and psychopathology: Looking up and down from the brain. *Psychoneuroendocrinology, 30,* 1050–1058.

Wallace, B. A. (2006). *Contemplative science: Where Buddhism and neuroscience converge.* New York: Columbia University Press.

Walsh, R., & Shapiro, S. L. (2006). The meeting of meditative disciplines and Western psychology: A mutually enriching dialogue. *American Psychologist, 61,* 227–239.

Wells, A. (2002). GAD, metacognition, and mindfulness: An information processing analysis. *Clinical Psychology: Science and Practice, 9,* 95–100.

11

Mindfulness and Obsessive-Compulsive Disorder: Developing a Way to Trust and Validate One's Internal Experience

Fabrizio Didonna

Not through actions, not through words
do we become free from mental contaminations,
but seeing and acknowledging them over and over
        – Anguttara Nikaya, 557–477 B.C.

Introduction

Obsessive-compulsive disorder (OCD) is a chronic and often severe psychiatric disease. It is characterized by recurrent, intrusive and distressing thoughts, images, or impulses (obsessions) and/or repetitive mental or overt acts (compulsions or neutralizing behaviors) performed to reduce or remove distress and anxiety caused by these obsessive thoughts and to prevent any perceived harmful consequences (American Psychiatric Association, 2000). This disorder has a lifetime prevalence of approximately 2–3 percent worldwide (Weissman et al., 1994) and often begins in adolescence or early adulthood, usually with a gradual onset (American Psychiatric Association, 2000). OCD is the fourth most common psychiatric disorder, following phobias, substance use disorders, and depression (Germer, Siegel & Fulton, 2005; Robins et al., 1984; Rasmussen & Eisen, 1992), and the tenth leading cause of disability in the world (World Health Organization, 1996). It is associated with high health care costs (Simon, Ormel, VonKorff, & Barlow, 1995) and leads to significant impairment in quality of life.

 OCD is also sometimes considered a thought disorder. This is why in OCD intrusive cognitions and obsessions are often, although not always, both the core feature and the trigger of the syndrome. However, OCD is not only a thought disorder. If the clinical features and phenomenology of this psychological condition are more carefully observed, it becomes clear that many OCD patients have a dysfunctional relationship with their entire private experience: sensory perceptions, emotional states, feelings and thoughts. Furthermore, we know that some people with obsessive problems (in particular chronic ones) may have no awareness of any cognitions during compulsive actions so that their rituals have became over time automatic behaviors with no need for conscious thought.

Cognitive-behavioral therapy (CBT) has long been recognized as an effective treatment for OCD, both in children and adults. In particular, exposure and response prevention (ERP) is the most widely supported psychological treatment for OCD; indeed, about 75% of patients treated with this method improve significantly and stay so at follow-up (Menzies & De Silva, 2003). Pharmacotherapy is also an effective treatment for this disorder, in particular serotonergic antidepressants, with a 40–60% response rate.

In spite of these effective interventions, a substantial number of patients who suffer from OCD do not respond well to the standard protocols of CBT and serotonergic medication and in the longer term, pharmacotherapy is associated with a high relapse rate on full discontinuation (80–90%; Pato, Zohar-Kadouch & Zohar, 1998). Furthermore, ERP can be associated with a significant dropout rate (25%) because of the highly anxiety-inducing nature of the treatment, and it is not very effective with individuals with obsession without overt compulsions (pure obsessive) and in patients with overvalued ideas (Kyrios, 2003). In addition to being refractory to current treatments, OCD patients very often share comorbidity with a range of DSM Axis I and II disorders that contribute to a compromised quality of life. This make therapies difficult to apply or reduces their effectiveness. OCD also has such a diverse, idiosyncratic clinical presentation that is not possible to consider the disorder as a single homogeneous diagnostic entity. In fact, different sub-types of the disorder have been identified that may differ in the psychological processes and fear structure that maintain the obsessive symptoms (Clark, 2004).

By definition, mindfulness (see Chapters 1 and 2) is a state which may be conceptualized, in some ways, as the antithesis of many obsessive mechanisms and phenomena and, in this sense, obsessive syndrome can be defined as a *state of mindlessness*.

This leads clinicians to wonder how and if it is possible to integrate the current treatments for OCD with "third wave approaches" (mindfulness- and acceptance-based interventions) in order to deal with these challenges, with the heterogeneity of the disorder, and to improve the effectiveness and application of already established treatment programs.

The aims of this chapter are to analyze the particular features of the relationship OCD patients have with their inner states (thoughts, emotions and sensory perception), using a mindfulness-based perspective, and to understand how this relationship might play an important role in activating and maintaining the obsessive problem. Furthermore, the author hypothesizes how mindfulness-based interventions may intervene to change and improve the relation of these patients with their private experience and consequently help them to deal with their specific *mindfulness deficits* (attention deficits, thought-action fusion, non-accepting attitude, self-invalidation of perception, interpretation bias for private experience, etc.), which invariably lead to the obsessive phenomenology. Preliminary research data and clinical observation suggest that mindfulness-based training and/or mindfulness techniques may be a helpful and effective intervention for individuals with OCD, in particular if integrated with other empirically supported treatments. Integrating more traditional treatments with mindfulness-based interventions may offer a more holistic approach for obsessive individuals – that is, one that deals with more than just the primary symptoms of the disorder and treats the "whole" person. This in turn might be of greater benefit because OCD affects so many areas and functions of a patient's life and experience, and because obsessive symptoms are quite possibly only the most evident manifestation of a more general dysfunction.

Why Can Mindfulness Be Effective for OCD? Rationale for the Use of Mindfulness for Obsessive Problems

It is better to fret in doubt than to rest in error
      Alessandro Manzoni (1785–1873), Italian novelist, poet, dramatist

A mindfulness-based approach to anxiety disorders and OCD is based on changing the way in which individuals relate to their own private experience. Within the framework of a cognitive-behavioral approach, various authors have made hypotheses which are consistent in some points with such a perspective. Salkovskis (1996) pointed out that the aim of CBT is not to persuade people that their present manner of interpreting situations is wrong, irrational or excessively negative; the objective is rather to allow them to identify where they are trapped or stuck in their way of thinking and to let them discover other ways of looking at their situation.

A cognitive-behavioral technique, called the tape-loop technique (Salkovskis, 1983), developed for individuals with pure obsessions (without overt rituals), consists in helping patients to provoke, listening repeatedly to and staying in touch with their obsessive thoughts (recorded with a tape-loop recorder). The aim is to simply observe them without reacting to them with overt or covert rituals, considering them just as thoughts, refraining from any evaluation, interpretation, or neutralization. This technique may be considered a powerful mindfulness exercise in which patients learn to see thoughts as just thoughts.

Other authors have highlighted the fact that most forms of psychopathology are characterized by an intolerance toward aspects of inner experience and also by consequent modes of avoidance aimed at removing oneself from such an experience. The most effective forms of psychotherapy tend to reduce experiential avoidance, helping patients to accept exposure to various aspects of their inner states which they fear, both in a behavioral manner and by offering encouragement to remain in contact with the painful or frightening thoughts and emotions which emerge during the course of treatment (Hayes, Wilson, Gifford, Follette, & Strosahl, 1996). As is described in other chapters of this book, experiential avoidance has been conceptualized as "the phenomenon that occurs when a person is unwilling to remain in contact with particular private experiences (e.g., bodily sensations, emotions, thoughts, memories, images) and takes steps to alter the form or frequency of these experiences or the contexts that occasion them" (Hayes et al., 1996). As is the case for other anxiety disorders, experiential avoidance is a central problem for OCD, taking the form of a number of strategies such as safety seeking behavior, rituals, seeking reassurance, and so forth. The practice of mindfulness encourages patients to suspend the "struggle" they engage in with their thoughts and emotions and renounce the ineffective experiential avoidance strategies with which, up until that time, they have defended themselves against the content of their experience. Furthermore, the clinical relevance of mindfulness in the treatment of various forms of pathology, and for OCD too, may stem from its intervening at a "radical" and *hierarchically superordinate* level in the process of activation and maintenance of the disorder. If we take into consideration the problem-formulation models of the cognitive theories, we see that mindfulness can intervene at the point of transition between activating factors and an individual's metacognitive processes (cf. Figure 11.3). Thus, the mindful state can be considered a *pre-metacognitive attitude* or *mode* that prevents patients from falling into the specific evaluations, judgments, and biases that maintain and/or overactivate the psychopathological problems. More specifically, the practice of mindfulness allows patients to acquire and develop the capacity to consciously recognize and accept undesired thoughts and emotions as an alternative to the activation of habitual, automatic and preprogrammed modes that tend to perpetuate difficulties. Moreover, it teaches patients how to "observe" their experience without entering into the mode of meta-evaluation.

The fact that disturbing cognitions in OCD are generally accompanied by *insight* (i.e., the recognition that one's symptoms are excessive and inappropriate) renders the disorder particularly amenable to mindfulness-based methods. In fact, the symptoms themselves can be easily made natural subjects of observation on the part of the patient, who is induced to view them with greater clarity and awareness (mindfulness) and initiate a process of *decentering* and *disidentification* from inner states.

OCD Phenomenology and Mindfulness Dimensions

There are two ways to slide easily through life:
To believe everything or to doubt everything.
Both ways save us from thinking.

Alfred Korzybski (1879–1950)

The core features and the source of distress of OCD are recurrent cognitive intrusions (obsessions) that create an awareness of alarm or threat (e.g., "Have I accidentally run over someone with my car? Did I lock the door?"). Individuals with OCD typically engage in some safety seeking behaviors (avoidance or escape response) in reaction to the obsessive threat. Obsessive thoughts normally take the form of either a perceived threat of physical damage to oneself or others or, in some cases, more of a moral or spiritual threat to oneself, others, or a divinity.

Considering the enormous heterogeneity and phenomenological differences that can be found in individuals suffering from OCD, clinical observation and several studies on information processing (Amir & Kozak, 2002) and obsessive belief domains (OCCWG, 1997) suggest that OCD patients may have a general problem of mistrust and lack of confidence in their private experience that leads them to continuously do something in order to prevent the feared outcomes. This particular way of relating to internal states might also be conceptualized, using a mindfulness-based perspective, as a deficit of mindfulness.

In a recent exploratory study (Didonna & Bosio, manuscript in preparation) with a sample of 21 OCD patients (mean total severity score at the Yale-Brown Obsessive-Compulsive Scale was 22 – moderate symptoms), the authors investigated the relationships between obsessive-compulsive phenomenology and mindfulness components and skills, using several clinical scales and a multifactorial mindfulness scale called the Five-Facets Mindfulness Questionnaire (FFMQ, see Baer et al., Chapter 9 of this volume; Baer, Smith, Hopkins, Krietemeyer, & Toney, 2006). The FFMQ measures a trait-like general tendency to be mindful in daily life, which is defined through five factors: *observing, describing, acting with awareness, nonjudging of inner experience*, and *nonreactivity to inner experience*. Preliminary data show that OCD patients scored significantly lower ($p < 0,001$) than the control group, a non-clinical sample, in three of the five factors plus the total score. These three dimensions found in OCD sample were *acting with awareness, nonreactivity to inner experience, and nonjudging of inner experience. Acting with awareness* includes attending to the activities of the moment. It contrasts with automatic pilot, behaving mechanically without awareness of one's actions (cf. rituals and neutralizations in OCD). *Nonreactivity to inner experience* is the tendency to allow thoughts and feelings to come and go, without getting carried away by them or caught up in them (cf. ruminations and neutralizations in OCD). *Nonjudging of inner experience* refers to taking a non-evaluative stance toward private experience (cf. cognitive biases and belief domains and assumptions in OCD). Furthermore, with respect to this latter factor, a negative correlation between Y-BOCS scores and *Nonjudging* sub-scale scores was found: the more the obsessive symptoms increase, the greater the tendency to judge the inner experience becomes. Further investigation is needed to confirm these relationships, but this data suggests that OCD may be associated with deficits in mindfulness skills which are clearly connected with some clinical features of OCD.

In what follows, the relationships and effects of mindfulness training and practice with respect to some typical OCD phenomenological features will be analyzed.

Rumination and Mindfulness

To believe with certainty we must begin with doubting
                                        – Stanislaw Leszczynski (1677–1766)

As has been observed by several authors (De Silva, 2000; Salkovskis, Richards, & Forrester, 2000b), the term *obsessional rumination* has been used in the literature indiscriminately to describe both obsessions and mental neutralizing. Interestingly, however, with respect to the contents and scope of this chapter and book, the meaning of the word "rumination" given by the *Oxford English Dictionary* (1989) is paradoxically *meditation*. Since "to ruminate" is defined as "to revolve, to turn over and over again in the mind," it is not a passive experience, and for this reason obsession cannot be a rumination (de Silva, 2003). Following the definition of de Silva (2003) "an obsessional rumination is (more likely) a compulsive cognitive activity that is carried out in response to an obsessional thought. The content of the intruding thought determines the question or the theme that the person will ruminate about." Some examples of rumination are "Am I a homosexual?," "Will I go to hell?," and "Am I going mad?"

Mindfulness training may affect processes common to many disorders (Teasdale, Segal, & Williams, 2003). Rumination is a mental behavior that characterizes several mental diseases, among them Generalized Anxiety Disorder, Social Anxiety Disorder, Depression, and OCD. Although the contents and behavioral and emotional consequences of rumination may be quite different depending on the disorder, the starting point or the trigger of the process and the clinical mechanisms of it are similar. There is a lot of agreement that rumination is a normal and adaptive process at least to some degree (in creativity, problem-solving, as a response to stress, etc.), but if this cognitive process fails to reach a natural closure, it can be maladaptive (Field, St-Leger & Davey, 2000). Rumination in both normal and clinical samples is used as a problem-solving strategy in order to decrease the discrepancy between actual state and desired state – the "doing mode" (Segal, Williams, Teasdale, 2002). For obsessive individuals, rumination is an attempt to pass from a feeling of discomfort or anxiety to calmness, or from an inflated sense of responsibility to feeling free from it. Since this strategy is related to self-states, in OCD patients, as is the case for other disorders, it is disastrously counterproductive because it maintains the undesired state (see Figure 11.3).

Several factors have been associated with iterative thinking and rumination, among them: *mood* (low mood influences cognitive perseveration; Schwarz & Bless, 1991); *perfectionism* (Bouchard, Rhéaume & Ladouceur, 1999) and *inflated responsibility* (Rhéaume, Ladouceur, Freeston & Letarte, 1994; Wells & Papageorgiu, 1998). In general, what above indicates that rumination is a reactive metacognitive process. Mindfulness-based interventions are a form of *mental training* aimed at reducing cognitive vulnerability to *reactive modes of mind* (e.g., rumination), which can intensify an individual's level of stress and emotional malaise or which can perpetuate the disorder (maintenance factors) (Segal et al., 2002). Mindfulness training (such as MBCT or MBSR) is an anti-ruminative intervention because it trains patients to shift from a "doing mode" (motivated to reduce discrepancies between actual and desired states) to a "being mode" (characterized by direct, immediate, intimate experience of the present, non-goal oriented, accepting and allowing what is) (Segal et al., 2002). In a mindful state, patients learn to have a direct experience of inner states by directly *living* the thoughts, emotions and sensations, rather than *thinking about* the experience. The anti-ruminative effect of mindfulness has been well described by Jon Kabat-Zinn (1990) in his illustration of the effects of his MBSR programme, which is also a definition of the cognitive process of *decentering*:

It is remarkable how liberating it feels to be able to see that your thoughts are just thoughts and they are not "you" or "reality. . ." For instance, if you have the thought that you have to get a certain number of things done today and you don't recognize it as a thought but act as if it's "the truth," then you have created a reality in that moment in which you really believe that those things must all be done today .... On the other hand, when such a thought comes up, if you are able to step back from it and see it clearly, then you will be able to prioritize things and make sensible decisions about what really does need doing. You will know when to call it quits during the day. So the simple act of recognizing your thoughts as thoughts can free you from the distorted reality they often create and allow for more clear sightedness and a greater sense of manageability in your life. (pp. 69–70).

Mindfulness practice is training that can help prevent ruminative processes because it uses intentional control of attention to establish a type of alternative information processing or cognitive mode that is incompatible with the factors that maintain the disorder (see Figure 11.3). During mindfulness practice patients are invited to intentionally maintain awareness of a particular object of attention, such as the physical sensations in the body while breathing, moment by moment (Teasdale, 1999). Whenever the mind wanders (and this is a normal condition) to thoughts, emotions, sounds or other physical sensations, the contents of awareness are noted. One then raises the intention to gently, but firmly bring awareness back to the original focus of attention. This focus, which is normally an internal experience that is always available, such as breathing, can be a clear and firm "anchor" for patients that brings their awareness back to the present moment limiting the extent to which they become lost in the reality created by the thought streams they are so often immersed in (rumination) (Teasdale, 1999). This process is repeated continuously on a regular basis through several moments of daily practice of mindfulness. This practice provides repeated experiences in which the ability to relate to thoughts as passing and impermanent events in the mind is facilitated by choosing a non-cognitive (frequently bodily) primary focus of attention, against which the experience of thoughts can be registered as simply another event in awareness rather than as the primary "stuff" of the mind or the self (Teasdale, 1999), which is a common mode of processing for OCD sufferers. As patients observe the content of thoughts as they arise and then to let go of them and return to the original focus of attention, they learn to develop a *decentered* and *detached* perspective with respect to every kind of cognitions. Several studies (Jain et al., 2007; Kocovski, Fleming, & Rector, 2007) carried out with non-clinical and clinical samples (social anxiety, depression) have showed that mindfulness- and acceptance-based interventions lead to decreases in rumination and that these decreases in rumination account for reductions in depressive and anxious symptoms (see also Chapter 5 of this volume for more details).

To conclude, mindfulness training may be an effective intervention to prevent or neutralize the tendencies to ruminate that obsessive individuals have, allowing them to learn to stay in touch with their intrusive (normal) thoughts without reacting to them in dysfunctional and counterproductive ways.

Inflated Responsibility and Mindfulness

> Move, but don't move the way fear moves you.
> Rumi

In the last few decades, many authors (Salkovskis, 1985; Salkovskis, Shafran, Rachman & Freeston, 1999; Rachman & Shafran, 1998, Obsessive Compulsive Cognitions Working Group-OCCWG, 1997) have highlighted the problem of an inflated sense of responsibility in OCD patients. Salkovskis

(1985) considers an exaggerated sense of responsibility to be a cardinal feature of the disorder. It is particularly common among patients whose main problem is checking and it tends to generate intense guilt. Inflated responsibility is defined by OCCWG (1997) as the "belief that one is especially powerful in producing and preventing personally important negative outcomes. These outcomes are perceived as essential to prevent. They may be actual problems, or perceived moral dilemmas. Such beliefs may pertain to responsibility for doing something to prevent or undo harm, and responsibility for errors of omission and commission." An example of this kind of belief is: "If I don't act when I foresee danger, I am to blame for any bad consequences."

OCD patients tend to misinterpret the meaning of responsibility, because for them, this concept can only suggest "duty" or "rules." They then mindlessly impose these rules upon themselves, most likely because they have been told that this is the "right" and "proper" way to live or because some particular experiences (in certain cases even traumatic ones) gave them an inflated sense of responsibility. However, authentic responsibility means being *aware* of the impact of our actions and being willing to *feel* how our behavior *really* affects ourselves and others. Responsibility means "*response-ability*" – the ability to be present in each moment and respond appropriately to each event we are confronted with (Trobe, T. & Trobe, G. D., 2005); this is, in fact, a definition of mindfulness. When people are accountable in this way, they are able to more deeply respect and trust themselves (*mindful self-validation*). This is because in a mindful state (paying attention to the present moment without judgement), patients are more able to clearly understand their own real involvement in the problematic situation. Therefore, mindfulness-based therapy may intervene in order to give patients a more functional and realistic meaning of the sense of responsibility, which is so seriously distorted in people suffering from obsessive problems.

Attentional Bias and Mindfulness

There is good evidence that OCD patients show disorder-specific attentional bias for threat (Lavey, van Oppen, & van den Hout, 1994; Foa, Ilai, McCarthy, Shoyer, & Murdock, 1993). This problem seems to involve both a general inability to inhibit processing of irrelevant information as well as distraction by threat relevant cues (Amir & Kozak, 2002). These individuals may be paying particular attention to threatening information relevant to their current concerns. Furthermore, because of their attentional biases, OCD patients are not able to attend to information that would disconfirm their fears (Didonna, 2003). OCD sufferers also show both deficits in orienting attention (how attention is placed) and conflict attention (the process of inhibiting an automatic response to attend to a less automatic response; Fan, McCandliss, Sommer, Raz, & Posner, 2002). These biases in information processing might be also conceptualized as *mindfulness deficits*. In fact, by definition, mindfulness is a state of mind in which individuals pay *attention* in a particular way: to the present moment, on purpose and without judgement (Kabat-Zinn, 1994). This definition can easily allow us to understand how mindfulness training and practice may intervene to change the way in which

OCD patients pay attention to their internal and external experience because mindfulness is a practice in which individuals learn and train themselves to direct attention in a wholesome, productive and efficient manner.

A group of leading authors (Bishop et al., 2004) in the field of mindfulness highlighted that the first component of mindfulness involves the *self-regulation of attention* so that it is focuses on the immediate experience, thereby allowing for increased recognition of mental events in the present moment. Mindfulness begins by bringing awareness to current experience – observing and attending to the ongoing stream of thoughts, feelings, and sensations from moment to moment – by regulating the focus of attention. This leads to a feeling of being very alert to what is occurring in the here-and-now (Bishop et al., 2004). It is hypothesized that self-regulation of attention involves two specific skills and components: *sustained attention* and *skills in switching*. *Skills in sustained attention* refer to the ability to maintain a state of vigilance over prolonged periods of time (Parasuraman, 1998; Posner & Rothbart, 1992) as is required to maintain an awareness of current experience. *Skills in switching* allow the patient to bring attention back to a mindful focus (e.g., the breath) once an internal experience has been acknowledged. *Switching* involves flexibility of attention so that one can shift the focus from one object to another (Posner, 1980). Patients with OCD lack both these abilities, and in fact, have a selective attention to threatening stimuli. But they are not really aware of the current experience and are unable to switch attention to another focus.

The self-regulation of attention also creates a non-elaborative awareness of private experience as it arises. Rather than getting caught up in ruminative, elaborative thought streams about one's experience and its origins, implications, and associations, mindfulness involves a direct experience of events in the mind and body (Teasdale, Segal, Williams, & Mark, 1995). This could be considered the opposite of what OCD patients normally do.

Clinical observation suggests that normally checking compulsions are mindless behaviors in which attention is paid to the checking actions rather than to the real perceptions and outcomes derived from the rituals or to what the individual learns through the behavior. Therefore, OCD sufferers are not able to bring mindful attention to their inner experience and then to the rituals, which are aimed at changing or avoiding that experience. The development of mindfulness can be associated with improvements in sustained attention and switching, which can be objectively measured using standard vigilance tests (e.g., Klee & Garfinkel, 1983) and tasks that require the subject to shift mind-set (Rogers & Monsell, 1995).

Recent studies (Zylowska, Ackerman, Yang, et al., 2008; Jha, Krompinger & Baime, 2007) which investigated the effects of a mindfulness meditation approach for Attention Deficit Hyperactivity Disorder (ADHD) and also for non-clinical samples showed that this kind of training can lead to significant cognitive changes, in particular those related to a reduction in various measures of attentional processes including alerting, orienting, conflict attention and attentional set-shifting (see Chapter 17 of this volume). These early findings suggest that mindfulness training might be effective to improve attentional deficits in OCD too, in which these biases may be relevant activating and maintenance factors for obsessive symptoms.

Thought-Action Fusion, Level of Insight and Mindfulness

Thought-action fusion is a cognitive bias, often found in OCD, in which a fusion or confusion between thought and action arises (Rachman, 1993). It may take two forms: (1) probability bias, in which the individual believes that having an unwanted thought concerning harm increases the risk of actual harm occurring to someone, and (2) morality bias, in which the person believes that having the unwanted intrusive thought is morally equivalent to carrying out the repugnant act (Rachman & Shafran, 1998). In this mental process, individuals tend to create a sort of identification with an aspect of their own private experience. In some way they say: "This thought is me," or "I am this thought," or "This thought is something real," creating a sort of reification of cognitive experience.

In mindfulness practice the thinking mind is considered similar to one of the five senses that registers (but does not cause) visual, auditory, and other incoming stimuli. Negative thoughts are similarly registered and noticed as transient "thought stimuli" that occur in the mind. As such, negative thoughts are not overpersonalized and do not serve as dictators of subsequent feelings and activities (e.g., rituals, neutralizations). Cognitions are accepted as the natural and normal behavior of the mind, but not as inherently defining the self (Marlatt & Kristeller, 1999; Epstein, 1996).

The mindfulness practice of *self monitoring* thoughts and other mental events trains individuals to become less identified with their own private experience ("thoughts without a thinker" – see Epstein, 1996), no matter how upsetting or entertaining they may be. Through meditation, individuals can learn to develop a sense of equanimity or balance without being absorbed into their own mental processes. This process has been called "mental disidentification" (Marlatt & Kristeller, 1999). As Goleman (1988) suggests, "The first realization in meditation is that the phenomena contemplated are distinct from the mind contemplating them." When individuals enter into this process of disidentification from mental states, they begin to see that these thoughts and feelings are not them. They happen accidentally and are neither an organic part of the patients nor are they obliged to follow them (Snelling, 1991. p. 55).

It has been ascertained that mindfulness training leads to a significant shift in perspective (Shapiro, Carlson, Astin, & Freedman, 2006; see also the Chapter 5 of this volume) and several concepts have been coined over the past few years to define these metacognitive processes in which patients learn to become a non-attaching and non-reacting observer and witness of their own inner states: *decentering* (Safran & Segal, 1990), *deautomatization* (Deikman, 1982; Safran & Segal, 1990), *reperceiving* (Shapiro et al., 2006) and *detachment* (Bohart, 1983). Safran and Segal (1990) define *decentering* (also called distancing) as the ability to "step outside of one's immediate experience, thereby changing the very nature of that experience" (p. 117). Decentering is also defined as the ability to observe one's thoughts and feelings as temporary events in the mind rather than reflections of the self that are necessarily true (see also Baer et al., Chapter 9 of this volume; Fresco et al., 2007). Decentering involves awareness of experiences without identifying with them or being carried away by them, and includes taking a present-focused, non-judgemental stance toward thoughts and feelings, accepting them as they are (Fresco, Segal, Buis, & Kennedy, 2007). As Segal et al. (2002) have suggested, mindfulness-based interventions, such as Mindfulness-Based Cognitive Therapy, may lead to clinical change not so much through the alteration of thought content, as through "decentering," by which individuals learn to switch from a perspective that thoughts represent reality to a perspective in which their thoughts are viewed as only an internal event. Deikman describes *deautomatization* as "an undoing of the automatic processes that control perception and cognition" (p. 137). *Reperceiving* (Shapiro et al., 2006) is conceptualized as a *metamechanism* in which individuals are able to disidentify from the contents of consciousness (thoughts, emotions, and body sensations) as they arise, and simply be with them instead of being defined (i.e., controlled, conditioned, or determined) by them. Through reperceiving patients realize: "this pain is not me," "this depression is not me," "these thoughts are not me," as a result of being able to observe them from a meta-perspective (Shapiro et al., 2006). Another related cognitive process, in which the focus is on changing individual's relationship to thought rather than attempting to alter the content of thought itself, is the concept of *cognitive defusion* (Hayes, Strosahl, and Wilson's, 1999). The authors noted that the ability to pay attention to private experience and becoming a detached observer of it is often associated with a *shift in the self-sense*. Through defusion, which is considered a change in perspective, identity begins to shift from the contents of awareness to awareness itself. Hayes et al. (1999) define this process as the shift from "self as content" (that which can be observed as an object in consciousness) to "self as context" (that which is observing consciousness itself). Individuals may develop a sense of the "self" as an ever-changing system of constructs, concepts, sensations, images and beliefs that are eventually seen to be as impermanent and transient conditions rather than a stable entity. One final related concept is the process of *detachment* (Bohart, 1983), which "encompasses the interrelated processes of gaining distance, adopting a phenomenological attitude, and the expansion of attentional space" (Martin, 1997).

As has been well stated by Schwartz & Beyette (1997), "there is an observing aspect of the mind that can really maintain its independence even though the contents of the consciousness are being flayed around by the disease process. We are really training the mind to not identify with those experiences but to see ourselves as separable from those experiences."

All the metacognitive processes illustrated above, developed through the practice of mindfulness, can have a significant clinical relevance for obsessive pathology. The problem in OCD is that individuals often tend to *reify* their rapport with cognitions and consider thoughts as something real, as a true and permanent representation of reality or *self* (in particular in patients with poorer insight). Such "real" thoughts are then given inflated importance (OCCWG, 1997). When obsessive sufferers realize the impermanence of all mental states, they are more able to relate to private experience with a sense of *non-attachment*, developing a higher level of tolerance for unpleasant inner states and disengaging themselves from the automatic behavioral patterns (neutralizations, compulsions, reassurance seeking) which maintain the obsessive syndrome. Thus it can be assumed that for OCD patients, these mechanisms may lead to an improvement and increase in the level of insight and ego-dystonicity (referred to the degree that the content of the obsession is contrary to or inconsistent with a person's sense of self as reflected in his or her core values, ideals, and moral attributes, (Purdon, 2001; Purdon & Clark, 1999). This, in turn, may decrease both the tendencies to judge and to react (with compulsive behavior) to the cognitive, emotional and sensory experience and to activate thought-action fusion bias. Furthermore, in mindfulness- and acceptance-based interventions, the therapist often makes use of metaphors or guided visualization exercises (see Chapter 7) that have the purpose of allowing patients to internalize and indirectly incorporate various elements of outer reality (connected in some way with mindfulness principles – e.g., *lake meditation*, see Appendix A), which may be subsequently be transformed into powerful resources. Metaphor is also proposed as a therapeutic tool to develop and improve decentering, detachment and defusion processes.

Acceptance and OCD

A core problem for obsessive individuals is *acceptance*. For them it is very difficult, or often impossible, to accept several experiences connected with their problem: intrusive or obsessive thoughts, imagined and feared consequences of not preventing harm or doing things in a wrong way, negative emotions (anxiety, guilty, shame, disgust), physical sensations. Therefore, OCD individuals are not able to accept potentially normal and nonthreatening experiences (see also the section on problem formulation and Figure 11.3).

As it is well illustrated in other chapters of this book, acceptance is one of the main components of mindfulness-based approaches and it is defined as a moment by moment process by which one moves away from viewing thoughts and feelings as reality or things that need to be changed, and toward embracing them simply as internal events that do not need to be altered without unnecessary attempts to change their frequency or form, especially when doing so would cause psychological harm (Hayes et al., 1999). Through acceptance, individuals can notice internal events they experience while simultaneously renouncing any effort to avoid or change these events and responding to the facts which actually occurred rather than the inner experience elicited by such events (Hayes et al., 1996). The use of acceptance for OCD patients implies a conscious abandonment of behavior that functions as experiential avoidance and a willingness to experience one's emotions and cognitions as they arise, without any secondary elaborative processing (judgement, interpretation, appraisal, meta-evaluation).

Mindfulness is a training process through which patients learn to calmly observe their inner experience with a feeling of clarity and without responding to it (Schwartz & Beyette,1997). The process of observing in and of itself helps people increasingly come to the realization that they can change their responses to those thoughts in very adaptive ways. In order to help OCD individuals to observe and analyze their level of acceptance toward private experience, in particular thoughts, and to develop and cultivate this attitude, it may be useful to give patients a task to carry out on their

Thoughts, Emotions, Sensations	Am I trying to cultivate acceptance now towards these internal experiences? (Yes/No)	Was I able to allow and accept this state (Emotion, sensation, thought) and stay in touch to it, without react? If not why?	*COMMENTS* How do I feel now if I was able to accept? How do I feel now if I was not able to accept? What are the consequences?

Figure. 11.1. Homework table of acceptance.

own (see Figure 11.1) in which they are asked to fill in a form as nega- tive internal experiences arise, noticing the private experience (emotions, sensations, thoughts) during critical situations and whether or not they are willing accept that state, if they are able to cultivate acceptance toward it, and if not why, and what the consequences of doing or not doing this are. This exercise can improve the metacognitive awareness of patients' attitude toward private experience and allow them to realize what the consequences of this attitude are on their cognitive and emotional experience and dis- ease.

Obsessive Doubt and Self-Invalidation of the Perceptive-Sensorial Dimension

> We do not see things as they are, we see them as we are.
>   The Talmud

Several studies have found that OCD patients, in particular checkers, lack *confidence* in their memory (Sher, Frost, & Otto, 1983; McNally & Kohlbeck, 1993) and are less satisfied with the vividness of their memories (Constans, Foa, Franklin, & Matthews, 1995). Empirical observation and some studies have suggested that this lack of confidence is only related to OCD-related stimuli (Foa et al., 1997) and threatening situations, and is significantly lower or often absent in normal or safe conditions (e.g., during a psychotherapy session).

More specifically, Hermans, Martens, De Cort, Pieters, & Eelen (2003) showed that this low cognitive confidence in OCD patients is present on at least three different levels: low confidence in their memory for actions, low confidence in their ability to discriminate actions from imaginations, and low confidence in their ability of keeping attention undistracted.

According with the already discussed attentional bias hypothesis (Lavey et al., 1994; Amir & Kozak, 2002), Hermans et al. (2003), in order to explain this lack of confidence, suggested that individuals suffering from OCD would mistrust the accuracy or completeness of previous avoidance behavior (checking, washing) because important elements of this behavior might have been missed due to distraction or moments of lessened attention.

It has also been suggested (Didonna, 2003, 2005) that this low confidence in cognitive experience in patients suffering from OCD – and "checkers" in particular – may depend on a cognitive bias in processing and/or using relevant sensory information regarding situations that tend to generate obsessive cognitions. This bias can be conceptualized as a *self-invalidation of perceptive experience*. It is hypothesized that this problem may play a decisive role in the activation of pathological doubt and in the relationship between the patient's conscious perceptive experience and the obsessive phenomenology.

Clinical observation (Didonna, 2005) suggests that, during psychotherapy sessions, obsessive patients are usually able to recall the perceptive experience they felt during the anxiety-evoking events that activated obsessions. Nevertheless, we also find that during an obsessive crisis they experience considerable difficulty in voluntarily recovering and trusting their own sensorial information relating to that event. They then become unsure of their own experience. If this information were used instead of being discounted, it might, neutralize obsessive doubt. On account of the vicious-cycle phenomenon in which the patient becomes ensnared (cf. Figure 11.2), this initial validation deficit consequently leads to an over-evaluation of the doubt, which tends to *invalidate* and/or increasingly "scotomizes" (to cover or exclude some elements in the perceptual and experiential field) and obscure the objectivity of their own perceptive experience. As was stated by Pema Chodron (2002), an American buddhist nun, "Whether we experience what happens to us as an obstacle and enemy or as teacher and friend depends entirely on our perception of reality. It depends on our relationship with ourselves."

In the following case example, a 23-year-old man performed "checking rituals" consisting in returning home up to 15–20 times to check whether he had closed the Venetian blinds of his apartment on the eight floor of the condominium where he lived. He feared that a burglar might break into the apartment while he was out and steal all of his possessions. During therapy, the patient was able to recall a visual memory of the blinds fully closed and the darkened rooms; he could visualize his hands moving as he manipulated the strap beside the window to roll down the shutters and he had an auditory memory of the noise that it made. Both the visual and auditory memories were related precisely and with considerable detail. The problem was that during the obsessive crisis, the patient did not use these memories at all.

To comprehend the underlying cause of the development of the obsessive phenomenon it may be useful to ask a seemingly obvious question: why do most people *not* present obsessive symptoms? The hypothesis proposed by the author – also useful in terms of the process of *normalization* of the obsessive phenomenon with patients – is that in people who do not have

OCD symptoms, an obsessive doubt concerning actions or events is not activated because they automatically use, and simultaneously *self-validate* their
own experience in the various situations they encounter, rendering such
consciousness salient and affording it due priority. Even obsessive patients
(in particular those with good insight) would have, in their *episodic memory
store*, a substantially clear memory of sensorial experiences. Awareness or
use of this memory could neutralize the doubt activation, but these patients
are not able to validate this information.

To validate one's own perceptive experience means that one considers it
as real and objective: the awareness of the perceptive experience is hierarchically superordinate in the activation of the emotions and the behavior of an
individual. For example, if after leaving their home, people wonder whether
they have switched off the light or not, they may immediately recover the
memory of the visual experience of seeing a dark room or recall a vision of a
finger as it presses down on the light switch. Although the image may not be
perfectly clear, such a recollection is usually sufficient in itself to prevent the
activation of doubt. In obsessive patients as well, and especially in those with
good insight, we may presume that a clear memory of sensory experiences
(visual, auditive, tactile, etc.) is present in the episodic memory store, the
awareness and use of which would allow them to see their recurrent doubts
as groundless. However, these patients are unable to validate the information
available to them. The patient's experience would thus in fact eventually be
relegated to a secondary position with respect to the obsessive doubt. The
patient may for example say, "I know I turned off the tap. I remember doing
it, but I am not absolutely certain that I did and I really need to be sure!" This
type of phenomenon only occurs when the patient has to face a situation that
can be associated in some way with the feared event. Moreover, its occurrence is facilitated by a dysfunctional evaluation of the *gravity* of the event,
rather than its likelihood. Consequently, an event can be evaluated by the
subject as being so "serious" (even if highly unlikely) that even the slightest
risk of its occurrence is unacceptable. This lack of confidence in one's sensorial experience is hypothesized to be linked to a fear found in OCD patients –
should a personal error actually occur – of being excluded, marginalized, and
humiliated by their social group (Guidano & Liotti, 1983; Didonna, 2003,
2005). A mindfulness-based treatment would thus have an important influence on the capacity of obsessive patients to validate the recollection and
awareness of their perceptual experience moment by moment. In this way,
the practice of mindfulness would serve as an antidote to the activation of
obsessive ideation, thereby managing to neutralize pathological doubts.

One of the problems in OCD sufferers is that in anxiety-evoking situations
and during obsessive crises, they may very well enter in a different state of
mind. Insight into the unreasonable or senseless nature of a person's obsessions is situation bound (Kozak & Foa, 1994; Steketee & Shapiro, 1995). In
fact, in clinical practice it has often been observed that the level of insight
is lowest in OCD patients during critical situations compared with "normal,"
nonthreatening conditions. For this reason these patients might benefit from
cultivating a regular mindfulness practice, which has the effect, among the
others, of stabilizing and normalizing one's states of mind and metacognitive
processes (see also Chapter 4 of this book).

A Mindfulness-Based Technique: The Perceptive Experience Validation Technique (PEV)

> Trust is intimately connected to the correspondence between our perceptions and reality.
>
> – *Matthieu Ricard*

The hypothesis illustrated in the previous section forms the *rationale* of a therapeutic technique called the Perceptive Experience Validation (PEV). This technique is aimed at training OCD patients, in particular checkers, to pay attention mindfully to their own perceptive experience and to *validate* as much as possible the memory and consciousness of it, using them as an "antidote" against the activation of obsessive ideation. As was stated above, during obsessive crises, patients' information processing skills can be compromised. They often experience significant difficulties in believing their own memory of the perceptual experiences they have had. Normally, OCD patients who don't have a totally incapacitating disorder and who have good insight also have good awareness of their decision making processes, successfully making decisions numerous times each day in situations unconnected with the disorder. To accomplish this, they must be fully aware of the perceptual information that informed those decisions. The problem arises in situations that evoke anxiety. In such situations, OCD patients are not able to validate (or are not used to validating) their perceptions and cannot, therefore, fight the doubt, which eventually takes over.

Based on this hypothesis, the author (Didonna, 2003, 2005) developed a procedure whose goal is to help patients to validate their perceptual experience during critical situations in order to credit this memory as objective and real, and consequently, to minimize the importance of the doubt. The basic idea, supported by clinical experience with dozens of clinical cases, is that helping and training patients to pay attention to the ongoing stream of their own experience in a mindful way and to validate it continuously can function as an *antidote* to the doubt. This initially takes place during the session and the patient learns to develop a continuous and persistent habit to do the same in vivo, first in normal (non-anxiety inducing) and then in critical situations. This activity may favor a reduction in or elimination of the deficit in working memory and the *self-invalidating* cognitive bias. It is hypothesized that a regular practice of a mindful, sustained attention to ordinary stimuli during daily life, and actively giving those perceptions a clear and intentional validation, can also create an improvement in the self-regulation of attention.

The technique is a process involving several different steps (see Figure 11.2). The first one is to have the patients write a precise description of an intrusive thought (doubt, obsession, image) they would like to work on, and indicate how convinced they are (%) that the feared event will happen, has happened, how serious it is, or that they could be responsible for it, and the level of discomfort or anxiety they experience thinking of it (0–100). The patients are then asked to divide the paper into two columns. On the left, they are to write down all of the information they remember about their perceptive experience in a given situation that are incompatible or conflicting with the obsessive doubt (e.g., I *saw* that the window was closed). On the right side of the paper, the patients are to write down anything and everything that keeps the obsessive doubt active (inferences, suppositions, hypotheses, selective reasoning, etc.) and that are not in any way based on their experience (e.g., "I could have done it without realizing it"). It is important that the patient understand that they are not to write on the left-hand side anything that comes from external reassurances or any rituals that would just be reinforced by being placed there. The next step has two aspects: On the one hand, there must be an intervention of *validation of the perceptive experience* of the patients (the left-hand side). The therapist confirms through verbal and non-verbal behavior that he/she believes that what the patient claims he/she has perceived is real, objective and indisputable. On the other hand, the therapist has to try to help the patients learn to observe the experience in a mindful way and to *self-validate* the experience, not only during a session, but more importantly, outside as well. This will automatically, and often immediately, lead the patients to place less importance on the elements that "feed" the doubt. One sentence often used with OCD patients in order to help them in this process is "Your senses don't lie."

Indeed, following a series of exercises, these elements (on the right side of the paper) will tend to be less and less present. It is important that the patients understand that they shouldn't put too many perceptive elements on the left-hand side of the page since this would lead to useless ruminating and be counterproductive. A single element related to the perceptual experience should be considered enough with most people to neutralize the doubt and put an end to the obsessive ritual. They need to be aware that this is what they actually do in situations not related to the obsessive problem. For example, one of the following recollections can be considered necessary and enough: "I did not *hear* a crash," "I *saw* that the room was dark when I left the house," "I didn't *hear* any sounds of a newborn coming from that rubbish heap," and so forth. At the end of the exercise, the patients are asked to identify again the degree to which they are convinced that the thought they are having in that moment related to the feared event is true and realistic, and compare the initial level, of discomfort to the present level.

In a single case study (Didonna, 2003) (see Figure 11.2), a 28-year-old patient was obsessed with the idea that when she had been driving her car she might have hit another vehicle – *without realizing it* – and that the ensuing damage would have later subsequently cause the death of the other driver. Analyzing the patient's recollection of her actual experience during the feared event, it was discovered during a treatment session that she possessed a very clear memory of her sensory experience which would have neutralized and prevented any obsessive doubt (e.g., "I didn't hear the sound of an impact" or "I didn't feel that I was losing control of the vehicle"). What the patient was incapable of doing was to simply validate and utilize those sensory experiences during her obsessive crisis. The therapist helped the patient validate the recollection, which was quite clear, of her actual experience, giving increased credibility to here experience (column on the left). This led the patient to automatically place less importance on the subjective elements that had previously fed her obsessive doubt (right-hand column). At the end of the exercise, both her level of conviction with respect to the obsessive thought and her level of discomfort decreased. The patient stated: "Today I understood that continuously seeking all of the elements that feed my doubts and obsessions (right-hand column) only leads to new doubts and

Intrusive thought: *"I'm afraid I hit a truck that was behind me when I was driving out of my parking space."*

Level of conviction: 75%

Level of anxiety/distress (0-100): 80

Information coming from my own perceptive experience	Information not coming from my own perceptive experience
(What did I **see, hear, smell, feel, touch, taste** in that situation?)	(What am I **worried** about? What do I **think** happened?)
• *I didn't hear* any noise on my car	• *I think* I moved backwards
• When I looked in the rear view mirror *I saw* that the truck was far enough away not to cause me any problems	• The driver *might not* have realised I hit him
• When I left I *heard* a noise, but it wasn't the typical noise you hear when you hit a car it	• *I think* I was at the right angle to have hit it
• *I saw* that the bumper wasn't damaged	
• *I saw* the truck pull out into the road without any problem	

Level of conviction at the end of the exercise: 10%

Level of anxiety/distress (0-100): 20

Figure. 11.2. Example of the use of the perceptive experience validation (PEV) technique.

obsessions; from now on I want to place more importance on my actual experience."

This procedure was repeated during other sessions and by the end, the patient only needed one "objective" element in the left-hand column to neutralize the obsessive doubts on the other side of the paper. The patient was also asked to conduct the same procedure at home each time obsessive ideations occurred and to try and maintain a mindful and validating attitude toward her own experience throughout the day even when she wasn't in an anxiety-evoking situation. Treatment gains were maintained at 3-month follow-up.

More than a therapeutic technique, it might be more appropriate to say that PEV is a mindful mental style or attitude. It is an alternative way for OCD patients to relate to themselves and their experience, helping them see that certainty is unnecessary because the information that they already possess is sufficient.

OCD Problem Formulation and Mindfulness

As has been pointed out by Teasdale et al. (2003), when a mindfulness-based intervention is provided for individuals with specific disorders, it is particularly important to share with patients, both in individual and group settings, a clear problem formulation explaining the potential role of the mindful state in order to prevent the maintaining mechanisms of the disorder. Mindfulness training is effective when it is linked to coherent alternative views of patients' problems, views that are shared with patients and reinforced through the mindfulness practices (Teasdale et al., 2003).

Anxiety disorders are activated and maintained by dysfunctional metacognitions about normal and innocuous mental events. Following the standard cognitive conceptualizations of psychological disorders, the clinical relevance of mindfulness for several diseases, and for OCD too, might lie in its intervening at a radical and hierarchically superordinate level, in particular, at a point between inner and outer activating stimuli and the metacognitive processes and maintaining mechanisms conducive to psychological distress (Figure 11.3). Mindfulness, which is a *being mode* (see Chapter 1), can be cultivated to prevent or deactivate the metacognitive processes which lead patients into the vicious, self-perpetuating cycles of obsessions and the associated counterproductive behaviors. (Didonna, 2006, 2008).

If we compare OCD with a related diagnosis such as panic disorder, we can observe that in both disorders the problem stems from how some normal experiences are perceived (Figure 11.3). Looking at a standard cognitive model of these problems, in the case of the obsessive-compulsive syndrome, the trigger is normally an intrusive cognition, while in panic disorder, in the trigger is one or more normal physical sensations. Subsequently, the patient starts to interpret these normal experiences as dangerous (metacognition), which in the case of OCD may involve a pervasive idea of responsibility for harm or damage, while in panic disorder it will involve a thought of imminent catastrophe. These two meta-evaluations then activate the maintenance mechanisms of the two disorders: "Doing mode" (neutralization, rituals, seeking reassurance, rumination) and cognitive biases (perceptive self-invalidation, attentional biases, thought-action fusion, non-acceptance bias) on the one hand and *safety seeking behavior* on the other (avoidance, flight, etc.), but also emotional states, anxiety, guilt, shame, disgust, depression in OCD and anxiety in Panic, which will reinforce the initial metacognitions that maintain the disorder. Compulsions, neutralizations, and safety behaviors are acts that are performed in an attempt to reduce

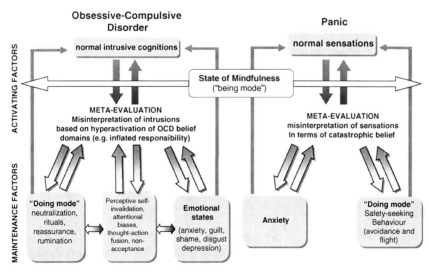

Figure. 11.3. A cognitive formulation of the role and effects of mindfulness state and practice with respect to the activating and maintenance factors in OCD and panic disorder.

the perceived threat and the anxiety and distress caused by the metacognitions, but the relief is only temporary: indeed, these behaviors increase, rather than reduce, the anxiety. These reactions maintain the problem and prevent habituation to the anxiety and disconfirmation of the patient's fears (Didonna, Salkovskis, 1996, 2006, 2008).

The activation of a mindful state (a "being mode") intervenes at an early stage in the activation of the symptoms of these disorders, allowing the patient to take a different attitude toward "normal" internal initial experiences (thoughts, sensations) from the moment he/she becomes aware of them, by means of an accepting, self-validating, and non-judgmental attitude. Such an attitude, cultivated through mindfulness practice, prevents the activation of those meta-evaluational processes that would otherwise give rise to the anxious syndrome (Figure 11.3).

Mindfulness training can help OCD patients inhibit secondary elaborative processing of the thoughts, feelings, and sensations that arise in the stream of consciousness and may cause improvements in cognitive inhibition, particularly at the level of stimulus selection (Bishop et al., 2004). This effect can be objectively evaluated using specific tests that involve the inhibition of semantic processing (e.g., emotional Stroop; Williams, Mathews, & MacLeod, 1996).

Integrating CBT and Mindfulness

Always do what you are afraid to do!
Ralph Waldo Emerson

Unlike standard CBT, in mindfulness-based interventions the main goal is not to change the content of the patient's system of cognitions but rather to change his or her way of relating to it. During mindfulness training, patients are helped to shift from a focus on the past and on the future (conditioned by memories and rumination) to a focus on the present moment, developing a process of *decentering* and *disidentification* from personal experience (Segal et al., 2002). Mindfulness-based treatments focus on altering the *impact* of and *response* to thoughts, emotions and sensations. It can thus be particularly effective for a disorder like OCD in which intolerance of negative inner experience and consequent behavioral avoidance play a central role.

Nevertheless, carrying out mindfulness interventions with obsessive patients is not always easy, especially in the case of patients with severe or chronic suffering. Such patients normally have rigid schemata and attitudes toward their inner experience. One solution to this challenge also suggested by other authors (Schwartz & Beyette, 1997; Hannan & Tolin, 2005; Wilhelm & Steketee, 2007; Fairfax, 2008), and that is adopted at the Mood and Anxiety Disorders Unit in Vicenza, is to integrate CBT with a mindfulness-based intervention. This integration may be usefully provided in three phases, summarized as follows:

(1) *Problem formulation*. This may be done during some preliminary sessions in which therapist and patient reach a clear and shared conceptualization of the activating and maintaining factors of OCD (Salkovskis, 1985) and the possible role and effects of mindfulness in this process (see Figure 11.3). This allows the patient to understand how

his/her problem works and how mindfulness training might challenge the dysfunctional mechanisms highlighted by the problem formulation. Mindfulness may ameliorate OCD deficits, change the modes and the maintaining factors of the disorder, help the patient modify how he/she relates to the entire experience (inner and outer), and develop a new *way of being*.

(2) *Training* patients in Mindfulness skills. For this purpose it is useful to provide patients with an already established and structured mindfulness-based group, such as MBCT or MBSR, that has been adapted for OCD patients. In this group, the importance and effects of exposure are highlighted, psychoeducational materials provided, and an explanation given of how obsessive individuals relate to their thoughts, emotions and perceptions. The mechanisms by which mindfulness can alter dysfunctional OCD attitudes are also illustrated.

(3) *Integrating Exposure and Response Prevention (ERP) techniques and mindfulness* using *mindful exposure*. Unlike classical ERP techniques, in this form of exposure, the patient is continuously invited to stay directly in touch with his/her private experience, carefully noticing, moment by moment, the real cognitive, sensory and emotional experience which arises during exposure, without judgement, evaluation or reaction to it, preventing on purpose any metacognitive processes on the real experience, or seeing any metacognitions as simply thoughts, and passing through it.

Anecdotal clinical experience with dozens of patients with OCD has suggested that sessions (in individual or group setting) should follow the following format (see Figure 11.4):

Practice of mindfulness
(Mindfulness of breath/body)

Exposure (in vivo or imagery) to anxiogenic stimuli
"Breath as an anchor"

Awareness of thoughts, sensations, feelings and emotions
and actively observing and describing private experience without judgment

Using allowing, 'letting be', acceptance attitudes towards
thoughts, sensations and emotional states
Using decentering, defusion and disidentification strategies;
'thoughts as impermanent mental facts'
Using metaphors (e.g. "thoughts like clouds in the sky")

Response Prevention – avoiding any overt and covert reaction to private
experience
(neutralizations, rituals, reassurance seeking)

Short mindfulness exercise (e.g. Breathing space)

Figure. 11.4. Example of an integrated model of exposure and response prevention procedure and mindfulness-based intervention.

(A) The session should start by inviting the patient to practice a mindfulness exercise which allows him/her to enter into a stable, balanced and wakeful state of mind (e.g., sitting meditation, body scan – see Appendix A), fully opening attentive and sensory processes.

(B) The patient should be exposed (in vivo or imaginal exposure) to anxiety-provoking or distressing situations or triggers. In each moment of this phase, it is important to invite the patient to bring attention to an "attentional anchor" or "mindfulness center" (e.g., the body or a sensory input such as breathing) in order to be centered in the present moment ("breathing as an anchor") observing whatever happens in the inner and outer experience.

(C) The patient should pay attention and bring awareness to any thoughts, sensations, feelings and emotions that may arise and actively observe and describe this private experience over and over again without judgment. For example, anxiety may be described by the patient as an array of innocuous physical sensations and thoughts whose increase cannot lead to any dangerous consequences.

(D) The attitudes to be used are allowing, "letting be," and acceptance attitudes (learned at the mindfulness training) toward thoughts, sensations and emotional states. Decentering, defusion and disidentification strategies are used and for this purpose it might be useful to use particular phrases or sentences utilized during the mindfulness groups (e.g., "thoughts are mental events, not facts," "thoughts and emotions are transient and impermanent events") or to invite the patient to use specific metaphors related to mindfulness (e.g., "thoughts like clouds in the sky"; see also Chapter 7 of this volume). The aim in this phase is not to change the content of the thoughts, but to change the way in which the patient relates to them.

(E) For the duration of the entire session, it is particularly important to invite and help the patient to prevent any overt or covert neutralization through rituals or compulsions by asking him/her on a regular basis what he/she is thinking he/she will do in that moment or after the session (rituals) or if he/she is using any neutralizing thoughts in order to deal with anxiety and distress. If so, the patient is invited to let go of the neutralization and to bring his/her attention back to the real physical sensations or sensory experience in the present moment, rating how the level of distress changes (on a scale 0–100) moment by moment. The patient is also invited to notice how discomfort is expressed by specific physical sensations and be aware of where they are located in the body.

(F) The session should end with a short mindfulness exercise (e.g., Breathing space – Segal et al., 2002) aimed at allowing the patient to recover a sense of balance, stability, and presence.

Outcome Research

At present there are no randomized and controlled trials that have investigated the effectiveness of a mindfulness-based treatment with OCD. However, there are some studies that have suggested a positive and significant outcome using various adapted forms of Mindfulness-based approaches or meditation with this disorder.

In a clinical case study, Singh, Wahler and Winton (2004) present the case of a patient who learned improved her quality of life by reframing her OCD as a strength and enhancing her mindfulness so that she was able to incorporate her OCD in her daily life. Results showed that she successfully overcame her debilitating OCD and was taken off all medication within 6 months of intervention. Three year of follow-up showed that she was well adjusted and had a full and healthy lifestyle and that although some obsessive thoughts remained, they did not control her behavior.

In another case report, Patel, Carmody, and Blair Simpson (2007) present an OCD patient who refused treatment with medication or EX/RP and was treated using an adapted Mindfulness-Based Stress Reduction (MBSR) program. After an 8-week adapted MBSR program, the endpoint evaluation revealed clinically significant reductions in symptoms of OCD as well as an increased capacity to evoke a state of mindfulness.

Schwartz, Stoessel, Baxter, Martin & Phelps (1996) investigated the effects of a cognitive-behavioral intervention integrated with mindfulness-based components (the Four Step Program) for a group of OCD patients. This study, which used brain-imaging methods (PET), showed that mindfulness-based treatments were associated with significant structural and functional change in the cerebral dysfunctions in the areas connected to the disorder (*self-directed neuroplasticity*; Schwartz & Beyette, 1997; Schwartz & Begley, 2002; Schwartz, Gullifor, Stier, & Thienemann, 2005a). Some neuroimaging research shows that patients with OCD would be capable of "reconstructing" the neuronal circuits associated with the disorder (Schwartz & Beyette, 1997; Schwartz, 1998) when mindfulness-based methods are adopted. Consciously directed attention may cause a cerebral re-organization, which leads to more adaptive cerebral and behavioral functioning (the *quantum zeno effect*) (Graybiel, 1998; Graybiel & Rauch, 2000; Beauregard, Levesque & Bourgouin, 2001; Ochsner, Bunge, Gross, & Gabrielli, 2002; Paquette et al., 2003; Schwartz, 1999). More specifically, these authors hypothesized that repeated acts of mindfulness, regularly practiced, could lay down circuitry in the habit-forming part of the brain in the *basal ganglia* (Graybiel, 1998). *Prefrontal cortex mechanisms* would be directly influenced in highly adaptive ways by wilfully instituting the mindful cognitive reframing perspective (Beauregard et al., 2001; Ochsner et al., 2002; Paquette et al., 2003). Regular practice of mindfulness would rewire the brain in ways that tend to calm the pathologically overactive orbital-frontal cortex, anterior cingulate gyrus, and caudate nucleus circuitry through *self-directed neuroplasticity* (Schwartz, 1999). These studies also show that brain metabolism in the orbital-frontal cortex changes in a significant manner when OCD patients apply mindfulness-based approaches (Schwartz & Begley, 2002).

Furthermore, in a recent pilot study (Didonna & Bosio, work in progress) the authors investigated the effect of an adapted form of MBCT for a group of six OCD patients (Y-BOCS mean total score 21). Preliminary data on this open trial showed that 4 out of 6 patients had a significant improvement in the Y-BOCS and Padua Inventory scores at the end of treatment and that they maintained this outcome at a 6-month follow-up (three of them were fully remitted). From the beginning of the MBCT group until the follow-up, the patients didn't receive any other kind of psychological treatment and those who were on medication had no changes in their dose from 4 months before MBCT GROUP until the follow-up. The 4 patients who made improvements maintained a medium-high level of mindfulness practice during the group and after 6 months. An interesting correlation between a significant improvement in OCD symptoms (post treatment and follow-up) and a significant improvement in Mindfulness skills at post treatment and follow-up (assessed using FFMQ, see Baer et al., Chapter 9 of this volume) was also observed .

These findings are encouraging, but further investigation using controlled and randomized trials with large samples is needed to confirm the effects and mechanisms illustrated above, and to understand to what degree mindfulness components affect and improve therapy outcomes.

Conclusions and Future Directions

> The true voyage of discovery is not in seeking new landscapes but in having new eyes.
>
> – Marcel Proust.

The introduction of mindfulness-based interventions into the psychological treatment of OCD is a relatively recent application even though the progress that these approaches have attained in the last two decades is noteworthy. From a mindfulness-based perspective, OCD can be conceptualized as a deficit in mindfulness skills. A Mindfulness-based approach seems to be a promising intervention that may improve some of fundamental mindfulness skills that are involved in the phenomenology of obsessive patients. More specifically, Mindfulness practice may strengthen exposure experiences and, since it is an antiavoidant strategy and an antirumination process, improve the attentional deficit in OCD. Furthermore, it has been hypothesized that Mindfulness may teach patients to validate private experience and prevent the secondary elaborative processing that is one of the main activating factors in the obsessive syndrome. Self-validation and acceptance are proposed as therapeutic attitudes that can modify the constant ongoing obsessive self-invalidation of one's own private experience and memory of it. The perception experience validation technique (PEV), described in this chapter, is a mindfulness procedure that may help patients with obsessive problems enhance their ability to acquire mindful attention and use the memory of their own sensorial experience in order to deal with doubt and rumination.

Mindfulness can help patients realize the *impermanence* of experience (using acceptance, allowing, "letting be" attitudes, and metaphors), developing a sense of *not-self* and *non-attachment* (using detachment, disidentification and defusion processes), with no need to control or react to thoughts. Mindfulness training may also be a valuable intervention for improving metacognitive skills and increase patients' insight, reality testing, and general functioning. It may also help patients learn to avoid activating the maintaining factors of OCD that lead to the chronic and self-reinforcing vicious cycles of the disorder (see Figure 11.3).

Mindfulness is a less specific intervention than standard behavioral techniques because it is aimed at teaching patients a different attitude, mental style, and way of being present to their entire private experience. This may have positive implications with respect to the intervention with OCD since it is such a heterogeneous nosographic entity with numerous comorbidities.

These patients, in fact, might need a therapeutic integration with a more comprehensive approach to their dysfunctional way of relating to thoughts, emotions and sensations, integrating in this way mindfulness for OCD into a complete view of the emotional suffering and disease of these patients.

Mindfulness practice can feasibly be integrated into traditional interventions for OCD. Such data as are currently available, as well as clinical observation, suggest that the effectiveness of established treatment programs for obsessive problems may be increased by adding mindfulness training or mindfulness-based components. In some cases, integration is associated with an improvement in therapy outcome in individuals who were previously described as refractory or resistant to traditional interventions. Furthermore, mindfulness offers an effective and less frightening integration with CBT, and in particular ERP, reducing the risk of drop-out, which is high for OCD patients who start a cognitive-behavioral intervention based on exposure techniques. Mindfulness may enhance motivation to use these anxiety-inducing, but effective, strategies.

A question for further exploration is whether or not there are any contraindications for mindfulness-based treatments of some kinds of severe OCD patients. Clinical experience and observation at my Unit for Mood and Anxiety Disorder suggests that, in general, there are no particularly significant contraindications for these approaches, or for integrating them into already existing protocols – even for challenging problems and with different types of obsessive domains. Moreover, the author has noticed that this kind of treatment may be more effective with obsessive checkers and cleaners, and that there could be a poorer response with people with poor insight and lower egodistony (e.g., individual with overvalued ideation). In any case, methods, strategies, and forms of meditation (mindfulness practice) that are specifically tailored for the heterogeneity of OCD and for comorbid disorders such as depression, personality disorder, and dissociation, need to be found. For example, perhaps patients with severe symptoms should be prepared gradually for the practice of mindfulness, and interventions should be integrated with CBT. With severe problems it is very helpful to provide mindfulness training in which patients can shift *gradually* from external sensory awareness (e.g., walking meditation) to inner mindfulness experiences (e.g., body scan), from short to long exercises, and from informal mindfulness practice to formal meditation (see also Chapter 24).

At present too few studies have investigated the therapeutic ingredients of Mindfulness for OCD to draw firm conclusions about the precise mechanisms of change. However, a number of tentative observations can be made. From the available data and clinical observation it seems that mindfulness-based interventions may lead to changes in some specific *mindfulness deficits* such as attentional biases, rumination, thought-action fusion, inflated responsibility, and self-invalidation of private experience. A central issue that requires further investigation is whether or not there are particular brain processes associated with the clinical conditions of OCD that mindfulness practice either alters (Farb et al., 2007; Schwartz et al., 1996; Lazar et al., 2005). There is a need to understand the cognitive, emotional, behavioral, biochemical, and neurological factors that contribute to the state of mindfulness (See also Chapter 3 of this volume), and to investigate the mechanisms through which mindfulness training may create clinical change in OCD.

It is important to conduct methodologically sound empirical evaluations of the effects of mindfulness interventions for OCD, both in comparison to other well-established interventions, and as a component of treatment packages, employing sizable samples and established protocols. A further aim of investigation would be to determine the differential effectiveness of mindfulness interventions with different types of OCD patients (checkers, cleaners, orders, etc., and to explore how improved mindfulness skills correlates with clinical change in obsessive individuals.

It is the hope of the author that this chapter will stimulate treatment advances and the empirical study of mindfulness-based interventions for OCD that can allow clinicians to deal effectively with it and better understand the clinical mechanisms of change for this chronic and challenging problem.

References

American Psychiatric Association (APA). (2000). *Diagnostic and statistical manual of mental disorders* (4th ed., Text Rev.). Washington, DC: Author.

Amir, N. & Kozak, M. J. (2002). Information processing in obsessive compulsive disorder. In R. O. Frost, & G. Steketee, (Eds.), *Cognitive Approaches to Obsessions and Compulsions: theory, assessment, and treatment*. Elsevier Science Ltd.

Baer, R. A., Smith, G. T., Hopkins, J., Krietemeyer, J., & Toney, L. (2006). Using self-report assessment methods to explore facets of mindfulness. *Assessment, 13*, 27–45.

Beauregard, M., Levesque, J. & Bourgouin, P. (2001). Neural correlates of the conscious self-regulation of emotion. *Journal of Neuroscience, 21*, RC165, 1-6.

Bishop, S., Lau, M., Shapiro, S., Carlson, L., Anderson, N., Carmody, J., Segal, Z. V., et al. (2004). Mindfulness: A proposed operational definition. *Clinical Psychology: Science and Practice, 11* (3), 230–241.

Bohart, A. (1983). Detachment: A variable common to many psychotherapies? Paper presented at the 63rd Annual Convention of the Western Psychological Association, San Francisco, CA.

Bouchard, C., Rhéaume, J., & Ladouceur, R. (1999). Responsibility and perfectionism in OCD: An experimental study. *Behaviour Research and Therapy, 37*, 239–248.

Clark, D. A. (2004). *Cognitive-bahavioral therapy for OCD*. New York: Guilford Press.

Constans, J. I., Foa, E. B., Franklin, M. E., & Matthews, A. (1995). Memory for actual and imagined events in OC checkers. *Behaviour Research and Therapy, 33*, 665–671.

Deikman, A. J. (1982). *The observing self*. Boston: Beacon Press.

De Silva, P. (2000). Obsessive-Compulsive Disorder. In L. Champion & M. Power (Eds.), *Adult psychological problems. An introduction, 2nd edn*. Hove: Psychology Press.

De Silva, P. (2003). Obsessions, ruminations and covert compulsions. In R. G. Menzies, & P. de Silva (Eds.), *Obsessive-compulsive disorder: Theory, research and treatment*. New York: Wiley

Didonna, F. (2003). *Role of the Perceptive-Sensorial Experience in Activating Obsessive Doubt: The Perceptive Experience Validation Technique (PEV)*. Paper presented at the XXXIII International Congress Of Cognitive And Behavioural Psichotherapy – EABCT. Prague (Czech Republic) 10-13 September 2003. Abstract Book.

Didonna, F. (2005). Ruolo dell'invalidazione dell'esperienza sensoriale nell'attivazione e mantenimento del dubbio ossessivo: La tecnica della Validazione dell'Esperienza Percettiva. *Psicopatologia Cognitiva, 2*(2).

Didonna, F. (2006). *Mindfulness-based training for clinical problems*. Meet the Expert Session, Lecture presented at the XXXVI International Congress of European Association for Behaviour and Cognitive Therapy. Paris. France, 21 September 2006, Abstract Book.

Didonna, F. Mindfulness and its clinical applications for severe psychological problems: conceptualization, rationale and hypothesized cognitive mechanisms of change (submitted for publication).

Didonna, F., & Bosio, V. Mindfulness facets in a sample of Obsessive-Compulsive Disorder patients (manuscript in preparation).

Epstein, M. (1996). *Thoughts without a thinker: Psychotherapy from a Buddhist perspective*. New York: Basic Books.

Fairfax, H. (2008). The use of mindfulness in obsessive compulsive disorder: suggestions for its application and integration in existing treatment. *Clinical Psychology & Psychotherapy, 15*(1), 53-59.

Farb, N. A. S., Segal, Z. V., Mayberg, H., Bean, J., McKeon, D., Fatima, Z., & Anderson, A. K. (2007). Attending to the present: mindfulness meditation reveals distinct neural modes of self-reference. *Social Cognitive and Affective Neuroscience Advance*.

Fan, J., McCandliss, B. D., Sommer, T., Raz, A., & Posner, M. I. (2002). Testing the efficiency and independence of attentional networks. *Journal of Cognitive Neuroscience, 14*(3), 340-347.

Field, A. P., St-Leger, E. & Davey, G. C. L. (2000). Past- and future-based rumination and its effect on catastrophic worry and anxiety (manuscript under review).

Foa, E. B., Amir, N., Gershuny, B., Molnar, C., & Kozak, M. J. (1997). Implicit and explicit memory in obsessive-compulsive disorder. *Journal of Anxiety Disorders, 11*, 119-129.

Foa, E. B., Ilai, D., McCarthy, P. R., Shoyer, B., & Murdock, T. B. (1993). Information processing in obsessive-compulsive disorder. *Cognitive Therapy and Research, 17*, 173-189.

Fresco, D. M., Moore, M. T., van Dulmen, M., Segal, Z. V., Teasdale, J. D., Ma, H., & Williams, J. M. G. (2007). Initial psychometric properties of the Experiences Questionnaire: Validation of a self-report measure of decentering. *Behavior Therapy, 38*, 234-246.

Fresco, D. M., Segal, Z. V., Buis, T., & Kennedy, S. (2007). Relationship of posttreatment decentering and cognitive reactivity to relapse in major depression. *Journal of Consulting and Clinical Psychology, 75*, 447-455.

Germer, C. K., Siegel, R. D., Fulton, P.R. (2005). *Mindfulness and Psychotherapy*. New York: Guilford Press.

Goleman, D. (1988). *The meditative mind*. Los Angeles: J. P. Tarcher.

Graybiel, A. M. (1998). The basal ganglia and chunking of action repertoires. *Neurobiology of Learning and Memory, 70*, 119-123.

Graybiel, A. M., & Rauch,S. L. (2000). Toward a neurobiology of obsessive-compulsive disorder. *Neuron, 28*, 343-347.

Guidano, V. & Liotti, G. (1983). *Cognitive processes and emotional disorders*. New York: Guilford Press

Hannan, S. E., & Tolin, D. F. (2005). Mindfulness and acceptance based behavior therapy for obsessive-compulsive disorder. In S. M. Orsillo & L. Roemer (Eds.), *Acceptance and mindfulness-based approaches to anxiety: conceptualization and treatment* (pp. 271-299). New York: Springer.

Hayes, S. C., Strosahl, K. D., Wilson, K. G. (1999). *Acceptance and Commitment Therapy*. New York: Guilford Press

Hayes, S. C., Wilson, K. G., Gifford, E. V., Follette, V. M., & Strosahl, K. (1996). Experiential avoidance and behavioral disorders: A functional dimensional approach to diagnosis and treatment. *Journal of Consulting and Clinical Psychology, 64,* 1152–1168.

Hermans, D., Martens, K., De Cort, K, Pieters, G., & Eelen, P. (2003). Reality monitoring and metacognitive beliefs related to cognitive confidence in obsessive-compulsive disorder. *Behaviour Research and Therapy, 41,* 383–401.

Kabat-Zinn, J. (1990). *Full catastrophe living.* New York: Delacorte.

Kabat-Zinn, J. (1994). *Wherever you go, there you are: Mindfulness meditation in everyday life.* New York: Hyperion.

Kocovski, N. L., Fleming, J., & Rector, N. A. (2007). Mindfulness and acceptance-based group therapy for social anxiety disorder: Preliminary evidence from four pilot groups. Poster accepted for presentation at the 41st Annual Convention of the Association for Behavioral and Cognitive Therapies (ABCT), Philadelphia, November 15–18, 2007.

Kozak, M. J., & Foa, E. B. (1994). Obsessions, overvalued ideas, and delusions in obsessive-compulsive disorder. *Behaviour Research and Therapy, 32,* 343–353.

Kyrios, M. (2003). Exposure and response prevention for obsessive-compulsive disorder. In R. G. Menzies, & P. de Silva (Eds.). *Obsessive-compulsive disorder: Theory, research and treatment.* New York: Wiley

Klee, S. H., & Garfinkel, B. D. (1983). The computerized continuous performance task: A new measure of inattention. *Journal of Abnormal Psychology, 11,* 487–495.

Jain, S., Shapiro, S. L., Swanick, S., Roesch, S. C., Mills, P. J., Bell, I. et al. (2007). A randomized controlled trial of mindfulness meditation versus relaxation training: Effects on distress, positive states of mind, rumination, and distraction. *Annals of Behavioral Medicine, 33,* 11–21

Jha, A. P., Krompinger, J., & Baime, M. J. (2007). Mindfulness training modifies subsystems of attention. *Cognitive, Affective, & Behavioral Neuroscience, 7*(2), 109–119.

Lavey, E. H., van Oppen, P., & van den Hout, M. A. (1994). Selective processing of emotional information in obsessive-compulsive disorder. *Behaviour Research and Therapy. 32,* 243–246.

Lazar, S. W., Kerr, C. E., Wasserman, R. H., Gray, J. R., Greve, D. N., Treadway, M. T., et al. (2005). Meditation experience is associated with increased cortical thickness. *Neuroreport, 16*(17), 1893–1897.

Marlatt, G. A., & Kristeller, J. L. (1999). Mindfulness and Meditation. In W. R. Miller (Ed), *Integrating spirituality into treatment.* Washington, D.C.: American Psycological Association.

Martin, J. R. (1997, April). Limbering across cognitive-behavioral, psychodynamic and systems orientations. In J. R. Martin (Chair), Retooling for integration: Perspectives on the training of post-licensed psychotherapists. Symposium presented at the 13th annual conference of the Society for the Exploration of Psychotherapy Integration, Toronto, Canada.

McNally, R. J., & Kohlbeck, P. A. (1993). Reality monitoring in obsessive-compulsive disorder. *Behaviour Research and Therapy, 31,* 249–253.

Menzies, R. G., & de Silva, P. (Eds.) (2003). *Obsessive-compulsive disorder: theory, research and treatment.* New York: Wiley

Obsessive Compulsive Cognitions Working Group (1997). Cognitive assessment of obsessive-compulsive disorder. *Behaviour Research and Therapy, 35,* 667–681.

Ochsner, K. N., Bunge, S. A., Gross, J. J., & Gabrielli, J. D. E. (2002). Rethinking feelings: An fMRI study of the cognitive regulation of emotion. *Journal of Cognitive Neuroscience, 14*(8), 1215–1229.

Oxford English Dictionary, 2nd edn. (1989). Oxford: Clarendon Press.

Paquette, V., Levesque, J., Mensour, B., Leroux, J. M., Beaudoin, G., Bourgouin, P., & Beauregard, M. (2003). Change the mind and you change the brain: Effects of cognitive-behavioral therapy on the neural correlates of spider phobia. *Neuroimage, 18*, 401–409.

Parasuraman, R. (1998). *The attentive brain.* Cambridge, MA: MIT Press.

Patel S. R., Carmody, J., & Blair Simpson, H. (2007). Adapting mindfulness-based stress reduction for the treatment of obsessive-compulsive disorder: A case report. *Cognitive and Behavioral Practice, 14*(4), 375–380.

Pato, M. T., Zohar-Kadouch, R., & Zohar, J. (1998). Return of symptoms after discontinuation of clomipramine in patients with obsessive compulsive disorder. *American Journal of Psychiatry, 145*, 1521-1522.

Pema Chodron (2002) *The Places that Scare You : A Guide to Fearlessness in Difficult Times.* Shambhala Classics.

Posner, M. I. (1980). Orienting of attention. *Quarterly Journal of Experimental Psychology, 32*(1), 3-25.

Posner, M. I., & Rothbart, M. K. (1992). Attentional mechanisms and conscious experience. In A. D. Milner & M. D. Rugg (Eds.), *The neuropsychology of consciousness* (pp. 91-111). Toronto: Academic Press.

Purdon, C. (2001). Appraisal of obsessional thought recurrences: Impact on anxiety and mood state. *Behaviour Therapy, 32*, 47-64.

Purdon, C. L., & Clark, D. A. (1999). Metacognition and obsessions. *Clinical Psychology and Psychotherapy, 6*, 102-110.

Rachman, S. (1993). Obsessions, responsibility and guilt. *Behaviour, Research and Therapy. 31*, 149-154.

Rachman, S., & Shafran, R. (1998). Cognitive and behavioural features of obsessive-compulsive disorder. In R. P. Swinson, M. M. Antony, S. Rachman & M. A. Richter (Eds), *Obsessive-compulsive disorder: Theory, research, and treatment.* New York: Guilford.

Rasmussen, S. A., & Eisen, J. L. (1992). The epidemiology and clinical features of obsessive compulsive disorder. *Psychiatric Clinics of North America, 15*, 743-758.

Rhéaume, J., Ladouceur, R., Freeston, M. H. & Letarte. H. (1994). Inflated responsibility and its role in OCD. II Psychometric studies of a semi-idiographic measure. *Journal of Psychopathological Behaviour, 16*, 265-276.

Robins, L., Helzer, J., Weissman, M., Orvaschel, H., Gruengerge, E., Burge, J., et al. (1984). Lifetime prevalence of specific psychiatric disorders in three sites. *Archives of General Psychiatry, 41*, 949-958.

Rogers, R. D., & Monsell, S. (1995). Costs of a predictable switch between simple cognitive tasks. *Journal of Experimental Psychology, 124*, 207-231.

Safran, J. D., & Segal, Z. V. (1990). Interpersonal process in cognitive therapy. New York: Basic Books.

Salkovskis, P. M. (1983). Treatment of an obsessional patient using habituation to audiotaped ruminations. *British Journal of Clinical Psychology, 22*, 311-313.

Salkovskis, P. M. (1985). Obsessional-compulsive problems: A cognitive-behavioural analysis. *Behaviour Research and Therapy, 23*, 571-583.

Salkovskis, P. M. (1996). The cognitive approach to anxiety: Threat beliefs, safety seeking behavior, and the special case of health anxiety and obsession. In P. M. Salkovskis, (Ed.) *Frontiers of Cognitive Therapy* (49-74). New York: Guilford.

Salkovskis, P. M., Richards, C., & Forrester. E. (2000b). Psychological treatment of refractory obsessive-compulsive disorder. In W. K. Goodman, M. V. Rudorfer & J. D. Maser (Eds.), *Obsessive-Compulsive Disorder: Contemporary Issues in Treatment.* Mahwah, NJ: Elbaum.

Salkovskis, P. M., Shafran, R., Rachman, S., & Freeston, M. H. (1999). Multiple pathways to inflated responsibility beliefs in obsessional problems: possible origins and implications for therapy and research. *Behaviour Research and Therapy, 37*, 1055-1072.

Shapiro, S. L., Carlson, L. E., Astin, J. A., & Freedman, B. (2006). Mechanisms of mindfulness. *Journal of Clinical Psychology, 62*, 373-386.

Sher, K. J., Frost, R. O., & Otto, R. (1983). Cognitive deficits in compulsive checkers: An exploratory study. *Behaviour Research and Therapy, 21*, 357-363.

Schwartz, J. M. (1998). Neuroanatomical aspects of cognitive-behavioral therapy response in obsessive-compulsive disorder: An evolving perspective on brain and behavior. *British Journal of Psychiatry, 173, Supplement 35*, 39-45.

Schwartz, J. M. (1999). A role for volition and attention in the generation of new brain circuitry: Toward a neurobiology of Mental force. Special issue of Journal of Consciousness Studies, Libet, B., Freeman, A. & Sutherland, K. (Eds.): The Volitional Brain: Towards a neuroscience of free will. *Journal of Consciousness Studies, 6*(89), 115-142.

Schwartz, J., & Begley, S. (2002). *The mind and the brain: Neuroplasticity and the power of mental force* (1st ed.). New York: Regan Books.

Schwartz, J. M., & Beyette, B. (1997). *Brain lock: Free yourself from obsessive-compulsive behavior*. New York: Harper Collins.

Schwarz, N. & Bless, H. (1991). Happy and mindless, but sad and smart? The impact of affective states on analytic reasoning. In J. Forgas (Ed.), *Emotion and social judgements*. 55-71. London: Pergamon.

Schwartz, J., Gullifor, E. Z., Stier, J., & Thienemann, M. (2005a). *Mindful awareness and self directed neuroplasticity: Integrating psychospiritual and biological approach to mental health with focus on obsessive compulsive disorder*. Haworth Press.

Schwartz, J. M., Stoessel, P. W., Baxter, L. R., Martin, K. M., & Phelps, M. E. (1996). Systematic changes in cerebral glucose metabolic rate after successful behavior modification treatment of obsessive-compulsive disorder. *Archives of General Psychiatry, 53*, 109-113.

Segal, Z. V., Williams, J. M., & Teasdale, J. D. (2002). *Mindfulness-based cognitive therapy for depression: A new approach to preventing relapse*. New York: The Guilford Press.

Simon, G., Ormel, J., VonKorff, M., & Barlow, W. (1995). Healt care costs associated with depressive and anxiety disorders in primary care. *American Journal of Psychiatry, 152*, 352-357.

Singh, N. N., Wahler R. G., & Winton, A. S. W. (2004). A mindfulness-based treatment of obsessive-compulsive disorder. *Clinical Case Studies, 3*(4), 275-287.

Snelling, J. (1991). *The Buddhist* handbook. Rochester, VI: Inner Traditions.

Steketee, G., & Shapiro, L. J. (1995). Predicting behavioural treatment outcome for agoraphobia and obsessive compulsive disorder. *Clinical Psychology Review, 15*, 317-346.

Teasdale, J. D. (1999). Metacognition, mindfulness and the modification of mood disorders. *Clinical Psychology and Psychotherapy, 6*, 146-155.

Teasdale, J. D., Segal, Z. V., Williams, J. M. G., & Mark, G. (1995). How does cognitive therapy prevent depressive relapse and why should attentional control (mindfulness) training help? *Behavior Research and Therapy, 33*, 25-39.

Teasdale, J. D., Segal, Z. V., & Williams, J. M. (2003). Mindfulness training and problem formulation. *Clinical Psychology: Science and Practice, 10*, 157-160.

Trobe, T., & Trobe, G. D. (2005). *From fantasy trust to real trust*. Amsterdam: Osho Publikaties.

Weissman, M. M., Bland, R. C., Canino, G. J., Greenwald, S., Hwu, H. G., Lee, C. K., et al. (1994). The cross-national epidemiology of obsessive-compulsive disorder. *Journal of Clinical Psychiatry, 55*, 5-10.

Wells, A., & Papageorgiu, C. (1998). Relationships between worry, obsessive-compulsive symptoms and meta-cognitive beliefs. *Behaviour Research and Therapy, 36*, 899-913.

Wilhelm, S., & Steketee G. (2007). Recent Advances in the Assessment and Cognitive Treatment of Obsessive Compulsive Disorder. Workshop presented at the World Congress of Behavioural and Cognitive Therapy. Barcelona, July, 2007.

Williams, J. M. G., Mathews, A., & MacLeod, C. (1996). The emotional Stroop task and psychopathology. *Psychological Bulletin, 120*(1), 3-24.

World Health Organization (1996). *The Global burden of disease*. Geneva: WHO

Zylowska, L., Ackerman, D. L., Yang, M. H., Futrell, J. L., Horton, N. L., Hale, T. S., C. Pataki, and S.L. Smalley (2008). Mindfulness Meditation Training in Adults and Adolescents With ADHD:A Feasibility Study. *Journal of Attention Disorders, 11* (6), 737-746

Mindfulness-Based Cognitive Therapy for Depression and Suicidality

Thorsten Barnhofer and Catherine Crane

I find hope in the darkest of days, and focus in the brightest. I do not judge the universe.

XIV Dalai Lama

Introduction

Major depression is one of the most prevalent and most disabling emotional disorders. Its impact is pervasive, affecting social, individual, and biological functioning. For individuals with depression, negative thinking pervades views of the personal past, the current self and the personal future while lack of interest and anhedonia reduce engagement in activities that used to be experienced as enjoyable. These psychological symptoms are accompanied by dysregulations in a number of physical systems, with symptoms such as fatigue and difficulties concentrating undermining the ability to deal actively with the challenges of everyday life. Individuals experience the state of depression as painfully discrepant from their usual or desired level of functioning and depressed mood is often perpetuated by the responses it evokes: attempts at coping that often remain passive and a tendency to engage in either avoidance or repetitive and analytical, ruminative thinking, which further increase the likelihood of deteriorations in mood. In a significant number of cases the hopelessness associated with this condition escalates into suicidal ideation and behavior.

The prevalence of depression in Western countries is extremely high. Current estimates of 1 year prevalence for major depression in Europe are around 5% (Paykel, Brugha, & Fryers, 2005), similar to recent estimates from North America, where the 2001–2002 replication of the National Comorbidity Survey showed a 1-year prevalence of 6.6% (Kessler et al., 2003). These rates are projected to increase even further as demographic studies have shown consistent increases in rates over the past decades (Compton, Conway, Stinson, & Grant, 2006), with major depression predicted to become the second leading cause of disability worldwide by the year 2020 (Murray & Lopez, 1996). In about 25% of depressed individuals in the community (Goldney, Wilson, Del Grande, Fisher & McFarlane, 2000) and 50% of depressed inpatients

(Mann, Waternaux, Haas, & Malone, 1999) depression is accompanied by *suicidal ideation* or behavior.

What makes these high rates of prevalence particularly concerning is that for most of those affected, an episode of depression is not a singular event. Individuals who have suffered from one episode of depression are very likely to suffer from further episodes. For example the collaborative depression study (CDS; Katz & Klerman, 1979) identified rates of recurrence of 25–40% after 2 years, increasing to 60% after 5 years (Lavori et al., 1994), to 75% after 10 years, and to 87% after 15 years (Keller & Boland, 1998), suggesting that risk for relapse remained even after prolonged periods of recovery. For individuals who become suicidal when depressed the picture is equally concerning. Perhaps the best predictor of death by suicide is a history of prior suicidal behavior and where suicidality has been a feature of one episode of depression it is very likely to recur as depression recurs (Williams, Duggan, Crane, & Fennell, 2006). Treating depression in general and suicidal depression in particular therefore requires a focus not only on alleviating current symptoms but also on reducing risk of relapse in those who have experienced depression in the past.

Mindfulness-based cognitive therapy (MBCT), developed by Zindel Segal, Mark Williams, and John Teasdale (2002), was specifically designed to target vulnerability processes that cognitive research has identified as playing a causative role in depressive relapse. The eight-week program combines training in mindfulness meditation, following the approach developed by Jon Kabat-Zinn (1990), with interventions from cognitive-behavior therapy (CBT) that have been used successfully in the treatment of acute depression. In common with other "third-wave" cognitive-behavioral therapies the emphasis of treatment is on acceptance as well as change, its general aim being to help participants become more aware of and respond differently to negative thoughts and emotions that might trigger downward cycles of thinking and mood. More recently research has begun to adapt MBCT for use specifically with patients who experience serious suicidal ideation or suicidal behavior when depressed. The aim of this overview is to describe the rationale for MBCT and explore how treatment is delivered. We then briefly review current research on the effectiveness of MBCT and present a case example to illustrate the treatment approach. Finally we describe why MBCT may be particularly suitable for patients with a history of suicidal depression and outline some initial adaptations to the programme for this high-risk group.

Theoretical Rationale

As discussed, risk of relapse to depression increases dramatically with numbers of previous episodes (e.g., Solomon et al., 2000). It is now generally assumed that risk for relapse after a first episode of depression is approximately 50%, rising to about 70% with a second, and about 90% with a third lifetime episode (DSM-IV TR). This has important implications both for the understanding of the factors which determine vulnerability to depression and the development of effective treatments, because models of depression must take into account the increase in risk of recurrence across episodes either by assuming changes in factors meditating risk, or at least changes in their relative contribution to determining risk. One example of this is the observation that the relationship between negative life events and onsets of depression is much stronger for first as compared to later episodes (for an overview see Monroe & Harkness, 2005). This research suggests that across episodes, depression is more likely to be triggered either autonomously or by increasingly minor or idiosyncratic stressors. Why might this occur and what might its treatment implications be?

From a cognitive science perspective these findings have been explained within the framework of differential activation (Segal, Williams, Teasdale, Gemar, 1996). The theory of differential activation suggests that across depressive episodes associations are formed between low mood and other emotions (e.g., anger, hopelessness), cognitions (e.g., dysfunctional attitudes), and behaviors (e.g., passivity, risk taking), which occur in depressed states. Although these patterns of response are likely to differ from individual to individual, forming the individual's unique "relapse signature," it is suggested that they will nevertheless be relatively stable for the same individual over time. Indeed across episodes of depression the associations between these different aspects of the depressed "mode" are thought to be strengthened (due to co-activation), such that they become increasingly coherent, with a reduced threshold for activation. Thus depressive episodes are more and more easily triggered, increasing the likelihood of recurrence and reducing the association between major negative life events and depressive onsets.

Another factor that has been found to be of particular importance with regard to vulnerability to depression is rumination. Research over the last decades has shown that those who are at risk for depression tend to respond to symptoms, negative cognitions and unpleasant body states by engaging in repetitive, abstract-analytical thinking (Nolen-Hoeksema, 2004). While initially instigated as a means to solve problems and reduce self-discrepancies, this ruminative thinking, in particular aspects characterized by brooding, has a range of negative effects (e.g., Treynor, Gonzalez, & Nolen-Hoeksema, 2003). Rumination causes further deterioration in mood, increases biases in negative thinking and undermines cognitive functions crucial for effective coping including the ability to retrieve specific memories of autobiographical events (Raes et al., 2006) and the ability to solve interpersonal problems (Watkins & Moulds, 2005). Paradoxically, previously and currently depressed individuals report predominately positive beliefs about its usefulness as a coping strategy (Papageorgiou & Wells, 2004), which are likely to contribute to the fact that ruminative thinking often persists despite its deleterious consequences.

As current mood worsens, individuals may oscillate in their attempts at coping between ruminative monitoring and avoidance of negative thoughts and body states. As with rumination, the effects of avoidance are predominately negative. Attempts to suppress negative thoughts, for example, have been shown to paradoxically increase the frequency of intrusions rather than reduce them (Wenzlaff & Wegner, 2000). Furthermore, avoidance precludes both engagement in more active forms of problem solving and habituation to distressing mental content. Teasdale, Segal, and Williams have argued that it is these and other processes that lead to a situation in which the very responses depression evokes serve to perpetuate the condition, a mechanism which they refer to as "depressive interlock."

Mindfulness-Based Cognitive Therapy: Overview

MBCT was developed specifically to target the above vulnerability processes. It teaches as its core skill the ability "to recognize and to disengage from mind states characterized by self-perpetuating patterns of ruminative, negative thought" (Segal et al., 2002, p. 75) and to adopt a stance toward experience, which is characterized by openness, curiosity and acceptance, rather than experiential avoidance. Like cognitive therapy, MBCT aims to give patients the ability to see thoughts as mental events rather than facts, to decouple the occurrence of negative thoughts from the responses they would usually elicit and, eventually, to change their meaning. However, while cognitive therapy maintains a strong focus on the content of thoughts and the re-evaluation of their meaning, the main aim in MBCT is to teach patients to take a different perspective on thinking and awareness itself. By consistently practicing bringing awareness to present moment experience, participants shift into a mode of functioning that is incompatible with the self-focused and analytical cognitive processes that perpetuate depressive states. Segal et al. (2002) describe this as change from a "doing" mode, in which the main focus is on the reduction of discrepancies between the current state and ideas of how things should be or ought to be through problem-solving behavior, to a mode of "being," in which the individual is in immediate and intimate contact with present moment experience, whatever that experience might be.

Mindfulness has been described as "paying attention in a particular way: on purpose, in the present moment and non-judgmentally" (Kabat-Zinn, 1994, p. 4). As such mindfulness is both a means of becoming aware of and switching from "doing" to "being" mode as well as a central characteristic of the "being" mode itself. In the MBCT program, participants train mindfulness through regular formal meditation practice and through exercises designed to generalize the effects of meditation to everyday life. In the early stages of the program participants are taught to become aware of and recognize the doing mode in its different manifestations and to cultivate the being mode as an alternative state. The increased awareness this facilitates is an essential foundation for the prevention of depressive relapse since without it individuals are poorly equipped to spot the relatively subtle changes in mood and body state that signal the activation of depressive modes of mind. In the later stages of the programme, as this foundation strengthens, the focus of the training moves toward recognizing the occurrence of negative emotions, negative cognitions (for example self-criticism and judgment) and triggers of negative moods in daily life. Practice during this stage cultivates the abilities to disengage from responses such as rumination which characterize the doing mode, and to be with difficult and aversive thoughts and emotions in more skillful ways, adopting an attitude of acceptance rather than avoidance. The final sessions emphasize the integration of learned skills to prevent future relapse.

MBCT is first and foremost a training of skills. A regular formal meditation practice between sessions and the practice of mindfulness in everyday life are essential components of the program. During the eight weekly sessions the focus is, as much as possible, experiential rather than didactic, apart from some psychoeducational elements in which participants learn about the symptoms of depression and vulnerability mechanisms leading to relapse. Most of the time in sessions is spent in the practice of meditation and subsequent enquiry, primarily reflections on current practice, but also on difficulties that participants may have encountered with their meditation practice during the week. The role of the instructor, in general, is that of a facilitator and a model, inviting participants to open to and reflect on their experiences. Through this dialogue and reflection MBCT encourages both the development of greater metacognitive *awareness*, for example an increased ability to observe the occurrence of mental events such as thoughts, emotional responses, bodily sensations "online"; and the arising of metacognitive *insight*, into the nature of the mind, the relationship between thoughts, emotions and bodily states, and the experience of suffering. The attitude the instructor brings to this enquiry is one of curiosity, and particularly one in which difficult thoughts and feelings are observed and accepted without having to resort to problem solving and "fixing." The instructor incorporates in the class process the same principles of openness and compassion that participants are taught to bring to their own meditation practice. In this way, enquiry serves as a continuation of the meditation practices. It is both because of the need to guide meditations from within, that is, from own meditation experience, and because instructors need to be able to bring their own ability to relate differently to negative affect into the class, that a developed regular mindfulness meditation practice is a prerequisite for teaching MBCT classes.

The Programme

MBCT consists of eight weekly sessions of 2 hours length, each of which follows its own theme and curriculum. Prior to the first class participants meet individually with the class instructor to give time for the instructor to orient them toward the treatment approach, develop an understanding of the participant's presenting problems, establish realistic expectations for treatment, and answer any questions the participant might have. Class sizes vary according to facilities but are often of around 12 participants. Sessions 1–4 emphasize learning to pay attention. Participants become aware of how their minds often take them away from present moment awareness and increase concentration and awareness of thoughts, feelings and bodily sensations as a means to being in the moment. Sessions 5–8 shift emphasis toward dealing with difficult thoughts and feelings. Participants learn to decenter as a means of becoming aware of their thoughts, feelings, and body sensations, to bring acceptance and kindly awareness to their sensations and to let go of thoughts, reducing the tendency to get entangled in ruminative thinking, ultimately leading to a general shift toward functioning in present moment awareness. Across the eight sessions different guided meditation practices, including an eating meditation, "body scan," yoga stretches, walking meditation, and sitting meditations are introduced to participants. Toward the end of the treatment participants are encouraged to develop a home practice which fits their needs and which can be maintained in the longer term. Table 12.1 outlines the meditation practices and CBT components introduced in each session, the skills developed and insights supported by these components and the activities suggested to participants as homework.

The Eight Sessions: A Case Example

We outline the progression of the eight classes of the program with a case example: Fiona, a 37-year-old single woman with one daughter, worked as a retail assistant. She referred herself to MBCT having read information about an ongoing programme of mindfulness research in the local newspaper. She had experienced several prior episodes of major depression accompanied by suicidal ideation and was still experiencing periodic episodes of anxiety, low mood and more fleeting suicidal thoughts. She described a typical "downward spiral" of depression. This would usually be triggered by a perceived rejection, either by someone at work or a social acquaintance and would lead to feelings of abandonment, agitation, depression and worthlessness, as well as physical reactions such as tightness in the chest and crying. Fiona reported that she would tend to withdraw from social situations as these feelings developed, reinforcing her sense of isolation, instead spending time on her own ruminating about her current situation and past rejections. As depression and worthlessness escalated she would experience thoughts of suicide, feeling that no one would care if she died. These sometimes progressed to specific plans for suicide, but she had never acted on these thoughts.

At her pre-class interview the instructor asked Fiona questions about her previous experiences of depression and factors that might be involved in relapse and maintenance. Fiona learned more about the general background of MBCT and how, more specifically, mindfulness meditation could help with her recurrent problems. Potential benefits discussed included the possibility of becoming more aware of the sequence of events and experiences which typically led to suicidal ideation and to respond differently; for example noticing her tendency to respond to social interactions with feelings of abandonment and to choose an alternative response rather than withdrawal. Other aspects touched on were how, through mindfulness, Fiona might be able to learn to disengage from the rumination that became habitual when she felt depressed and how she might be able to develop a different relationship to the bodily symptoms of anxiety, which bothered her a great deal and contributed to the escalation of her negative mood. Fiona stated as her general intention that she wanted to improve her well-being and become more engaged with life, rather than struggling from one crisis to the next.

The theme of the first session is "Automatic Pilot." Through exercises and meditation practice participants explore and become more aware of how oftentimes we function in ways that are mechanical or automatic, what this means for our experience of life, and how bringing mindful attention to whatever we do can change the nature of the experience of it. Although the class instructor discussed with Fiona the fact that learning meditation was challenging and would not lead to immediate results she started the classes with a lot of optimism that this would be "the cure" for her depression. Her initial experience of the group, having heard each participant introduce him- or herself briefly, was positive and she found the exercises in the first class

Table 12.1. A week-by-week summary of the practices introduced in MBCT, their aims, the skills developed and insights supported through the practices, and the activities participants are encouraged to complete at home.

Session theme	Practices and exercises	Skills learned	Insights supported by practices	Home practice
				Mindfulness of everyday activities
1. Automatic Pilot Aim: to make participants more aware of how often we function in automatic pilot and what the effects of being mindful are.	*Raisin Exercise* A meditation in which participants spend several minutes exploring the sensory features (sight, smell, taste, touch) of one raisin.	To begin to experience the shift from 'doing' mode to 'being' mode. To experience the qualities of mindful attention.	Experiences can be richer if we pay full attention. Much of our everyday experience is missed because the mind is elsewhere.	Participants choose a routine activity and attend to it mindfully.
	Body Scan A 45 minute guided meditation in which participants move their attention through the body attending to any sensations that arise in each area and breathing into each area	Sustained practice in engaging, disengaging and shifting attention to different objects of awareness. Practice at returning the mind repeatedly to the intended object of concentration when it wanders.	Mind wandering is habitual. It is possible to develop greater awareness of bodily sensations (which may be associated with emotional states)	*Body Scan* Participants practice a 45-minute body scan supported by CDs, on at least 6 days, noting their experiences.
2. Dealing with Barriers Aim: to explore initial experiences of the practice of meditation and to introduce the metacognitive perspective.	*Body Scan* As above	To observe mind wandering, to practice letting go of thoughts and bringing attention repeatedly back to the intended object.	We have a tendency to judge our experiences as pleasant or unpleasant, to avoid unpleasant experiences and seek those that are pleasant.	*Body Scan* Participants practice a 45-minute body scan supported by CDs, on at least 6 days, noting their experiences.

(Continued)

Table 12.1 (*Continued*).

Session theme	Practices and exercises	Skills learned	Insights supported by practices	Home practice
	Thoughts and Feelings Exercise Participants imagine an ambiguous scenario (not being noticed by an acquaintance) and explore their reactions to such an event, as well as how these might vary as a function of mood.	To begin to reflect on the associations between thoughts, feelings, body sensations and behaviours from a metacognitive perspective.	Our mood influences our interpretation of events, and our interpretation of events influences subsequent emotions, cognitions, bodily sensations and behaviours.	*Noticing Pleasant Events* Participants are asked to notice events or moments they experience as pleasant and observe the thoughts, feelings and bodily sensations that arise on these occasions.
3. *Mindfulness of Breath* Aim: To introduce the breath as a vehicle for reconnection with present moment awareness when the mind has wandered to difficult thoughts, emotions or bodily sensations.	*Sitting Meditation* A 30–40 minute guided sitting meditation in which participants are invited to attend to the constantly changing sensations of the breath, to observe with curiosity wherever the mind wanders and then to gently return attention to the breath. In the final stages of the practice attention is broadened to the body as a whole.	To attend to the breath, to notice mind wandering and to become familiar with the habits of the mind.	Increasing awareness of habitual patterns of the mind (e.g. the occurrence of self-critical thoughts, or difficult bodily sensations)	*Stretch and Breath* A sequence of standing yoga stretches followed by a shorter sitting meditation focusing on the breath, completed on days 1, 3, 5.
To explore reconnection with the breath and staying with difficult experiences as an alternative to engaging in conceptual thought and attempts at problem solving.		To begin to use the breath as a vehicle to reconnect with present moment awareness when the mind has wandered.	The breath is a route to present moment awareness.	*Yoga* (2, 4, 6) A longer sequence of Yoga postures guided by CD, completed on days 2, 4, 6.

(*Continued*)

Table 12.1 (*Continued*).

Session theme	Practices and exercises	Skills learned	Insights supported by practices	Home practice
	Yoga Stretches/Mindful Walking Participants are guided through a series of *gentle yoga stretches* and are encouraged to observe changing bodily sensations during and after each stretch.	To become aware of the body in movement, to observe mind wandering during practice and learn to reconnect with bodily sensations.	Bodily sensations are richer and more changeable if observed with full attention.	*Scheduled Breathing Spaces* Participants practice the 3-minute breathing space on three pre-determined occasions each day.
	Participants are instructed in the practice of *walking meditation*, attending to the sensations arising from the movement and placement of the feet and legs. Pace is usually slow. Attention is redirected to the body when the mind wanders			
	3-Minute Breathing Space A 3-minute practice in which participants first become aware of present moment thoughts, feelings and bodily sensations, then shift their attention to the breath and finally expand their attention to the body as a whole.	To begin to generalize the practice of meditation into everyday life.	It is possible to shift perspective and reconnect with the present moment through the use of the breathing space.	*Noticing Unpleasant Events* Participants are asked to notice events or moments they experience as unpleasant and observe the thoughts, feelings and bodily sensations that arise on these occasions.

(*Continued*)

Table 12.1 (*Continued*).

Session theme	Practices and exercises	Skills learned	Insights supported by practices	Home practice
4. Staying Present Aim: to explore new ways of relating to intense or emotionally charged thoughts, feelings and sensations	*Seeing Meditation/Hearing Meditation* A short meditation practice in which participants focus attention on either sights or sounds, returning gently to these sensations whenever the mind wanders. *Sitting Meditation* A sitting meditation in which the focus is initially on the breath, moving then to the body as a whole. Participants are encouraged to explore intense sensations with an attitude of openness and curiosity, rather than immediately changing position to alleviate discomforts. Attention then moves to sounds, and to thoughts and finally to whatever is salient in awareness from moment to moment ('choiceless awareness').	To include sights or sounds as the object of awareness. To practice shifting out of automatic pilot and tuning in to different aspects of moment to moment experience. To begin to explore the possibility of staying with difficult sensations, adopting an attitude of curiosity, openness and acceptance.	It is possible to use awareness of sights and sounds to step out of automatic pilot and reconnect with the present moment. Attention to sights or sounds can be particularly 'grounding'. When one chooses to stay with difficult sensations rather than trying to eradicate them it is possible to notice their qualities in more detail. Sometimes difficult sensations spontaneously change.	*Sitting Meditation* A 40 minute sitting meditation in which the object of attention shifts from breath, to body, to sounds, to thoughts and finally to a choice-less awareness. *Breathing Spaces* Participants are encouraged to take 3-minute breathing spaces on three scheduled occasions but also at times when they notice stress or emotional pressure mounting.

(Continued)

Table 12.1 (*Continued*).

Session theme	Practices and exercises	Skills learned	Insights supported by practices	Home practice
	Automatic Thoughts Questionnaire Participants read through the questionnaire to explore the most common dysfunctional and negative thoughts that occur in depression. They also review the DSM-IV symptoms of major depression.	To recognize negative and dysfunctional thoughts. To reflect on these symptoms from a meta-cognitive perspective.	The negative thoughts and experiences that accompany depression are recognized symptoms, not signs of personal weakness or unique to the individual.	
5. *Allowing/ Letting Be* Aim: To begin to develop a radically different relationship to experience in which all experiences are allowed and accepted.	*Sitting Meditation* A 40 minute meditation in which participants bring attention first to the breath, to body sensations, to sounds and then to thoughts. Participants are invited to notice wandering of the mind and if the mind returns repeatedly to certain thoughts, feelings or bodily sensations to bring a curiosity and openness to these. Participants are encouraged to explore how difficulties that arise during meditation are expressed in the body, to become aware of tensions or other bodily sensations associated with difficulty and to use the breath as a vehicle to stay with these experiences in an open way, 'breathing into and out of' regions where the difficulties are manifesting themselves. Once thoughts or sensations no longer pull for attention, participants are encouraged to come back to whatever the current focus of the meditation is. Towards the end of the meditation practice participants are invited to practice this by deliberately bringing a difficulty to mind.	To begin to explore the possibility of staying with and accepting difficult thoughts, images, memories, emotions and body sensations. To observe how difficulties manifest themselves in the body.	Difficult experiences may have bodily manifestations that can be observed. By staying with difficulties rather than attempting to avoid them or change them, change sometimes occurs spontaneously.	*Guided Sitting Meditation* A 40 minute guided meditation following the format of the sitting meditation practiced in the class. *Sitting in Stillness* An unguided 40-minute sitting meditation in which patients guide their own practice, moving through different objects of attention, to choiceless awareness.

(*Continued*)

Table 12.1 (*Continued*).

Session theme	Practices and exercises	Skills learned	Insights supported by practices	Home practice
		To observe our usual tendency to attempt to suppress or avoid unpleasant experiences or to try to fix difficulties and to practice an alternative approach.		*Breathing Spaces* Participants continue to practice both scheduled breathing spaces and spontaneous breathing spaces at times of stress or difficulty.
6. *Thoughts are not facts* Aim: to encourage participants to reduce their identification with thoughts and to begin to relate to thoughts, including difficult thoughts, as mental events.	*Sitting Meditation* A meditation in which thoughts form the object of awareness. Thoughts are observed arising and passing away, rather than being sought. This process is supported through the use of metaphors – imagining thoughts as images on a cinema screen, or as clouds passing in the sky, or leaves on a river. Participants are then invited to deliberately bring to mind a difficult thought and to adopt the same attitude of openness and non-judgmental awareness. If this proves too difficult, because the thoughts that arise are extremely distressing, participants are encouraged to bring awareness to the impact of the thoughts on the body; and to stay with and observe these sensations, before returning to the experience of passing thoughts.	To further develop the ability to stay with difficult thoughts that arise during meditation practice.	It is possible to stay with difficult thoughts rather than engaging in habitual, but unhelpful, reactions.	*Shorter Guided Meditations* Participants are given a series of shorter guided meditations and are encouraged to mix and match these to build up a flexible practice that they can maintain in daily life. Yoga practice and walking meditation can also be incorporated into these routines if participants find them to be helpful.

(*Continued*)

Table 12.1 (*Continued*).

Session theme	Practices and exercises	Skills learned	Insights supported by practices	Home practice
		To practice becoming aware of the bodily responses to difficult thoughts and to attend to these as a form of grounding, rather than resorting to attempting to suppress or challenge the content of difficult thoughts.	Remaining with difficult thoughts and observing them from a de-centered perspective, can, over time, lead to a reduction in their capacity to evoke emotions.	*Breathing Spaces* Participants are encouraged to continue using breathing spaces at regular intervals and at times of stress. The breathing space is emphasized as a response that introduces greater choice and flexibility in responding to difficulty.
	Ambiguous Scenarios Participants are introduced to a further ambiguous scenario – someone being too busy to talk to them – and are asked to explore the different reactions they would have if they had just had a quarrel with someone at work as compared to if they had just had a positive appraisal from their boss.	To take a meta-cognitive perspective, reflecting on the impact that internal and external contexts have on reactions to events and experiences.	Interpretations of events can be heavily influenced by context and the mental state we bring to the event. Mindful awareness can allow us to see events and their contexts more clearly and as a result increase flexibility of responding.	

(Continued)

Table 12.1 (*Continued*).

Session theme	Practices and exercises	Skills learned	Insights supported by practices	Home practice
7. *How can I best take care of myself?* Aim: To explore how awareness can be used to guide skillful action	*Sitting Meditation* This follows the format outlined above	To further develop the ability to attend to, stay with and be open to experiences as they arise during meditation practice.		*Self-Directed Practice* Participants choose from all the formal meditation practices they have learned and settle on one or more to use on a daily basis.
	Reflection on Daily Activities Participants list daily activities and divide them into those that lift mood, give energy and are nourishing and those which dampen mood and drain energy. Working in small groups participants explore how to increase the occurrence of nourishing activities (including very small events) and reduce the occurrence of depleting activities, whilst holding difficult aspects of their lives in mind, rather than simply trying to avoid them. Participants then reflect on nourishing activities identifying those that lift mood by providing a sense of mastery and those that do so by providing a sense of pleasure.	To reflect on the consequences of different activities for mood and well-being To use a breathing space at times of low mood to explore whether the wisest response to a difficult situation is to adopt mindful awareness of ongoing experience or to take skillful action. If appropriate to deliberately increase the occurrence of activities that lift mood and provide a sense of mastery or pleasure at times of low mood.	An awareness of the balance of nourishing to depleting activities in our lives and how this can be modified without simply avoiding difficulties. An awareness of the differences between reacting and responding wisely at times of low mood.	*Breathing Spaces* Participants continue to use scheduled and spontaneous breathing spaces to integrate mindfulness into daily life and as a means of responding wisely to challenging experiences. *Relapse Planning* Participants elaborate their relapse prevention plan that includes information about other people who may be able to provide help or support.

(Continued)

Table 12.1 (*Continued*).

Session theme	Practices and exercises	Skills learned	Insights supported by practices	Home practice
	Relapse Signatures Participants work in groups to identify their own warning signs for depressive relapse. Once identified participants discuss what to do when relapse threatens	To become familiar with one's own warning signs of depressive relapse and develop a plan to implement in such situations which includes taking a breathing space, reflecting on how things are in the moment and making a conscious choice about how to respond.		
8. *Using what has been learned* Aim: To reflect on what has been learned and how it can be maintained	*Body Scan* As described above	To focus attention on different body sensations. To remain open to whatever arises in awareness.	Experiences and responses to the practice may have changed over time in the light of new learning.	
	Reflection Participants reflect either, alone or in pairs, on their initial intentions in coming to classes, what they have learned and potential obstacles for continuing practice.	Participants are encouraged to aim for daily practice, even if only for very brief periods of time, and are introduced to the idea of beginner's mind – that it is always possible to restart practice, even after a long break.		
	Feedback Participants give written feedback on their experiences in the class.			
	Reminder Object At the close of the class participants are each given a small object such as a stone, marble or bead as a symbolic reminder of the experiences shared in class, their hard work and their intention to continue the practice they have begun. The class closes with a short meditation in which these objects are explored in a similar way to which the participants explored the raisin in session 1.			

illuminating, noticing the difference between her usual experience of eating raisins by the handful with the intensity of flavors and textures she experienced when, as instructed in the first exercise of the class, eating one raisin mindfully, bringing attention to how each of her senses was involved in doing this. The first class finished with the "body scan," a lying down meditation in which participants bring attention to every part of the body in turn.

Doing the body scan during the first week of homework proved challenging for Fiona. At the second class she reported that she "could not do" the body scan. She said she had been crying more during the week after the first class and it emerged that she had experienced feelings of panic on several occasions during the body scan, finding it extremely unpleasant. The instructor explored with Fiona the bodily sensations she had noticed during the body scan at the start of the second class. However she was unable to clearly describe them, simply repeating that she felt "panicky." The instructor encouraged Fiona to approach the sensations with curiosity should they arise again, looking in detail at what she experienced in her body during these periods. He also emphasized to the class that there was no right or wrong way to feel during the body scan. In the second session of the program, themed "Dealing with Barriers," addressing reactions to the first week of practice such as Fiona's is an important feature. Many participants have questions about whether they are doing the practice right, or expect to find the meditation relaxing, getting bored and frustrated when this is not their experience. At this point in the classes it is necessary to emphasize to participants that just doing the practice and observing their experiences whatever they are, is all that is required. It is also critical at this stage that the instructor models an openness and curiosity toward participants' experiences, in order to encourage them to maintain their practice of the body scan for a second week. The second session is also used to introduce the cognitive model in order to demonstrate the strong relation between interpretations and emotions.

During the third class participants were introduced to both sitting meditation, and to walking meditation and yoga. Fiona had continued to experience unpleasant sensations during the body scan meditation but also reported what she was beginning to relax to some degree in her attempts to control her emotions. During exploration of her experiences during the sitting meditation in class, Fiona was more able to describe the qualities of the sensations she experienced (tension in her chest, irregular breathing, sadness). However after her initial enthusiasm she also reported increasing doubts about the helpfulness of the classes as she was not yet starting to feel "better." This response is not unusual as participants, through their practice, tend to experience negative thoughts, feelings and body states more clearly or more strongly. At the same time, they begin to realize how their usual ways of responding often entail avoidance or ruminative thinking. In contrast to these habitual tendencies, MBCT teaches participants to become more aware of difficult aspects of experience. In the third session, themed "Mindfulness of the Breath," the focus is on learning how attention to the breath and body sensations can serve to stabilize the mind and return the focus to the experience of what is present, even when the mind is drawn toward difficulties.

A big shift came for Fiona as she began to practice the sitting meditation. She described a period of sitting meditation during which she felt a great sense of relief in response to the occurrence of the thought "its ok to be me." She said that she had realized that she had previously avoided spending time alone and so had tried to surround herself with other people because she did not like herself. This contributed to her sense of anxiety and abandonment in the face of perceived rejections. Through the sitting meditation she began to explore her experiences of "being with herself" in this new way. Spontaneous insights like this frequently arise as the MBCT classes progress and participants begin to observe the workings of their mind and their reactions to events from a new perspective. Up to session 3, participants are instructed to respond to mind wandering by noticing where their mind has gone and then simply returning attention to the object of the meditation. From session 4 onwards, there is a change in emphasis in that participants are instructed more explicitly to turn toward difficult experiences and explore them with gentleness, curiosity and interest. Fiona's greater sense of compassion for herself nicely reflects this shift in emphasis. The focus in session 4 is on "Staying Present" with difficult experience. Session 5, themed "Allowing/Letting Be," explores ways of bringing a sense of acceptance to such experiences, particularly through staying with and exploring the body sensations that come with negative thoughts. Session 6 makes explicit the core theme of the program, that "Thoughts are Not Facts," and that they occur as transient mental events which individuals can choose to attend to or not. As part of the sitting meditations in these sessions, participants deliberately bring to mind a difficulty in order to practice these different ways of relating. Fiona, at first, found it difficult to see the benefit of deliberately approaching difficulties. However, over time it became possible for her to stay with the distress she experienced when bringing a difficulty to mind, focusing her attention on the bodily sensations accompanying what she experienced (tightness in the chest, difficulty breathing, sadness) and the gradual change in these as she continued to observe them. Hearing other participants of the class talk about similar experiences helped her to develop compassion both for herself and others. Many of the participants reflected on the way that they judged themselves and the consequences this had for their mood and well-being. The instructor encouraged participants to bring mindfulness to the occurrence of difficult thoughts during their meditation practice, for example noting "here is guilt," "here is judgement" when familiar thoughts arose. Participants were also encouraged to experiment with techniques to facilitate de-centering including imagining thoughts as leaves gliding down a stream, or projected on a cinema screen.

The theme of session 7 is "How Can I Best Take Care of Myself." In this session, participants reflect on the balance of nourishing and depleting activities in their lives. As often occurs, Fiona realized that she spent very little time on activities that lifted her mood or improved her well-being, often being so concerned to meet the needs of others and avoid rejection that she failed to meet her own needs adequately. In common with other members of the group Fiona recognized a typical spiral of depression in which, as her mood deteriorated, she increasingly gave up activities that might give her a sense of mastery or pleasure. A key part of her relapse planning was therefore to identify the early warning signs of this process, to take a breathing space and reflect on an appropriate course of action, and to deliberately engage in nourishing activities at times of low mood.

Session 8, themed "Using What Has Been Learned to Deal with Future Low Mood," is used to both look back at what has been learned and forward to how what has been learned can be maintained and used to prevent relapse and increase well-being. Fiona identified several areas in which she had made progress. She was more able to recognize her tendency to react to social stressors "online" and was able to use meditation, including short 3-minute breathing spaces, to become aware of her reactions and make choices. For example Fiona described a situation in which she had been sitting on a train and had smiled at the person opposite who promptly got up and walked away. Her initial reaction was to assume that the person opposite had thought her strange and that others had also noticed the situation and his departure, leading to feelings of embarrassment. However, rather than triggering a cycle of rumination Fiona was able to stay with her immediate experiences and observe her thoughts and bodily reactions in response to the event. Shortly after the person opposite returned to their seat from the restroom! This experience and others illustrated to Fiona the benefits of staying in the present moment. and allowing events and experiences to unfold, rather than getting trapped in habitual but unhelpful patterns and reaction.

Research Findings

Two randomized controlled trials have evaluated the effectiveness of MBCT for recurrent depression. In an initial multi-center trial by Teasdale et al. (2000), 145 recovered depressed patients were randomized to MBCT or treatment as usual and followed up over a period of 60 weeks. MBCT significantly reduced relapse rates in patients with three or more previous episodes of depression, with 66% of those in the treatment as usual group compared to 40% of those in the MBCT group suffering from relapse. A later study by Ma and Teasdale (2004) replicated this finding in a smaller sample of 73 recovered patients, 55 of whom had suffered from three or more previous of depression. Of this latter group, 78% of those who had continued treatment as usual relapsed within the one-year follow-up compared to only 36% in the MBCT group.

The results from both of these trials advocate the use of MBCT to help reduce risk of relapse in individuals with recurrent depression. The fact that MBCT reduced relapse rates to about half in individuals with three or more episodes of depression, but did not produce significant effects in those with one or two previous episodes, is consistent with its focus on cognitive reactivity and rumination and the assumption that through associative learning these processes come to be increasingly relevant for relapse as individuals go through repeated episodes.

Studies explicitly investigating effects on relevant cognitive parameters and hypothesized mechanisms of action are only beginning to emerge. Williams, Teasdale, Segal and Soulsby (2000) found that MBCT can reduce deficits in autobiographical memory specificity, a phenomenon that has been shown to be play a central etiological role in depression. In a pre-post comparison study, Ramel, Goldin, Carmona, McQuaid (2004) found that mindfulness-based stress reduction (MBSR), the generic mindfulness program developed by John Kabat-Zinn, reduced ruminative tendencies in previously depressed patients, (2007).

While specifically developed for preventing relapse to depression, the programs' focus on changing cognitive reactivity and rumination suggests that it may also have some beneficial effects for patients currently suffering from depression. Some preliminary evidence that this may be the case comes from a pre-post comparison of MBCT (Kenny and Williams, 2007), which found significant reductions in symptoms in individuals with treatment-resistant depression who were treated with MBCT after CBT. The possibility of delivering MBCT to patients with ongoing symptoms of depression is welcome since individuals with highly recurrent depression may experience significant residual symptoms and fail to meet the strict recovery criteria that have been imposed in existing clinical trials (12 weeks symptom free). However, further randomized controlled trials exploring the use of MBCT for individuals with current depressive symptoms will be required before we can have confidence in the suitability of the approach for this group.

MBCT for Individuals with a History of Suicidal Depression

There are several reasons to suspect that the skills acquired during MBCT may be particularly suitable for patients who become suicidal when depressed (Williams et al., 2006; Lau, Segal & Williams, 2004). First, avoidance tendencies, targeted by MBCT, appear to be critically important in understanding suicidal ideation and behavior. The desire to escape from an unbearable situation is one of the most commonly reported motivations for suicidal behavior (e.g., Hjelmeland et al., 2002) and prominent psychological theories of suicidality converge on the suggestion that suicidality can be understood as an attempt to escape, from aversive self-consciousness (e.g., Baumeister, 1990), unbearable "psychache" (e.g., Schneidman, 1997) or intolerable circumstances in which the opportunity to escape by other means or to be rescued is perceived to be remote (e.g., Williams & Pollock, 2000; Williams, 2001). Thus the capacity to remain open to and stay with difficult experiences, responding with self-compassion and acceptance may be critically important. Additionally clinical experience suggests that some individuals spend considerable amounts of time ruminating about suicidal plans and fantasies, with suicidal ideation eliciting both distress and comfort and occurring in the context of broader deficits in effective problem solving (Schotte, Cools & Payvar, 1990). Thus the ability to disengage from ruminative thinking, and as a result to see suicidal thoughts and fantasies, like other thoughts and fantasies, simply as mental events, has the potential to be extremely beneficial for suicidal patients. Finally suicide-related cognitions and behavioral deficits appear to be subject to the same cognitive reactivity processes as other features of depression (Williams, van der Does, Barnhofer, Crane & Segal., in press; Williams, Barnhofer, Crane & Beck, 2005). As such, developing the ability to spot early warning signs of suicidal crisis and to remain mindful and make wise choices about how to respond may be critical in determining whether crises become suicidal crises, or whether individuals experiencing suicidal ideation go on to engage in suicidal behavior.

Pilot work in Oxford suggests that MBCT is acceptable to formerly suicidal patients, and a number of modifications have been incorporated into pilot groups to tailor MBCT more closely to the needs of individuals with a history of suicidality. These include (1) a greater emphasis on orienting participants' attention outward, through formal meditation practices (e.g., seeing, hearing meditations) and through encouragement to attend to and notice small things in everyday life (e.g., the sight of a bird, the sound of traffic). The aim of this is to enhance participants' ability to ground themselves in the present moment at times of intense negative affect, intrusive thoughts or memories, (2) a greater emphasis on the use of active meditation practices (yoga, stretching, walking) for participants experiencing difficulty with sitting meditation practices, for example due to agitation or overwhelming intrusive cognitions, (3) reflection in class on the cognitions which accompany suicidal states of mind and participants' own relapse signatures for suicidal crisis, to increase metacognitive awareness of these, (4) development of a crisis plan to enable participants to take wise action in the event that their mood deteriorates in the future, incorporating action to take in the event of suicidal ideation, (5) limited individual contact outside of classes (by telephone or face-to-face) between the instructor and any participants who are experiencing particular difficulties, to discuss how these might be managed through modification of the meditation practice or use of alternative strategies.

In running groups for individuals who had experienced suicidal ideation or behavior, there was an initial reticence about directly exploring suicidal cognitions in class, for fear of "giving people ideas." However the experience has been that the effects of raising these issues directly in class are positive, helping to reinforce an attitude of openness to *all* experiences, and the benefits of taking a metacognitive approach to even those thoughts which are perceived to be most powerful, shameful, dangerous or compelling. The pilot classes have been encouraging, suggesting that MBCT may hold benefit for at least some individuals with a history of suicidal depression. Whilst there is very little data in this area one recent pilot study from our group has suggested that MBCT may exert protective effects on prefrontal alpha asymmetry in resting EEG in formerly suicidal patients, a neurophysiological indicator of emotional functioning (Barnhofer et al., 2007). Interestingly the study by Kenny & Williams (2007) which examined MBCT in currently depressed patients also found equivalent results for patients whose depression had suicidal features as for those whose did not.

Summary and Conclusions

Mindfulness-based cognitive therapy is a skills training programme which teaches participants "to recognize and to disengage from mind states characterized by self-perpetuating patterns of ruminative, negative thought" (Segal et al., 2002, p. 75) and to adopt a stance toward experience which is characterized by openness, curiosity and acceptance, rather than experiential avoidance. Meditation practice, exercises from cognitive therapy and guided enquiry facilitate this process. Further research is needed to explore the mechanisms of action of MBCT and to examine its efficacy when compared to plausible alternative psychotherapeutic interventions, but initial findings suggest that it is a promising treatment for individuals with recurrent depression and may also be applicable to those whose depression has suicidal features and those with ongoing symptoms.

Acknowledgements: This work was supported by a grant from the Wellcome Trust, GR067797.

References

Barnhofer, T., Duggan, D. S., Crane, C., Hepburn, S., Fennell, M., & Williams, J. M. G. (2007). The effects of meditation of frontal alpha-asymmetry in previously suicidal individuals. *NeuroReport, 18,* 709-712

Compton, W. M., Conway, K. P., Stinson, F. S., & Grant, B. F. (2006). Changes in the prevalence of major depression and comorbid substance use disorders in the United States between 1991-1992 and 2001-2002. *American Journal of Psychiatry, 163,* 2141-2147.

Goldney, R. D., Wilson, D., Del Grande, E., Fisher, L. J., & MacFarlane, A. C. (2000). Suicide ideation in a random community sample: Attributable risk due to depression and psychosocial and traumatic events. *Australian and New Zealand Journal of Psychiatry, 34,* 98-106.

Hjelmeland, H., Hawton, K., Nordvic, H., Bille-Brahe, U., De Leo, D., Fekete, S., et al. (2002). Why people engage in parasuicide: a cross-cultural study of intentions. *Suicide and Life-Threatening Behaviour, 32,* 380-393.

Kabat-Zinn, J. (1990). *Full catastrophe living.* New York: Dell Publishing.

Kabat-Zinn, J. (1994). *Wherever you go, there you are: Mindfulness meditation in everyday life.* New York: Hyperion.

Katz, M., & Klerman, G.L. (1979). Introduction: Overview of the clinical studies program. *American Journal of Psychiatry, 136,* 49-51.

Keller, M. B., & Boland, R. J. (1998).Implications of failing to achieve successful long-term maintenance treatment of recurrent unipolar Major Depression. *Biological Psychiatry, 44,* 348-360.Katz & Klerman (1979)

Kenny, M. A., & Williams, J. M. G., (2007). Treatment-resistant depressed patients show a good response to Mindfulness-based cognitive therapy. *Behaviour Research & Therapy, 45,* 617-625.

Kessler, R. C., Berglund, P., Demler, O., Jin, R., Koretz, D., Merikangas, K. R. et al. (2003). The epidemiology of major depressive disorder: results from the national comorbidity survey replication (NCS-R). *JAMA: The Journal of the American Medical Association, 289,* 3095-3105.

Kessler, R. C., Mcgonagle, K. A., Zhao, S. Y., Nelson, C. B., Hughes, M., Eshleman, S. et al. (1994). Lifetime and 12-month prevalence of DSM-III-R psychiatric- disorders in the United-States – results from the national comorbidity survey. *Archives of General Psychiatry, 51,* 8-19.

Lau, M. A., Segal, Z. V., & Williams, J. M. G. (2004). Teasdale's differential activation hypothesis: Implications for mechanisms of depressive relapse and suicidal behavior. *Behaviour Research & Therapy, 42,* 1001-1017.

Lavori, P. W., Keller, M. B., Mueller, T. I., Scheftner, W., Fawcett, J., & Coryell, W. (1994). Recurrence after recovery in unipolar MDD- an observational follow-up-study of clinical predictors and somatic treatment as a mediating factor. *International Journal of Methods in Psychiatric Research, 4,* 211-229.

Ma, S. H., & Teasdale, J. D. (2004). Mindfulness-based cognitive therapy for depression: Replication and exploration of differential relapse prevention effects. *Journal of Consulting and Clinical Psychology, 72,* 31-40.

Mann, J. J., Waternaux, C., Haas, G. L., & Malone, K. M. (1999). Towards a clinical model of suicidal behaviour in psychiatric patients. *American Journal of Psychiatry, 156,* 181–189.

Monroe, S. M., & Harkness, K. L. (2005). Life stress, the "Kindling" hypothesis, and the recurrence of depression: Considerations from a life stress perspective. *Psychological Review, 112,* 417–455.

Murray, C. J. L. & Lopez, A. D. (1996). *The global burden of disease.* Cambridge, MA: Harvard University Press.

Nolen-Hoeksema, S. (2004). The response styles theory. In Papageorgiou, C., & Wells, A. Eds. *Depressive Rumination: Nature, theory and treatment*, pp. 107–124, Wiley, Chichester, UK.

Papageorgiou, C., & Wells, A. (2004). Nature, functions and beliefs about depressive rumination. In Papageorgiou, C., & Wells, A. Eds. *Depressive Rumination: Nature, theory and treatment*, pp. 3–20, Wiley, Chichester, UK.

Paykel, E. S., Brugha, T., & Fryers, T. (2005). Size and burden of depressive disorders in Europe. *European Neuropsychopharmacology, 15,* 411–423.

Raes, F., Hermans, D., Williams, J.M.G., Beyers, W., Brunfaut, E, Eelen, P (2006). Reduced autobiographical memory specificity and rumination in predicting the course of major depression. *Journal of Abnormal Psychology, 115,* 699–704.

Ramel, W., Goldin, P. R., Carmona, P. E., & McQuaid, J. R. (2004). The effects of mindfulness meditation on cognitive processes and affect in patients with past depression. *Cognitive Therapy & Research, 28,* 433–455.

Segal, Z. V., Williams, J. M. G., & Teasdale, J. D. (2002). *Mindfulness-based cognitive therapy for depression: a new approach to preventing relapse.* New York: Guilford.

Segal, Z. V., Williams, J. M. G., Teasdale, J. D., & Gemar, M. (1996). A cognitive science perspective on kindling and episode sensitization in recurrent affective disorder. *Psychological Medicine, 26,* 371–380.

Schneidman, E., (1997). The suicidal mind. In R. Maris, M.M. Silverman, & S. S. Canetto (Eds). *Review of Suicidology*, pp. 22–42. Guilford Press, New York.

Schotte, D. E., Cools, J., & Payvar, S. (1990). Problem-solving deficits in suicidal patients – trait vulnerability or state-phenomenon. *Journal of Consulting & Clinical Psychology, 58,* 562–564.

Solomon, D. A., Keller, M. B., Leon, A. C., Mueller, T. I., Lavori, P. W., Shea, M. T. et al. (2000). Multiple Recurrences of Major Depressive Disorder. *American Journal of Psychiatry, 157,* 229–233.

Teasdale, J. D., Segal, Z. V., Williams, J. M. G., Ridgeway, V. A., Soulsby, J. M., & Lau, M. A. (2000). Prevention of relapse/recurrence in major depression by mindfulness-based cognitive therapy. *Journal of Consulting and clinical Psychology, 68,* 615–623.

Treynor, W., Gonzalez, R., & Nolen-Hoeksema, S. *(2003). Rumination reconsidered: A psychometric analysis.* Cognitive Therapy and Research *(Special Issue on Rumination), 27, 247–259.*

Watkins, E., & Moulds, M. (2005). Distinct modes of ruminative self-focus: Impact of abstract versus concrete rumination on problem solving in depression. *Emotion, 5,* 319–328.

Wenzlaff, E. M., & Wegner, D. M. (2000). Thought Suppression. *Annual Review of Psychology, 51,* 59–91.

Williams, J. M. G. (2001). *Suicide and attempted suicide: understanding the cry of pain.* Penguin Books, London, UK.

Williams, J. M. G., Barnhofer, T., Crane, C. & Beck, A. T. *(2005).* Problem solving deteriorates following mood challenge in formerly depressed patients with a history of suicidal ideation. *Journal of Abnormal Psychology,* 114, 421–431.

Williams, J. M. G., Duggan, D. S., Crane, C., & Fennell, M. J. V. (2006). Mindfulness-based cognitive therapy for prevention of recurrence of suicidal behaviour. *Journal of Clinical Psychology, 62,* 201–210.

Williams, J. M. G., & Pollock, L. (2000). The psychology of suicidal behaviour. In K. Hawton & K. Van Heeringen (Eds). *The international handbook of suicide and attempted suicide.* pp. 79–93. John Wiley & Sons, Chichester, UK.

Williams, J. M. G., Teasdale, J. D., Segal, Z. V., & Soulsby, J. (2000). Mindfulness-based cognitive therapy reduces overgeneral autobiographical memory in formerly depressed patients. *Journal of Abnormal Psychology, 109,* 150–155.

Williams, J. M. G., Van der Does, A. J. W., Barnhofer, T., Crane, C., & Segal, Z. V. (in press). Cognitive reactivity, suicidal ideation and future fluency: preliminary investigation of a differential activation theory of hopelessness/suicidality. *Cognitive Therapy and Research.*

13

Mindfulness and Borderline Personality Disorder

Shireen L. Rizvi, Stacy Shaw Welch, and Sona Dimidjian

Borderline personality disorder (BPD) is a severe personality disorder characterized by prominent and pervasive dysregulation of emotion, behavior, and cognition. Current diagnostic criteria for BPD include difficulties with interpersonal relationships, affective instability, problems with anger, destructive impulsive behaviors, frantic efforts to avoid abandonment, problems with self-identity, chronic feelings of emptiness, transient dissociative symptoms and/or paranoid ideation, and suicidal behaviors (American Psychiatric Association, 2000). In order for a diagnosis to be made, at least five of these nine criteria must be present beginning in early adulthood and lasting for several years.

Of all psychiatric disorders, BPD represents one of the more challenging to manage and treat within the mental health system for several reasons. First, individuals with BPD utilize mental health treatment at highly disproportionate rates. Although prevalence rates indicate that 1–2% of the general population meet criteria for BPD, it is estimated that between 9 and 40% of high inpatient services utilizers have a diagnosis of BPD (Surber et al., 1987; Swigar, Astrachan, Levine, Mayfield, & Radovich, 1991). Second, a diagnosis of BPD is associated with a number of "therapy interfering behaviors" which makes administration of consistent treatment difficult. High dropout rates of up to 60% are not uncommon in treatment studies for BPD and usually occur within the first three to six months of treatment regardless of actual planned treatment length (Kelly et al., 1992; Skodol, Buckley, & Charles, 1983; Waldinger and Gunderson, 1984). Other behaviors that interfere with therapy and may lead to therapist burn-out are storming out of sessions early or not leaving when the session is over, throwing objects, not showing up for appointments or showing up extremely late, not paying for therapy, or not doing assigned tasks (Linehan, 1993a; Stone, 2000). Third, individuals with BPD often carry diagnoses for several disorders at the same time. Mood disorders, especially major depression, are most commonly observed, but rates of other Axis I disorders, including eating disorders, substance use disorders, and PTSD are also quite high (Lieb, Schmahl, Linehan, & Bohus, 2004; Skodol et al., 2002). Finally, BPD is associated with high risk of lethality. BPD is the only DSM-IV diagnosis for which chronic attempts to harm or kill oneself is a criterion and studies have demonstrated up to 8% of individuals with BPD ultimately commit suicide (Linehan, Rizvi, Shaw Welch, & Page, 2000).

Fortunately, recent advances in the field have led to promising treatments for BPD. Dialectical Behavior Therapy (DBT), originally developed by Linehan for suicidal individuals with BPD (Linehan, 1993a, b), has received the most empirical support thus far, with nine randomized clinical trials demonstrating its efficacy (see Linehan & Dexter-Mazza, 2007, for a review). DBT is also one of the first psychosocial treatments for any disorder to incorporate mindfulness as a core component.

Overview of DBT for BPD

DBT is a cognitive-behavioral therapy infused with acceptance strategies. The central "dialectic" in DBT exists in the tension between accepting the client exactly as he/she is in that moment and simultaneously pushing toward change and creating a life worth living. Change is achieved through standard cognitive-behavioral strategies, such as functional analyses, contingency management, cognitive restructuring, exposure, and skills training. Acceptance is an active process, demonstrated through the use of validation strategies (Linehan, 1997).

In its standard form, four components comprise the treatment: weekly individual psychotherapy, weekly group skills training sessions, as-needed telephone consultation, and weekly consultation team meetings involving all DBT therapists. Guidelines for conducting individual sessions specify that treatment should address clearly prioritized targets. These targets include, in order of priority: life threatening behaviors including suicidal/self-harm and homicidal urges and actions, behaviors that interfere with or threaten therapy, severe Axis I disorders, and patterns that preclude a reasonable quality of life. In addition, sessions are structured to begin with a review of the diary card, which is a monitoring form that the client completes daily to record urges, behavior, skills use, and emotional experiences that arose in week since the preceding session. Skills training sessions function similar to a class and follow a particular agenda each week designed to enhance skills capabilities in four domains: mindfulness, interpersonal effectiveness, emotion regulation, and distress tolerance (Linehan, 1993b).

Biosocial Theory and the Development and Maintenance of BPD Symptomatology

Linehan's biosocial theory of BPD posits that the disorder is primarily a dysfunction of the emotion regulation system. From this perspective, BPD criterion behaviors can be seen as either attempts to regulate negative emotions or inexorable consequences of dysregulated emotions. Furthermore, the theory states that this emotion regulation dysfunction develops over time. The theory posits that there is a transaction between a biological tendency toward intense emotionality and an "invalidating environment" (see Linehan, 1993a), which often punishes, corrects, or ignores behavior independent of its actual validity. Through interactions with this environment, the individual learns to discount the validity of their own emotional responses and often looks to external cues for information on how to respond. In addition, the individual learns to form unrealistic goals and expectations for themselves and others. As a consequence of this learning over time, a person with BPD tends to oscillate between emotional inhibition (shutting down emotional responses) and extreme emotional styles. Furthermore, Linehan theorized that a central problem in individuals with BPD is that their experience of emotions is different than individuals without BPD in three specific domains. First, individuals with BPD have lower thresholds to emotional cues. Second, BPD individuals have higher reactivity to emotional cues, meaning that their responses are more extreme more quickly than other individuals. Third, in BPD, a slower return to baseline following an emotion episode is theorized to be evident. These three characteristics are a result of both the biological deficit and the invalidating environment, proposed in the biosocial theory, and inevitably lead to a life filled with intense emotions, interpersonal difficulties, coping problems, and dysfunctional behaviors, which often function (no matter how short-lived) to ease the pain and suffering of such intolerable emotional states.

Addressing Emotion Dysregulation Through Mindfulness in DBT

The core mindfulness skills in DBT are designed to help individuals focus more on the present moment, letting go of memories of the past and worry about the future. The seven concrete skills also target the difficulties that are inevitable consequences of the pervasive emotion dysregulation described above. These difficulties include problems that occur under highly aroused states with processing new information vital to learning, longstanding patterns of self-invalidation, and impulsive behavior that occurs in the context of emotional arousal and that functions to decrease emotional suffering in the short-term. Mindfulness skills, described below, are taught routinely in group skills training.

In addition to the teaching of mindfulness in skills groups, the individual therapist also frequently incorporates mindfulness into individual therapy. Therapy is an opportunity (though often an unwelcome one!) during which individuals with BPD are put into direct contact with emotional cues that they generally try to avoid. Being asked to describe a recent negative interaction with a partner or recount their latest self-injurious act about which they feel intense shame can cause highly dysregulated states. A goal of DBT is to have the individual learn to be skillful in all relevant contexts, including during times of difficulty. Mindfulness skills are used within sessions, then, to help the individual begin to regulate his or her emotions in an effective manner. Mindfulness practice helps a client with BPD in four overlapping ways: (1) increasing attentional control, (2) increasing awareness of private experience, (3) decreasing impulsive action, and (4) increasing self-validation (Lynch, Chapman, Rosenthal, Kuo, & Linehan, 2006).

Increased attentional control occurs through an emphasis on full participation in each moment. This focus on the current moment initially requires constant effort as most individuals report that they very infrequently do this. Clients in distress might be asked to focus on their breath as it comes in and out of their nostrils as a way of drawing awareness to this one moment. This focus of attention also allows for a client to begin to practice experiencing and attending to their own states (emotions/urges/thoughts) without doing anything to eliminate them. By doing so, clients become more aware of their private experience and can begin to label a thought as a thought, a feeling as a feeling without judgment. An added benefit of these skills is an increase in insight of possible precipitants and consequences of maladaptive behavior (e.g., "I realize that the thought 'I'm a horrible person' went through my mind before I had the urge to harm myself" or "I noticed a decrease in anger immediately after I injured myself"). This insight helps in contributing to comprehensive behavioral assessment of maladaptive behavior, which is the foundation of all cognitive-behavioral treatment.

Furthermore, this greater awareness also leads to more effective solutions in that the individual learns to "ride out" impulsive urges. By just noticing physiological sensations or thoughts without doing anything to try to overtly change them, individuals learn to accept and tolerate them through mindfulness. The behavioral conceptualization of destructive behaviors characteristic of BPD (e.g., substance use, suicidal behavior) specifies that such behaviors are frequently negatively reinforced due to the immediate reduction in emotional distress that follows such behavior. Because individuals have learned to engage in such behaviors over time, they have typically *not* learned that emotional distress will dissipate on its own.

Finally, mindfulness targets the self-invalidating behavior so common to clients with BPD. According to the biosocial theory, individuals with BPD have often grown up in environments that consistently modeled invalidation. Thus, many have learned to self-invalidate over time. Such self-invalidation typically presents in treatment through the often repeated words of "I can't" and "I shouldn't" as they apply to what clients think, what they feel, and who they are. The ubiquity of self-invalidation among clients with BPD is particularly troubling given the research on the effects of thought suppression and avoidance. These studies demonstrate a clear pattern in which thought suppression and avoidance have the paradoxical consequence of *increasing* the very thoughts and feelings one attempts to decrease (Gross & John, 2003; Wegner, 1994). One of the functions of mindfulness interventions in DBT is to target explicitly self-invalidation among clients with BPD. Mindfulness teaches clients to approach experience with a nonjudgmental and accepting stance. Through practice, clients learn to apply these skills to thoughts and feelings that they may have learned through past experience to invalidate automatically. In these ways, mindfulness strategies can help to interrupt the cycle of intense emotion and the paradoxical effects of invalidation.

DBT Mindfulness Skills

In DBT, mindfulness is conceptualized as the experience of entering fully into the present moment, at the level of direct and immediate experience. In order to accomplish this, a set of seven concrete skills is taught and practiced on a regular basis. These skills are considered "core" skills in that they are directly relevant to effective practice of all other DBT skills and are therefore repeated frequently in instruction. These seven skills are wise mind, observe, describe, participate, nonjudgmentally, one-mindfully, and effectively.

In DBT, it is assumed that all people have innate access to wisdom. This state of wisdom, or "wise mind," represents the synthesis of two other abstract "states of mind": "emotion mind" and "reasonable mind." Emotion mind refers to the state in which emotions are experienced as controlling thoughts and behavior. Commonly, clients with BPD who start treatment describe feeling like they are continually in emotion mind because they constantly feel under the control of their emotions. In contrast, reasonable mind refers to the state in which logic and reason control thoughts and behavior. Whereas emotion mind is hot and impulsive, reasonable mind is cool and calculating. Wise mind is considered to be a blend of the best parts of these states of mind in addition to the quality of an intuitive sense of *knowing* something deep within. Accessing wise mind allows one to take action with ease even though the action itself may be challenging. For instance, wise mind may guide one to enter a burning house to save a child, an action that is clearly difficult but is accompanied by clarity of intuitive knowing. An assumption in DBT is that everyone is "in wise mind" some of the time; through practice, wise mind can be experienced on a more regular basis and more readily accessed when desired.

The other six mindfulness skills are categorized into *what* skills and *how* skills. *What* skills describe the actions that one takes when practicing mindfulness. These include: *observing, describing*, and *participating*. The *what* skills can only be practiced one at a time; for example, it is not possible to observe and describe or to describe and participate in the same moment. The how skills include *nonjudgmentally, one-mindfully*, and *effectively*. The how skills can be practiced individually when learning and, as skill increases, can be brought to bear simultaneously as one practices particular *what* skills.

The first what skill, *observing*, is direct perception of experiences, without the addition of concepts or categories. This can be extremely unfamiliar and difficult for many clients (and many therapists!). It is useful to think of the five senses when practicing the observe skill because sounds, touch, taste, sight, and smell provide constant opportunity for observation. The instruction invites clients to bring their attention to the level of direct sensation and to *just notice*. Frequently when teaching this skill, clients report automatically attending to conceptual descriptions. For instance, a client might observe a sound of "chirp chirp" outside the window and ascribe a label to it (e.g., "that's a bird"). The therapist helps to identify the categorization that has occurred and redirect the client back to the sensations of sound. Often, categorization will be quickly followed by judgmental evaluation (e.g., "I hate birds; this place is too noisy; I can't practice this stupid homework thing anyway"). Practice with the observing skill helps clients to return again and again to direct sensation, including those judged to be unpleasant. Observations can also be applied to internal experiences, such as the sensations of a particular emotion. By just noticing what anger feels like, for example, without doing anything to change it, one can observe the physical sensations and, over time, recognize that the emotion itself is not threatening.

Describing involves adding a descriptive label to what is observed. When individuals are asked to recount what they observed aloud to the therapist or the group, they are being asked to describe. For instance, if the client described above had been practicing describing, she might have been instructed to note "thinking," as in "I had the thought that a bird is going 'chirp chirp"' or "judging," as in "the judgment 'this is stupid' went through my mind." Many clients experience thoughts as literal and objective facts. While many thoughts that are assumed to be facts are relatively harmless (e.g., "that sound is being made by a bird"), other thoughts assumed to be facts can be associated with significant negative consequences. For example, clients report that they "know" that somebody doesn't like them based on a facial expression or a comment that they interpret as malicious. Recognizing that the *thought* "she doesn't like me" is different than the *fact* "she doesn't like me" is an important step in learning new behavior. If it is just a thought, then it is open to supporting evidence of falsification. Practicing the skill of describing allows clients to begin to experience thoughts as mental events that arise and pass away in the mind. Clients can practice describing using external experiences (e.g., sounds, colors) or internal experiences (e.g., thoughts, emotions).

Participating refers to entering fully and completely into an experience. When participating, the separation between self and activity falls away. It is a state of full engagement, similar to the state of flow described by other authors (e.g., Csikszentmihalyi, 1991). It is also void of self-consciousness, as self and activity are experienced in a united state. Clients can often call to mind some activities in which they participate fully and naturally; this varies widely, but examples include sports activity, dancing, or participating in conversations that captivate interest. However, practicing participation in a greater number of daily activities can be very difficult for clients with BPD, who frequently struggle with high levels of self-consciousness. Both individual and group therapy can be opportunities for practice of this skill and clients are often asked to throw themselves into the activity of participating in therapy. Participating can also be a valuable practice for clients who are sensation seeking or likely to judge certain activities as mundane/boring.

In many ways, the first how skill, n*onjudgmentally*, is the most radical skill taught in DBT. It involves letting go of all judgments, including both good and bad judgments, about self and others. Often clients object to this skill because they assume that to give up judgment means to give up preference or approval. For instance, clients often assume that being judgmental means that they cannot hate something very painful. It is important to clarify that being nonjudgmental does not mean giving up strong emotional responses. Moreover, it does not mean giving up values and preferences in the world. A client can prefer to live in a world without prejudice against people with mental illness, can in fact hate instances of prejudice when they occur, and still be nonjudgmental. Being nonjudgmental involves emphasizing observable facts (e.g., who, what, when, and where) and describing consequences, as opposed to making evaluations and interpretations. Clients are asked to practice the nonjudgmental skill by just describing, without adding on their interpretations. They are also challenged to restructure judgmental cognitions in the moment and to repeat a phrase or statement nonjudgmentally.

One-mindfully simply means attending to one thing at a time. It is the opposite of multi-tasking and doing one thing while thinking about another. Clients are encouraged to think that everything can be done one-mindfully. A well-used example is referencing Thich Nhat Hanh's description of washing dishes (1991). He writes "Washing the dishes is at the same time a means and an end – that is, not only do we do the dishes in order to have clean dishes, we also do the dishes just to do the dishes, to live fully in each moment while washing them" (1991, p. 27). When taught this skill, clients often respond by saying that they get more done when they are doing many things at once and that doing one thing at a time is inefficient. Here it is useful to cite the research that suggests that multi-tasking is associated with more time spent on each task (e.g, Foerde, Knowlton, & Poldrack, 2006). Personal anecdotes about how multi-tasking creates more problems are also useful demonstrations of the negative consequences of doing more than one thing at a time (e.g., talking on a cell phone while driving led to a near-accident, having a conversation with someone while thinking about something else led to an embarrassing moment in which you didn't know what the person just asked you). Positive consequences of practicing one-mindfully include increased attentional control and decreased rumination, which can often reduce emotional distress.

The skill of *effectively* asks clients to practice giving up being "right" in favor of doing "what works." The maxim "Don't cut off your nose to spite your face" is appropriate here. Practicing effectively means doing just what is needed in the moment to achieve one's desired goals, no more and no less. Clients with BPD often struggle with this skill due to the strong emphasis on proving that they are "right" and that things "should" be a certain way. Clients are taught that whether they are right or wrong is not at question, but rather the focus is on getting what they want. DBT with clients with BPD frequently provides a multitude of opportunities for clients to practice being effective; interactions with family members, friends, and treatment providers are all valuable contexts in which to practice. Being effective, thus, is highlighted throughout treatment and therapists frequently ask clients "what is the effective thing to do in this situation?" as a way of guiding and structuring client behavioral responses.

It is important to note that throughout DBT therapy, the therapist is modeling the use of all these skills. The DBT therapist one-mindfully participates in therapy in a nonjudgmental and effective manner. The therapist practices with the client and shares his or her own experience of mindfulness practice. Ideally, the therapist demonstrates that mindfulness is not easily acquired but with practice and diligence, the use of these skills will lead to an overall improvement in quality of life.

Case Example

As previously mentioned, mindfulness is taught to all clients in DBT skills groups, and is considered to be the basis for many other skills. The degree to which mindfulness is emphasized by the individual DBT therapist depends on the client's goals, therapy targets, and case formulation. The following case example will illustrate how mindfulness skills are woven into the individual therapy mode of DBT. "Mia"[1] was a 22-year-old woman who met criteria for BPD. She reported a history of suicide attempts and non-suicidal self-injury, typically cutting, which she had engaged in between 10–30 times per month since she was 17. Mia attended a local community college and lived

---

[1] Names and details have been altered to protect confidentiality.

with her boyfriend, with whom she had a tumultuous relationship that often included intense arguments followed by temporary break-ups. He would typically leave the apartment they shared for several days, sometimes getting involved with other women, before returning and re-engaging in the relationship. Mia would typically cut herself or take non-lethal overdoses of pain medication after fights with her boyfriend. Detailed analyses indicated that the typical pattern was that after a conflict, she would take enough pain medication to put herself to sleep, with the thought that "if it kills me, fine." Upon waking, she would cut herself until she felt "soothed" and would then skip classes and spend the day alone. This pattern occurred 1–5 times per month, and had also resulted in academic struggles and threat of suspension, despite the fact that Mia was an extremely bright, dedicated student who did very well academically despite this pattern and hoped to attend medical school one day.

The initial stages of therapy focused on helping Mia stop all self-injurious behavior, and teach her other more skillful means of regulating her affect. Mindfulness skills were conceptualized as essential throughout the treatment for Mia. Main areas of emphasis included (1) helping her use "Wise Mind" to make more effective decisions about her life that were based on her values, rather than on avoidance of immediate negative affect, and (2) increasing her ability to observe her private experiences without judgment, self-invalidation, or avoidance, so that she could (a) tolerate negative affect more skillfully, and (b) more mindfully choose an effective response (thereby decreasing impulsive, destructive behavior).

The focus on mindfulness was primarily achieved by emphasizing the seven mindfulness skills in individual therapy. This was not done in a formal protocol, but in response to the problems and issues Mia brought up each week in treatment. Practicing the skills in the treatment session was a priority, as the skills were novel and difficult for Mia. Simply describing them and assigning them for homework would have set her up for failure. Examples of how the skills were incorporated into the treatment session are given below.

Wise Mind

Mia, like the majority of clients with BPD, immediately identified herself as someone who *"lives in emotion mind"* and had difficulty acting mindfully based on her values/internal wisdom. The following is an example of how wise mind was used in a conversation about giving up self-injury as an option.

T: OK, so what did you cut yourself with?
C: A razor blade...
T: but I thought you got rid of all of them last week...did you go out and buy one?
C: No...I had to keep one, just in case. I kept one saved. It's a special one to me. I guess I'm really not ready to do this. I won't give this up. All I can say is that cutting works for now and to be honest I really don't think I want to give it up. It made sense when we were talking about it last week but now I know this is just not for me.

T: So you've been thinking about this a lot.

C: yes…

T: Ok. So did you go over Wise Mind in group last night?

C: Yes…

T: So here is what I want to do, is go over this decision of whether or not to give up cutting but use Wise Mind, really practice that skill here. Here's why; when we were talking about it last week, you had all the reasons to stop cutting, you had the logic, what state of mind would you call that?

C: Reason mind.

T: Right, yes, because you're using reason. Now it strikes me that when you got home and threw out all those razor blades except one, I am betting that you made that decision from emotion mind. Do you know what I mean?

C: Yeah, I agree. I should do it but it feels like I can't. That's like the story of my life.

T: Well, right, for many people that is true, we can think about something logically before we're tempted with something but when we're upset we think with our emotions. Using the Wise Mind skill is trying to use mind-ful awareness to get out of that trap, to really go inside yourself and access your own wisdom, and that has both logic and emotion. So I want to actually practice that right now and just see what your wise mind says about this decision with cutting. Because even if my Wise Mind wants you to do this and you agree when you're with me, ulti-mately it's true that you have to know in your own Wise Mind. So, what practice did you find the most helpful in group in terms of finding wise mind?

C: I liked the one where we pretended we were a flake of rock, floating to the bottom of a lake and the bottom was wise mind.

T: Ok, so lets do that now. Just notice your breath and then imagine the rock…when you get to the bottom, I want you to see if you can just notice what your Wise Mind says about letting go of that last razor. Don't force anything. Just notice what comes.

Following this exercise, Mia said that she felt that her wise mind was telling her that she needed to close the door on cutting and that it was the right thing to do, but that her fear of "going crazy" without the outlet of cutting was holding her back from fully committing to abstinence. This realization facilitated a discussion about ways to tolerate intense emotion, and also a plan to agree to give up cutting for three months with the understanding that her fear was valid, and that if help from the therapist and the DBT skills did not work, she could always go back to cutting later.

Observe and Describe

Observing and describing were used to help Mia begin to experience moments of intense negative affect, and to mindfully chose her responses instead of reacting impulsively. Emphasis was placed on observing the "wave" of emotions and allowing them to peak and decrease without engag-ing in avoidance behaviors. During sessions, the therapist frequently asked

Mia to observe and describe her emotions and tolerate them for increasingly lengthy periods of time (30 seconds, 2 minutes, etc.) without engaging in efforts to avoid. Instead of "becoming" her emotion, Mia learned to step back and observe the thoughts, physiological sensations, and urges she was having. She also began asking "can I tolerate this moment?" or "can I tolerate this for the next 5 minutes?" She would then use the describe skills to either describe to herself what was happening *("I notice the thought that I can't stand this...there are tears in my eyes and I feel the urge to run out of the room...my chest is tight...I feel hot...")*. The difficulty of this task for Mia (and many clients with BPD) cannot be overstated. However, practicing these mindfulness skills in this manner was extremely useful and she began to recognize that her emotions *"may hurt but won't kill me...and they do go down on their own even if I don't do anything to stop them."*

Other Mindfulness Skills

The other mindfulness skills were also incorporated into the treatment often; space precludes detailed transcripts of each. Working on decreasing self-judgments, which were frequent for Mia and tended to increase her emotional vulnerability, was a frequent topic in treatment. In therapy, the following types of interactions occurred numerous times:

C: I'm just so STUPID! Why do I do these things...
T: Could you please tell me what you mean and lose the judgment?
C: I can't believe I...did something...so stupid...
T: So stupid doesn't tell me anything...what is the thought? Use the describe skill...
C: I'm so mad at myself that I avoided class.
T: Wonderful! So you noticed anger at yourself for avoiding. So that was great, now I know what's happening and you and I can work on solving this problem...

The key to interactions such as this one is a light, nonjudgmental (even gently teasing or irreverent) tone, and coaching where needed. Mia worked on observing judgments, and mindfully choosing to either reframe them, noticing them and letting them go, or building empathy.

Mia incorporated the participate skills in several ways. First, she would use this skill often to throw herself into whatever skillful behavior she chose as an alternative to cutting; for instance, she would often go walking and mindfully observe her feet touching the ground, all physical sensations, and so forth. She was often prompted by the therapist to practice the participate skill during sessions, as well, especially when she was tempted to avoid difficult content. Finally, she began participating in routine household tasks, such as washing dishes and doing laundry. Mia also used the "one-mindful" skill in similar ways, to help her engage fully in skillful alternates to self-injury. She also used this skill to help herself "slow down" in highly emotional moments, and it appeared to both her and the therapist that this was extremely useful in decreasing impulsive behavior.

Over the course of treatment, Mia showed remarkable improvement. By the end of treatment, she had stopped all self-injurious behavior, was much less judgmental of herself, and was steadily attending classes and doing well. She eventually ended the relationship with her boyfriend in a highly skillful manner, and moved into a house with female roommates. It appeared to both the therapist and Mia that the mindfulness skills had been of paramount importance to her. The most striking example was her use of the observe and describe skills; once Mia learned that she could tolerate emotional pain and that it would not last forever *without her doing anything about it*, avoidance behaviors such as self-injury decreased dramatically. It also appeared that the practice of these skills, along with participating and wise mind, resulted in her increased sense of self. The practice of the nonjudgmental and effective skills was also very helpful to her in increasing her behavioral control.

Specific Mindfulness Exercises

What follows are some specific mindfulness exercises that we use in our practice of therapy with BPD clients. This list should be considered illustrative rather than exhaustive. As one practices DBT, one quickly realizes that there is no limit to the possibilities for mindfulness practice! Remembering that the *how* skills are incorporated into the practice of wise mind and the what skills, we did not include specific exercises for them. Rather, the DBT therapist is mindful of a client's judgment, engagement in more than one thing at a time, use of "should statements" throughout the practice, and the presence of willfulness (as opposed to effective willingness to engage in the process). There are also many written sources available for mindfulness practice ideas. The DBT skills are heavily influenced by the writings of Thich Nhat Hanh and many of his published books contain valuable practice exercises. Another source for exercises is Jon Kabat-Zinn's *Full Catastrophe Living* (1990) and *Whereever you go, There you are* (1994). Furthermore, the Linehan skills manual (1993b), recent publications of a book on adaptations of DBT in clinical settings (Dimeff & Koerner, 2007), and a book on DBT for adolescents (Miller, Rathus, & Linehan, 2007) contain additional DBT practice exercises.

Wise Mind

- Clients are asked to use imagery and imagine that they are a flake of rock drifting to the bottom of a deep and clear lake. The therapist guides the imagery by instructing with some statements as: "Imagine that you are a little flake of rock skipping across a lake, out into the water. As this flake of rock, you begin to go down in the water, floating in circles, deeper in the clear, cool water containing you. Slowly, you circle further down and then you reach the bottom. As you rest there at the bottom, you experience being centered and at peace."
- Ask clients to follow the feeling and cadence of their breath with a simple practice or whatever practice has already been learned. After a few moments, ask clients if they can experience or connect with a wise, centered place within them.

Observe

- The therapist can say a word like "elephant" and ask clients to just notice that word going through their mind. Clients are instructed not to push it away or to hold on to it, but rather to just watch the word come and go.
- The therapist can bring in something small to eat like a raisin, piece of fruit, mint, or small chocolate. Clients are asked to observe the sensations of eating, such as taste, texture, smell, and the physical sensation of swallowing.
- The therapist can play music that is quite dissonant, or might be experienced as unpleasant by many. Clients are instructed to observe the sound, and also observe any thoughts, emotions or sensations that arise.

Describe

- Pictures of people making emotional expressions (e.g., anger, fear, joy) can be brought in and clients asked to describe what they see. Often clients will say "she's really angry" or "he's scared" and the therapist can point out that anger and fear are not directly observable and therefore cannot be described. Rather, "lips turned down," "brow furrowed," "squinted eyes," and others are examples of describe statements.
- Following an observe exercise like the ones above, clients can be asked to describe their experience, without adding on judgments, interpretations, and so forth.

Participate

- Activities can be brought into group sessions and clients asked to fully participate in them. For example, using a word puzzle or a maze, clients can be asked to throw themselves completely into the solving of the puzzle for a certain period of time. After the exercise is over, they can be asked if judgments went through their mind about themselves or the exercise.
- Any activity that tends to prompt self-consciousness offers abundant opportunity for practicing the skill of participate. Popular choices include singing (e.g., typical rounds such as "Row Row Row Your Boat"), dancing, or laughing out loud in a "laugh club."
- Another interesting participate exercise is to do an exercise that will likely draw self-consciousness, like those listed above. Afterwards, ask clients to imagine what they would have looked like doing the exercise had they done it with no self-consciousness. Then repeat the exercise, allowing them additional opportunity to practice throwing themselves into participating.

References

American Psychiatric Association (2000). *Diagnostic and statistical manual of mental disorders* (4th Ed.). Washington, DC: Author.

Csikszentmihalyi, M. (1991). *Flow: The psychology of optimal experience*. New York: Harper Perennial.

Dimeff, L. A., & Koerner, K. (Eds.), *Dialectical Behavior Therapy in clinical practice: Applications across disorders and settings*. New York: Guilford Press.

Foerde, K., Knowlton, B. J., & Poldrack, R. A. (2006). Modulation of competing memory systems by distraction. *Proceedings of the National Academy of Sciences, 103*, 11778-11783.

Gross, J. J., & John, O. P. (2003). Individual differences in two emotion regulation processes: Implications for affect, relationship, and well-being. *Journal of Personality and Social Psychology, 85*, 348-362.

Hanh, T. N. (1991). *Peace is every step*. New York: Bantam Books.

Kabat-Zinn, J. (1990). *Full catastrophe living*. New York: Delta.

Kabat-Zinn, J. (1994). *Whereever you go, there you are: Mindfulness meditation in everyday life*. New York: Hyperion Press.

Kelly, T., Soloff, P. H., Cornelius, J., George, A., Lis, J. A., & Ulrich, R. (1992). Can we study (treat) borderline patients? Attrition from research and open treatment. *Journal of Personality Disorders, 6*, 417-433.

Lieb, K., Schmahl, C., Linehan, M. M., & Bohus, M. (2004). Borderline Personality Disorder. *The Lancet, 364*, 453-461.

Linehan, M. M. (1993a). *Cognitive behavioral treatment for borderline personality disorder*. New York: Guilford Press.

Linehan, M. M. (1993b). *Skills training manual for treating borderline personality disorder*. New York: Guilford Press.

Linehan, M. M. (1997). Validation and psychotherapy. In A. Bohart & L. Greenberg (Eds.), *Empathy reconsideration: New directions in psychotherapy* (pp. 353-392). Washington, DC: American Psychological Association.

Linehan, M. M., & Dexter-Mazza, L. (2007). Dialectical Behavior Therapy for borderline personality disorder. In D. H. Barlow (Ed.), *Clinical handbook of psychological disorders* (4th ed.). New York: Guilford Press.

Linehan, M. M., Rizvi, S. L., Shaw Welch, S., & Page, B. (2000). Psychiatric aspects of suicidal behaviour: Personality disorders. In K. Hawton & K. v. Heeringen (Eds.), *The International Handbook of Suicide and Attempted Suicide* (pp. 147-178). New York: John Wiley & Sons.

Lynch, T. R., Chapman, A. L., Rosenthal, M. Z., Kuo, J. R., & Linehan, M. M. (2006). Mechanisms of change in Dialectical Behavior Therapy: Theoretical and empirical observations. *Journal of Clinical Psychology, 62*, 459-480.

Miller, A. L., Rathus, J. H., & Linehan, M. M. (2007). *Dialectical behavior therapy with suicidal adolescents*. New York: Guilford Press.

Skodol, A. E., Buckley, P., & Charles, E. (1983). Is there a characteristic pattern to the treatment history of clinic outpatients with borderline personality? *Journal of Nervous and Mental Disease, 171*, 405-410.

Skodol, A. E., Gunderson, J. G., Pfohl, B., Widiger, T. A., Livesley, W. J., & Siever, L. J. (2002). The Borderline diagnosis I: Psychopathology, comorbidity, and personality structure. *Society of Biological Psychiatry, 51*, 936-950.

Stone, M. H. (2000). Clinical guidelines for psychotherapy for patients with Borderline Personality Disorder. *Psychiatric Clinics of North America, 23*, 193-210.

Surber, R. W., Winkler, E. L., Monteleone, M., Havassy, B. E., Goldfinger, & Hopkin (1987). Characteristics of high users of acute psychiatric inpatient services. *Hospital and Community Psychiatry, 38*, 1112-1114.

Swigar, M. E., Astrachan, B., Levine, M. A., Mayfield, V., & Radovich (1991). Single and repeated admissions to a mental health center: Demographic, clinical and use of service characteristics. *International Journal of Social Psychiatry, 37*, 259-266.

Waldinger, R. J., & Gunderson, J. G. (1984). Completed psychotherapies with borderline patients. *American Journal of Psychotherapy, 38*, 190-202.

Wegner, D. M. (1994). *White bears and other unwanted thoughts: Suppression, obsession, and the psychological of mental control*. New York: Guilford Press.

14

Mindfulness-Based Approaches to Eating Disorders

Ruth Q. Wolever and Jennifer L. Best

Worries go down better with soup

~Jewish Proverb

Introduction

Eating disorders (ED) are complex multidimensional behavioral syndromes characterized by pervasive core deficits in the self-regulation of food intake, affect, and cognition (Dalle Grave, Di Pauli, Sartirana, Calugi & shafran, 2007; Deaver, Miltenberger, Smyth, Meidinger & Crosby, 2003; Shafran, Teachman, Kerry, & Rachman, 1999; Spoor, Bekker, Van Heck, Croon, & Van Strien, 2005). Disturbance in self-regulation of food intake is linked to difficulty in recognizing physiological signals of hunger and satiety as well as in discerning these signals from somatic signals of emotion. Disturbance in emotion regulation reflects deficits in identifying, managing and adaptively utilizing emotion. Disturbance in cognition reflects extreme rigidity seen in cognitive restraint around eating behaviors, perfectionism and distorted thinking about weight and shape. ED frequently persist even in the face of significant deterioration in psychological and physiological wellness. Given their increasing prevalence, and the associated high risk of relapse and concurrent psychopathology, greater attention is warranted to improve the efficacy of existing treatments. Mindfulness approaches can intervene by improving self-regulation and the emerging evidence demonstrates the potential utility of these approaches.

Eating Disorders: An Overview of Diagnostic Characteristics, Epidemiology, Course and Outcome

Individuals suffering from ED are typically driven by an intense desire to achieve a thin body ideal (Thomsen, McCoy, & Williams, 2001) and are frequently characterized by distorted body images (Cash & Deagle, 1997), preoccupations with thoughts related to food (Powell & Thelen, 1996), and self-concepts that are overly invested in body weight and shape (APA, 2000). Additionally, recovery from ED is often further complicated by comorbid Axis I and/or Axis II pathology (Fernandez-Aranda et al., 2008). Development of ED is related to the confluence of biopsychosocial factors: dominant sociocultural values and peer influences (Hutchinson & Rapee, 2007), family of origin interpersonal dynamics (Felker & Stivers, 1994), and individual differences in temperament and personality style (Franco-Paredes, Mancilla-Diaz, Vazquez-Arevalo, Lopez-Aguilar, & Alvarez-Rayon, 2005), in conjunction with established biological vulnerabilities (Becker, Keel, Anderson-Fye, & Thomas, 2004). Prevalence of clinically significant eating disturbances now traverse socioeconomic and demographic lines (e.g., ethnic minorities, males, middle-aged women: Brandsma, 2007; Harris & Cumella, 2006; Striegel-Moore, Wilfley, Pike, Dohm, & Fairburn, 2000). The three primary ED recognized in the clinical and scholarly communities include anorexia nervosa (AN), bulimia nervosa (BN) and binge eating disorder (BED) (APA, 2000).

Anorexia Nervosa

A diagnosis of AN reflects: (1) a rigid refusal to maintain body weight of at least 85% of the expected weight based on age and height; (2) an overriding fear of weight gain or becoming fat; (3) the undue influence of body weight or shape on self-evaluation; and (4) the absence of at least 3 consecutive menstrual cycles in post-menarcheal females (APA, 2000). Individuals diagnosed with AN may be further classified as either a restricting type or as a binge eating/purging type (APA, 2000). The current point prevalence of AN is estimated to be 0.3% in the United States and Western Europe (Hoek, & van Hoeken, 2003) with a lifetime prevalence of roughly 0.5–3.7% among women (APA Work Group on Eating Disorders, 2000). AN has an average age of onset occurring between ages 14 and 18 (APA, 1994), although symptoms of disordered eating and poor body image are emerging at an alarming rate in pre-pubescent cohorts (Rohinson, Chang, Haydel, & Killen, 2001).

Due to its hallmark clinical features of extreme weight loss and chronic malnutrition, AN poses significant long-term health risks (Office on Women's Health, 2000; NIMH, 2001) and is considered among the most lethal psychiatric disorders (Sullivan, 1995). Long-term prognosis is equivocal (see Berkman, Lohr, & Bulik, 2007 for an extensive review); for instance, ten-year recovery rates range from 27% in a US sample (Halmi, Eckert, Marchi, Sampugnaro et al., 1991) to 69% in a German sample (Herpertz-Dahlmann, Muller, Herpertz, & Heussen, 2001). Given this grim picture, a recent systematic review of randomized controlled trials (RCTs) underscored the considerable need to enhance the modest support for efficacy of cognitive-behavioral therapy and family therapy in preventing relapse among weight-restored adults with AN and in resolving AN symptoms in adolescent samples respectively (Bulik, Berkman, Brownley, Sedway, & Lohr, 2007).

Bulimia Nervosa

BN is defined by (1) recurrent episodes of binge eating (consuming large quantities of food within a discrete period of time coupled with the perception of loss of control); and (2) recurrent inappropriate compensatory behaviors with the intent to avoid weight gain. Such behaviors may include self-induced vomiting, fasting, excessive exercising and/or the misuse of laxatives, diuretics or other medications that promote weight loss (APA, 2000). The binge-compensatory behavioral cycle must occur on average at least twice a week for three months in order to reach diagnostic severity. Although both patients with AN and BN tend to develop self-concepts principally based on body weight and shape, BN patients by definition must not be underweight (APA, 2000).

The current prevalence of BN is roughly 1% in women and 0.1% in men in the Western world (Hoek, & van Hoeken, 2003) with a lifetime prevalence estimated between 1.1 and 4.2% in women (APA Work Group on Eating Disorders, 2000). However, a significantly higher proportion of the population suffers from subclinical symptoms of the disorder (i.e. 5.4% partial syndrome; Hoek, & van Hoeken, 2003). Onset tends to occur in adolescence or young adulthood (e.g., among college-aged samples) and a substantial number of individuals with AN subsequently develop BN following weight restoration (Office on Women's Health, 2000). Health consequences of BN center on complications of chronic purging behavior, with the most serious potential complication being cardiac arrest (Office on Women's Health, 2000). Average mortality rate has been reported as < 1% (Keel & Mitchell, 1997; Steinhausen, 1999). Recovery rates are variable, ranging from 22 to 77%, with a high probability of relapse (Fairburn, Cooper, Doll, Norman, & O'Connor, 2000; see Quadflieg and Fichter, 2003 for a review).

Treatment of BN typically involves psychopharmacological agents (e.g., fluoxetine) and/or some form of psychotherapy (e.g., CBT) or self-help-based approach. An extensive qualitative review of RCTs published between 1980 and 2005 (Shapiro et al., 2007) cited robust evidence for both medical and behavioral interventions for significantly reducing core BN symptoms and promoting relapse prevention, but also highlighted the major challenge of retaining participants in all therapeutic technologies (Shapiro et al., 2007).

Binge Eating Disorder

Individuals meeting diagnostic criteria for BED endorse recurrent episodes of uncontrollable eating binges in the absence of inappropriate compensatory behaviors (APA, 2000). Secondary features involve eating more rapidly than usual during the binge episode, eating when not feeling physically hungry, eating to the point of being uncomfortably full, feeling guilty, depressed and/or embarrassed due to excessive food intake and experiencing significant distress in reaction to the eating binge (APA 2000). These symptoms must occur on at least two days per week over a 6 month period of time with no more than two weeks of abstinence (APA, 2000). Although not a requirement for diagnosis, a majority of individuals with BED tend to be overweight or obese (Hudson, Hiripi, Pope, & Kessler, 2007; Reichborn-Kjennerud, Bulik, Sullivan, Tambs, & Harris, 2004). BED remains a research diagnosis and officially is classified as a form of Eating Disorder Not Otherwise Specified (ED-NOS; APA, 2000).

BED is the most prevalent of the three primary ED affecting between 0.7 and 4% of individuals. U.S. community-based studies cite somewhat higher rates (2–5%; Bruce & Agras, 1992) and BED rates as high as 30% have been reported among obese persons seeking weight loss treatment (Spitzer et al. 1992; 1993). Though BED appears to be on the rise across diverse groups, some data suggests that racial disparities in rates of BED are lower than have been published in previous reports (Striegel-Moore et al., 2003). Risk for obesity and related medical consequences are central physical health outcomes relevant to chronic BED pathology (Fairburn et al., 2000). Like BN, and in contrast to the earlier average age of onset of AN, BED more typically emerges in late adolescence or young adulthood (Office on Women's Health, 2000). The natural course of BED has received less attention in comparison to other ED. Based on the limited literature available, it would seem that rates of relapse are low at longer-term follow-up (Fairburn et al., 2000; Fichter, Quadflieg, & Gnutzmann, 1998) though more equivocal outcomes were observed in the short-term (Cachelin et al., 1999).

While the treatment of BED runs the similar gamut of pharmacological, CBT and self-help based interventions, this smaller evidence base of RCTs has yielded inconclusive findings (see Brownley, Berkman, Sedway, Lohr, & Bulik, 2007 for an extensive review). One of the ongoing debates in managing BED in overweight and obese samples is whether to prioritize regulating eating before targeting weight loss efforts (see Brownley, Berkman, Sedway, Lohr, & Bulik, 2007 for a discussion). Regarding this challenge, CBT has been effective in producing significant and enduring positive shifts in binge eating pathology but has not been consistently effective in promoting appreciable weight loss (see Brownley, Berkman, Sedway, Lohr, & Bulik, 2007 for an overview).

Eating Disorders as Attempts to Self-Regulate: Problem Formulation and Theoretical Rationale for the Use of Mindfulness

Over the last several decades, a compelling body of research has suggested that the core deficits in ED stem from ineffective attempts to self-regulate (e.g., Davis & Jamieson, 2005; Overton, Selway, Stongman, & Houston, 2005; Whiteside et al., 2007). Severe caloric restriction, binge eating and inappropriate compensatory behaviors are conceptualized as attempts to regulate aversive aspects of experience and may be considered products of stress reactivity. Viewing ED from a functional self-regulatory perspective, four conceptual models serve as cornerstones: emotion regulation theory (e.g., Gross, 1998; Heatherton & Baumeister, 1991; Wilson, 1984), cognitive-behavioral restraint theory (Herman and Polivy, 1980; Polivy & Herman, 1985); cognitive avoidance (Heatherton & Baumeister, 1991) and mental control theory (Wegner, 1994). These theories posit that ED symptoms attempt to regulate: (1) emotion through behavior; (2) behavior through cognition; and (3) cognition through behavior (mental control). Physiological processes confound each step of this attempt.

Attempts to Regulate Emotion through Behavior

Individuals with ED have marked deficits in adaptive emotional self-regulation; that is, they have difficulty accurately identifying emotions, managing them, and using them adaptively (Bydlowski et al., 2005; Carano et al., 2006; Gilboa-Schechtman, Avnon, Zubery, & Jeczmien, 2006; Wheeler, Greiner, & Boulton, et al, 2005). Higher levels of alexithymia (difficulty identifying and describing emotional experience) are both self-reported

(Bydlowski et al., 2005; Wheeler, Greiner, & Boulton, et al, 2005) and observed (Berthoz, Perdereau, Godart, Coros, & Haviland, 2007) in individuals with ED compared to normative samples. Furthermore, higher levels of alexithymia are related to more disturbed body attitudes, poorer self-esteem, higher depression ratings and more severe binge eating pathology among BED patients (Carano et al., 2006). Importantly, tendencies toward alexithymia commonly occur in those with an externally oriented, concrete thinking style (Sifneos, 1996).

Accurate identification of emotion requires an internal orientation, refined attention to the physiological component of emotional experience and discernment between true emotions versus other physical states (e.g., hunger, fatigue). Poor interoceptive awareness is a hallmark of ED (Fassino, Piero, Gramaglia, & Abbate-Daga, 2004; Spoor, Bekker, Van Heck, Croon, & Van Strien, 2005) and physiological signals of emotion are often confounded with appetite regulation cues. Those who practice strict dieting do not respond to hunger signals; eventually, hunger becomes paired and confounded with negative emotion.

Those more prone to binge eating not only have trouble reading hunger signals, but also have difficulty discriminating the somatic signaling of gastric satiety as well as taste-specific satiety (Allen & Craighead, 1999; Hetherington & Rolls, 1988). In all types of ED, this considerable dysregulation in the experience of hunger and fullness is not only related to emotional dysregulation, but also to dysregulation in the physiology of hunger and fullness. Individuals with AN may not perceive hunger due to dysregulated processing of insulin signals (Nakai & Koh, 2001). In addition, disturbed activation patterns have been observed in the neurophysiological correlates of somatosensory and attentional processing of food stimuli on fMRI (Santel, Baving, Krauel, Munte, & Rotte, 2006). Furthermore, subjective hunger ratings are negatively correlated with preoccupation with eating, weight and shape (Spoor, Bekker, Van Heck, Croon, & Van Strien, 2005).

Skills in emotion identification not only rely on a highly attuned sense of interoceptive awareness, but are also facilitated by acceptance of emotional experience. Conversely, when emotions are labeled as pathological, individuals tend to binge eat, use substances or dissociate in an attempt to reduce awareness of emotion (e.g., Leahy, 2002). Moreover, individuals with ED may avoid emotion in part because they hold inaccurate beliefs about the nature and consequences of emotions (Linehan, 1993a; Corstorphine, 2006).

Individuals with ED have difficulty managing and utilizing emotion adaptively. They tend to use eating as a way to avoid or escape negative emotional states and to create more positive states. For example, stress, pain and negative affect are common antecedents to binge eating (Agras & Telch, 1998; Davis & Jamieson, 2005; Gluck, Geliebter, Hung, & Yahav, 2004; Lynch, Everingham, Dubitzky, Hartman, & Kasser, 2000; Stein et al., 2007). When faced with negative emotion, those with ED have a limited range of emotion regulation strategies available (e.g., binge eaters in a college sample Whiteside et al., 2007); binge eating and compensatory behaviors are used to escape aversive experience by escaping self-awareness altogether (Heatherton & Baumeister, 1991). Attention is narrowed, focused externally, and inhibitions against bingeing or purging are reduced. This is consistent with the finding that alexithymia commonly occurs in those with an externally oriented, concrete thinking style (Sifneos, 1996).

Difficulty regulating emotion is further complicated by the fact that individuals with ED may be prone to greater stress reactivity in light of identified biological vulnerabilities (e.g., elevated cortisol, cardio-vagal abnormalities: Faris et al., 2006; Gluck et al., 2004; Kollai, Bonyhay, Jokkel, & Szonyi, 1994; Petretta et al., 1997). In addition, they have greater difficulty accepting and managing distress (Corstorphine, Mountford, Tomlinson, Waller, & Meyer, 2007). In fact, emotional eating has emerged as a more general avoidant coping style in a broad range of clinical and non-eating disordered samples (Lindeman & Stark, 2001; Spoor, Bekker, Van Strien, & van Heck, 2007). Individuals with ED may also use eating and compensatory behaviors to produce a more positive emotional state (Overton et al., 2005). Purging, for example, is often enacted to relieve the overwhelming emotional distress experienced following an eating binge (Corstorphine, Waller, Ohanian, & Baker, 2006).

Rationale for Mindfulness Approaches Based on Emotion Regulation

Mindfulness offers a strong opportunity to improve emotion regulation. It trains individuals to focus inwardly in a highly externally oriented culture, cultivates an acceptance of emotion as a part of human experience, and allows individuals to practice identifying and experiencing emotion without reacting to it. At the same time, mindfulness techniques applied specifically to eating allow individuals to tease apart physiological cues of emotion with those of hunger or satiety.

Interplay of Behavior and Cognition in Self-Regulation

Attempts to Regulate Behavior through Cognitive Rigidity

> *My body started to shut down. I got really, really ill. When you're starving yourself, you can't concentrate.*
> *I was like a walking zombie, like the walking dead.*
> *I was just consumed with what I would eat, what I wouldn't eat.*
> ~Tracey Gold, Actor

ED populations are characterized by rigid and distorted cognition in relation to eating patterns, perfectionism, and appearance-related thinking. They attempt to regulate behavior through a rigid cognitive-behavioral orientation of restraint (Herman & Polivy, 1980; Polivy & Herman, 1985). Such restraint with respect to eating is obvious in anorexia, but is also prominent in those with bulimia and binge eating disorder. Individuals who diet in order to lose weight internalize a set of stringent dietary rules that result in highly restricted caloric intake that deprives the body of essential nutrients and energy. In response to this chronic state of "starvation," some individuals experience the urge to binge as too overwhelming to avoid (Polivy & Herman, 1985). Inflexible dietary rules are overridden by this physiological urge and the abstinence-violation effect often results in a full blown eating binge (Agras & Telch., 1998). Consequently, dieting and related thought patterns are inherent in the emergence and maintenance of eating pathology.

Behavioral restraint in the form of dieting has also been longitudinally predicted by appearance-related beliefs in structural equation modeling

(Spangler, 2002). Similarly, appearance-related beliefs predicted body dissatisfaction and other vulnerabilities to eating pathology across time points in an ethnically diverse group of adolescent females. Furthermore, statistical modeling failed to support a bi-directional relationship over time (Spangler, 2002), suggesting that distorted appearance-related cognitions lead to behavioral restraint (e.g., dieting), which then leads to eating pathology.

Such appearance-related thoughts are one form of perfectionistic thinking common in ED (see Bardone-Cone et al., 2007 for a review). In perfectionism, individuals hold extraordinarily high standards for performance, appearance and/or achievement and tend to have poor tolerance for outcomes that are not consistent with meeting personal standards (see Bardone-Cone et al., 2007 for a review). Ironically, since measures of success tend to be inordinately unrealistic, perfectionistic individuals with ED are chronically dissatisfied due to holding unattainable eating, weight, and shape-related goals (Steele, Corsini, & Wade, 2007) and are known to frequently experience feelings of shame (Swan & Andrews, 2003; Lawson, Waller & Lockwood, 2007).Residual perfectionistic beliefs observed in recovered ED patients are seen as indicators of risk for relapse (Lilenfeld et al., 2000).

Clinical severity of ED is also related to severely distorted, rigid and even magical cognitions about the relationship of food-related thoughts to eating, body weight and shape (Shafran et al., 1999; Shafran & Robinson, 2004; Spangler, 2002). Termed thought-shape fusion (TSF), this cognitive characteristic reflects beliefs that merely thinking about foods considered "forbidden": (1) increases the likelihood that the individual has gained weight, (2) is morally equivalent to actually consuming such problematic foods, and (3) leads to the individual experiencing him or herself as feeling heavier (Shafran et al., 1999). Thus, thoughts about difficult foods are fused with the belief that such thoughts can directly influence weight or shape as well as impact one's self-evaluation as immoral and somatically fatter. From a self-regulatory standpoint, TSF has been associated with the urge to engage in compensatory behaviors including body checking, exercise and even purging (see Shafran & Robinson., 2004 for a discussion).

Attemps to Regulate Cognition through Behavior (Mental Control)

I eat merely to put food out of my mind.
    ~N.F. Simpson, Playwright

As some models posit that cognition is used to manage behavior, others suggest that behavior is used to manage cognition. One well-accepted theory posits that ED behaviors are maintained through avoidance of aversive self-awareness (e.g., Heatherton et al., 1991); mental control theory (Wegner, 1994) further informs this approach. Preoccupation with body image, negative self-concept and food is strongly related to eating pathology (Dobson & Dozois, 2004; Eldredge & Agras, 1996; Faunce, 2002; Lazarus & Galassi, 1994; Lingswiler, Crowther, & Stephens, 1989; Marcus, Wing, & Hopkins, 1988; Nauta, Hospers, Kok, & Jansen, 2000; Phelan, 1987; Powell & Thelen, 1996; Ricciardelli, Williams, & Finemore, 2001; Shafran, Lee, Cooper, Palmer, & Fairburn, 2007). In fact, eating pathology is often rooted in a narrow and rigidly held (or highly accessible) self-concept centered on body weight and shape (e.g., APA, 2000; Dunkley & Grilo, 2007; Farchaus Stein, 1996; Hrabosky, Masheb, White & Grilo, 2007). Individuals with ED are known to have low self-esteem (e.g., Jacobi et al., 2004) and tend to hold maladaptive core beliefs about the self and interpersonal relatedness (Dingemans, Spinhoven, & van Furth, 2006; Hughes, Hamill, van Gerko, Lockwood, & Waller, 2006; Leung & Price, 2007). To complicate this tendency, those with BN and BED demonstrate a selective attentional bias for cues threatening to self-concept (Jansen, Nederkoorn, & Mulkens, 2005; Meyer, Waller, & Watson, 2000). With attention consistently directed toward undermining thoughts, they are subsequently inclined to binge or purge as a means of avoiding or escaping prolonged exposure to them (Lingswiler et al., 1989, Powell & Thelen, 1996; Spranger, Waller & Bryant-Waugh, 2001). This is true even in at-risk samples, and even when the threat to self-concept is subliminal (e.g., Waller & Mijatovich, 1998; Meyer & Waller, 1999). Furthermore, physiological states appear to impact these avoidance tendencies; the degree of fasting influenced selective attentional biases in women with greater self-reported eating pathology. They showed a greater attentional bias for low calorie words when in a non-fasting state and demonstrated an opposite attentional pattern when food deprived (Placanica, Faunce & Soames Job, 2002).

Explanation of the above findings is most easily understood through the paradoxical relationship of rumination and thought suppression. Rumination is a perseverative cognitive process in which attention is focused on replaying upsetting events in the mind and/or on a repetitive stream of negative self-critical cognitions (Nolen-Hoeksema, 2000) in an often unsuccessful attempt to avoid intense negative affect (see Gross, 1998 for a discussion) and make meaning out of situations when important goals have not been attained (Martin, Tesser, & McIntosh, 1993). Thought suppression is a covert self-regulatory behavior used to limit exposure to upsetting thoughts and images (Wegner, 1994). However, chronic attempts to suppress unwanted private events ironically elicit a rebound effect whereby the disturbing image or thought becomes more intrusive (i.e., the white bear phenomenon; Wegner, 1994). In such cases, rumination may be characterized as a "failure" of thought suppression wherein attention becomes fixated on the very unpleasant cognitions one would prefer to avoid. Hence, the more one suppresses thoughts of food or negative self-concept, the more one focuses on food or negative self-concept. Presumably, this impaired ability to consciously shift attention toward or away from certain cognitive content is mediated by being overly invested in the believability of such thoughts. Binge eating and compensatory behaviors thus appear to function as behavioral attempts to suppress and control upsetting or negative thoughts. However, no research to date has directly examined a mental control model of eating pathology.

Rationale for Mindfulness Approaches Based on the Cognition-Behavior Interplay

Mindfulness is clearly appropriate to address the entrenched interplay (release the rigid lock) between rigid cognitive processes and dysfunctional behavior seen in ED. Mindfulness training can simultaneously: (1) cultivate a nonjudgmental and accepting attitude (Kabat-Zinn, 1994); (2) provide more conscious control of attention (Jha, Krompinger & Baime, 2007); and (3) demonstrate that thoughts are just thoughts. Mindfulness is a quality of attention, in which a person intentionally brings nonjudgmental awareness to his or her present moment experience (i.e., thoughts, feelings and physical sensations) with willingness, curiosity and acceptance of what is (Kabat-Zinn, 1994). Theoretically, the more one practices, the more one develops this nonjudgment or acceptance. Acceptance is conceptualized as a dynamic process of self-affirmation or self-validation composed of cognitive, affective and behavioral components (Linehan, 1993a; Wilson, 1996; Hayes, Strosahl, & Wilson, 1999). When an individual is consciously accepting of his or her internal experience, this "discerning wakefulness" ironically provides enhanced control over responding to experience flexibly and adaptively rather than impulsively or rigidly (Kabat-Zinn, 1994).

Most recently, Bishop and colleagues have proposed a two-component model in operationalizing mindfulness which includes adopting an accepting orientation to experience as well as self-regulation of attention (Lau et al., 2006). This training in attention can help individuals with ED shift their attention from food, body image and negative self-concept to more adaptive content by helping them to disengage from such content rather than suppress it. Mindfulness practice teaches one to observe thoughts from a distance, and recognize that thoughts are just thoughts, mental events that may or may not have any basis in reality. Self-critical automatic thoughts thus become "mental events" to be neutrally observed rather than truths to be automatically believed.

Consistent with a stress reactivity model (Kabat-Zinn, 1990), mindfulness provides a rich opportunity for learning. Enhanced by taking a nonjudgmental, observer stance, individuals are taught to unbundle the wealth of information about the stress experience obtained from emotions, thoughts, and physical sensations that drive behavior. They have the opportunity to separate each component of the stress reaction (e.g., physiological cue about mood versus appetite cue) and develop an internal guide ("inner compass") as to how to use the information gained in a conscious and adaptive way (Wolever, Ladden, Davis, Best, Greeson, & Baime, 2007).

In addition, when mindfulness is directly applied to eating, participants are trained to direct attention to the full sensory experience of eating and satiety. They learn to approach eating in a more relaxed, nonjudgmental way, and improve registration of appetite regulation cues. The latter involves both reducing the misappraisal of internal physical states and becoming more attuned to utilizing physiological appetite cues for initiating and ending the eating period. Finally, mindfulness-based approaches may further lay the ground work for adopting a more fluid and expansive sense of self and for engaging in more self-accepting behaviors among patients with ED.

Thus, mindfulness is viewed as a self-regulatory process through which individuals hone their *capacity to attend to* the constant stream of thoughts, emotions and physical sensations as well as hone their capacity to alter their *orientation and relationship to their experience*. This self-regulatory process actually functions as a powerful learning paradigm in which individuals become their own empowered experts in interrupting personal dysfunctional self-regulatory processes, allowing a shift in entrenched patterns. This promising rationale is now being tested empirically in an emerging body of research that has found preliminary evidence for the efficacy of mindfulness-based programs in reducing the core symptoms of ED. That said, empirical clarification of the mechanisms of action in these approaches is still in its infancy.

Mindfulness-based Interventions for Eating Disorders: The Current State of the Evidence

Eating disorders are complex syndromes representing both specific and generalized deficits in self-regulation. These conditions frequently persist even in the face of significant deterioration in psychological and physiological wellness. Given the increasing prevalence of ED coupled with the associated high risk of relapse and concurrent psychopathology, greater attention is warranted to improve the efficacy of existing treatments. In response to this growing need, four innovative mindfulness-based therapeutic approaches have been blended with traditional cognitive-behavioral theory: Dialectical Behavior Therapy (DBT; Linehan, 1993a), Acceptance and Commitment Therapy (ACT; Hayes et al., 1999), Mindfulness-based Cognitive Therapy (MBCT; Segal, Williams, & Teasdale, 2002; Baer, Fischer, & Huss, 2006), and Mindfulness-Based Eating Awareness Training (MB-EAT; Kristeller, Baer, & Quillian-Wolever, 2006; Kristeller & Hallett, 1999).

Dialectical Behavior Therapy (DBT)

DBT was first introduced in the early 1990's to improve the self-regulation deficits in borderline personality disorder (BPD) (Linehan, 1993a). DBT helps patients cultivate core mindfulness abilities in conjunction with other emotion regulation, interpersonal effectiveness, and distress tolerance skills (Linehan, 1993b).From an empirical standpoint, DBT has had an encouraging impact on improving clinical symptomatology in BPD (Linehan, Armstrong, Suarez, Allmond et al., 1991; Linehan, 1993a) and is the most extensively studied mindfulness-based approach within eating disorder samples. In a seminal analysis, Telch (1997) presented an in-depth case study of adapting DBT for an obese woman with BED. The 23-session intervention (i.e., 19 weekly meetings and 4 monthly meetings) was structured to include three phases: (1) theoretical rationale of the program, (2) teaching principal components of DBT and (3) reinforcing and generalizing gains (Telch, 1997). This approach yielded significant improvements in binge eating though weight and mood symptoms did not stabilize (Telch, 1997). Telch and collaborators then tested the efficacy of the approach in a group DBT program for BED in an initial uncontrolled trial (Telch, Agras, & Linehan, 2000); eighty-two percent of the sample attained binge-free status by the end of the 18-session program (Telch et al., 2000; see Wiser & Telch, 1999 for a detailed description of the intervention) and abstinence rates remained high three (i.e., 80%) and six months (i.e., 70%) post-treatment. (Telch et al., 2000). Eating, weight and shape concerns also improved, as did self-reported emotional eating urges and negative mood regulation (Telch et al., 2000).

In a more rigorous RCT (Telch, Agras, & Linehan, 2001), 44 women with BED reduced objective binge eating behaviors in both a DBT and wait-list control condition (Telch, Agras, & Linehan, 2001). However, among the 18 that completed treatment, those in DBT showed significantly higher abstinence rates by the end of treatment relative to controls (i.e., 89% versus 12.5%), though sustained improvements were more modest (i.e., 56% abstinent at 6-month follow-up). DBT-completers were also characterized by less weight, shape and eating concerns and on average reported a weaker urge to eat in response to anger than wait-list participants (Telch, Agras, & Linehan, 2001). Subsequent post-hoc analysis of women who completed DBT across both trials (N = 32) indicated that early onset of binge eating (prior to age 16) and higher restraint scores at baseline predicted poorer outcome (Safer, Lively, Telch, & Agras, 2002).

The application of DBT to treating BN and AN is less well-developed. Safer et al. (2001a) provided the first clinical account of adapting DBT for treatment-resistant BN with positive results (Safer et al., 2001a). In addition, one RCT of women with BN showed greater reductions in binge eating and purging for DBT participants compared to wait-list controls (Safer, Telch, & Agras, 2001b). Regarding AN, McCabe and Marcus (2002) discuss the effectiveness of DBT from a clinical standpoint, though virtually no research has empirically tested whether DBT is useful for treating AN. The one exception is a current uncontrolled pilot study being conducted in Germany of inpatient adolescents with AN and BN (Salbach et al., 2007).

Three directions for future DBT research with ED would supplement the promising findings thus far: (1) testing the manualized, integrative approach against or as a complement to traditional CBT, Interpersonal Therapy (IPT) and family-based interventions; (2) testing DBT for AN; and (3) exploring the generalizability of the findings by including males and ethnically diverse samples.

Acceptance and Commitment Therapy (ACT)

The second mindfulness-based approach that can be easily adapted for ED is ACT (Hayes et al., 1999). Conceptualized for treating a wide range of psychiatric and behavioral disorders, its core philosophy holds that maladaptive behaviors are purposefully or habitually performed to reduce or control aversive experience (e.g., self-critical cognitions, negative emotions, painful bodily sensations; Hayes et al., 1999). Ongoing distress and dysfunction are maintained by this experiential avoidance as well as by cognitive fusion (i.e., holding thoughts to the level of absolute truths such as "I think I'm fat; therefore I am"). The adaptation of ACT as a treatment for ED is theoretically appropriate given its excellent fit with the prominent models explaining eating pathology (restraint, emotion regulation, and escape theories).

ACT utilizes mindfulness skills, metaphor, and cognitive defusion techniques to reduce cognitive-behavioral rigidity, improve self-regulation and overall quality of life (Hayes et al., 1999). ACT further emphasizes clarification of important life values as a continuous form of motivation for sustaining adaptive behavior change (Hayes et al., 1999). In essence ACT exposes patients to the very aspects of their experience they deem problematic, but from a de-centered, mindful and accepting vantage point. This exposure-based component along with values clarification assists patient in more creatively engaging in and adapting to a wide range of life circumstances.

Although ACT has received noteworthy support for improving symptoms across a spectrum of clinical disorders (Hayes, Luoma, Bond, Masuda, & Lillis, 2006), there is a dearth of such work conducted in eating disordered samples. The existing literature is comprised of single case studies in AN (Bowers, 2002; Hayes & Pankey, 2002; Heffner, Sperry, Eifert, & Detweiler, 2002; Orsillo & Batten, 2002). Wilson and Roberts (2002) provide an important overview of issues to consider in assessing and treating AN from an ACT perspective. Clearly, clinical trials of ACT-based approaches for improving core eating pathology symptoms are one promising area of further scientific inquiry.

Mindfulness-Based Cognitive Therapy (MBCT)

MBCT is an extension of Jon Kabat-Zinn's pioneering Mindfulness-Based Stress Reduction (MBSR; Kabat-Zinn, 1990) program aimed at the enduring cognitive vulnerability in chronic, treatment-resistant depression (Segal et al., 2002). MBCT applies core mindfulness skills from MBSR (e.g., body scan meditation, sitting meditation, walking meditation, awareness of the breath, mindful yoga) to reduce the believability of persistent depressogenic thoughts and to improve the pervasive affect avoidance style (Segal et al., 2002). However, in contrast to existing cognitive therapeutic change techniques, MBCT, much like ACT, does not attempt to change the *content* of experience; rather, it challenges the individual to alter the *context* of experience through practicing acceptance and "letting be" (Segal et al., 2002). Baer and collaborators evaluated MBCT for treating binge eating in subclinical and clinical BED (Baer, Fischer, & Huss, 2005; Baer et al., 2006). They used MBCT to reduce reactivity toward automatic thoughts and emotions that precede binge eating rather than reducing the thoughts and emotions themselves. Unlike other mindfulness-based approaches to eating disorders, (e.g., MB-EAT, DBT and ACT), there is a stronger emphasis placed on training in pure mindfulness strategies in the absence of directly applying mindfulness to eating, physical activity, or CBT approaches such as problem-solving or assertiveness skills (Baer et al., 2005).

In the original case analysis, MBCT was associated not only with both immediate and sustained improvements in binge eating pathology but it also led to significant increases in self-reported mindfulness (Baer et al., 2005). Similarly, a more recent uncontrolled trial of a 10-session MBCT showed positive effects for objective binge eating, self-reported binge eating severity, and eating concerns (Baer et al., 2006). Women in this trial also demonstrated notable increases in self-observation and nonjudgment of these private events following treatment (Baer et al., 2006). These preliminary findings are encouraging, and set the stage for RCT evaluation of this approach.

Mindfulness-Based Eating Awareness Training (MB-EAT)

Also informed by MBSR, the first mindfulness-based approach created specifically for treating an eating disorder (Kristeller & Hallett, 1999) applied mindfulness to CBT and guided imagery developed to address weight, shape and eating-related self-regulatory processes. The approach, later named

MB-EAT (Kristeller et al., 2006) is consistent with affect regulation models (e.g., Wilson, 1984), restraint theory (e.g., chronic dieting model of Herman & Polivy, 1980), the escape model (Heatherton & Baumeister, 1991) and mental control (Wegner, 1994) yet further expands these self-regulation explanations to include the science of food intake regulation including the role of hunger and satiety cues. Using a single group pre–post, extended baseline design, Kristeller and Hallett (1999) demonstrated reductions in self-reported symptoms of binge eating, binge severity, anxiety and depression in obese women with BED undergoing a six-week treatment. Importantly, correlational analyses indicated improvements in binge eating were associated with improvements in mindfulness, eating control and awareness of satiety signals Moreover, time spent practicing eating-related meditations predicted lower binge severity (Kristeller & Hallett, 1999). The original approach was then expanded to a 9-session treatment (MB-EAT: Kristeller, Baer, & Quillian-Wolever, 2006; Kristeller, Wolever & Sheets, 2008), informed by Craighead's appetite awareness training (Craighead & Allen, 1995; Allen & Craighead, 1999) and deeper levels of self-acceptance work using forgiveness and cultivation of inner wisdom for sustaining change. The efficacy of MB-EAT was then tested in a dual site RCT comparing it to an active CBT-informed psychoeducational approach, and a wait-list control (Kristeller, Wolever & Sheets, 2008) in an ethnically diverse sample of obese men and women with BED or subclinical binge eating patterns. Intent-to-treat analyses showed declines in objective binge eating, binge eating severity and depressive symptoms for both active treatments. However, only those randomly assigned to the MB-EAT condition exhibited lower levels of food locus of control, suggesting a greater internalization of change (Kristeller, Wolever & Sheets, 2008). Interestingly, significant improvements in post-prandial glucose metabolism (Wolever, Best, Sheets, et al., 2006; Wolever, Best, Sheets, & Kristeller, 2008) were also found solely in the MB-EAT group, and independent of weight change. This finding raises the possibility that the mindfulness-based approach also influences biological indices of self-regulation in a way that other behavioral approaches do not. The U.S. National Institutes of Health are currently funding additional testing of this hypothesis in conjunction with efficacy trials of this approach for weight loss (MB-EAT; NIH Grant 5U01 AT002550) and weight loss maintenance (EMPOWER: NIH Grants 5U01 AT004159 and 5 U01 AT004158). These grants have allowed the opportunity to further enhance and develop this approach, resulting in the current 15-week protocol (described below) called EMPOWER (Enhancing Mindfulness for the Prevention of Weight Regain; Wolever et al., 2007).

One additional approach merits mention. Preliminary findings from a non-clinical sample of community participants with binge eating tendencies suggest utility in an 8 week modified MBSR approach with psychoeducational components (Smith, Shelley, Leahigh, & Vanleit, 2006). Randomized, controlled testing of this model is certainly in order.

EMPOWER Exercises and Participant Experiences

Training in traditional mindfulness techniques (e.g., sitting meditation, body scan) provides a basic platform from which to nonjudgmentally learn about oneself. In addition, this learning platform appears to facilitate application of CBT and other traditional skills known to enhance recovery. In the EMPOWER approach (Wolever et al., 2007), there are at least 9 core skill sets, all of which are fundamental to recovery from eating disorders:

1. to nonjudgmentally observe the bundle of reactive thoughts, emotions and body sensations that drive behavior;
2. to separate emotions from this bundle of reactivity;

   a. that emotions are transient events that often do not require response;

3. to separate thoughts from this bundle of reactivity;

   a. that thoughts are just thoughts, transient events that often do not require response;

4. to separate and tolerate behavioral urges from this bundle of reactivity;
5. to clarify physiological signals of hunger and fullness (gastric satiety);
6. to attend to taste-specific satiety;
7. to discern the physiological signature of appetite regulation cues (5 and 6) from emotions (e.g., the difference in anxiety and hunger; the difference in peaceful and stuffed);
8. to discern the true need underlying the reactivity; and
9. to make a wise and informed decision about addressing this true need.

Skill Set 1: Nonjudgmental observation of reactivity - As a starting place, individuals with ED need to develop skills in shifting attention to internal states in order to observe emotion, cognition and sensation, and the way these interact to drive behavior. Most participants initially struggle to center their attention on internal states, and mindfulness training can best be described as a learning paradigm that allows individuals to become their own experts and advocates. Nonjudgment is seminal in creating this learning environment allowing individuals to explore their patterns with lowered defenses. They often express surprise when they sample nonjudgment. It is also common for participants to cry during their first practice of forgiveness meditation when asked to consider forgiving themselves for mistakes made, or unhealthy behaviors performed; many clients have just "never considered this." Some participants initially experience anxiety at the idea of forgiving themselves because they believe that sharp self-judgment gives them a greater sense of control. In addition, further attention is needed to explore the fine line between accountability and judgment when using mindfulness to support behavior change of any kind (Table 14.1).

Skill Set 2: Separating Out Emotions - Individuals need to demonstrate a willingness to accept emotional experience (including changes in physiological arousal) reassured by the understanding that emotions are transient events (Linehan, 1993b; Gratz & Gunderson, 2006) and that one does not have to react to them. It is actually the process of engaging emotions that can elongate their presence. Regular sitting meditation practice strengthens this learning and may include guidance such as:

> If you notice that your mind wanders away or your attention is pulled by an emotion, just observe what that is...whatever feelings are present are fine...and you don't have to do anything about them...just observing them without judging them...just noticing whatever you are experiencing...not

Table 14.1. Nine core skill sets enhanced by mindfulness approaches that are seminal to recovery from eating disorders.

Nine core skill sets in the EMPOWER approach

1. nonjudgmental observation of reactivity (bundle of thoughts, emotions, and body sensations that drive behavior)
2. separation of emotions from this bundle and learning that emotions are transient events that often do not require response
3. separation of thoughts from this bundle of reactivity, and learning that thoughts are just thoughts, transient events that often do not require response
4. separation and tolerance of behavioral urges from this bundle of reactivity
5. clarification of physiological signals of hunger and fullness (gastric satiety)
6. attention to taste-specific satiety
7. discernment of the physiological signature of emotions and appetite regulation cues
8. discernment of the true need underlying the reactivity
9. wise and informed decision making to address the true need

trying to change it, but just noticing it. . .whatever you experience is fine. . .just notice it, whatever it is. . .you may even find that emotions come and they go. . .like leaves in a river floating downstream. . .you can observe them arrive and pass without engaging them. . .and if you find yourself floating downstream with the leaves, you can climb back onto the bank of the river and watch again as the leaves float downstream. . .

The next step is then to sit with the emotion from a more accepting stance. Accurately registering such signals allows one to explore what true need exists that is driving unhealthy behavior (e.g., eating due to physical hunger, to self-soothe anxiety, or to stay awake because exhausted). For the past year, we have been teaching clients a tool called Stop-Breathe-Feel (Wolever et al., 2007), a tool that teaches them to recognize without judgment the emotion present and understand that eating (or compensatory behavior) will not address the real need. For example, if one eats to manage anxiety, the cues of hunger are less relevant because the goal of eating is to manage anxiety. We encourage clients to catch the information from the body early on and apply mindfulness; just notice the anxiety and recognize that the issue generating anxiety is not likely to be managed by eating. Rather, the emotion is just a tool in the decision-making process about how to handle the real need (whatever is triggering the anxiety). The more we become okay with recognizing the importance of emotions as tools in the decision-making process, the less afraid we will be when they arise in the moment. In fact, acceptance itself has been described as "actively responding to feelings by allowing or letting be before rushing in and trying to fix or change them. Allowing means that participants register their presence before deciding how to respond to them" (Segal, Williams, & Teasdale, 2002). Most clients experience this simple Stop-Breathe-Feel tool as powerful: just deciding to stop, breathe and allow oneself to feel whatever is present in that moment without avoidance strengthens confidence. We use the metaphor of riding on a train: one aim of this program is to develop a certain kind of attention so one can identify the right stop (e.g., directly observe the emotional cue from a nonreactive stance). However, when we miss our stop, we can still work back. So, when the emotional cue is missed, we may catch ourselves riding to another stop (e.g., bingeing or engaging in compensatory behavior) and retrace our steps in how we arrived there.

Skill Set 3: Separating Out Thoughts – Traditional mindfulness approaches are excellent at helping participants learn that thoughts are just thoughts, mental events that do not necessarily have any basis in reality. This is a powerful recognition for participants with ED whose thoughts are fused with behavioral and emotional patterns. One 33 year old obese female with BED felt significantly empowered when she, on her own, came to the realization that "I want to eat' is just a thought;" I don't have to respond to it." In addition to recognizing that thoughts are not truths, observations of the quality of thought can provide insight. For instance, participants with ED benefit from recognizing when their thinking becomes negative. In pure mindfulness, nonjudgmental observation of the negative thought is enough to reduce its power, but it remains an empirical question whether or not more support (e.g., additional tools) is needed to help counter life-long perceptual patterns. This question is of course confounded by the amount participants practice. Clinical experience suggests that many participants practice the shorter techniques and attain some shifts in perspective, but may not practice enough to re-pattern habitual thought patterns without the aid of additional tools.

Skill Set 4: Separation and tolerance of behavioral urges – The behaviors of ED participants fall along a compulsive-impulsive continuum (Claes, Vandereycken, & Vertommen, 2005; Lawson, Waller & Lockwood, 2007) and thus learning to sit through an urge to react is important. Participants strengthen their ability to sit with behavioral urges by learning to watch urges develop without responding to them. Instruction is woven into weekly EMPOWER sessions that encourage observation of small urges that are not enacted, building strength to tolerate stronger urges (Wolever et al., 2007). For example, during a sitting meditation, participants are asked to note any desires to fidget or readjust their body position as well as to observe what happens to the urge if not enacted. Similarly, during eating meditations, participants are asked to play with the urge to swallow in a similar way, pausing momentarily before biting or before swallowing to observe what happens. The learning is then reinforced through specific discussion about tolerating such urges. This tolerance serves to weaken the automatic link between urges and reaction. Participants then benefit from using minimeditation (Kristeller et al., 2006), the Stop-Breathe-Feel technique (Wolever et al., 2007), and eventually 20 minutes of regular sitting practice when experiencing the urge to binge or compensate. Tolerance, and subsequently confidence, is likely to develop further through nonjudgmental observation of these urges rather than the more traditional clinical (although also useful) approach of distracting oneself during an urge.

Skill Set 5: Recognition of hunger and fullness – Geneen Roth's early clinical work (e.g., Roth, 1984) was the first widespread approach to "compulsive eating" that drew attention to the importance of hunger and fullness. MB-EAT expanded this approach by incorporating additional training on fullness and by contextualizing the training within mindfulness, heavily emphasizing nonjudgment. Registering appetite regulation cues (and emotions for that matter) both require experience in sensing the body. This is challenging in ED because those with more restrictive ED report such paradoxical body sensations and those with more compulsive and impulsive ED are often dissociated from somatic experience. They have many thoughts and judgments about the body, but considerably less experience feeling its sensations. Traditional MBSR practices in body scanning techniques and gentle yoga are used to develop this essential core skill. Since it is very difficult for participants to maintain focus on the experience of the body, individuals with significant dieting and/or bingeing histories also tend to have more difficulty practicing the body scan than they do practicing sitting meditation. The experience of an obese 52-year-old woman with BED demonstrated how difficult it was to center her attention on physical experience during a guided body scan. Although she was extremely engaged in her treatment group, and volunteered verbal accounts of her experience often, she could only note, "I took this opportunity to do ankle circles (stretch her ankles)" when asked about her experience during the body scan.

In EMPOWER, MBSR body scan techniques are then adapted to focus an individual on sensations that cue hunger and gastric satiety (fullness). A seven point Hunger/Fullness scale informed by the work of Craighead & Allen (1995) provides participants the conceptual frame to rate their somatic experience of hunger and fullness. We have used the below exercises with BED and BN patients for the past 7 years, but have no experience using them with AN. Clinically speaking, AN clients tend to experience a sense of fullness in the absence of food in the stomach; it is unclear if participants with AN would benefit from this model of interoceptive awareness. They are likely to need adjustments to this approach that focus more on tolerating the sensation of food in the body and separating out judgments from actual sensations in the process (Figure 14.1).

BN and BED participants are reminded that the stomach is located right below and to the left of breastbone, as many people believe it is lower and incorrectly center attention on the intestinal area for cues. They are then taught to center themselves and carefully attend to areas of potential sensations with instructions such as:

> When you're ready you can move your awareness to the sensations in the stomach … Noticing whatever is there … You may even want to rest one of your hands on your stomach to help you notice whatever your body has to share with you … if it is giving you any sensations of hunger … Remembering that these may be very subtle, or they may be very intense and obvious … There are no right or wrong sensations … just noticing whatever physical sensations are taking place in your belly … your body … sensing what your body is telling

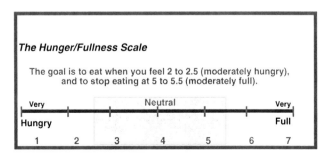

Figure. 14.1. Seven-point Hunger and Fullness Scale.

you, or not telling you in this moment . . . Noticing to yourself right now how hungry or full you are, with 1 being as hungry as possible, and 4 being neutral, and 7 being as full as you could possibly be.. [leave enough time for everyone to find a number] . . . Again remembering that these sensations may be very subtle or strong . . . making your best estimate of your hunger or fullness level. Any slight pangs from the stomach, mild hunger, at say a 3? Or slightly stronger signals, of moderate hunger, perhaps a 2.5 or a 2? Or are you too hungry? Feeling stronger discomfort, lower than a 2? Just taking a minute to notice what your stomach is telling you. No one knows this information better than you . . . So, as you become more aware of your hunger or fullness level, just asking yourself how you know this? . . . What experiences or sensations help you find the number/level?

You may also notice other sensations, feelings, or thoughts . . . Just noticing whatever you are experiencing. Not trying to change it, but just noticing it. Trying to separate out the emotion or thought from the sensations of physical hunger . . . Or perhaps you don't have any particular sensations, feelings, or thoughts. Just training yourself to reconnect with your body . . . whatever you experience is fine . . . just notice it, whatever it is . . . And with the next breath, or one soon after, you can begin to re-orient yourself to the room. And open your eyes.

Teaching participants to register fullness is similar. In the initial trainings, however, they are given fullness suggestions rather than hunger suggestions. For example:

Again remembering that these sensations may be very subtle or strong . . . making your best estimate of your hunger or fullness level. How physically satisfied are you feeling? Perhaps your stomach feels warm, moderately full – perhaps a 5.5. Or maybe it is earlier in the process. . . . . .perhaps sensing just the very first hint of stretch . . . a 5 or so. Or maybe it feels more stretch or a little distension, if you have eaten more than you needed – say a 6 or so. Whatever physical sensations you experience, just notice them. Also, noticing your emotions, and thoughts. And being aware of the difference between physically and emotionally satisfied. Perhaps you are bored, and want to get out of here. Or maybe you are surprised to learn something about yourself. Whatever you experience, just observe it, trying not to judge or criticize it.

Exercises in registering satiety are more easily accomplished in tandem with the intake of a moderate meal, particularly one of high fiber. Participants often say that they do not know what moderate fullness feels like; "I know when I'm hungry and when I'm stuffed, but I never paid attention to the in-between states." It's useful to remember that regaining this skill requires attention, patience, and practice. Clinically, most can identify episodes when they felt stuffed, and often report sedation at the same time. It is important for them to eventually uncouple the cognitive label "full" and sensations indicative of overeating. Some say they experience pain and others report deep comfort at this state. Either way, the experience of over-fullness serves to shift attention from thoughts or emotions to a set of sensations, and allows a continued mislabeling of experience.

Participants benefit from carefully listening to others' descriptions of hunger-fullness ratings, particularly noting the physical sensations that led them to choose that rating. Multiple examples are essential to learning this process. This is also an ideal time to point out potential confounds if participants mention emotions rather than physical signals (e.g. irritable, panicky, comfortable, happy), pointing out that physical rather than emotional signals are the most reliable indicators of when to eat. While physiology can sometimes lead to these (e.g. low blood sugar can make one irritable), there is a risk in using these to signal a need to eat since other things can also create such emotional states.

It is also not uncommon for participants with significant dieting and/or bingeing histories to say, "I feel nothing" when first asked to register hunger or fullness signals. It can take weeks of practice, particularly preceding, during and following meals; individuals that have been disconnected from their somatic experience for years need continual encouragement and practice to begin to register these cues again. In clinical practice, very few individuals have been unable to re-learn to sense these cues; these failures may have been due to complications of diabetes such as neuropathy.

Skill Set 6: Recognition of taste – Geneen Roth's early clinical work (e.g., Roth, 1984) also centered attention on taste; again, MB-EAT and EMPOWER expand this to add components of nonjudgment. A segment of such an exercise using chocolate reads:

> Begin by placing a single Hershey's kiss in front of you, out of your hands. Allow your eyes to close or find a downward gaze if closing your eyes feels too uncomfortable. Just resting your hands on your stomach, and inviting 4–5 deep, easy breaths. Not forcing the breath, but just inviting it all the way to the bottom of the lungs. You may feel your chest rise and fall. You may feel your ribs expand out to the sides and release. And as the breath gently reaches the bottom of your lungs, you may feel your abdomen expand on the inbreath, and contract on the outbreath. So just allowing the body to rest while you move your attention to the stomach and mouth. Just noticing what physical sensations you have at this time. Noticing any thoughts you have . . . any emotions. And being aware of the difference between physical sensations on the one hand and thoughts or emotions on the other. Whatever you experience, just observe it, trying not to judge or criticize it. Just noticing whatever you are experiencing. Not trying to change it, just noticing it. Or perhaps you don't sense any particular sensations, feelings, or thoughts. That's OK too. At this point, just notice it, whatever it is.
>
> In the next breath, or the one after that, just allowing your eyes to fully open but maintain a downward gaze, Taking the piece of chocolate in your hand, just unwrap it gently. Continuing to be aware of any thoughts or emotions that pass through your mind. Now just looking at the chocolate, holding it in your flat hand, noticing it as if this were the first time you had ever seen chocolate. If you were a painter, how would you paint it? Noticing the shape, the size, the colors, the way the light reflects on it . . . (long pause)
>
> Now moving your attention to the smell of the chocolate. Placing it under your nose and closing your eyes again . . . just noticing the scent. Where in your nose do you smell the chocolate? What aspects of it can you smell? Milk? Vanilla? Tobacco or an earthy scent? Just noticing all you can about the scent . . . (long pause)
>
> Now rubbing the kiss on your lips so you get just a hint of flavor. Allowing your eyes to remain closed . . . What do you taste? What do you notice about the texture? Is it smooth or gritty? Melting or not? Just being aware of all the intricacies in this one chocolate kiss.
>
> Now placing the chocolate on your tongue, and just holding it in your mouth, not biting it. What do you now notice about the flavor? Move it around

your mouth. Does it taste different in different parts of your mouth? Allow it to melt on your tongue. What do you notice as it melts? Just allowing yourself to be fully present with this bite. What do you notice about your saliva? About your mouth itself? Does the flavor change over time, as it melts? In what way? Just taking as long as you like to allow the chocolate to melt and to fully experience the sensations of eating it. Can you feel it move out of your mouth, into your throat? Down your throat toward your stomach? And being aware of any thoughts or emotions that pass through, distinguishing a thought or emotion from a sensation like taste ... What if you ate like this most of the time? ... Observing whatever is present for you now, without judging it ... (very long pause) ... and opening your eyes when ready.

Skill Set 7: Discernment of appetite regulation cues from other internal events – Appetite regulation cues (hunger, fullness and taste-satiety) need to be teased apart from emotions, thoughts, behavioral urges as well as other physical sensations (e.g., fatigue) in order to be well utilized. While learning this skill set requires the acquisition of the previous six skills, the learning is not a linear process. As such, the EMPOWER program layers skill training in each of these arenas. Each skill influences the other, and new contexts challenge existing skills. For example, once participants can sense an emotion, and can sense hunger, they can begin to compare them and develop personal ways to distinguish between the two. Refining that distinction further informs the identification of emotion and hunger, and so on. One female participant, for example, over time noted that her anxiety sensations are higher in the chest while hunger signals emanate from the stomach area right below the breastbone. Another participant who often ate to quell anxiety observed that she is most aware of sensations of anxiety (e.g., palpitations) at the bottom of the breath, after the exhale when she can feel her heartbeat most saliently. These powerful realizations gave these women mechanisms to use in distinguishing anxiety and hunger.

Skill Set 8: Identification of true needs – Once participants are proficient in observing and teasing out the components of their own experience, the EMPOWER approach encourages the next step; to make an informed decision to best address their true needs. Although reactivity is sometimes driven by habit alone, it often is an attempt to meet an underlying need. As participants gain skills in nonjudgmental self-observation, they are able to discern their true needs with greater clarity. For example, if the true need is boredom, participants may decide to find a better way to entertain themselves. If the true need is temporary fatigue, sleep may be a useful response. If the true need is frustration related to a specific incident, assertiveness or problem solving may be appropriate. In theory, once the true need is identified, wise mind then guides behavior choices. Many participants, however, also appear to benefit from having specific exercises to clarify their processes for decision making.

Skill Set 9: Addressing true needs – Clinical scientists have underscored the need to promote greater self-acceptance in individuals with ED while still fostering meaningful behavioral change (e.g., Wilson, 1996). EMPOWER participants appear better able to deal with this dialectic when needed changes are contextualized as attempts toward enacting their personal mission statements and visions for health. They are guided to reflect on and develop personal mission statements (similar to ACT approaches), as well as to spend time cultivating a long-term vision for health. Participants then use this context of what they really want for themselves in the long run to guide decisions in the moment. Stop-Breath-Connect is taught to encourage participants to take a momentary pause before behaviors they are trying to change; they mindfully center themselves and remember why the change matters in the long run (Wolever et al., 2007). This approach is further aided by strategies for setting Specific, Measurable, Action-oriented, Realistic and Time-bound (SMART) short and long-term goals. While it remains an empirical question, clinical experience suggests that these additional tools significantly augment the mindfulness approach and vice versa.

The choice to add additional tools to mindfulness treatment may depend in part on the level of mindfulness practice that individuals are willing to undertake, and their ability to create an environment conducive to internal listening. Given the practical reality of most clients' lives, and the fact that these approaches may benefit many people that are not drawn to meditation per se, it may be wise to use mindfulness to create a learning space to enhance wise decision making in a more active fashion as well. For example, when one is deciding whether or not to eat, it is useful to reference physiological hunger cues rather than external signals that it is time to eat (food is present, meal break begins, etc.). Similarly, when deciding to stop eating, it is useful to register physiological cues of moderate fullness rather than external cues that eating is complete (clean plate, time is up, etc.). However, Western culture is so externally driven and fast-paced, it is often not enough to teach clients to pay attention to hunger and fullness. They must also carefully plan to establish an environment in which they can register these signals; and this requires assertiveness and other traditional techniques. For instance, imagine that you are a nurse working a 12 hour shift without a meal break. While physiologically, it is important to eat during your shift, the health system does not build in time for this task. The nurse must use assertiveness skills to assure even a 15 minutes break to eat, as well as flexibility to sense the best time to take the break, as well as planning and preparation to ensure that nutritious food is available in small quickly-edible portions. Similarly, registering moderate hunger and moderate fullness signals after the work shift may help the nurse avoid overeating after work, but some nutritious intake during the shift will also help avoid overeating later.

In such situations, mindfulness helps participants to create an optimum learning space, and the introduction of concepts and tools from other traditional approaches may strengthen the intervention. For example, state of the art treatments for bulimia and BED (e.g., Apple & Agras, 1997; Fairburn, 1995) encourage participants to recognize and label thoughts and emotions that precede bingeing. Mindfulness, however, can facilitate this learning by applying a layer of nonjudgment to remove harsh criticism (from self or others), freeing up participants for more accurate self-observation. One significant difference in these approaches and mindfulness-informed approaches, however, is that CBT encourages direct intervention into the thoughts or behaviors whereas pure mindfulness suggests that just observing the thought, emotion, or sensation is enough; the mere process of nonjudgmentally attending to them allows for a shift from within the participant.

In sum, participants with ED are driven by deficits in the self-regulation of food intake, emotion and cognition. There is strong theoretical support for the application of mindfulness to this dysregulation, and an emerging literature on its efficacy. Some approaches use more traditional MBSR techniques while others apply these mindfulness techniques directly to eating and compensatory mechanisms characteristic of ED. The EMPOWER approach conceptualizes mindfulness as a strong self-learning tool in which individuals explore new ways to self-regulate; some ways are taught through pure mindfulness whereas others apply mindfulness to other behavior change techniques (e.g., goal-setting). Additional research will be important in evaluating the efficacy of various aspects of mindfulness-based treatments in treating specific issues.

Acknowledgements: The authors wish to thank and acknowledge Jean Kristeller, PhD, Sasha Loring, MEd, LCSW, Michael Baime, MD and Larry Ladden, PhD whose wise attention to the application of mindfulness has deeply informed our work.

References

Agras, W. S. & Telch, C. F. (1998). The effects of caloric deprivation and negative affect on binge eating in obese binge-eating disordered women. *Behavior Therapy, 29,* 491–503.

Allen, H. N. & Craighead, L. W. (1999). Appetite monitoring in the treatment of binge eating disorder. *Behavior Therapy, 30,* 253–272.

American Psychiatric Association. (1994). *Diagnostic and Statistical Manual of Mental Disorders* (DSM-IV, 4th ed.). Washington, D.C.: American Psychiatric Press.

American Psychiatric Association. (2000). *Diagnostic and Statistical Manual of Mental Disorders* (DSM-IV, 4th ed. Text revision). Washington, D.C.: American Psychiatric Press.

American Psychiatric Association Work Group on Eating Disorders. (2000). Practice guideline for the treatment of patients with eating disorders (revision). *American Journal of Psychiatry, 157*(1), 1–39.

Apple, R. F. & Agras, W. S. (1997). Overcoming Eating Disorders: A Cognitive-Behavioral Treatment for Bulimia Nervosa and Binge-Eating Disorder. Graywind Publications, Inc.

Baer, R. A., Fischer, S., & Huss, D. B. (2005). Mindfulness-based cognitive therapy applied to binge eating: A case study. *Cognitive and Behavioral Practice, 12,* 351–358.

Baer, R. A., Fischer, S., & Huss, D. B. (2006). Mindfulness and acceptance in the treatment of disordered eating. *Journal of Rational-Emotive & Cognitive-Behavior Therapy, 23,* 281–300.

Bardone-Cone, A. M., Wonderlich, S. A., Frost, R. O., Bulik, C. M., Mitchell, J. E., Uppala, S., & Simonich, H., et al. (2007). Perfectionism and eating disorders: Current status and future directions. *Clinical Psychology Review, 27,* 384–405.

Becker, A. E., Keel, P., Anderson-Fye, E. P., & Thomas, J. J. (2004). Genes and/or jeans?: Genetic and socio-cultural contributions to risk for eating disorders. *Journal of Addictive Diseases, 23,* 81–103.

Berkman, N. D., Lohr, K. N., & Bulik, C. M. (2007). Outcomes of eating disorders: A systematic review of the literature. *International Journal of Eating Disorders, 40,* 293–309.

Berthoz, S., Perdereau, F., Godart, N., Corcos, M., & Haviland, M. G. (2007). Observer- and self-rated alexithymia in eating disorder patients: Levels and correspondence among three measures. *Journal of Psychosomatic Research, 62,* 341–347.

Bowers, W. A. (2002). Cognitive therapy for anorexia nervosa. *Cognitive and Behavioral Practice, 9*, 247–253.

Brandsma, L. (2007). Eating disorders across the lifespan. *Journal of Women and Aging, 19*, 155–172.

Brownley, K. A., Berkman, N. D., Sedway, J. A., Lohr, K. N., & Bulik, C. M. (2007). Binge eating disorder treatment: A systematic review of randomized controlled trials. *International Journal of Eating Disorders, 40*, 337–348.

Bruce, B. & Agras, W. S. (1992). Binge eating in females: A population-based investigation. *International Journal of Eating Disorders, 12*, 365–373.

Bulik, C. M., Berkman, N. D., Brownley, K. A., Sedway, J. A., & Lohr, K. N. (2007). Anorexia nervosa treatment: A systematic review of randomized controlled trials. *International Journal of Eating Disorders, 40*, 310–320.

Bydlowski, S., Corcos, M., Jeammet, P., Paterniti, S., Berthoz, S., Laurier, C., Chambry, S., & Consoli, S.M. (2005). Emotion-processing deficits in eating disorders. *International Journal of Eating Disorders, 37*, 321–329.

Cachelin, F.M., Striegel-Moore, R. H., Elder, K. A., Pike, K. M., Wilfley, D. E., & Fairburn, C. G. (1999). Natural course of a community sample of women with binge eating disorder. *International Journal of Eating Disorders, 25*, 45–54.

Carano, A., De Berardis, D., Gambi, F., Di Paolo, C., Campanella, D., & Pelusi, L. (2006). Alexithymia and body image in adult outpatients with binge eating disorder. *International Journal of Eating Disorders, 39*, 332–340.

Cash, T. F. & Deagle, E. A. (1997). The nature and extent of body image disturbances in anorexia nervosa and bulimia nervosa: A meta-analysis. *International Journal of Eating Disorders, 22*, 107–125.

Claes, L., Vandereycken, W., & Vertommen, H. (2005). Impulsivity-related traits in eating disorder patients. *Personality and Individual Differences, 39(4)*, 739–749

Corstorphine, E. (2006). Cognitive-emotional-behavioral therapy for the eating disorders: Working with beliefs about emotions. *European Eating Disorders Review, 14*, 448–461.

Corstorphine, E., Mountford, V., Tomlinson, S., Waller, G., & Meyer, C. (2007). Distress tolerance in the eating disorders. *Eating Behaviors, 8*, 91–97.

Corstorphine, E., Waller, G., Ohanian, V., & Baker, M. (2006). Changes in internal states across the binge-vomit cycle in bulimia nervosa. *Journal of Nervous and Mental Disease, 194*, 446–449.

Craighead, L. W. & Allen, H. N. (1995). Appetite awareness training: A cognitive behavioral intervention for binge eating. *Cognitive and Behavioral Practice, 2*, 249–270.

Dalle Grave, R., Di Pauli, D., Sartirana, M., Calugi, S., & Shafran, R. (2007). The interpretation of symptoms of starvation/severe dietary restraint in eating disorder patients. *Eating and Weight Disorders, 12*, 108–113.

Davis, R. & Jamieson, J. (2005). Assessing the functional nature of binge eating in the eating disorders. *Eating Behaviors, 6*, 345–354.

Deaver, C. M., Miltenberger, R. G., Smyth, J., Meidinger, A., & Crosby, R. (2003). An evaluation of affect in binge eating. *Behavior Modification, 27*, 578–599.

Dingemans, A. E., Spinhoven, Ph., & van Furth, E. F. (2006). Maladaptive core beliefs and eating disorder symptoms. *Eating Behaviors, 7*, 258–265.

Dobson, K. S. & Dozois, D. J. A. (2004). Attentional biases in eating disorders: A meta-analytic review of Stroop performance. *Clinical Psychology Review, 23*, 1001–1022.

Dunkley, D. M. & Grilo, C. M. (2007). Self-criticism, low self-esteem, depressive symptoms, and over-evaluation of shape and weight in binge eating disorder patients. *Behaviour Research and Therapy, 45*, 139–149.

Eldredge, K. L. & Agras, W. S. (1996). Weight and shape overconcern and emotional eating in binge eating disorder. *International Journal of Eating Disorders, 19*, 73–82.

Fairburn, C. G. (1995). *Overcoming binge eating*. New York: Guildford Press.

Fairburn, C. G., Cooper, Z., Doll, H. A., Norman, P., & O'Connor, M. (2000). The natural course of bulimia nervosa and binge eating disorder in young women. *Archives of General Psychiatry, 57*, 659-665.

Farchaus Stein, K. (1996). The self-schema model: A theoretical approach to the self-concept in eating disorders. *Archives of Psychiatric Nursing, 10*, 96-109.

Faris, P. L., Eckert, E. D., Kim, S. W., Meller, W. H., Pardo, J. V., Goodale, R. L., & Hartman, B. K. (2006). Evidence for a vagal pathophysiology for bulimia nervosa and the accompanying depressive symptoms. *Journal of Affective Disorders, 92*, 79-90.

Fassino, S., Piero, A., Gramaglia, C., & Abbate-Daga, G. (2004). Clinical, psychopathological and personality correlates of interoceptive awareness in anorexia nervosa, bulimia nervosa and obesity. *Psychopathology, 37*, 168-174.

Faunce, G. J. (2002). Eating disorders and attentional bias: A review. *Eating Disorders, 10*, 125-139.

Felker, K. R. & Stivers, C. (1994). The relationship of gender and family environment to eating disorder risk in adolescence. *Adolescence, 29*, 821-834.

Fernandez-Aranda, F., Pinheiro, A. P., Thornton, L. M., Berrettini, W. H., Crow, S., Fichter, M. M., Halmi, K. A., Kaplan, A. S., Keel, D., Mitchell, J., Rotondo, A., Woodside, D. B., Kaye, W. H. & Bulik, C. M. (2008). Impulse control disorders in women with eating disorders. *Psychiatry Research, 157*, 147-157.

Fichter, M. M., Quadflieg, N., & Gnutzmann, A. (1998). Binge eating disorder: Treatment outcome over a 6-year course. *Journal of Psychosomatic Research, 44*, 385-405.

Franco-Paredes, K., Mancilla-Diaz, J. M., Vazquez-Arevalo, R., Lopez-Aguilar, X., & Alvarez-Rayon, G. (2005). Perfectionism and eating disorders: A review of the literature. *European Eating Disorders Review, 13*, 61-70.

Gilboa-Schectman, E., Avnon, L., Zubery, E., & Jeczmien, P. (2006). Emotional processing in eating disorders: Specific impairment or general distress related deficiency? *Depression and Anxiety, 23*, 331-339.

Gluck, M. E., Geliebter, A., Hung, J., & Yahav, E. (2004). Cortisol, hunger, and desire to binge eat following a cold stress test in obese women with binge eating disorder. *Psychosomatic Medicine, 66*, 876-881.

Gratz, K. L. & Gunderson, J. G. (2006). Preliminary data on an acceptance-based emotion regulation group intervention for deliberate self-harm among women with borderline personality disorder. *Behavior Therapy, 37*, 25-35.

Gross, J. J. (1998). The emerging field of emotion regulation: An integrative review. *Review of General Psychology, 2*, 271-299.

Halmi, K. A., Eckert, E., Marchi, P., Sampugnaro, V., Apple, R., & Cohen, J. (1991). Comorbidity of psychiatric diagnoses in anorexia nervosa. *Archives of General Psychiatry, 48*, 712-718.

Harris, M. & Cumella, E. J. (2006). Eating disorders across the life span. *Journal of Psychosocial Nursing, 44*, 20-26.

Hayes, S. C., Luoma, J. B., Bond, F. W., Masuda, A., & Lillis, J. (2006). Acceptance and commitment therapy: Model, processes and outcomes. *Behaviour Research and Therapy, 44*, 1-25.

Hayes, S. C. & Pankey, J. (2002). Experiential avoidance, cognitive fusion, and an ACT approach to anorexia nervosa. *Cognitive and Behavioral Practice, 9*, 243-247.

Hayes, S. C., Strosahl, K. D., & Wilson, K. G. (1999). *Acceptance and commitment therapy: An experiential approach to behavior change*. New York: Guilford Press.

Heatherton, T. F. & Baumeister, R. F. (1991). Binge eating as escape from self-awareness. *Psychological Bulletin, 110*, 86-108.

Heffner, M., Sperry, J., Eifert, G.H., & Detweiler, M. (2002). Acceptance and commitment therapy in the treatment of an adolescent female with anorexia nervosa: A case example. *Cognitive and Behavioral Practice, 9*, 232-236.

Herman, C. & Polivy, J. (1980). Restrained eating. In A. Stunkard (Ed.), *Obesity*. Philadelphia: Saunders.

Herpertz-Dahlmann, B., Muller, B., Herpertz, S., & Heussen, N. (2001). Prospective 10-year follow-up in adolescent anorexia nervosa—course, outcome, psychiatric comorbidity, and psychosocial adaptation. *Journal of Child Psychology & Psychiatry, 42*, 603-612.

Hetherington, M. & Rolls, B. (1988). Sensory specific satiety and food intake in eating disorders. In B. Walsh (Ed.), *Eating behaviors in eating disorders*. Washington, D.C.: American Psychiatric Press.

Hoek, H. & van Hoeken, D. (2003). Review of the prevalence and incidence of eating disorders. *International Journal of Eating Disorders, 34*, 383-396.

Hrabosky, J. I., Masheb, R. M., White, M. A., & Grilo, C. M. (2007). Overvaluation of shape and weight in binge eating disorder. *Journal of Consulting and Clinical Psychology, 75*, 175-180.

Hudson, J. I., Hiripi, E., Pope, H. G., & Kessler, R. C. (2007). The prevalence and correlates of eating disorders in the National Comorbidity Survey Replication. *Biological Psychiatry, 61*, 348-358.

Hughes, M. L., Hamill, M., van Gerko, K., Lockwood, R., & Waller, G. (2006). The relationship between different levels of cognition and behavioural symptoms in the eating disorders. *Eating Behaviors, 7*, 125-133.

Hutchinson, D. M. & Rapee, R. M. (2007). Do friends share similar body image and eating problems? The role of social networks and peer influences in early adolescence. *Behaviour Research and Therapy, 45*, 1557-1577.

Jacobi, C., Paul, T., de Zwaan, M., Nutzinger, D. O., & Dahme, B. (2004). Specificity of self-concept disturbances in eating disorders. *International Journal of Eating Disorders, 35*, 204-210.

Jansen, A., Nederkoorn, C., & Mulkens, S. (2005). Selective visual attention for ugly and beautiful body parts in eating disorders. *Behaviour Research and Therapy, 43*, 183-196.

Jha A. P., Krompinger J., & Baime M. J. (2007). Mindfulness Training Modifies Subsystems of Attention. *Cognitive, Affective & Behavioral Neuroscience, 7*(2):109-119.

Kabat-Zinn, J. (1990). *Full catastrophe living: Using the wisdom of your body and mind to face stress, pain, and illness*, New York: Delacorte.

Kabat-Zinn, J. (1994). *Wherever you go, there you are: Mindfulness meditation in everyday life*. New York: Hyperion.

Keel, P. K. & Mitchell, J. E. (1997). Outcome in bulimia nervosa. *American Journal of Psychiatry, 154*, 313-321.

Kollai, M., Bonyhay, I., Jokkel, G., & Szonyi, L. (1994). Cardiac vagal hyperactivity in adolescent anorexia nervosa. *European Heart Journal, 15*, 1113-1118.

Kristeller, J. L., Baer, R. A., & Quillian-Wolever, R. (2006). Mindfulness-based approaches to eating disorders. In R. A. Baer (Ed.), *Mindfulness-based treatment approaches*. Oxford, U. K.: Academic Press (Elsevier).

Kristeller, J. L. & Hallett, C. B. (1999). An exploratory study of a meditation-based intervention for binge eating disorder. *Journal of Health Psychology, 4*, 357-363.

Kristeller, J. L., Wolever, R., & Sheets, V. (2008). *Mindfulness-based eating awareness therapy (MB-EAT): A randomized clinical trial for binge eating disorder*. Manuscript submitted for publication.

Lau, M. A., Bishop, S. R., Segal, Z. V., Buis, T., Anderson, N., Carlson, L., Shapiro, S., Carmody, J., Abbey, S., & Devins, J. (2006). The Toronto Mindfulness Scale: Development and validation. *Journal of Clinical Psychology, 62*, 1445-1467.

Lawson, R., Waller, G., & Lockwood, R. (2007). Cognitive content and process in eating-disordered patients with obsessive-compulsive features. *Eating Behaviors, 8*(3), 305-310.

Lazarus, S. & Galassi, J. P. (1994). Affect and cognitions in obese binge eaters and non-binge eaters: The association between depression, anxiety, and bulimic cognitions. *Eating Disorders: The Journal of Treatment and Prevention, 2*, 141-157.

Leahy, R. L. (2002). A model of emotional schemas. *Cognitive and Behavioral Practice, 9*, 177-190.

Leung, N. & Price, E. (2007). Core beliefs in dieters and eating disordered women. *Eating Behaviors, 8*, 65-72.

Lilenfeld, L. R., Stein, D., Bulik, S. M., Strober, M., Plotnicov, K., Pollice, C., Rao, R., Merikangas, K. R., Nagy, L., & Aye, H. K. (2000). Personality traits among currently eating disordered, recovered and never ill first-degree female relatives of bulimic and control women. *Psychological Medicine, 30*, 1399-1410.

Lindeman, M. & Stark, K. (2001). Emotional eating and eating disorder psychopathology. *Eating Disorders, 9*, 251-259.

Linehan, M. M. (1993a). *Cognitive-behavioral treatment of borderline personality disorder*. New York, NY: Guilford Press.

Linehan, M. M. (1993b). *Skills training manual for treating borderline personality disorder*. New York: The Guilford Press.

Linehan, M. M., Armstrong, H. E., Suarez, A., Allmond, D., & Heard, H. L. (1991). Cognitive-behavioral treatment of chronically parasuicidal borderline patients. *Archives of General Psychiatry, 48*, 1060-1064.

Lingswiler, V. M., Crowther, J. H., & Stephens, M. A. P. (1989). Affective and cognitive antecedents to eating episodes in bulimia and binge eating. *International Journal of Eating Disorders, 8*, 533-539.

Lynch, W. C., Everingham, A., Dubitzky, J., Hartman, M., & Kasser, T. J. (2000). Does binge eating play a role in the self-regulation of moods? *Integrative Physiological and Behavioral Science, 35*, 298-313.

Marcus, M. D., Wing, R. R., & Hopkins, J. (1988). Obese binge eaters: Affect, cognitions, and response to behavioral weight control. *Journal of Consulting and Clinical Psychology, 56*, 433-439.

Martin, L. L., Tesser, A., & McIntosh, W. D. (1993). Wanting but not having: The effects of unattained goals on thoughts and feelings. In D. W. Wegner & J. W. Pennebaker (Eds.), *Handbook of mental control* (pp. 552-572). Englewood Cliffs, NJ: Prentice Hall.

McCabe, E. B. & Marcus, M. D. (2002). Is dialectical behavior therapy useful in the management of anorexia nervosa? *Eating Disorders, 10*, 335-337.

Meyer, C., & Waller, G. (1999). The impact of emotion upon eating behavior: The role of subliminal visual processing of threat cues. *International Journal of Eating Disorders, 25*, 319-326.

Meyer, C., Waller, G., & Watson, P. (2000). Cognitive avoidance and bulimic psychopathology: The relevance of temporal factors in a nonclinical population. *International Journal of Eating Disorders, 27*, 405-410.

Nakai, Y. & Koh, T. (2001). Perception of hunger to insulin-induced hypoglycemia in anorexia nervosa. *International Journal of Eating Disorders, 29*, 354-357.

National Institute of Mental Health. (2001). Eating disorders: Facts about eating disorders and the search for solutions. *NIH Publication NO. 01-4901*. Bethesda, MD: National Institute of Mental health, National Institutes of Health, U.S. Department of Health and Human Services.

Nauta, H., Hospers, H., Kok, G., & Jansen, A. (2000). A comparison between a cognitive and a behavioral treatment for obese binge eaters and obese non-binge eaters. *Behavior Therapy, 31*, 441-461.

Nolen-Hoeksema, S. (2000). The role of rumination in depressive disorders and mixed anxiety/depressive symptoms. *Journal of Abnormal Psychology, 109*, 504-511.

Office on Women's Health. (February 2000). Eating disorders. Washington, D.C.: National Women's Health Information Center, U.S. Department of Health and Human Services.

Orsillo, S. M. & Batten, S. V. (2002). ACT as treatment of a disorder of excessive control: Anorexia. *Cognitive and Behavioral Practice, 9,* 253-259.

Overton, A., Selway, S., Strongman, K., & Houston, M. (2005). Eating disorders—The regulation of positive as well as negative emotion experience. *Journal of Clinical Psychology in Medical Settings, 12,* 39-56.

Petretta, M., Bonaduce, D., Scalfi, L., de Filippo, E., Marciano, F. Migaux, M. L., Themistoclakis, S., Ianniciello, A., & Contaldo, F. (1997). Heart rate variability as a measure of autonomic nervous system function in anorexia nervosa. *Clinical Cardiology, 20,* 219-224.

Phelan, P. (1987). Cognitive correlates of bulimia: The Bulimic Thoughts Questionnaire. *International Journal of Eating Disorders, 6,* 593-607.

Placanica, J. L., Faunce, G. J., & Soames Job, R. F. (2002). The effect of fasting on attentional biases for food and body shape/weight words in high and low Eating Disorder Inventory scorers. *International Journal of Eating Disorders, 32,* 79-90.

Polivy, J. & Herman, C. P. (1985). Dieting and bingeing. *American Psychologist, 40,* 193-201.

Powell, A. L. & Thelen, M. H. (1996). Emotions and cognitions associated with bingeing and weight control behavior in bulimia. *Journal of Psychosomatic Research, 40,* 317-328.

Quadflieg, N. & Fichter, M. M. (2003). The course and outcome of bulimia nervosa. *European Child & Adolescent Psychiatry, 12*(1), 99-109.

Reichborn-Kjennerud, T., Bulik, C. M., Sullivan, P., Tambs, K., & Harris, J. R. (2004). Psychiatric and medical symptoms in binge eating in the absence of compensatory behaviors. *Obesity Research, 12,* 1445-1454.

Ricciardelli, L. A., Williams, R. J., & Finemore, J. (2001). Restraint as misregulation in drinking and eating. *Addictive Behaviors, 26,* 665-675.

Robinson, T. N., Chang, J. Y., Haydel, K. F., & Killen, J. D. (2001). Overweight concerns and body dissatisfaction among third-grade children: The impacts of ethnicity and socioeconomic status. *Journal of Pediatrics, 138,* 181-187.

Roth, G. (1984). *Breaking free from emotional eating.* New York, N. Y.: Plume.

Safer, D. L, Lively, T. J., Telch, C. F., & Agras, W. S. (2002). Predictors of relapse following successful dialectical behavior therapy for binge eating disorder. *International Journal of Eating Disorders, 32,* 155-163.

Safer, D. L., Telch, C. F., & Agras, W. S. (2001a). Dialectical behavior therapy adapted for bulimia: A case report. *International Journal of Eating Disorders, 30,* 101-106.

Safer, D. L., Telch, C. F., & Agras, W. S. (2001b). Dialectical behavior therapy for bulimia nervosa. *American Journal of Psychiatry, 158,* 632-634.

Salbach, H., Klinowski, N., Pfeiffer, E., Lehkuhl, U., & Korte, A. (2007). Dialectical behavior therapy for adolescents with anorexia and bulimia nervosa (DBT-AN/BN)—a pilot study. *Praxis der Kinderpsychologie und Kinderpsychiatrie, 56,* 91-108.

Santel, S., Baving, L., Krauel, K., Munte, T. F., & Rotte, M. (2006). Hunger and satiety in anorexia nervosa: fMRI during cognitive processing of food pictures. *Brain Research, 1114,* 138-148.

Segal, Z. V., Williams, J. M. G., & Teasdale, J. D. (2002). *Mindfulness-based cognitive therapy for depression: A new approach to preventing relapse.* New York: The Guilford Press.

Shafran, R., Lee, M., Cooper, Z., Palmer, R. L., & Fairburn (2007). Attentional bias in eating disorders. *International Journal of Eating Disorders, 40,* 369-380.

Shafran, R., Teachman, B. A., Kerry, S., & Rachman, S. (1999). A cognitive distortion associated with eating disorders: Thought-shape fusion. *British Journal of Clinical Psychology, 38,* 167-179.

Shafran, R. & Robinson, P. (2004). Thought-shape fusion in eating disorders. *British Journal of Clinical Psychology, 43*, 399-408.

Shapiro, J. R., Berkman, N. D., Brownley, K. A., Sedway, J. A., Lohr, K. N. & Bulik, C. M. (2007). Bulimia nervosa treatment: A systematic review of randomized controlled trials. *International Journal of Eating Disorders, 40*, 321-336.

Sifneos, P. E. (1996). Alexithymia: Past and present. *American Journal of Psychiatry, 153*, 137-142.

Smith, B. W., Shelley, B. M., Leahigh, L., & Vanleit, B. (2006). A preliminary study of the effects of a modified mindfulness intervention on binge eating. *Complementary Health Practice Review, 11*, 133-143.

Spangler, D. L. (2002). Testing the cognitive model of eating disorders: The role of dysfunctional beliefs about appearance. *Behavior Therapy, 33*, 87-105.

Spitzer, R., Devlin, M., Walsh, B., Hasin, D., Wing., D., Marcus, M., Stunkard, A., Yanovski, S., Agras, S., Mitchell, J., & Nonas, C. (1992). Binge eating disorder: A multisite field of the diagnostic criteria. *International Journal of Eating Disorders, 11*, 191-203.

Spitzer, R. L., Yanovski, S., Wadden, T., Wing, R., Marcus, M. D, & Stunkard, A., Devlin, M., et al. (1993). Binge eating disorder: Its further validation in a multisite study. *International Journal of Eating Disorders, 13*, 137-153.

Spoor, S. T. P., Bekker, M. H. J., Van Heck, G. L., Croon, M. A., & Van Strien, T. (2005). Inner body and outward appearance: The relationships between appearance orientation, eating disorder symptoms and internal body awareness. *Eating Disorders: Journal of Treatment and Prevention, 13*, 479-490.

Spoor, S. T. P., Bekker, M. H. J., Van Strien, T., & van Heck, G. L. (2007). Relations between negative affect, coping and emotional eating. *Appetite, 48*, 368-376.

Spranger, S. C., Waller, G., & Bryant-Waugh, R. (2001). Schema avoidance in bulimic and non-eating-disordered women. *International Journal of Eating Disorders, 29*, 302-306.

Steele, A., Corsini, N., & Wade, T. D. (2007). The interaction of perfectionism, perceived weight status, and self-esteem to predict bulimic symptoms: The role of 'benign' perfectionism. *Behaviour Research and Therapy, 45*, 1647-1655.

Stein, R. I., Kenardy, J., Wiseman, C. V., Zoler Dounchis, J., Arnow, B. A., & Wilfley, D. E. (2007). What's driving the binge in binge eating disorder?: A prospective examination of precursors and consequences. *International Journal of Eating Disorders, 40*, 195-203.

Steinhausen, H. C. (1999). Eating disorders. In H. C. Steinhausen & F. Verhulst (Eds.), *Risk and outcome in developmental psychopathology* (pp. 210-230). Oxford, U.K.: Oxford University Press.

Striegel-Moore, R. H., Dohm, F. A., Kraemer, H. C., Taylor, C. B., Daniels, S., Crawford, P. B., & Schreiber, G. B. (2003). Eating disorders in white and black women. *American Journal of Psychiatry, 160*, 1326-1331.

Striegel-Moore, R. H., Wilfley, D. E., Pike, K. M., Dohm, F. A., & Fairburn, C. G. (2000). Recurrent binge eating in black American women. *Archives of Family Medicine, 9*, 83-87.

Sullivan, P. F. (1995). Mortality in anorexia nervosa. *American Journal of Psychiatry, 152*, 1073-1074.

Swan, S., & Andrews, B. (2003). The relationship between shame, eating disorders and disclosure in treatment. *British Journal of Clinical Psychology, 42*, 367-378.

Telch, C. F. (1997). Skills training treatment for adaptive affect regulation in a woman with binge-eating disorder. *International Journal of Eating Disorders, 22*, 77-81.

Telch, C. F., Agras, W. S., & Linehan, M. M. (2000). Group dialectical behavior therapy for binge-eating disorder: A preliminary, uncontrolled trial. *Behavior Therapy, 31*, 569-582.

Telch, C. F., Agras, W. S., & Linehan, M. M. (2001). Dialectical behavior therapy for binge eating disorder. *Journal of Consulting and Clinical Psychology, 69,* 1061-1065.

Thomsen, S. R., McCoy, J. K., & Williams, M. (2001). Internalizing the impossible: Anorexic outpatients' experiences with women's beauty and fashion magazines. *Eating Disorders, 9,* 49-64.

Waller, G. & Mijatovich, S. (1998). Preconscious processing of threat cues: Impact on eating among women with unhealthy eating attitudes. *International Journal of Eating Disorders, 24,* 83-89.

Wegner, D. (1994). Ironic processes of mental control. *Psychological Review, 101,* 34-52.

Wheeler, K., Greiner, P., & Boulton, M. (2005). Exploring alexithymia, depression, and binge eating in self-reported eating disorders in women. *Perspectives in Psychiatric Care, 41,* 114-123.

Whiteside, U., Chen, E., Neighbors, C., Hunter, D., Lo, T., & Larimer, M. (2007). Difficulties regulating emotions: Do binge eaters have fewer strategies to modulate and tolerate negative affect? *Eating Behaviors, 8,* 162-169.

Wilson, G. T. (1984). Toward the understanding and treatment of binge eating. In R. C. Hawkins, W. J. Fremouw, & P. F. Clement (Eds.). *The binge purge syndrome* (pp. 264-289). New York, N. Y.: Springer.

Wilson, G. T. (1996). Acceptance and change in the treatment of eating disorders and obesity. *Behavior Therapy, 27,* 417-439.

Wilson, K. G. & Roberts, M. (2002). Core principles in acceptance and commitment therapy: An application to anorexia. *Cognitive and Behavioral Practice, 9,* 237-243.

Wiser, S. & Telch, C. F. (1999). Dialectical behavior therapy for binge eating disorder. *Journal of Clinical Psychology in Session: Psychotherapy in Practice, 55,* 755-768.

Wolever, R. Q., Best, J. L., Sheets, V. L., Davis, J., Psujek, J., Liebowitz, R., & Kristeller, J. L. (2006). *Bio-behavioral outcomes of a mindfulness-based intervention for binge eating disorder.* Paper presented at the North American Research Conference on Complementary and Integrative Medicine, Edmonton, Canada.

Wolever, R., Best, J. L., Sheets, V. L., & Kristeller, J. L. (2008). *Mindfulness-based intervention for binge eating disorder (BED) enhances post-prandial glucose metabolism independent of weight change.* Manuscript in preparation.

Wolever, R. Q., Ladden, L., Davis, J., Best, J., Greeson, J., & Baime, M. (2007). *EMPOWER: Mindful Maintenance Therapist Manual.* Unpublished treatment manual for NIH funded grants 5U01 AT004159 and 5 U01 AT004158). Duke University and University of Pennsylvania (respectively).

15

Paradise Lost: Mindfulness and Addictive Behavior

Thomas Bien

Whether the ground beneath our feet is heaven or hell depends entirely on our way of seeing and walking.

–Thich Nhat Hanh (2001)

In the Beginning was Paradise

According to the stories of many cultures, the human beginning was a time of ease and wonder, free from hard labor, struggle, strife, and the alienation and fragmentation we know today. Sometimes this perfection is projected into the future—a New Jerusalem descending upon the earth, the city of God, or a heaven we enter after death. Sometimes it is viewed as the possible result of human effort, a tradition spanning from Plato's Republic (ca. 360 B.C.E.; Hamilton and Cairns, 1969) and Thomas Moore's *Utopia* (1516), to James Hilton's Shangri-La, (1933) and B. F. Skinner's *Walden Two* (1948), among many others.

In a Buddhist context, paradise is always available, but it cannot be found in the future or in the past. It is only available in the present moment, in that brief moment of perception before we split the world into judgments of pleasure and pain, gain and loss, desire and aversion. With these comes the sense of I or ego, the feeling that "*I* like this and want more of that for myself," or "*I* dislike that, and want to avoid that." This sense of I is the flaming sword blocking our return to the garden. It is the sense that we are a separate, unchanging entity, cut off from everything and everyone else, a bit of flotsam and jetsam floating haphazardly in a meaningless universe.

In Buddhism, paradise is found the moment we reverse this process. Paradise is found when we re-enter the present moment deeply and clearly, without being caught in either desire or aversion, without the narrow point of view of the separate and alienated self that wants and wants and wants, without our habitual mental patterns of judgment or blame. This kind of perception is called mindfulness. And with mindfulness, paradise is available here and now. Indeed, it can only be found here and now—not in the mythic past, not in the eschatological future, and not even as the result of human social engineering—important as such efforts may be for other reasons.

This human tendency to seek pleasure and avoid pain is neither wrong nor evil. It even has a certain necessity about it, a certain utility. Life requires such a capacity. Only, when coupled with our large brains, it becomes a capacity that can easily run amok. It is impossible that this endless process of struggle can ever yield peace. For peace is not found by constructing a world that contains only pleasant experiences and avoids all pain. To find peace requires wisdom, and wisdom teaches us that the foundation of peace lies in acceptance of the fundamental nature of human life—that good and bad, pleasure and pain, gain and loss are both necessary and inevitable. When we accept this plain fact, avoiding the extremes of either futile struggle or nihilistic passivity, we can come into the present moment, and be fully alive.

Addiction as Avoidance

Addiction in the narrow sense entails the use of substances to create an altered state of consciousness, and to do so in a way that is both compulsive and destructive. But in the broadest sense, all human beings are addicted. We are addicted to compulsive patterns of pleasure seeking and pain avoidance. When the Buddha said that "all worldlings are deranged" (Goleman, 1988), this is exactly what he meant. Our non-acceptance of the nature of reality, the *suchness* (Sanskrit: *tathata*) of things, yields an endless struggle to create a world totally free of pain and full of pleasure. The addict just happens to go about this in particular way—with drugs and alcohol—or by extension, with behaviors like gambling or sex. This is just one form of the essential human problem of the aboriginal splitting of the perceptual world into opposites.

The addicted person is someone who hopes to find a simple solution to this existential dilemma. Life hurts, he feels, and he wants to avoid this pain. He likes pleasure very much, on the other hand, and wants to find more of it in an easy, reliable, readily repeatable way. Whatever the drug of choice, the intention is to avoid pain and increase pleasure.

And it works. Drugs do, at least temporarily and in the short term, provide pleasure. They also provide a rather complete respite from our worries and difficulties. Drug addiction would not be so great a problem if this were not the case. If this were not the case, no one would be very tempted by addictive substances. It is precisely because they work so effectively, in this sense, that drugs are so compelling.

I emphasize, however, that the effect is short term. On the one hand, one may take a drug initially to enhance a positive experience. The individual finds herself with friends, and wants to really let go and have fun with them. Or she wants to celebrate a success. On the other hand, she may use drugs to turn off pain. A friend said something insensitive. The anticipated salary increase was not offered. She uses to turn off the pain for a while. But as the tendency to use a drug for such purposes gradually increases, the drug at the same time comes to lose its positive effects. Because of physiological and psychological tolerance, she tries to use more and more of the same substance to try to get back to that original, appealing state of mind, that effortless and paradisiacal feeling that made the drug so attractive in the first place. But ultimately, this is a matter of quenching thirst with salt water, and the effort fails. Paradise cannot be re-entered in this way.

What is considered problematic use varies considerably across cultures. What Americans would consider serious alcoholism evokes puzzled looks from Australians, who might consider such a level of consumption at most heavy, social, nonproblematic drinking. Traditional Jewish culture incorporates wine into family rituals such as the Passover Seder, and Jews are traditionally low on rates of alcoholism until perspective on what constitutes normal wine drinking, while eastern Europeans are known for their love of vodka. But the clinical key to determining what constitutes problematic drinking within a cultural context is the impact it has on one's life, health, well-being, and life functioning.

However, the diagnosis is made of what constitutes abuse or dependence, once the pattern of dependence is established, drug use is far from a benignly altered state in which one takes temporary respite from one's problems or enhances a celebratory mood. Instead, as one seeks the drug with increasing frequency, one's life becomes centered on maintaining supply, the rituals of drug use, and recovering from the episodes of use. There are few resources left to invest in solving life problems. Work and relationships are neglected and financial resources are wasted. Increasingly, when the addicted person tries to cope with life, the life he encounters is one that is painful and out of control. In the face of these difficulties, he has only the one highly developed and overpracticed response: use.

At this point, drug use has little to do with pleasure. Many individuals who have been addicted for a long time report that there is actually very little that remains enjoyable any more about using their drug. One reason for this may be that the body becomes conditioned to anticipate introduction of the drug at certain times and places or under certain conditions. In the case of alcohol, for example, the body prepares for the introduction of the depressant drug by an anticipatory homeostatic adjustment in a direction opposite from the drug's effects. That is, whereas alcohol slows heart rate and respiration, and lowers blood pressure, for example, the body anticipating the introduction of alcohol raises heart rate, respiration and blood pressure even before the drug is introduced. Once such conditioning is established, the addicted person requires more of the drug to achieve the same effect.

When the pleasure of use is gone or at least largely diminished, what is left is simply a compulsive pattern. In terms of conditioning, it is now almost exclusively a matter of negative reinforcement or avoidance. Instead of using to enhance pleasurable states, now it is a matter of avoiding pain or discomfort, including the discomfort of physiological withdrawal. But even more important is avoiding the pain of a life that has deteriorated on all important fronts.

The destructive downward spiral is captured in the story of the Tippler in Saint-Exupery's *The Little Prince* (1943):

"Why are you drinking?" demanded the little prince.
"So that I may forget," replied the tippler.
"Forget what?" inquired the little prince, who already was sorry for him.
"Forget that I am ashamed," the tippler confessed, hanging his head.
"Ashamed of what?" insisted the little prince, who wanted to help him.
"Ashamed of drinking!" The tippler brought his speech to an end, and shut himself up in an impregnable silence.

If then drug abuse is an avoidance paradigm, if it is about forgetting, then it stands to reason that the solution lies in the direction of non-avoidance, of remembrance. An approach which helps a person to remember rather than to forget, to be more aware rather than less, which increases one's capacity to face the truth of the present moment, even in its unpleasant elements, might, prima facie, be the essence of cure. Mindfulness is just such an approach. Mindfulness teaches us to be present, even with what hurts. And indeed, when we learn to do this fully, we encounter many positive elements of the present as well, elements that we miss when we are so intent on avoiding pain. In this sense, mindfulness can ultimately be a way to re-enter paradise, to acquire the state of profound psychological balance which Buddhists call *nirvana*.

But it is not so easy for the addicted individual to see the trap that she has fallen into with sufficient clarity to change it. For one thing, the psychology of learning teaches us that we are more controlled by the immediate consequences of our behavior than by the longer term consequences. In the laboratory paradigm, if a hungry rat presses a lever, and the food pellet drops almost immediately, the rat quickly learns to do lever presses. But if that food pellet drops more slowly—if it drops, for example, an hour later—learning does not take place so readily. Likewise, it is precisely the early stages of drug use that are generally the most pleasant. The first two drinks feel very good. The initial rush of cocaine feels nice. Unfortunately, the unpleasant sequelae are less determinative of subsequent behavior.

A further complication here is that drug use affects memory. In the case of alcohol, memory problems occur across a continuum that begins with acute effects, such as a vagueness of fuzziness in the recall of events, increasing to actual alcoholic blackouts, in which the memory for an entire period of time is missing, and reaching the extreme and chronic effect of Korsakov's syndrome, in which no new information can be assimilated (Miller & Saucedo, 1983). A Korsakov's patient can be introduced anew to the same therapist day after day without remembering him, or may ask why a former political leader, long dead, is no longer in the papers, since the ability to remember new information ceases at the point of onset of the disorder.

But even in the less extreme cases, the negative consequences of drug use remain less salient since they are not remembered clearly if they are remembered at all. The user remembers the pleasant buzz and sense of well-being, but forgets the nasty confusion or anger or stupor or even, in some cases, arguments and physical violence which follow later.

Mindfulness of the Process of Change

If addiction involves unawareness and avoidance, then it stands to reason that what is needed is an increase in awareness and in the capacity to experience life clearly, as it is, with calmness and clarity, and without evasion. Mindfulness is just such a practice. It is a non-judgmental, moment-by-moment openness to experience. The role of the therapist then is to help facilitate a shift in awareness, to make the negative consequences of use more salient. This is particularly challenging, however, given the memory effects noted above, in addition to powerful conditioning effects.

The type of awareness required varies with the stage of change. Prochaska and DiClemente (1986) conducted factor analyses of the stages people go through in changing an addictive behavior.[1] In the full six factor model, these

---

[1] Subsequent research by these two revealed that these same stages are found in all kinds of change in human behavior they have investigated and not just addiction.

stages are: *precontemplation, contemplation, determination, action, maintenance*, and *relapse*. Understanding these stages, and knowing where the client is in this regard, can help the therapist be present in a helpful way, facilitating the kind of awareness required for progress. The procedures for helping the addicted individual through these stages of change have been detailed by Miller and Rollnick (1991) in a process they call *motivational interviewing*. For our purposes here, motivational interviewing is the art of increasing a person's awareness in a specific kind of way, making it a process of increased mindfulness

Precontemplation means unawareness. At this stage, a person simply does not know there is a problem. This is not to say they are in denial, since denial connotes that the individual knows, at some level, that a problem exists, but refuses to recognize it. If asked whether they have a substance abuse problem, people in this stage will express genuine surprise. For this reason, people in this stage of change are not often found in treatment, unless a spouse or concerned other has insisted on it. What is needed for people at this stage is clear evidence that there is a problem. The therapist's job here is not to lecture and convince, but to draw out whatever evidence is available to this person that a problem exists. A spouse's concern, for example, is reframed in this procedure to indicate that the person's drug use is causing relationship difficulties—without arguing about whether the perception of the spouse is veridical.

Contemplation. In this stage, the individual may be thought of as engaged in an inner dialog about whether or not the problem is real. "Well, I am spending a lot of money on cocaine, and I know it's not good for me...but, look at George, he does even more than I do, and he seems okay." Once again, the therapist working with someone in this stage seeks to make the problematic aspects of the individuals experience more salient, overcoming the normalizing effects of memory distortion and social context (drug users associate with drug users), taking care always to draw the concerns from the individual rather then telling them what they *should* be concerned about. For as every experienced therapist knows, lecturing elicits reactance rather than behavior change.

Determination is a stage that does not always emerge from factor analysis, but remains useful heuristically. In this stage, the person is ready to change. In order to move on into the next stage, the individual must perceive that there are options that make change possible. If the individual has heard about a support group, or about a useful book, or about a therapist who offers help, then she can move into the next stage. But if she has come this far, has recognized that there is a problem, and is ready to change, but sees no possible way to go about it, she is likely to return to the precontemplation stage.

The *action* stage is where the individual takes the actual steps involved in change. He might attend a group, seek out therapy, read a book, or make a plan of his own. Such a plan can involve elements such as setting a date to quit, disposing of the drug and paraphernalia, informing significant others about his plan, avoiding high risk situations, and so on. The action stage, however, involves skills differing from those required for the subsequent stage of *maintenance*, however, and this is in fact one of the most significant implications of the model. Put colloquially, quitting is different from staying quit. For this reason, it is important for the therapist to know which stage the client is in, and offer strategies appropriate to that stage. Staying quit involves skills such as anticipating difficult situations that may be coming up (such as a wedding where alcohol will be available), explaining the change of behavior to friends, managing stress without using, and so on. All of this requires a heightened awareness and clarity.

Most people are unsuccessful in their first attempt to alter addictive behavior, and thus enter the stage of *relapse*. In this stage, the individual requires a way of moving through the earlier stages again as expeditiously as possible, without getting lost in feelings of guilt, shame, or hopelessness: facing the unawareness of precontemplation, the ambivalence of contemplation, the readiness of determination, formulation a plan of action, and developing skills to stay on track. Once the individual has established a stable, new way of being in the world without the drug (or, alternatively, a stable state of moderation), they may be thought of as having exited this process entirely. Such an individual may no longer see herself as an addicted person, and may not have to struggle very much to persist in the changed behavior. What urges may arise from time to time are usually not very strong and are readily dealt with.

It can be quite helpful to the person trying to change an addictive pattern to be aware of these stages, and to understand the predictable processes and potential difficulties. One of the difficulties about changing drug use, particularly where abstinence is the preferred goal, is that the addicted person might be successful all day long, and succumb in one weak moment. For this reason, the skills involved in mindfulness may be very helpful, teaching the person to see thoughts and feelings as passing phenomena rather than unalterable truth, changing the way the person relates to these inner processes rather than struggling to alter their nature. Patients in therapy often seem proud to report to me that they are not experiencing any relapse urges, but I remind them that whether or not urges are present is actually of little significance. Urges arise or fail to arise, and we are not in control of this process. Since we are not in control, we deserve neither credit nor blame for their occurrence or lack. What matters is how we handle the urge to relapse when it does arise. Though it may seem counterintuitive, mindfulness suggests that we are in fact better off being aware of the relapse thoughts and feelings when they arise instead of trying to deny their arising.

Urge Surfing

In the urge surfing approach, one approaches the arising of relapse urges with mindfulness (Marlatt & Gordon, 1985). Instead of struggling against them, which often increases the power of whatever we are trying to suppress, one seeks to ride these feelings out, like a surfer riding a wave. In this approach, the necessity of the linkage between inner states and outer behavior is challenged. Many of us, in point of fact, have often had feelings about wanting to do something that we knew to be harmful, or wanting to avoid doing something that we knew to be beneficial, while discovering that we can still make the positive choice. On a dreary Monday morning, we may feel that we would rather stay in bed than go to work, but most of us go to work anyway.

Once the absolute link between inner states and behavior is challenged, once we see clearly that we do not, in fact, need to act in accord with passing

moods and emotions, we are then free to experience whatever arises without fear that it inevitably means relapse. The onset of an urge, in its cognitive, affective, and physiological dimensions, can be experienced clearly
without acting on it, especially since we also come to see all such inner
states as impermanent and transitory. Experience with meditation is helpful here, since in meditation one learns that every itch does not need to be
scratched, that we can think repeatedly of getting up from our cushion to
perform some "urgent" duty, while still remaining seated, looking into this
impulse calmly and clearly without succumbing to it. In such a way, the individual experiencing a relapse urge learns to ask: "What thoughts are arising
in me about this?" It is not even necessary to challenge them as one might in
cognitive-behavior therapy: it is enough to see them clearly *as thoughts*, arising and passing away. In the same way one can ask, "What are the emotions
coming up for me attached to this urge?" and "What does this feel like in
my body?," in each case inviting calm, accepting awareness of these passing
inner events. In urge surfing there is a meta-message that relapse thoughts
and feelings are not at all terrifying, since I can experience them without
giving in to them. Attempting to suppress such feelings, however, gives the
opposite kind of message: if we are afraid to even acknowledge such inner
states, they must be truly terrible, and if they are so dangerous, this can create a state of chronic guardedness and anxiety rather than free-flowing, open
awareness.

Mindfulness of Life Problems

The relationship between addiction and problems in living is bi-directional:
a person may abuse drugs in a problematic way in part due to difficult life
circumstances, while the abuse itself also creates more problems. Once an
individual begins to change problematic drug use, life problems, often long
avoided, tend to surface. For the person to succeed in establishing a new
pattern of behavior, she must do more than quit. She must also establish a
satisfying and happy life and an adequate way of dealing with problems. If
such a way of life is created, then the temptation toward problematic drug
use will not be overpowering. If not, however, the pull may seem irresistible.
  Often life problems are linked with inner states. The recovering person
may want to repair a relationship injured by unskillful speech and behavior during years of drug use, but his anger feels overwhelming, and so he
says something that causes the relationship further injury. An unemployed
person may know she should begin the search for work, but anxiety about
interviewing may inhibit the active and energetic pursuit of this goal.
  In order to face such life problems effectively, the individual needs ways
to take care of the emotional state underlying maladaptive behavior or avoidance. Mindfulness is an ideal practice for this, since, as discussed above in the
context of urge surfing, one see through practice that there is no essential
connection between inner states and behavior, and since one experiences
clearly and repeatedly that all inner states, no matter how uncomfortable,
arise and eventually pass away, if not always as quickly as one might prefer.
In this way, one comes to see anxiety is a normal and natural event, something that all people will experience intermittently. One need not compound

the problem by becoming anxious about being anxious, but instead, one can learn to experience anxiety with clarity while still pursuing desirable life goals. Though anxiety may indeed arise in a job interview, this does not mean that one has to avoid such situations. Not only would that create many problems, financial and otherwise, but also, avoidance tends to increase the anxiety. No one, for example, experiences as much anxiety as people who have agoraphobia. If avoidance were effective, such individuals would have extinguished the anxiety by staying within their zone of safety. Unfortunately, even while doing so, they still experience a great deal of anxiety, probably more than the person who accepts anxiety as a natural occurrence and faces the world anyway. In this way, teaching patients to work mindfully with their thoughts and feelings can have great value in helping them lean into their life problems and face them effectively, instead of trying to avoid and evade, the very processes that helped to create a pattern of drug abuse.

Mindfulness and the Therapist

I have suggested elsewhere (Bien, 2006) that the most important psychotherapeutic implication of mindfulness may lie not so much in techniques to teach clients—though these may be valuable—but in the capacity of the therapist to be truly present. Indeed, Siegel, Williams, and Teasdale (2002) found, contrary to initial expectation, that teaching mindfulness to clients was not really possible without practicing it themselves. Lambert and Simon (2008), for example, report that 30% of the variance in therapeutic outcome is attributable to common factors such as the therapeutic relationship, while only 15% of the variance is attributable to specific therapeutic technique. This is so despite the fact that therapists generally consider their specific technique to be of greatest importance. Miller, Taylor, & West (1980), found that rankings of therapist empathy, one of the important factors in a therapeutic relationship, correlated highly ($r=0.82$) with therapeutic outcome. Mindfulness, the practice of moment-to-moment, non-judgmental awareness, would seem exactly the kind of attention needed to facilitate empathy and a positive therapeutic relationship. And indeed, while more research is needed in this area, some initial studies have supported the notion that mindfulness practice increases empathy (Aiken, 2006; Wang, 2006; Shapiro, Schwartz, & Bonner 1998), and improves the quality of the therapeutic alliance (Wexler, 2006). This may be particularly important with a stigmatizing disorder such as addiction, in which the quality of the interpersonal relationship with the therapist (whether for example the therapist is empathic, on the one hand, or lecturing on the other) is more determinative of client reactance than any supposed trait of denial on the part of the client (Miller & Rollnick, 1991).

A therapist who practices mindfulness may be more able to track the moment by moment changes in a client's emotional state, to be aware of what stage of change the client is in (which may make minor swings even within one clinical session), and to accept whatever the client presents as natural and understandable including the very human tendency to resist change.

References

Aiken, G. A. (2006). The Potential Effect of Mindfulness Meditation on the Cultivation of Empathy in Psychotherapy, PhD Thesis, Saybrook Graduate School and Research Center, San Francisco, California

Bien, Thomas, (2006). *Mindful Therapy: A Guide for Therapists and Helping Professionals*. Boston: Wisdom.

Hamilton, E., & Cairns, H. (1969), Eds. *Plato: The collected dialogues* (pp. 575–844.) Princeton: Bollinngen.

Hilton, James. (1933). *Lost horizon: A novel*. New York: William Morrow.

Goleman, D. (1988). *The meditative mind: The varieties of meditative experience* (p. 132). New York: Tarcher/Putnam.

Lambert, M., & Simon, W. (2008). The therapeutic relationship: central and essential in psychotherapy outcome. In S. Hick & T. Bien, (Eds.), *Mindfulness and the therapeutic relationship*. New York: Guilford Press.

Marlatt, G. A., & Gordon, J. R. (Eds). (1985). *Relapse prevention: Maintenance strategies in the treatment of addictive behaviors*. New York: Guilford Press.

Miller, W. R., & Saucedo, C. F. (1983). Assessment of neuropsychological impairment and brain damage in problem drinkers. In W. R. Miller (Ed.), *Alcoholism: Theory research and treatment*, 2nd edition, Needham Heights, MA: 1989.

Miller, W. R., Taylor, C. A., & West, J. C. (1980). Focused versus broad-spectrum behavior therapy for problem drinkers. *Journal of Consulting and Clinical Psychology, 48*, 590–601.

Miller, W. R., & Rollnick, S. (1991). *Motivational interviewing: Preparing people to change addictive behavior*. New York: Guilford Press.

More, Sir Thomas. (1516). *Utopia*. Indianapolis: Hackett Publishing Co.

Nhat Hanh, Thich. (2001). *Transformation at the base: Fifty verses on the nature of consciousness*. Berkeley: Parallax Press, p. 198.

Prochaska, J. O., & DiClemente, C. C. (1986). Toward a comprehensive model of change. In W.R. Miller & N. Heather (Eds.), *Treating addictive behaviors: Processes of change* (pp. 3–27). New York: Plenum Press.

Saint-Exupery, de, Antoine. (1943). *The little prince*. Translated by Katherine Woods. New York: Harcourt Brace Jovanovich. pp. 50–52.

Segal, Z. V., Williams, J. M. G., & Teasdale, J. D. (2002). *Mindfulness-based cognitive therapy for depression: A new approach to preventing relapse*. New York: Guilford Press.

Shapiro, S. L., Schwartz, G. E., & Bonner, G. (1998). Effects of mindfulness-based stress reduction on medical or premedical students. *Journal of Behavioral Medicine, 21*, 581–599.

Skinner, B.F. (1948). *Walden Two*. (2005). Indianapolis: Hackett Publishing Co., Inc.

Wang, S. J. (2006). *Mindfulness meditation: Its personal and professional impact on psychotherapists*, doctoral thesis, Capella University.

Wexler, J. (2006). *The relationship between therapist mindfulness and the therapeutic alliance*, doctoral thesis, Massachusetts School of Professional Psychology.

16

Mindfulness for Trauma and Posttraumatic Stress Disorder

Victoria M. Follette and Aditi Vijay

The only way out is through.

– Robert Frost

As a result of events such as the terrorist attacks of September 11th, the bombings in Madrid in 2004, and multiple armed conflicts throughout the world, the word *trauma* and the term *posttraumatic stress disorder* (PTSD) have become a part of the popular lexicon. The word trauma comes from the Greek word for *wound* and in psychological terms it has come to refer to distressing experiences that overwhelm an individual's ability to function. Psychological trauma is associated with exposure to external events, which is considered painful and can impact internal psychological processes (Wilson, Friedman & Lindy, 2001). However, it is important to note that trauma does not occur in a vacuum or in an isolated context; other environmental factors impact the exposure to trauma and the subsequent responses or reactions. The effects of trauma are not limited to PTSD. Rather they can be multidimensional and impact numerous domains of life. These complex responses to trauma can affect an individual's relationships, level of functioning, and ability to engage and participate in one's own life. The exposure to a potentially traumatic event is a statistically normative experience with some estimates suggesting that the average person will be exposed to at least one potentially traumatic event over the course of a lifetime (Bonanno, 2005; Breslau, 2002). Trauma is defined as an event where someone "experiences, witnesses or confronts an event or events that involved actual or threatened death or serious injury, or a threat to the physical integrity of self or others" (APA, 1994, pp. 427–428). It is important to note that while some individuals exhibit signs of psychological distress following exposure to a traumatic event, others recover their prior level of functioning without external intervention. While labeled as "disorders," PTSD and acute stress are considered by many to be normal response patterns to extremely stressful life events (Wilson et al., 2001).

In response to the need for treatment for survivors of trauma, cognitive behaviorists have developed exposure based treatments that are effective in treating reactions to trauma (Foa & Meadows, 1997). Exposure based therapy targets the cognitions and emotional reactions associated with memories of the traumatic event. Cognitive processing therapy (CPT) is a related evidence-based treatment that incorporates elements of cognitive and exposure therapy. Although CPT was originally developed to intervene with victims of sexual assault, recent research indicates that CPT is effective in veterans with chronic PTSD (Monson et al., 2006).

While exposure based treatments have documented utility, the literature also indicates that a proportion of trauma survivors have difficulty engaging in exposure based treatments and therefore do not always fully experience the benefits (Becker & Zayfert, 2001). We propose that mindfulness enhanced behavioral treatments will prove to be a useful treatment that provides an alternative for approach for clients who are either unwilling or unable to engage in traditional therapies. Moreover, in that our treatment addresses a variety of domains that are beyond trauma-related symptoms, it can provide an approach that is more suitable for clients presenting with a wide range of problems associated with trauma exposure (Follette, Palm & Rasmussen-Hall, 2004; Follette, Palm & Pearson, 2006). This chapter will briefly present the literature on trauma and mindfulness and the utility of the construct of mindfulness within an integrative behavioral approach to treatment. The integrative behavioral approach draws from the theoretical foundations and practices associated with what has been called third wave behavior therapy. This "third wave" builds upon the earlier traditions of behavior therapy and provides a contextual approach for dealing with complex psychological problems. Traditional behavior therapy focused on problematic behavior and emotion and attempted to changes these behaviors through conditioning and behavioral principles (Hayes, 2004). The second wave of behavior therapy moved toward targeting faulty cognitions and pathological schemas and became known as cognitive-behavior therapy. Ineffective behavior was modified through the application of a cognitive model that targeted dysfunctional beliefs and/or information processing. Third wave behavior therapy integrates components of the first and second waves while also emphasizing constructs of mindfulness, acceptance, values, and dialectics. Third wave behavior therapy is based on an empirical, principle-focused approach that emphasizes function over form, where the underlying cause of behavior is targeted rather than the topography. These approaches tend to utilize experiential and contextual change strategies in conjunction with more traditional behavioral approaches. The treatment approaches that have emerged in association with this movement (acceptance and commitment therapy [ACT], functional analytic psychotherapy [FAP], and dialectical behavior therapy [DBT]) seek to enhance a client's existing repertoire by enhancing psychological flexibility, leading to more effective behavior (Hayes, 2004). Our integrative behavioral approach to the treatment of trauma draws on the third wave behavior therapy practices and to enable therapists to tailor treatment idiographically, while remaining theoretically and philosophically consistent. In order to demonstrate the application of this approach, a clinical illustration will be utilized to demonstrate how mindfulness exercises can be implemented with a trauma survivor and enhance overall treatment.

Trauma

A traumatic event is considered to be anything that overwhelms a person's ability to cope and subsequently impedes their ability to function effectively. Cloitre, Cohen & Koenen (2006) assert that trauma is defined as "any circumstance in which an event overwhelms a person's capacity to protect his or her psychic well-being or integrity, where the power of the event is greater than the resources available for effective response and recovery" (p. 3). Inherent within this conceptualization is the notion that a distressing event on its own is not considered traumatic; a critical part of determining the impact of an event is the individual reaction. Thus, trauma exposure represents a complex relationship between the traumatic event, the individual and their response. The impact of such an event can be shattering for some people, while others are able to resume life with seemingly few interruptions. Trauma-related distress can be compounded by the individual's desire to spend a great deal of time processing the event while at the same time avoiding reminders of the experience. The movement between seeming opposite poles in reacting to the experience is referred to as the central dialectic of trauma (Herman, 1992; Follette & Pistorello, 2007).

Initial definitions and conceptualizations of trauma assumed that any individual who was exposed to an event outside the range of normal human events would develop some form of psychological distress. Research now indicates that exposure to potentially traumatic events is far more "normal" than was originally assumed and that the development of psychological distress is not the necessary response to the event (Breslau, 2002; Bonanno, 2005). While there is some controversy about the precise figures, there is evidence that the rates of PTSD vary in relation a variety of factors including the population and the type of trauma exposure. Traumatic stress has been studied most often within the context of exposure to combat, interpersonal violence, and natural disasters. However, new data is also emerging in the domain of exposure to terrorist events. Epidemiological studies indicate that in veterans from the Vietnam War, 30.9 percent of male veterans and 21.2 percent of female veterans developed PTSD (Breslau et al., 1998). The experience of rape is highly associated with PTSD, with 65 percent of males and 45.9 percent of women who experience a rape developing PTSD. The literature indicates that 13–30 percent of the general population is exposed to a natural disaster during the course of their lifetime (Briere & Elliott, 2000). Overall, men are more likely to report witnessing injury or death while women are more likely to experience some sort of interpersonal violence (Fairbank, Ebert & Caddell, 2001). Gender is a moderating variable in developing PTSD with women being two times more likely than men to develop the disorder (Breslau et al., 1998). Finally, changes in technology and the geopolitical context have significantly increased the risk of exposure to terrorist events.

The Psychological Sequelae of Trauma

There is a range of adverse outcomes that are associated with psychological trauma that is not limited to the development of PTSD. Acute stress disorder (ASD) is a psychological disorder that is characterized by cluster of anxiety and dissociative symptoms that include derealization, depersonalization, dissociative amnesia, and a subjective sense of numbing (APA, 1994). In ASD, these symptoms manifest within the month following the traumatic event. This diagnostic category was introduced into the DSM in order to distinguish between time-limited reactions to trauma and longer term post-traumatic stress disorder. Specifically, distress that persists for longer than one month is labeled as posttraumatic stress disorder. The psychological distress that ensues following a traumatic event can also include depression, anxiety, eating disorders, substance abuse or self-harm behaviors in addition to PTSD (Polusny & Follette, 1995). Moreover, the resulting distress of trauma exposure can be associated with later difficulties in engaging in and maintaining personal relationships. This distress may manifest immediately following the traumatic incident or much later in life (Cloitre et al., 2006).

PTSD is the psychological disorder most commonly associated with trauma exposure and it is different from all other psychological disorders in that the etiology is specified within the diagnostic criteria. Specifically, in order to be eligible for this diagnosis, clients need to have been exposed to a traumatic event. However, as noted earlier, exposure to a distressing event is not sufficient to determine the psychological outcome. Rather it is the response of the individual and associated symptomatology that determines the classification of the event. PTSD is characterized by a constellation of symptoms that are clustered into the following categories: reexperiencing, avoidance of stimuli and hyperarousal. Individuals reexperience the trauma in various ways including recurrent or intrusive recollections, distressing dreams or extreme distress at exposure to cues that remind them of the trauma. The second cluster of symptoms includes persistent avoidance of anything that is a reminder of the trauma. This includes a general sense of numbness that may manifest as avoiding thoughts, feelings or conversations associated with the trauma. Hyperarousal symptoms include insomnia, irritability or angry outbursts, difficulty concentrating, hypervigilance and an exaggerated startle response (Fairbank et al., 2001). The clusters of PTSD symptoms are reciprocal in nature with symptoms from one cluster influencing the behavioral manifestations of the other symptom clusters (Wilson, 2004). When an individual reports symptoms from one of these clusters, it is probable that functioning in other areas is impacted and that they are experiencing symptoms from more than one cluster. For example, if an individual is reexperiencing the event, it likely that they are also having difficult concentrating at work or that they are not able to sleep properly. This underscores the importance of a comprehensive assessment in order to determine the range of disturbance and to get an accurate glimpse of what is going on with the client.

Complex PTSD is a category that is conceptualized as including symptoms in addition to those specified in the diagnostic criteria for PTSD. As research into trauma and PTSD evolved, researchers and clinicians noticed that the original DSM diagnosis of PTSD did not fully capture the symptoms that survivors of prolonged and extended trauma were reporting. In response to these observations the diagnosis of Complex PTSD was developed to refer to the symptomatology that follows "trauma that occurs repeatedly and cumulatively, usually over a period of time and within specific relationships and contexts" (Courtois, 2004, p. 412). The topic of complex trauma is the source of controversy within the field of traumatic stress. One important aspect of this discussion is whether complex PTSD is sufficiently different from current conceptualizations of PTSD, thereby warranting its own diagnostic criteria. At the present time, complex PTSD has not been included as a separate category in the DSM, but many clinicians and researchers find it useful to utilize this construct in their work with trauma survivors. Complex trauma is typically observed in situations where the victim is trapped, such as in prolonged instances of child abuse. In addition to the PTSD symptoms, complex PTSD includes interpersonal ineffectiveness and emotion regulation problems that are associated with survivors of prolonged trauma exposure. Follette, Iverson, & Ford (in press) note that complex trauma can influence the development of personality characteristics or poor generalized coping skills in survivors of early onset or long-term abuse. One of the distinguishing features of a complex PTSD diagnosis is interpersonal and emotion regulation difficulties. These difficulties can make it extremely difficult for the client to engage in exposure treatments in a safe manner (Ford, 1999). Further, some researchers suggest that there may be the possibility of iatrogenic effects if exposure is implemented with this population prior to mastering emotion regulation skills that would allow them to more fully engage in the treatment (Ford & Kidd, 1998).

Trauma symptomatology can result from a range of stressors and both clinicians and researchers are increasingly aware of clients presenting with multiple trauma experiences. Additionally, the salience of contextual factors on trauma-related symptoms, as well as resiliency, is now clearly documented in the literature. The context can moderate the outcomes associated with traumatic experiences and it is therefore important for clinicians and researchers to be aware of some of the more common environmental factors that may impact treatment. For our purposes, we will discuss the environmental factors associated with trauma by examining three frequently observed categories: interpersonal violence, combat, and natural disasters.

Interpersonal violence. The term interpersonal violence refers to forms of violence that are perpetrated by one individual toward another with the specific intent of causing harm or injury. Interpersonal violence includes physical or sexual abuse, sexual trauma or victimization. Child abuse (physical/sexual abuse or neglect) is a problem throughout the world and the consequences of the maltreatment and abuse of children is extensive. A child is vulnerable to abuse simply because they are dependent on adults for their overall safety and well-being. Further, when a child exists in an abusive environment, frequently there are other factors present (e.g., lack of adequate financial resources, lack of appropriate supervision) that are associated with poor psychological outcomes. One distinctive feature of childhood trauma is that it can be detrimental to a child's developmental trajectory in that he/she is denied access to variety of age appropriate learning experiences (Cloitre et al., 2006). When a child does not have the opportunity to access developmentally appropriate learning experiences it can lead to difficulties later in life such as attachment difficulties. Specifically, when the child did not develop in an environment in which the caretaker was safe, reliable and emotionally validating, difficulty with trust, intimacy, and boundaries can occur. Attachment problems have also been related to difficulties with affect regulation, emotion regulation, accurate expression and general psychological distress (Cloitre et al., 2006)

Sexual victimization and sexual revictimization are forms of interpersonal violence that impact a significant proportion of the population. Revictimization is one of the more frequently observed outcomes associated with child victimization (Polusny & Follette, 1995). There are several factors thought to be associated with increased rates of revictimization. Child sexual abuse (CSA) and adolescent sexual abuse (ASA) seem to be the most robust risk factors for future victimization (Classen, Palesh & Aggarwal, 2005; Desai, Arias, Thompson & Basile, 2002; Marx, Heidt & Gold, 2005). The severity, frequency and age at the time of the first incident, relationship to the perpetrator and the duration of the abuse all serve to increase the risk of revictimization. The nature of sexual contact also impacts future risk; the more invasive the sexual contact was in childhood, the greater the risk of revictimization. The extant literature indicates that woman who are revictimized are significantly more likely than women who have experienced a single incident of sexual assault to exhibit PTSD symptoms or suffer from anxiety disorders (Classen et al., 2005; Arata, 2002). In addition to experiencing psychological distress, women who are the victims of sexual abuse at any time during their lifespan tend to experience more health problems (Buckley, Green & Schnurr, 2004). If PTSD develops following the first incident of victimization, it greatly increases the possibility of further distress and revictimization (Chu, 1992). Victimization and revictimization put individuals with a trauma history at risk for affect regulation problems, interpersonal and intrapersonal difficulties and general forms of psychological distress (Cloitre & Rosenberg, 2006).

Repeated and prolonged victimization experiences increases the probability of developing more serious psychopathology and detracts from functioning in other domains. Moreover, some data suggests that the effects of trauma are cumulative; with increases in exposure to trauma increasing the likelihood of developing trauma symptomatology (Follette, Polusny, Bechtle & Naugle, 1996; Kaysen, Resick & Wise, 2003). Interpersonal violence has a different impact on the victim than other traumatic events (e.g., combat or natural disaster) as a function of the relational factors associated with the assault. For many survivors of childhood interpersonal violence, they have been perpetrated against by someone they knew and/or trusted and these are cases where it is likely that difficulty with affect regulation, emotion regulation and sense of self are a part of the presenting symptoms. A complex PTSD conceptualization may be especially appropriate and useful in these cases. Another salient construct to this population is betrayal, which suggests that outcomes such as amnesia are an adaptive response to childhood abuse because the child remains dependent on the caretaker for their basic needs and the resulting amnesia allows them to forget the betrayal of the abuse (Freyd, 1994). It is not in a child's best interest to behave in a way that would negatively impact attachment to their caregiver. This type of amnesia is in the service of maintaining this relationship in order to allow them to survive. Factors associated with interpersonal trauma, such as problems with trust and memory, have implications for the therapeutic relationship. Survivors of these experiences may not have had the opportunity to engage in safe and appropriate relationships. Thus, problems may arise in developing a therapeutic alliance. On the other hand, the benefits of the therapeutic relationship may be especially essential to this population, presenting clients with a model for healthy interpersonal relationships in the future.

Combat. Sadly, war and armed conflicts are a central part of both the current and historical, political and social landscape. Involvement in a combat situation has been cited as one factor that is very likely to lead to trauma symptoms, psychological distress, and/or PTSD (Fairbank et al., 2001). Veterans of war are different from other survivors of trauma due to the number and type of traumatic events they may have been exposed to such as a function of living in combat zones (Keane, Zimering & Caddell, 1985). The constellation of symptoms that are now recognized as PTSD were originally studied because of the psychological distress returning soldiers were reporting (Wilson, 2004). The lifetime prevalence of PTSD in military personnel is estimated to be 30.9 percent for men and 26.9 percent for women (Breslau et al., 1998). However, these numbers remain in question, and may be serious underestimates, because of the stigma of seeking mental health services and the potential career ramifications for military personnel.

The duration of time in a combat zone and the environment (e.g., living on the front line) were associated with higher rates of trauma symptomatology (Kaysen et al., 2003). In addition to the duration of time, soldiers who are in combat frequently remain hypervigilant as a result of exposure to chronic and unpredictable danger. This constant stress can be related to cognitive and biological changes that are frequently associated with later psychological distress. Moreover, combat veterans report the difficulty in returning to civilian life related to transitioning from "battlemind" thinking and a sense of disconnection from the normalcy of daily life. Epidemiological studies indicate that a significant proportion of military personnel are experiencing psychological distress (Fairbank et al., 2001). At the present time in the United States, there continue to be large numbers of military personnel who are returning from multiple deployments in Iraq and/or Afghanistan, who have served extended terms of duty and may be at significant risk for developing PTSD (Hoge, Castro & Messer, 2004). Finally, in a somewhat related vein, it should also be noted that exposure to the risk of terrorist activity remains a rather chronic stressor for both civilians and military personnel. Bonanno (2005) provides data on the impact of the events of September 11th which indicates that the US population was impacted by these attacks.

Natural disasters. Disasters such as earthquakes, fires, floods, hurricanes, and tornadoes are large-scale events that adversely affect a significant number of people throughout the world (Briere & Elliott, 2000). As with other extreme stressors, the psychological symptoms that have been associated with natural disasters include PTSD, depression, anxiety, anger, dissociation, aggression and antisocial behavior, somatic complaints, and substance abuse problems (Briere & Elliott, 2000). In addition to the distress resulting from the disaster, including injury and loss of loved ones, there is often stress associated with the loss of resources such as property and shelter. This can interfere with employment, school, and accessing necessary resources to rebuild their lives. Hurricane Katrina, which affected the southeast region of the United States in 2005, provides an iconic example of a natural disaster that resulted in extensive property loss with far reaching consequences for both individuals and the community at large. The conservation of resources model, which asserts that people attempt to keep, protect and build resources when there is imminent threat, is demonstrated in some of the impacts of Hurricane Katrina (Hobfoll, 1989; Hobfoll, Johnson, Ennis & Jackson, 2000). In the example of Hurricane Katrina survivors reported that the trauma of the hurricane was compounded by the loss of loved ones, the loss of their homes and the chaotic environment that resulted when people in the area were unable to access resources to replace the ones they had recently lost. Moreover, many survivors of that event were displaced and lost a variety of sources of social support as well as the more general sense of support that belonging to a community can provide.

Functional Analytic Assessment of PTSD

As we have stated several times, the contextual elements of trauma-related exposure are critical for analysis when assessing for trauma-related outcomes. Multiple factors affect the course of the disorder by exacerbating, maintaining, or improving the symptoms and overall course of the disorder (Wilson, 2004; Follette & Naugle, 2006). Therefore, a range of factors beyond the trauma per se becomes significant in treatment planning. A functional analytic clinical assessment is a process that identifies potentially relevant controlling variables and allows for an individualized understanding of the client (Follette & Naugle, 2006). A functional analysis examines the relevant behavior, its antecedents and the consequences. When conducting such an analysis, the clinician is working to determine what the relevant controlling factors are for an individual client, as well as what might influence the probability of behavior change. The purpose of this analysis is to select and investigate the relationships between variables that are observable and changeable, in that we cannot change historical factors such as the exposure to the trauma itself. Focusing only on the traumatic event, ignoring other significant proximal and distal variables could lead to inappropriate case conceptualization with a resulting misapplication of treatment components. A functional analytic assessment allows the clinician to get an idiographic picture of the client so that treatment can be tailored in a manner that is most likely to lead to a positive outcome.

Learning Theory and the Development and Maintenance of PTSD

Mowrer's Two-Factor theory offers a widely accepted model to explain the way PTSD is developed and maintained. The Two-Factor theory asserts that psychopathology is a function of classical conditioning and instrumental learning (Mowrer, 1960). A behavioral formulation of two-factor theory provides a framework through which to conceptualize the development and maintenance of PTSD (Keane, Zimering & Caddell, 1985). The first factor proposes that fear is learned through classical conditioning. The traumatic event serves as an unconditioned stimulus that is conditioned and subsequently associated with intense feelings of fear. Through the process of classical conditioning, the feeling of fear is sustained through emotional learning despite naturally occurring consequences that would typically extinguish it. The second factor of the model details the avoidance behaviors that ensue to prevent coming into contact with the conditioned cues, therefore reducing the possibility of extinguishing the behavior. Through the process of instrumental learning, individuals avoid conditioned cues that evoke anxiety. The individual feels that their anxiety has been lessened by the avoidance of the aversive stimulus thus reinforcing their avoidant behaviors. In individuals with PTSD, symptoms from any of the clusters (avoidance, reexperiencing or hyperarousal) can serve to help the individual avoid cues that evoke anxiety or distress. The two-factor theory explains the development and maintenance of PTSD, and the behavioral principle of stimulus generalization explicates the phenomenon of the complex reactions to a variety of stimuli. It is a common observation that for some individuals PTSD is exacerbated over time. Stimulus generalization is the process that occurs when a novel stimulus evokes stronger reactions in an individual because it is similar to an already conditioned stimulus. This process of stimulus generalization can occur in trauma survivors whereby they react to a range of stimuli by attempting to avoid an increasing number of potentially anxiety evoking situations. Classical conditioning is critical in the development of PTSD while instrumental learning and the reinforcement of avoidance, reexperiencing and hyperarousal behaviors are critical in maintaining PTSD (Keane et al., 1985; Fairbank et al., 2001).

Third Wave Behavior Therapy

A contextual behavioral approach underlies third wave treatments, which contends that the only way to truly understand behavior is to examine it within the context in which it occurs. A notable feature of third wave approaches is the emphasis on the distinction between the function and form of behavior. The ability to identify and then target the underlying causes of behavior has powerful implications for treatment. Experiential avoidance is one construct that has been proposed as a framework for which conceptualizing the functionally similar behaviors that are associated with trauma (Hayes, Wilson, Gifford, Follette, & Strosahl, 1996).

Experiential Avoidance

Experiential avoidance is a process that occurs when an individual is reluctant or unwilling to experience unpleasant thoughts, feelings or emotions (Hayes et al., 1996). This avoidance is conceptualized as a functional diagnostic dimension that organizes behavior by function rather than topography and encompasses a large and varied class of behaviors associated with a range of psychopathologies. Trauma-related symptoms represent a class of cases in which the initial presentation of behaviors is varied, but the function that they serve is similar. Therefore in order to affect the most significant gains, the primary goal is to target the function of the behavior in the client's life. For example, a client may present with severe substance use issues and reports of frequent self-harm. While these behaviors appear to be different on the surface, it is frequently observed that the underlying cause and the function are similar. We see both these strategies as ones that are utilized to avoid unpleasant thoughts and feelings associated with prior trauma. Thus, it is the avoidance itself that becomes the target of treatment. Of course, it is important to note that experiential avoidance is not always harmful. Avoidance can be utilized strategically, thus enabling an individual to function in an adaptive manner when coping with competing environmental requirements. Experiential avoidance becomes clinically relevant when it interferes with the client's ability to live life fully and in a valued manner.

Avoidance is increasingly recognized as a central component in the maintenance of trauma symptoms by a range of trauma researchers (Briere & Runtz, 1991; Foa, Riggs, Massie & Yarczower, 1995; Plumb & Follette, 2006). The experiential avoidance paradigm represents one conceptualization that is useful when working with survivors of trauma, however others have developed clinical approaches that also include a focus on avoidance. While EA may not *always* be maladaptive, continuous attempts to avoid a range of thoughts and feelings can lead to disruptions across a range of domains that can include but is not limited to psychological distress (Follette et al., 2004). In a review of problems associated with a history of sexual abuse, Polusny & Follette (1995) posit that trauma survivors attempt to avoid their distress in a variety of ways, including substance abuse, self-harm, and intimacy avoidance. While these behaviors provide some short-term relief, in the long term they are related to other difficulties and increased general distress. Higher levels of experiential avoidance have been shown to be associated with increased trauma symptomatology as well as other forms of psychopathology (Plumb, Orsillo & Luterek, 2004).

The behavioral conceptualization of PTSD contends that avoidance of feared stimuli serves to maintain trauma symptoms or PTSD. The process of experiential avoidance provides a deeper look into the ways that a variety of behaviors (e.g., substance use, self-harm, reexperiencing, etc.) can function as avoidant behaviors because they do not allow the individual to remain in contact with the present moment, thus avoiding contact with important areas of their lives. These avoidant behaviors serve to maintain trauma symptomatology over an extended period of time. This chapter proposes an integrative behavioral approach to treatment that incorporates techniques, mindfulness, from third wave therapies to target experiential avoidance.

Psychological flexibility, which is increasingly considered to be related to EA, is a construct that is operationalized as "contacting the present moment as a conscious human being, and, based on what that situation affords, acting in accordance with one's chosen values" (Hayes, Strosahl, Bunting, Twohig & Wilson, 2004; Bond & Bunce, 2003). Psychological flexibility enables an individual to persist in changing his/her actions in accordance with important life values. Elements of contemporary behavior therapy seek to increase psychological flexibility by broadening the individual's repertoire through the incorporation of mindfulness and acceptance techniques which allow individual's to live a values consistent life. Our approach targets experiential avoidance, in a variety of ways, in order to increase psychological flexibility.

Treatment of Trauma

The majority of current treatments for trauma focus on reducing trauma symptoms, which is appropriate for a large number of clients (Becker & Zayfert, 2001; Follette, Palm & Rasmussen-Hall, 2004). There is compelling evidence to indicate that exposure therapy, based on Mowrer's two-factor theory, is effective in the treatment of trauma (Rothbaum, Meadows, Resick & Foy, 2000). Specific techniques for exposure (in vivo vs. imaginal) can vary depending on a variety of theoretical and practical considerations. Exposure therapy is thought to function in a number of ways, including activation of the fear structure, change in the relationship to the thoughts and feelings associated with the trauma memories, and establishing more accurate cognitions about the trauma. Exposure also helps to demonstrate that anxiety does not remain constant when either imagining or being in a feared situation and that simply experiencing anxiety, distress or PTSD symptoms does not automatically lead to loss of control (Foa & Meadows, 1997).

Although there is evidence in support of the efficacy of exposure, many clinicians are apparently reluctant to utilize it because of lack of training or concerns about the client's ability to tolerate the work. Moreover, some clients actually do refuse this treatment, either at intake or early in the therapy process. Clinical concerns include increases in suicidal thoughts, dissociation, self-harm, and premature termination in clients who begin exposure based therapies for trauma (Becker & Zayfert, 2001). There is evidence to suggest that many trauma survivors adopt an avoidant coping strategy to manage the distress evoked by the trauma and memories of the trauma (Rosenthal, Rasmussen-Hall, Palm, Batten & Follette, 2005). While exposure targets the distressing and unpleasant feelings associated with the traumatic event, a limited repertoire of coping skills, including an unwillingness to engage in the exposure work, may limit the utility of this approach for some individuals. Additionally, in cases of complex PTSD, individuals may not have developed normative regulation skills that are necessary to engage in this type of treatment. We believe that mindfulness enhanced exposure offers clinicians a way in which to target the avoidance that is a barrier to effective trauma therapy. Additionally, an alternative therapy approach can be useful in treating the myriad of trauma symptoms that are not directly related to the PTSD.

Mindfulness

As it has been already well explained in the first part of the book, the origins of mindfulness practice are in Eastern philosophies and principles (Follette, Palm & Pearson, 2006; Baer, 2003). Marlatt and Kristeller (1999) define mindfulness as "bringing one's complete attention to the present experience on a moment to moment basis" (p. 68). Kabat-Zinn defines mindfulness as "paying attention in a particular way: on purpose, in the present moment and nonjudgmentally" (Kabat-Zinn, 1994, p. 4). Despite the slight variability in definitions, the core components of mindfulness involve coming into contact with the present moment and observing that moment in a nonjudgmental way. While there are many ways to develop one's mindfulness practice, one widely recognized way to do this is through meditation. Several of the mindfulness-based interventions teach individuals a range of skills that help them to attend to internal experiences that are occurring in the moment. While the skills that are taught and the methods used to teach them vary, the majority of these interventions promote a nonjudgmental attitude to one's internal experiences. (Baer, 2003) Extant literature indicates that mindfulness-based interventions are effective in the treatment of a variety of psychological and physical disorders (Baer, 2003; Shapiro, Carlson, Astin & Freedman, 2006). Mindfulness has been shown to be effective with reducing pain and in treating depression (Kabat-Zinn, Lipworth, & Burney, 1985; Segal, Williams & Teasdale, 2002).

Data suggests that the capacity to self-regulate emotions is related to mindfulness and overall psychological well-being (Brown & Ryan, 2003). Many clients report deficits in the ability to notice, label, and regulate internal experiences associated with emotions. Mindfulness is one potential strategy to help individuals learn skills that will enhance their ability to self-regulate thereby allowing them to manage distress. The preliminary data establishing the utility of mindfulness with psychological difficulties has important and positive implications for treatment of trauma and PTSD.

Mindfulness and Trauma

Research on the incorporation of mindfulness into existing treatments for trauma is promising (Becker & Zayfert, 2001; Cloitre, Cohen & Koenen, 2006). Mindfulness encourages acceptance rather than avoidance and can provide a tool in facilitating exposure to feared stimuli. We do not consider mindfulness to function as a form of control but rather to increase psychological awareness and flexibility when responding to emotional experiences (Follette et al., 2006). In part, mindfulness is a way to provide a client with skills to help them manage the distress that occurs when engaging in exposure work.

For some individuals who have experienced trauma, there might have been behaviors or strategies such as dissociation that were utilized as a sort of survival mechanism. While these behaviors may have been adaptive in that context, they are no longer useful in the current context and may even be dangerous, by putting the client at risk for revictimization. In some cases these behaviors are characterized as obvious avoidance strategies while in other situations they manifest as hypervigilance symptoms, which we would conceptualize as another form of avoidance. Both of these classes of behaviors share an "unawareness" of the environment in common, whether it is misreading potentially threatening situations or an inability to accurately label their own feelings. The goal of mindfulness is to facilitate individuals ability to become aware of their experiences in the present moment in order to build the foundation to fully engage in not only therapy but also their lives (Follette & Pistorello, 2007).

Integrative Behavioral Approach

Our approach to treatment is guided by a contextual behavioral approach; with the fundamental assumption that it is most effective to understand the function of behavior rather then merely its topography. This approach is not aimed solely at targeting symptoms and reducing distress, but is also aimed at addressing the mechanism that mediates the distress. The additional goal of this work is in helping the client move forward and to identify values and goals associated with a meaningful life. A contextual behavioral approach examines relevant historical and environmental variables, as described in a functional analytic clinical assessment, in relation to the development and maintenance of psychological distress (Follette et al., 2004). The integrative behavioral approach utilizes an experiential avoidance paradigm to conceptualize distal and proximal factors that are also related to current stressors and long-term consequences of trauma (Hayes et al., 1996; Follette et al., 2004). This approach has ACT at its core, however it also incorporates techniques from DBT and FAP. We believe the similar theoretical foundations of these approaches, makes this integration coherent in fundamental principles (Follette et al., 2004). As noted above, this integrative behavioral approach utilizes different aspects of treatment from contemporary behavior therapies in order to be able to tailor the treatment to the particular needs of the client. The integrative behavioral model seeks to avoid theoretical eclecticism by combining the approaches of DBT (Linehan, 1993), ACT (Hayes, Strosahl & Wilson, 1999), and FAP (Kohlenberg & Tsai, 1991). However, we should also note that both ACT and DBT have described coherent treatment approaches that do not involve any integration (cf. Walser and Hayes, 2006 and Wagner and Linehan, 2006).

In the initial stages of therapy, the primary goal is to assist the client in building and enhancing a skill set that will be useful in engaging the difficult work to follow. Various acceptance strategies, mindfulness practice, distress tolerance, and interpersonal skills are at the core this early work (Hayes, Strosahl & Wilson, 1999; Linehan, 1993). The overarching goal of mindfulness practices in this context is to begin to get the client to let go of the agenda of controlling internal experiences. Skills such as emotion regulation and accurate expression of emotions serve to enrich the individual's behavioral repertoire to cope with negative emotions. Once it has been established that a client is willing to experience increased levels of distress, treatment will move toward mindfulness-enhanced exposure.

DBT was originally developed to treat individuals with BPD who exhibited suicidal and parasuicidal behaviors (Linehan, 1993). It is based on the concept that self-injurious behavior is associated with the emotion dysregulation that is related to avoiding or escaping difficult thoughts and feelings. As with ACT, this treatment embraces the dialectic of acceptance and change in order to live the life that is desired. DBT uses concepts such as self-validation to help clients accept themselves as they are while working toward changes they want in their lives. For many trauma survivors, self-acceptance can be a difficult step and mindfulness is one way to work toward it.

FAP is a key behavioral treatment that provides important strategies for dealing with the relationship factors associated with a history of trauma. FAP asserts that the therapeutic relationship can be utilized as an agent of change (Kohlenberg & Tsai, 1991) and provides necessary foundational work for clients with what has been described as complex PTSD. At its core, FAP targets clinically relevant behaviors that occur in session such as difficulty in developing a sense of trust and safety in relationship to another person. Therapists are able to respond contingently to behaviors in order to reinforce adaptive and appropriate behaviors. One reason we consider FAP to be so essential in trauma therapy is that it helps the client to build a repertoire for developing an alliance with the therapist that can lead to doing the difficult work of letting go of previous strategies of control and avoidance. The integrative behavioral approach integrates constructs of mindfulness and skill development to help the client learn to accept distressing thoughts and feelings as they build a more fulfilling life. As treatment progresses, the concept of acceptance is also incorporated to help the client begin to engage in new behaviors that may be anxiety provoking but are associated with the client's valued life directions. The integration of these treatment approached allows us to tailor treatment to the individual clients needs without sacrificing the theoretical integrity.

Clinical Vignette

In order to demonstrate the incorporation of mindfulness practices within an integrative behavioral paradigm, we will use a clinical vignette. Consider for a moment the following description of a trauma survivor:

> *Helen is a 32-year-old woman who presents for treatment to work on the guilt she experiences as a result of sexual abuse that occurred over a period of six years, beginning at the age of eleven. While she had a close relationship with her biological father, he passed away suddenly after being involved in a motor vehicle accident when she was seven. Her mother remarried three years later. Her stepfather began to abuse her approximately one year after his marriage to Helen's mother.*
>
> *When describing her reasons for seeking treatment at this time, Helen describes feeling as though she "did something" to precipitate the abuse and that she has difficulty concentrating at work or sleeping through the night. She reports that these difficulties have made it difficult to remain in a relationship, which is something that she wants. Helen indicated that over the past fifteen years she has used alcohol and self-harm to try to cope with difficulties in her life. Additionally, she reports that it is extremely difficult to remain in treatment because therapists ask her to do things that are very difficult for her, so she has terminated therapy twice before.*

At this initial stage of treatment, the goal is to help the client develop a skill set to deal with distressing thoughts and feelings without engaging in self injury. It is also clear that building a strong therapeutic relationship will be necessary in order for her to tolerate the work. In keeping with the integrative behavioral approach, we would suggest beginning with a combination of mindfulness and distress tolerance skills. In a sense, we use the distress tolerance skills as a bridge to safety for the client, with the longer term goal being "radical acceptance" in a way that moves beyond emotion management. As stated earlier, the mindfulness exercises will serve to allow the client to experience the present moment as it is not what it seems to be. That is, in this moment the trauma is over, has been survived, and the client is in a safe place. Thoughts and feelings are accepted, not as a reality, but as learned reactions to prior experiences. The client does not have to run, hide, self injure, or do any other behavior to get rid of her internal experiences. Rather, she can just sit with this moment and notice the range of her thoughts and feelings, noticing that they cannot kill or harm her-learning to just be in this present moment. In order to provide a context for this work, we are also discussing values with the client with respect to the life they would like to live. This work is helpful in investing the client in the therapeutic process and in providing a rationale for the importance of the work they are doing. This orientation to living a valued life is a critical step in that treatment for trauma is difficult work and it is important that the client have a sense of the direction of the work.

During the preliminary stages of mindfulness practice it is important to begin with more basic exercises as a foundation. A mindful breathing exercise can be a good place to start.

Let's start by closing your eyes and simply noticing your breath. It has been noted that sometimes trauma survivors are reluctant to close their eyes and that is fine, they can do these exercises with their eyes open, direct them to look at a neutral point somewhere in the room.) Notice the air as it comes into their body and through their lungs. Notice the inhalation and exhalation of your breath. Notice how you feel when you are taking in air and how you feel as you expel your breath. You are not changing how you breathe, you are simply noticing your breath and how your body feels. It is ok to notice when you are distracted or your attention is elsewhere. Simply notice this and return your attention to your breathing.

(Follette and Pistorello, 2007)

This is an example of a basic mindfulness exercise for clinicians to use with clients, especially in the early stages of treatment. Returning to the breath is at the core of most mindfulness practices and provides a fundamental skill that can always be used. As with all behaviors, mindfulness is a skill that can be developed and like any other skill it needs to be practiced.

The therapist can introduce different forms of mindfulness exercises, always with the goal of bringing clients attention to the present moment. It is often easiest to start with mindfulness exercises that target bodily or physical sensations. In addition to the breathing mindfulness, mindfulness exercises involving external stimuli such as colors in the room, the taste of food, and sounds in the environment can be useful. These exercises address the physical aspects of the environment and provide a tangible starting place for the client. As the client demonstrates mastery of these concepts, the therapist can introduce the concept of mindfulness in relation to noticing internal thoughts and feelings. As therapy progresses to exposure based work, it is important to integrate mindfulness and other self-regulation strategies as appropriate. We assert that the incorporation of these skills will facilitate the rapport between the client and therapist and allow the clients to learn how to care for themselves. These are important steps toward taking care of the client throughout the process while simultaneously working toward changing her life in a direction she wants.

We believe that for a client like Helen, these exercises will help to invest her in the process of therapy, which has been a barrier to treatment in the past. Additionally they will help her to better assess her current life situation and identify what she wants her life to be about. This part of the process will help her to determine the steps she needs to take to move in that direction. We contend that incorporating mindfulness practice and values exercises target the experiential avoidance that many trauma survivors experience and exhibit in their lives. These are powerful methods to help bring the client into contact with his/herself and the present moment therefore allowing full investment in the therapeutic process.

Final Thoughts

Experiencing a traumatic event is difficult for any individual and managing the psychological effects can be hard as well. One common reaction is to avoid any reminders or references to the trauma, but this way of living can be ultimately maladaptive. A contextual behavioral approach offers a way to conceptualize a case through an experiential avoidance paradigm that encompasses a range of behavior problems and deficits that are related to a trauma history. It emphasizes the examination of proximal and distal factors related to the presenting complaints such that the clinician will take into account all relevant factors. This approach incorporates principles of mindfulness and acceptance to help bring a client into contact with the moment and then to begin to move their life in a direction they value. These core principles work toward increasing psychological flexibility that ultimately will broaden their ability to respond effectively. In addition to working with clients from a technically valid context, it is also imperative that therapists approach this work with compassion for both the client and themselves. The work is difficult but the rewards are significant. Building on what has already been established in the cognitive-behavioral therapies; we believe that the use of mindfulness and acceptance strategies will enhance the repertoire of clinical tools for trauma therapists.

References

American Psychiatric Association. (1994). *Diagnostic and statistical manual of mental disorders* (4th Ed.). Washington DC: Author.

Arata, C. M. (2002). Child sexual abuse and sexual revictimization. *Clinical Psychology: Science and Practice, 9*, 135–164.

Baer, R. A. (2003). Mindfulness training as a clinical intervention: A conceptual and empirical review. *Clinical Psychology: Science and Practice, 10*(2), 125–143.

Becker, C. B. & Zayfert, C. (2001). Integrating DBT-based techniques and concepts to facilitate exposure treatment for PTSD. *Cognitive and Behavioral Practice, 8*, 107–122.

Bonanno, G. A. (2005). Resilience in the face of potential trauma. *Current Directions in Psychological Science, 14*, 135–138.

Bond, F. W., & Bunce, D. (2003) The Role of Acceptance and Job Control in Mental Health, Job Satisfaction, and Work Performance. *Journal of Applied Psychology, 88*(6), 1057–1067.

Breslau, N. (2002). Epidemiologic studies of trauma, posttraumatic stress disorder and other psychiatric disorders. *The Canadian Journal of Psychiatry, 47*(10), 923–929.

Breslau, N., Kessler, R. C., Chilcoat, H. D., Schultz, L. R., Davis, G. C. & Andreski, P. (1998). Trauma and posttraumatic stress disorder in the community. *Archives of General Psychiatry, 55*, 626–632.

Briere, J. & Elliott, D. (2000). Prevalence, characteristics and long-term sequelae of natural disaster exposure in the general population. *Journal of Interpersonal Violence, 13*(4), 661–679.

Briere, J. & Runtz, M. (1991). Childhood sexual abuse: Long term sequelae and implications for psychological assessment. *Journal of Interpersonal Violence, 8*, 312–330.

Brown, K. W. & Ryan, R. M. (2003). The benefits of being present: Mindfulness and its role in psychological wellbeing. *Journal of Personality and Social Psychology, 8*(4), 822–848.

Buckley, T. C., Green, B. L. & Schnurr, P. P. (2004). *Trauma, PTSD and physical health: Clinical Issues*. In J. P. Wilson & T. M. Keane (Eds) *Treating psychological trauma and PTSD*. New York: Guilford Press.

Chu, J. A. (1992). The revictimization of adult women with histories of childhood abuse. *Journal of Psychotherapy Practice and Research, 1*, 259-269.

Classen, C. C., Palesh, O. G. & Aggarwal, R. (2005) Sexual revictimization: A review of the empirical literature. *Trauma, Violence and Abuse, 6*(2), 103-129.

Cloitre, M., Cohen, L. R. & Koenen, K. C. (2006). *Treating survivors of Childhood Abuse: Psychotherapy for the interrupted life*. New York: Guilford.

Cloitre, M. & Rosenberg, A. (2006). Sexual revictimization: Risk factors and prevention. In V. M. Follette & J. I. Ruzek (Eds) *Cognitive-behavioral therapies for trauma*, (pp. 321-361). New York: The Guilford Press.

Courtois, C. (2004). Complex trauma, complex reactions: Assessment and treatment. *Psychotherapy: Theory, Research, Practice, Training, 41*(4), 412-425.

Desai, S., Arias, I., Thompson, M. P., & Basile, K. C. (2002). Childhood victimization and subsequent adult revictimization assessed in a nationally representative sample of women and men. *Violence and Victims, 17*, 639-653.

Fairbank, J. A., Ebert, L. & Caddell, J. M. (2001). Posttraumatic stress disorder. In H. E. Adams & P. B. Sutker (Eds) *Comprehensive handbook of psychopathology*, (p. 183-209). New York: Springer.

Foa, E. B. & Meadows, E. A. (1997). Psychosocial treatments for posttraumatic stress disorder: A critical review. *Annual Review of Psychiatry, 48*, 449-480.

Foa, E. B., Riggs, D. S., Massie, E. D. & Yarczower, M. (1995). The impact of fear activation and anger on the efficacy of exposure treatment for posttraumatic stress disorder. *Behavior Therapy, 26*, 487-499.

Follette, V. M., Iverson, K. M. & Ford, J. D. (in press). Contextual behavioral treatment for complex PTSD. In C. C. Courtois & J. D. Ford (Eds) *Complex traumatic stress disorders: An evidence-based clinician's guide*. New York: Guilford.

Follette, V. M., Palm, K. M. & Pearson, A. N. (2006). Mindfulness and trauma: Implications for treatment. *Journal of Rational-Emotive & Cognitive-Behavior Therapy, 24*(1), 45-61.

Follette, Palm & Rasmussen-Hall (2004). Acceptance, mindfulness and trauma. In S. C. Hayes, V. M. Follette & M. M. Linehan (Eds) *Mindfulness and Acceptance: Expanding the Cognitive-Behavioral Tradition*, (pp. 192-208). New York: Guilford Press.

Follette, V. M. & Pistorello, J. (2007). Finding life beyond trauma: Using acceptance and commitment therapy to heal from post-traumatic stress and trauma-related problems. Oakland, CA: New Harbinger Publications.

Follette, V. M., Polusny, M. A., Bechtle, A. E. & Naugle, A. E. (1996). Cumulative trauma: The impact of child sexual abuse, adult sexual assault and spouse abuse. *Journal of Traumatic Stress, 9*(1), 25-35.

Follette, W. C. & Naugle, A. E. (2006). Functional analytic clinical assessment in trauma treatment. In V. M. Follette & J. I. Ruzek (Eds). *Cognitive-behavioral therapies for trauma, 2nd Ed.*, (pp. 17-33). New York: The Guilford Press.

Ford, J. D. (1999). PTSD and disorders of extreme stress following war zone military trauma: Comorbid but distinct syndromes? *Journal of Consulting and Clinical Psychology, 67*, 3-12.

Ford, J. D. & Kidd, P. (1998). Early childhood trauma and disorders of extreme stress as predictors of treatment outcome with chronic PTSD. *Journal of Traumatic Stress, 11*, 743-761.

Freyd, J. J. (1994). Betrayal trauma: Traumatic amnesia as an adaptive response to childhood abuse. *Ethics & Behavior, 4*(4), 307-329.

Hayes, S. C. (2004). Acceptance and commitment therapy, relational frame theory, and the third wave of behavioral and cognitive therapies. *Behavior Therapy, 35*, 639-665.

Hayes, S. C., Strosahl, K. D. & Wilson, K. G. (1999). *Acceptance and Commitment Therapy: An Experiential Approach to Behavior Change*. New York: Guilford Press.

Hayes, S. C., Strosahl, K. D., Bunting, K., Twohig, M. & Wilson, K. G. (2004). What is Acceptance and Commitment Therapy? In S. C. Hayes & K. D. Strosahl (Eds.), *A practical guide to Acceptance and Commitment Therapy* (pp. 3-29). New York: Springer-Verlag.

Hayes, S. C., Wilson, K. G., Gifford, E. V., Follette, V. M., Strosahl, K. D. (1996). Experiential avoidance and behavioral disorders: A functional dimensional approach to diagnosis and treatment. *Journal of Consulting and Clinical Psychology, 64(6)*, 1152-1168.

Herman, J. L. (1992). Complex PTSD: A syndrome in survivors of prolonged and repeated trauma. *Journal of Traumatic Stress, 5*(3), 377-391.

Hobfoll, S. E. (1989). Conservation of resources: A new attempt at conceptualizing stress. *American Psychologist, 44*, 513-524.

Hobfoll, S. E., Johnson, R. E., Ennis, N. & Jackson, A. P. (2000). Resource loss, resource gain and emotional outcomes among inner city women. *Journal of Personality and Social Psychology, 84*(3), 632-643.

Hoge, C. W., Castro, C. A., Messer, S. C. (2004). Combat duty in Iraq and Afghanistan, mental health problems and barriers to care. *New England Journal of Medicine, 350*, 13-22.

Kabat-Zinn, J. (1994). *Wherever you go, there you are: Mindfulness meditation in everyday life*. New York: Hyperion.

Kabat-Zinn, J., Lipworth, L. & Burney, R. (1985). The clinical use of mindfulness meditation for the self regulation of chronic pain. *Journal of Behavioral Medicine, 8*, 163-190.

Kaysen, D., Resick, P. A. & Wise, D. (2003). Living in danger: The impact of chronic traumatization and the traumatic context on posttraumatic stress disorder. *Trauma, Violence and Abuse, 4*(3), 247-264.

Keane, T. M., Zimering, R. T. & Caddell, J. M. (1985). A behavioral formulation of posttraumatic stress disorder in Vietnam veterans. *The Behavior Therapist, (8)*, 9-12.

Kohlenberg, R. J. & Tsai, M. (1991). *Functional Analytic Psychotherapy*. New York: Plenum Press.

Linehan, M. M. (1993). *Cognitive-Behavioral Treatment of Borderline Personality Disorder*. New York: Guilford Press.

Marlatt, G. A. & Kristeller, J. L. (1999). Mindfulness and meditation. In W. R. Miller (Ed) *Integrating Spirituality into Treatment: Resources for Practitioners*, (p. 67-84). Washington, D. C.: American Psychological Association.

Marx, B. P., Heidt, J. M. & Gold, S. D. (2005). Perceived uncontrollability and unpredictability, self-regulation and sexual revictimization. *Review of General Psychology 9*(1), 67-90.

Monson, C. M., Schnurr, P. P., Resick, P. A., Friedman, M. J., Young-Xu, Y. & Stevens, S. P. (2006). Cognitive processing therapy for veterans with military-related posttraumatic stress disorder. *Journal of Consulting and Clinical Psychology, 74*(5), 898-907.

Mowrer, O. H. (1960). *Learning theory and behavior*. New York: Wiley.

Plumb, J. C. & Follette, V. M. (2006). Acceptance and Commitment Therapy for Surviving Trauma. In A. Maercker & R. Rosner (Eds), *Psychotherapy for posttraumatic stress disorder: Illness models and therapy practice*, (pp. 128-140).Germany: Thieme.

Plumb, J. C., Orsillo, S. M. & Luterek, J. A. (2004). A preliminary test of the role of experiential avoidance in post-event functioning. *Journal of Behavior Therapy and Experimental Psychiatry, 35*, 245-257.

Polusny, M. & Follette, V. M. (1995). Long term correlates of child sexual abuse: Theory and review of the empirical literature. *Applied and Preventive Psychology, 4(3)*, 143–166.

Rosenthal, Z. M., Rasmussen-Hall, M., Palm, K., Batten, S. & Follette, V. M. (2005). Chronic avoidance helps explain the relationship between the severity of child sexual abuse and psychological distress in adulthood. *Journal of Child Sexual Abuse, 14*(4), 25–41.

Rothbaum, B. O., Meadows, E. A., Resick, P. & Foy, D. W. (2000). Cognitive-behavioral therapy. In E. B. Foa, T. M. Keane & M. J. Friedman (Eds). *Effective treatments for PTSD.* New York: The Guilford Press.

Segal, Z. V., Williams, J. M. G. & Teasdale, J. D. (2002). *Mindfulness-based cognitive behavior therapy for depression: A new approach to preventing relapse.* New York: Guilford Press.

Shapiro, S. L., Carlson, L. E., Astin, J. A. & Freedman, B. (2006). Mechanisms of mindfulness. *Journal of Clinical Psychology, 62*(3), 373–386.

Wagner, A. W. & Linehan, M. M. (2006). Applications of DBT to PTSD and related problems. In V. M. Follette & J. I. Ruzek (Eds) *Cognitive-Behavioral Therapies for Trauma,* (pp. 117–145). New York: The Guilford Press.

Walser, R. D. & Hayes, S. C. (2006). Acceptance and commitment therapy in the treatment of posttraumatic stress disorder: Theoretical and applied issues. In V. M. Follette & J. I. Ruzek (Eds) *Cognitive-Behavioral Therapies for Trauma,* (pp. 146–172). New York: The Guilford Press.

Wilson, J. P. (2004). PTSD and complex PTSD: Symptoms, syndromes, and diagnoses. In J. P. Wilson & T. M. Keane (Eds) *Assessing Psychological Trauma and PTSD.* New York: The Guilford Press.

Wilson, J. P., Friedman, M. J. & Lindy, J. D. (2001). *Treating psychological trauma and PTSD.* New York: Guilford Press.

17

Mindful Awareness and ADHD

L. Zylowska, S.L. Smalley, and J.M. Schwartz

The faculty of voluntarily bringing back a wandering attention over and over again, is the very root of judgment, character, and will. No one is compos sui (master of himself) if he have it not. An education which should improve this faculty would be the education par excellence. But it is easier to define this ideal than to give practical instructions for bringing it about.

William James, 1890

Introduction

One of our most important faculties is attention. It is a doorway into our experience and a foundational quality of our awareness. Where and how we place our attention or where and how other things grab our attention determines our daily experiences, relationships with ourselves and others, and the quality of our lives. This connection between the ability to regulate attention and well-being is profoundly exemplified in mindfulness or mindful awareness, and a neuropsychiatric condition called attention-deficit hyperactivity disorder (ADHD). In both, the role of attention is thought to be crucial to the self-regulation of cognition, emotion, and behavior, and while ADHD may be considered a disorder characterized by difficulties in self-regulation, mindful awareness training maybe considered a tool of enhancing self-regulation. This chapter outlines the theoretical framework for how mindful awareness training can be applied to treat different facets of ADHD as informed by cognitive-affective neuroscience and our own experiences with a mindfulness-based program for ADHD, appropriate for adults and teens, called mindful awareness practices (MAPs) for ADHD.

Attention Deficit Hyperactivity Disorder

ADHD is a behaviorally defined condition characterized by a clustering of symptoms of inattention (e.g., "difficulty following tasks," "forgetful") and/or hyperactivity and impulsivity (e.g., "fidgety," "difficulty remaining seated") with onset by seven years of age and impairment in at least two settings (APA, 1994). Currently, three subtypes of ADHD are recognized: primarily inattentive (50–75%), primarily hyperactive/impulsive (20–30%), and a combined subtype (less than 15%) (Wilens, Biederman, & Spencer, 2002). Prevalence rates vary from 2 to 16% but with a majority of estimates falling between 5 and 10% of children and adolescents and 4% of adults (Kessler et al., 2006;

Skounti, Philalithis, & Galanakis, 2007). From early age, diagnosis of ADHD is associated with a wide variety of comorbid conditions including disruptive behavior disorders (oppositional defiant and conduct disorder), anxiety and/or mood disorders, and substance abuse/dependence (Cantwell, 1996; McGough et al., 2005). In addition to psychiatric comorbidity, individuals with ADHD often have comorbid disorders of learning and social–emotional development, including dyslexia, executive function deficits, and social problems (including elevated rates of autism spectrum disorders) (Biederman et al., 2004; Clark, Feehan, Tinline, & Vostanis, 1999; Loo et al., 2007).

Etiology of ADHD

The disorder is heterogeneous in presentation and etiology: genetic, neurobehavioral, psychosocial and environmental influences have all been identified as influential in the development and variability of ADHD. While environmental risk factors such as low birth weight, maternal smoking during pregnancy, lead exposure, and socioeconomic status are important, a biological predisposition is perhaps most salient (Nigg, 2003; Zuddas, Ancilletta, Muglia, & Cianchetti, 2000). Family, twin, and adoption studies show that ADHD and its component behaviors of inattention, hyperactivity, and impulsivity are highly heritable, with estimates of heritability on the order of 76% (Faraone et al., 2005). Genes involved in brain neurotransmission (e.g., dopamine, serotonin, norepinephrine, and cannabinoids) (Faraone, Biederman, & Mick, 2006; Lu et al., 2008) are implicated. Several brain regions (e.g., prefrontal cortex, amygdala, cerebellum, basal ganglia) show functional and/or structural differences in ADHD individuals as compared to non-ADHD controls (Bush, Valera, & Seidman, 2005). Certain brain regions involved in ADHD are also implicated in self-control or self-regulation (Berger, Kofman, Livneh, & Henik, 2007; Nigg & Casey, 2005). Increasingly, ADHD is understood as a disorder with varied genetic, developmental and environmental underpinnings that results in difficulties in self-regulatory abilities.

It should be noted that although ADHD is a categorically defined condition (i.e., either the diagnosis is present or absent), the continuous nature of the behavioral dimensions of inattention and hyperactivity-impulsivity is well recognized (Smalley, 2008a; Swanson et al., 2001). It may be appropriate to think of ADHD as an extreme along a population continuum of variability along these behavioral dimensions, much in the same way that we now recognize dyslexia as an extreme along a continuum of reading ability, or diabetes as an extreme along a continuum of glucose tolerance. Neurobiological research over the last several decades has led to an improved understanding of the likely etiological factors that contribute to liability in ADHD. Three inter-related broad areas—attention/cognition, affect, and stress reactivity show differences in ADHD and likely play a role in its etiology. These areas are likely to underlie many of the observed self-regulatory difficulties in ADHD and are discussed as mechanisms by which mindful awareness training may be helpful in this condition (reviewed subsequently).

Current Treatment Modalities in ADHD

A variety of treatments have been investigated in ADHD including: psychotropic medications (stimulants and non-stimulants), psychosocial treatments (behavioral therapy, cognitive-behavioral therapy, family therapy, social skills training), individual psychotherapy, coaching, and complementary and alternative approaches (neurofeedback, dietary changes, supplements, and mind-body interventions) (Arnold, 2001). The standard treatment for ADHD, involves medications, behavioral therapy or both (Jensen et al., 2007). Stimulant medications are considered "best practice" in the treatment of ADHD across the lifespan (Dodson, 2005). While clearly helpful for many ADHD individuals, as many as 20–30% of children and adolescents and perhaps 50% of adults are considered non-responders because of insufficient reduction in symptoms or intolerable side effects (Shekim, Asarnow, Hess, Zaucha, & Wheeler, 1990; Wender, 1998). Importantly, many parents or adults with ADHD dislike the use of medication for various reasons, and desire alternative forms of treatment.

Novel Self-Regulatory Approaches

Novel non-pharmacological treatment strategies that target neurocognition and/or build self- awareness and self-regulatory capacities are of increasing interest in ADHD. Although still limited, recent studies of such treatments support the utility of such approaches. In children and adults, examples of such studies include a working memory training program (Klingberg et al., 2005), and attention training programs including ones using neurofeedback (Beauregard & Levesque, 2006). In adults, additional approaches that build greater "self-awareness" capacities include individual psychotherapy (Rostain & Ramsay, 2006), cognitive-behavioral therapy (Safren et al., 2005), metacognitive training (using metaphors to describe ADHD brain and behavior patterns) (Wasserstein & Lynn, 2001), Cognitive Remediation Program (remediation of skill deficits in planning and organization) (Stevenson, Whitmont, Bornholt, Livesey, & Stevenson, 2002) and coaching (ADDA, 2002).

Meditation has been proposed as a promising complementary/alternative treatment for ADHD (Arnold, 2001) and a few early studies investigated its effectiveness in this population. Two unpublished pilot studies ($n = 23$–24) looked at the use of meditation in children 12 years of age and younger (type of meditation unspecified). Both studies supported the utility of meditation for improving behavior in ADHD (Kratter, 1983; Moretti-Altuna, 1987). Another pilot study ($n = 8$) with ADHD adults investigated effects of a structured skills training program based on the principles of dialectical behavioral therapy (Hesslinger et al., 2002) which includes teaching in mindfulness skills (done without a formal meditation training). Improvements in ADHD and depression symptoms as well as attentional tests were found in the treatment group compared to a wait list control; however, interpretation of findings is limited due to small sample size and high drop out rate. Little is yet know regarding how meditation or mindfulness practices can be used in the ADHD population across the lifespan. Our group recently completed a feasibility study of a mindfulness-based training in a group of ADHD adults ($n = 25$) and adolescents ($n = 8$). An 8-week training called mindful awareness practices for ADHD (MAPs for ADHD; see description in section to follow) was tested in an open label study with pre- and post-assessments of ADHD symptoms, symptoms of mood and anxiety, perceived stress, mindfulness and measures of neurocognition (attention, inhibition, and working memory). Several of the self-report scales (ADHD, anxiety, depression, stress and mindfulness measures) were also collected at 3 months after the training. The study and its initial results are described in detail elsewhere (Zylowska et al., 2008). Overall, the study found good program adherence rate and high satisfaction among the participants. Pre-post training comparisons showed significant ($p < 0.01$) reductions in self-reported ADHD, anxiety, and depressive symptoms as well as measures of conflict attention and attentional set-shifting. In addition, (unpublished data) significant ($p < 0.01$) improvements were found in measures of perceived stress and mindfulness. At a 3-month follow-up, additional improvements were reported in ADHD symptoms with no changes (e.g., no additional improvement or loss of improvement) in anxiety, depression, mindfulness, or stress. The study demonstrated that mindfulness-based training is a feasible intervention in a subset of ADHD adults and adolescents and may improve behavioral and neurocognitive impairments.

Mindful Awareness: Overview

The term *mindful awareness* or *mindfulness* has been used in different contexts and can denote different things: a quality of awareness or attention, a mental mode or process, a psychological trait, a specific meditative technique, a collection of techniques, or an outcome of the practice itself (Bishop et al., 2004; Brown & Ryan, 2003; Hayes & Shenk, 2004; Schwartz & Begley, 2002; Segal, Williams, & Teasdale, 2002). In discussing the application of mindfulness to ADHD, we focus on "mindful awareness" as meta-awareness, (Teasdale et al., 2000) a quality of consciousness that has a regulatory (observing and correcting) function on the rest of the one's experience and leads to improved cognitive-emotional and behavioral self-regulation (Brown & Ryan, 2003; Brown, Ryan, & Creswell, 2007). We believe that mindful awareness can be fostered in diverse ways (meditation or non-meditation tools) and in our program we use psychoeducation and formal (sitting and walking meditation) and informal (mindfulness in daily life) practices as ways to train mindful awareness.

There are many definitions of self-regulation, either as a unitary concept, or as its components of emotional regulation, cognitive regulation or behavioral regulation. Terms such as impulse control, inhibition, self-control, self-management, self-correction or independence have been used to describe aspects of self-regulation. It can be said that self-regulation is central to being a human being, a mark of one's ability to execute a choice, self-correct and over-ride pre-potent responses that can come from genetics/biology, intrauterine environmental influences, and/or or early learning. While self-regulation capacities are a result of a combination of temperament, cognitive processing styles, parenting, and environment, humans can learn to self-regulate through active (or effortful) engagement of higher cortical functions involved in cognitive and emotional regulation (Ochsner & Gross, 2005; Schwartz, Gullifor, Stier, & Thienemann, 2005a). In this context, mindful awareness could be seen as a specific quality of attention and intention (Bishop et al., 2004; Brown & Ryan, 2003; Shapiro, 1982) that leads to monitoring and modulation of cognition, emotion and behavior resulting in improved awareness and flexibility in responding. The processes involved in this regulatory function have been diversely described including de-centering, de-automatization (Teasdale, Segal, & Williams, 2003), exposure (Baer, 2003), attention regulation to the present moment and adoption of open and accepting attitude (Bishop et al., 2004; Hayes, Follette, & Linehan, 2004; Kabat-Zinn, 1990), and an impartial spectator stance (Schwartz & Beyette, 1997).

Below we outline how training in mindful awareness may impact aspects of self-regulation in ADHD namely attention/cognition, emotion, and stress management and potentially lead to functional/structural brain changes. While we recognize that 1) emotional regulation involves conflict or executive attention or cognitive control (Hariri, Bookheimer, & Mazziotta, 2000; Ochsner & Gross, 2005); 2) affective states or stress can influence attention (Davidson, Amso, Anderson, & Diamond, 2006); and 3) stress response is likely related to one's cognitive-emotional regulation capacities (Urry et al., 2006), we discuss these domains separately to emphasize affect and stress as the so far under-emphasized dimensions in ADHD and targets for mindfulness-based approaches.

Mindful Awareness as an Attention/Cognition Regulation Tool in ADHD

In ADHD, impairments in four cognitive processes are fairly consistently found to show deficits: language processing (e.g., verbal fluency, reading, spelling), working memory, inhibition (the ability to inhibit a response), and attention (Barkley, 1997; Nigg, Blaskey, Stawicki, & Sachek, 2004; Seidman, 2006; Verte, Geurts, Roeyers, Oosterlaan, & Sergeant, 2006). Several of these cognitive processes are known to work together in forming executive function, defined as the ability to plan ahead, set goals, and execute upon such goals. Executive function (a concept closely related to the idea of cognitive control) is frequently compromised in ADHD and it also a key component in development of self-regulation; a process that begins to emerge at around 3 years of age and continues development through adolescence into early adulthood (Davidson et al., 2006; Diamond, 2002). Reviews of imaging studies investigating brain differences in ADHD (Bush et al., 2005) show underactive prefrontal cortical functioning on executive function tasks along with differences in structures related to attention (e.g., anterior cingulate). Individuals with ADHD often show deficits on various measures of attentional processes including alerting, orienting and/or conflict attention. Alerting refers to how attention is readied and sustained; Orienting defines how attention is placed (disengaged and reengaged) and conflict attention is defined as the process of inhibiting an automatic response in order to attend to a less automatic response (Fan, McCandliss, Sommer, Raz, & Posner, 2002). While most research supports deficits in conflict attention in ADHD (Loo et al.,

2007; Seidman, Biederman, Faraone, Weber, & Ouellette, 1997) neural processing differences in alerting and orienting are also found (Konrad, Neufang, Hanisch, Fink, & Herpertz-Dahlmann, 2006).

Given the multiple attention/cognitive impairments in ADHD, mindful awareness training can be seen as either a remediation (compensatory) or rehabilitation (reversal) approach in this condition. The diverse processes involved in formal and informal mindfulness practice are likely to repeatedly engage executive function (attention, working memory and inhibition) potentially leading to strengthening of these abilities and broad changes in self-regulatory abilities. As attention is at the core of mindfulness practice (i.e., "paying attention to attention") all attentional systems (alerting, orienting, and conflict) (Fan et al., 2002) are likely to be involved. In formal practice (sitting or walking meditation) attention is continually engaged in the following steps: (1) bringing attention to an "attentional anchor" (usually a sensory input such as breath); (2) noting that distraction occurs and letting go (or non-grasping) of the distraction; (3) re-focusing or re-orienting attention back to the "attentional anchor." Attentional monitoring and attentional conflict as well as orienting attention may be particularly critical in carrying out this process. Other mindfulness meditation exercises train flexibility of attentional focus by varying focus from narrow to broad and engendering the so-called open awareness or "receptive attention" (Jha, Krompinger, & Baime, 2007). Mindful awareness in daily life (or informal practice) in which the individual checks his/her awareness/attention throughout the day may continue to engage the same attentional networks as in formal practice but perhaps offer modalities to generalize from the educational or clinical setting where the practices may be introduced.

Emerging empirical research is demonstrating that attention and their networks can be modified by meditation training in different non-clinical or clinical populations. A study by Jha (2007) showed that intensive (1-month retreat) training with long-term meditators improved alerting attention but less-intensive (8-week non-retreat setting) training with novices impacted orienting attention. At the same time, long-term meditators appeared to have better conflict attention abilities than novices at the beginning of the study. A review of different meditation studies implicate activation of the anterior cingulate (ACC) and the prefrontal cortex (Cahn & Polich, 2006) structures that are involved in the development of conflict attention and self-control/self-regulatory capacities and the modulation of cognition and emotion in adults (Creswell, Way, Eisenberger, & Lieberman, 2007; Lieberman et al., 2007). Pagnoni and Cekic (2007) demonstrated that long-term meditators when compared to healthy controls did not show typical age-related declines in attentional performance and had less age-related gray matter volume reduction in several brain regions, particularly the putamen. Additionally, improvements in response on an attentional blink test, or more effective allocation of attentional resources, were noted after in experienced meditators after an intensive 3-month training (Slagter et al., 2007).

Overall, what specific attentional processes are most affected by mindful awareness training may depend on the type and duration of mindfulness practice or pre-existing cognitive strengths or vulnerabilities. Future research with ADHD individuals—an extreme along the attention/cognitive spectrum—will further shed light on these questions.

Mindful Awareness as an Emotional Regulation Tool in ADHD

A relatively new line of emerging ADHD research is an interest in affect regulation and aspects of temperament and character traits with ADHD (Lynn et al., 2005; Panzer & Viljoen, 2005; Plessen et al., 2006). High rates of comorbidity of mood, anxiety, substance abuse and behavioral disorders in ADHD have been noted for a long time (Cantwell, 1996; McGough et al., 2005) indicating potential vulnerability to affect dysregulation in ADHD. Deficits in inhibition and impulse control have also been proposed to relate to difficulties in emotional regulation (Barkley, 1997; Nigg & Casey, 2005). An increasing number of studies are investigating affective processing in ADHD and differences in affect recognition and labeling (Braaten & Rosen, 2000; Pelc, Kornreich, Foisy, & Dan, 2006; Rapport, Friedman, Tzelepis, & Van Voorhis, 2002; Yuill & Lyon, 2007). Recent neuroimaging studies suggest that brain regions associated with affect regulation (amygdala, ventralmedial prefrontal cortex) may differ in structure and function in ADHD (Cardinal, Winstanley, Robbins, & Everitt, 2004; Plessen et al., 2006). In addition, Novelty-seeking (NS)—a temperament trait that impacts affect regulation and potentially stress reactivity is elevated in ADHD (Lynn et al., 2005; Stadler, 2007; Tyrka, 2006).

The emotional regulation differences in ADHD support the hypothesis that affect regulation is a key continuum underlying ADHD liability and provides further rationale for using mindfulness as a complementary treatment in ADHD. Mindfulness training teaches engagement in emotional states in a way that is neither avoidant, flooding, nor dissociative, but rather "mindfully observing and staying present with the emotion." This framing brings curiosity, openness and acceptance/willingness toward emotional experiences as well as a degree of distancing or dis-identifying from the emotion that can be helpful in cases of emotional over-engagement (depression or anger problems) as well emotional avoidance (e.g., anxiety disorders) (Teasdale et al., 2003). Attention on breathing, used in both formal and informal exercises, can induce relaxation and lower physiological arousal, a core aspect of emotional experience. Shifting attention to a neutral focus (e.g., breath, soles of the feet, or an external object) can be used to disengage from particularly intense emotional states. Mindfulness training has been shown to prevent relapse in chronic depression (Teasdale et al., 2001), improve impulsive behavior in patients with borderline personality disorder (Bohus et al., 2004), reduce aggressiveness in adolescents with conduct disorder (Singh et al., 2007), and improve outcomes in substance abuse (Marlatt et al., 2004), and generalized anxiety disorder (Roemer & Orsillo, 2007). Induction of a mindful awareness state was shown to reduce negative affect in response to aversive pictures (Arch & Craske, 2006) and emotionally provocative events (Broderick, 2005). Higher levels of a dispositional mindfulness correlated with buffering of amygdala response to negative affect via the prefrontal cortex in an affect labeling task (Creswell et al., 2007). In the course of mindfulness training, the processes likely to be invoked—engagement of the conflict attention, a reappraisal of emotional states (i.e., detachment from and observation of emotions), and training in equanimity and appropriate self-compassion promote adaptive emotional regulation (Leary, Tate, Adams, Allen, & Hancock, 2007b; Mauss, Cook, Cheng, & Gross, 2007). Overall, the body of literature supports mindfulness training as a tool for enhancing emotional regulation with likely efficacy in ADHD.

Mindful Awareness as a Stress Regulation Tool in ADHD

In addition to having alterations in cognitive-emotional regulation, ADHD individuals may differ from non-ADHD individuals in their stress response or stress load. There is a large body of research suggesting that stress—such as parental conflict or prenatal/perinatal insults—can increase the risk of ADHD or impairment associated with ADHD (Pressman et al., 2006; Talge, Neale, & Glover, 2007). High rates of family conflict, relationship or marital discord, academic or job underachievement, and lower health-related quality of life are reported in ADHD (Adler, 2004; Escobar et al., 2005; Pressman et al., 2006). Several studies show abnormal HPA axis response in ADHD (Blomqvist et al., 2007; Kaneko, Hoshino, Hashimoto, Okano, & Kumashiro, 1993; King, Barkley, & Barrett, 1998; Sondeijker et al., 2007). Furthermore, an elevated rate of post-traumatic stress disorder is also found in ADHD (Kessler et al., 2005; Smalley et al., 2007) and supports the hypothesis that ADHD may be associated with alterations in stress response or stress (allostatic) load. Mindfulness training and other mind-body approaches may impact ADHD via induction of the relaxation response (Benson, 1997; Kabat-Zinn, 1990).

Mindful Awareness and Neuroplasticity—Implications for ADHD

A growing number of studies suggests that brain activity can be modulated by repeated behavior or experience (Draganski et al., 2004; Schwartz, Stapp, & Beauregard, 2005b) including mental training such as meditation (Lazar et al., 2005; Pagnoni & Cekic, 2007). This neuroplasticity effect—lasting functional and/or structural changes in the corresponding neural circuitry after a repeated behavior—has been demonstrated in animal (Nudo et al., 1996) and human (Draganski et al., 2006; Maguire et al., 2000; Mechelli et al., 2004) research, including a study of cognitive training in ADHD (Olesen, Westerberg, & Klingberg, 2004). With initially more effortful practice, prefrontal cortical regions are likely to be repeatedly engaged and thus their function may be improved. In addition, as repeated practice continues, automatization of a mindful stance and a corresponding shift from prefrontal cortex to basal ganglia may occur (Graybiel, 1998). This automatization of mindful awareness may help bring present-moment awareness "on line" more easily (Schwartz et al., 2005a). In ADHD (as well as non-ADHD individuals), this could lead to a more automatic disruptions of periods of "daydreaming" or "spacing out" or "being caught in thinking" and improved ability to "step back" during periods of intense emotional response.

Mindful Awareness Practices for ADHD (MAPs for ADHD)

The MAPs for ADHD program was developed in the course of a feasibility study over a 2 year period by Drs. Zylowska and Smalley. The program was informed by Mindfulness-Based Stress Reduction (MBSR) (Kabat-Zinn, 1990), Mindfulness-Based Cognitive Therapy (MBCT) (Segal et al., 2002) and the tradition of vipassana meditation. Other mindfulness and acceptance-based approaches as well as ADHD psychosocial approaches provided more distal influence. The consultants on the study included several experts in mindfulness including Ms. Diana Winston (a Buddhist teacher), Dr. Jeffrey Schwartz (co-author) and Dr. Alan Wallace (a Buddhist scholar). The mindful awareness training was adapted to meet the unique challenges of ADHD symptoms and includes psychoeducation about ADHD (Smalley, In Press a).

Overview of the Program Structure

The MAP program is an 8-week training in Mindful Awareness delivered in a group format. The program consists of once per week sessions lasting 2.5 h and daily at-home practice. The at-home practice consists of gradually increasing sitting meditation (i.e., formal practice) and daily life exercises (i.e., informal practice). Walking meditation can be substituted for sitting meditation. The participants receive a CD containing guided meditations ranging in length from approximately 5 min (weeks 1–2), to 10 min (weeks 3–5) and 15 min (weeks 6–8). At each session, the participants receive a weekly practice form that lists their weekly practice "assignment" and they are asked to use the form as a visual reminder by placing it in a frequently visited area (i.e., the refrigerator). The MAPs program for ADHD differs from other mindfulness-based programs in that it includes (1) a psychoeducation component on the clinical symptoms, neurobiology and etiology of ADHD; (2) sitting or walking meditation periods that are shorter than in other similar programs (e.g., in MBSR program 45 min of at-home practice is recommended); (3) didactic visual aids explaining mindful awareness concepts; (4) strategies from ADHD cognitive-behavioral therapy or coaching to help with mindful awareness practice; and (5) a loving-kindness meditation (an exercise of wishing-well to self and others) at the end of each session to address the low-self esteem problems often associated with ADHD. While body awareness is practiced throughout the training in diverse ways (walking, short movement and stretching exercises, body-breath-sound meditation, and mindfulness of emotions), longer (45 min) body scan and yoga poses typically used in MBSR and MBCT are not included. These latter modifications, as well as omission of a half-day retreat typically included in MBSR or MBCT were motivated by our desire to balance the intensity of the training and the ease of delivery within diverse clinical or research settings. Overall, the program was designed to provide a beginner-level instruction in mindful awareness, make the training ADHD-friendly and foster a life-long engagement with the approach.

Overview of the Program Content

The program begins with a session devoted to introduction of the participants, overview of ADHD and mindful awareness, and basic sitting meditation instructions. The introduction involves a "Getting to know you" exercise in which everyone (including the trainers) are asked to share a playful aspect of themselves with the group (e.g., "Tell us about your hobby"). The participants are also asked to reflect on their intention for being in the class. The initial introductions set the tone of the class as both a playful and a reflective process. The ADHD psychoeducation is provided in the first two sessions and re-frames the impairment or "deficit" aspects of ADHD by highlighting ADHD as a "neurobiological difference." Thus, ADHD represents one extreme on a spectrum of functioning which can come with both non-adaptive and potentially adaptive aspects (Jensen et al., 1997; Smalley, 2008). This framework de-stigmatizes ADHD and fosters openness and curiosity in observing one's own ADHD characteristics. Visual aids explaining some of the concepts are used to reinforce learning and to accommodate diverse information processing styles that may be more common in ADHD. The rationale for using mindful awareness in ADHD is presented by discussing common self-regulation difficulties found in this condition. The emerging neuroscience of mindful awareness is reviewed to highlight the potential of mental training to change brain function and structure with long-term practice. We believe that a review of the scientific rationale reinforces the motivation to engage in this kind of training. The raisin exercise (Kabat-Zinn, 1990) and a basic 5-min sitting meditation on mindfulness of the breath are used to experientially introduce mindful awareness practice. Formal meditation is de-mystified and basic sitting meditation instructions are provided using either a meditation cushion or a chair. The 5-min sitting meditation (done with a CD) plus the "Telephone breath" (taking a mindful breath every time the phone rings) are the at-home practice for week 1.

Session II: Difficulties in practicing meditation such as distractibility, restlessness, and boredom are discussed and emphasized as common for everyone but also with recognition that they may be particularly difficult for those with ADHD. The approach of returning to the framing of ADHD as an extreme along a normal continuum of functioning discourages the feelings of separateness often voiced by ADHD individuals and appears to foster increased self-compassion by recognition of difficulties we all face as part of the "human condition" (Leary, Tate, Adams, Allen, & Hancock, 2007a). While difficulties are explained and validated, participants are encouraged to work with the difficulties as much as they can and take responsibility for their actions. This is similar to the attitude used in ADHD coaching where gentle yet firm support is used to help with quick discouragement, lack of persistence or inconsistent effort often reported in ADHD. In dealing with difficulties with distraction, it is emphasized that "it is not about staying with your breath but returning to your breath" to encourage persistence even in the context of frequent distractions. Mindful observation includes maladaptive habits frequently associated with ADHD such as being oppositional, irritable, overly reactive, procrastinating or avoidant of attention requiring tasks.

Session III. Mindful awareness of sound is introduced using a short musical piece during which the participants are asked to observe their experience of listening including shifts of attention to different instruments, evoked feel-ings, imagery or thought associations. This is followed by a meditation dur-ing which the participants are asked to pay attention to the predominant present-moment experiences of body sensation (e.g., pain, feeling or rest-lessness), breath or a sound. While attentional movement from one stimulus to the next is often familiar to the ADHD individual, being aware of the "grab-bing" and changing of attention from an "impartial observer" stance is often a new experience. The participants are asked to practice mindful awareness throughout the week by using using cueing questions of "where is my atten-tion right now?" or "what am I doing right now?" and bringing yourself back to the intended task. Visual reminders such as sticker dots or a frame with a word "breathe" are recommended as environmental reminders to connect with the present-moment awareness (Safren, 2006)

Session IV: Counting the breath meditation is introduced as an alternative way to train concentration. Body awareness is fostered through gentle body movement, mindfulness of pleasant/unpleasant and neutral sensations and ways to work mindfully with pain. Mindful awareness of a daily activity are reinforced by an exercise such as putting on or taking off shoes mindfully, or practicing mindfulness when placing important items such as one's keys or wallet.

Session V: Mindful awareness of thoughts is introduced by using a picture of sky and clouds to contrast the concept of meta-awareness (represented as the blue sky) versus present-moment experiences (represented by clouds with different labels such as "thought," "feeling," "image," "sound," or "body sensation"). As many individuals with ADHD feel their minds are constantly "on the go," we also suggest that the numerous thoughts and feelings they experience (probably more than the "average" individual) may provide them with a greater capacity for practicing awareness. Overly negative or criti-cal thoughts are explored using an exercise in a dyad and reporting self-judgments to the partner. In clinical practice, ADHD individual often report low-self esteem and endorse overly critical self-judgments. The difference between being judgmental or judging (as in discerning) is discussed and non-judgmental awareness is explained as a step in the learning process that leads to discernment, choice and mindful action. As part of at-home practice, the participants are asked to count moments of being hypercritical or judgmental (to self or others) throughout one typical day.

Session VI: Mindful awareness of emotions is fostered via a short didactic on function and acceptance of emotions. Common difficulties in regu-lating emotional states in ADHD are discussed and a RAIN mnemonic (Winston, 2003) is introduced to help establish mindful awareness during emotional responses. The mnemonic stands for R (recognize), A (accept), I (investigate), and N (non-identify/not-personalize). A sitting mediation using imagery of a recently emotionally evoking event is used as an exercise in applying the mnemonic to evoked emotions. A longer loving-kindness medi-tation, starting with an imagery of a loved person is used to practice cultiva-tion of positive emotional states. The participants are asked to pay attention to positive and negative emotions throughout their week.

Session VII: Open awareness of all present-moment experiences is prac-ticed. Parallels are drawn to different attentional aspects (e.g., alerting, ori-enting, conflict attention) and participants are asked to notice the quality of their attention frequently throughout the day (fostering "meta-attention"). As difficulties in social interactions and social awareness are frequently found in ADHD including not listening, interrupting, talking too much, blurting out answers, or being distracted in a conversation, this session also teaches mindful listening and mindful speech. In one exercise, one partner is the sole speaker while the other one is the sole listener bringing awareness to one's automatic responses or impulsive urges to interrupt. The participants are asked to practice mindful listening with a friend or a spouse.

Session VIII: The mindful awareness concepts and practices are reviewed and resources for a continuous mindful awareness practice are provided. Participants comment on what they learned in the process of the class during a "speaking council" exercise in which everyone has a chance to comment about their experience. Learning mindfulness is framed as life-long process of checking in with one's attention, renewing the intention to return to the present moment, and applying the acceptance-change dialectic in each day. Environmental modifications derived from ADHD coaching and CBT approaches are reviewed to help remember to be mindful or practice loving-kindness such as visual reminders, using a habitual activity as a reminder to be mindful (e.g., associating the act of turning on a computer with becoming mindful), e-mail reminders to be mindful, using electronic organizers as reminders, having a friend or a spouse as a mindfulness-coach, and attending an on-going meditation group or periodic workshops/retreats. We encourage practice by highlighting "how long it takes to develop a new skill" in general (e.g., it takes 50 h to learn harmonica or 1,200 h to learn play a violin) (Strayhorn, 2002).

Case Studies of Participants in the MAPs for ADHD Program

Mrs. X is a writer in her forties. Diagnosed with ADHD as a young child, she was briefly treated with the stimulant medication Ritalin but her parents, weary of using medications, discontinued the stimulant after several months. Since then, she coped without treatment and was able to finish college (although she took a two extra years to do so). She worked from home and was able to pursue a writing career, but frequently doubted her abilities as a writer and suffered from intermittent depression and anxiety. She complained of difficulties with concentration, had problems organizing her day, was forgetful, and frequently did not follow-through on projects. She reported having many exciting ideas but not being able to organize her thoughts enough to produce a screenplay. She frequently felt overwhelmed by attention requiring tasks. When unable to accomplish what she set out to do in a day, she often berated herself for being lazy or inept. She was re-motivated for treatment after her 10-year-old son was diagnosed with ADHD. She was diagnosed with generalized anxiety disorder, major depression and likely ADHD-inattentive subtype. The initial treatment with an anti-depressant helped with depression and anxiety but she continued to complain of disorganization and inattentiveness. Several ADHD medications were tried but they either exacerbated Mrs. X's anxiety or were ineffective. Consequently, Mrs. X decided to pursue non-medication approaches to help with her ADHD symptoms and she enrolled in the MAPs for ADHD program. During the training she was relieved to learn that he could start with 5 min of sitting practice and bring mindful awareness to any experience including distractions or impatience. She found loving-kindness exercises particularly helpful and when reactive self-criticisms arose during her ADHD-related difficulties she was able to distance herself from the criticisms. She found that when she did not over-react, she could problem-solve and organize her work more effectively. After the training, she also reported a better ability to concentrate and to accomplish tasks. She stated "the idea that you can see yourself getting distracted and then you can bring yourself back was probably the most pivotal thing, just like the experience of practicing it in the meditation—going off and then coming back. So, when I'm aware now that I'm distracting myself from a task, I'm able to see it better and get back to it sooner."

Mr. Y is a 16-year-old teenager diagnosed with ADHD-Combined Type (i.e., both inattentive and hyperactive symptoms) at age 10 y/o. He has been taking stimulants such as amphetamine or methylphenidate since the diagnosis, which he reported as helpful for paying attention in school and doing his homework. However, even when taking his medications, he still endorsed having periods inattention and restlessness, and frequently needed to get up out of his seat. He also described "freaking out" when he forgot to take his medication because he couldn't seem to focus at all and felt especially irritable and moody as a side effect of discontinuing the medication. During the MAP training sessions, he found himself needing to get up even during 5-min meditations but learned to use walking meditation as a way to continue the formal practice for the required duration. He attended most MAPs for ADHD sessions and reported that while his formal practice at home was irregular (5–10 min twice per week) he had been frequently applying mindful awareness throughout his day. He gave examples of being mindful of his body moving during a soccer practice and being more aware of his emotions and thoughts during an argument with his friend. He was noticing his hypercritical thoughts more readily and found that without berating himself, he was more motivated to "try again." He kept a post-it note at his computer reminding him to "breathe" and used a cell phone reminder at lunchtime to "eat more mindfully." Overall, he felt more empowered to be able "to do something for my ADHD." He found that it was easier to regulate his mood and his attention when he forgot his medication. She stated: "whenever I get distracted. . .I can put myself back in the thing. . .whenever I can feel my mind wandering, I am able to realize that it's wandering and let go of the feeling."

Future Directions

ADHD is a complex trait that arises in childhood but continues throughout the lifespan in a majority of individuals. It is highly heritable but the likely interactions of genes and environmental influences that shape its development are only now beginning to be understood. ADHD may be thought of as an extreme along continua of variability of affect and cognitive processes in the population that alone, or in combination, result in self-regulation impairment associated with ADHD. We believe mindful awareness training (such as our MAPs for ADHD) can strengthen self-regulatory capacities and potentially alter the neurobiological impairments of individuals affected with ADHD as well as those "at risk" for it (based on familial loading of ADHD or in the future, detectable risk genes). Overall, mindful awareness training can be a valuable approach in a comprehensive treatment of ADHD across the lifespan by balancing medication treatment of biological vulnerability with tools to enhance individual ability for self-regulation.

References

ADDA. (2002). The Attention Deficit Disorder Association Guiding Principles for Coaching Individuals with Attention Deficit Disorder. September 17, 2007, from http:www.add.org/articles/coachingguide.html

Adler, L. A. (2004). Clinical presentations of adult patients with ADHD. *Journal of Clinical Psychiatry, 65 Suppl 3*, 8–11.

APA. (1994). *Diagnostic and Statistical Manual of Mental Disorders* (Fourth ed.). Washington, D.C.: American Psychiatric Association.

Arch, J. J., & Craske, M. G. (2006). Mechanisms of mindfulness: Emotion regulation following a focused breathing induction. *Behaviour Research and Therapy, 44(12)*, 1849–1858.

Arnold, L. E. (2001). Alternative treatments for adults with attention-deficit hyperactivity disorder (ADHD). *Annals of the New York Academy of Sciences, 931*, 310–341.

Baer, R. A. (2003). Mindfulness training as a clinical intervention: a conceptual and empirical review. *Clinical Psychology Science and Practice, 10*, 125–143.

Barkley, R. A. (1997). Behavioral inhibition, sustained attention, and executive functions: constructing a unifying theory of ADHD. *Psychological Bulletin, 121*(1), 65–94.

Beauregard, M., & Levesque, J. (2006). Functional magnetic resonance imaging investigation of the effects of neurofeedback training on the neural bases of selective attention and response inhibition in children with attention-deficit/hyperactivity disorder. *Applied Psychophysiology and Biofeedback, 31*(1), 3–20.

Benson, H. (1997). The relaxation response: therapeutic effect. *Science, 278*(5344), 1694–1695.

Berger, A., Kofman, O., Livneh, U., & Henik, A. (2007). Multidisciplinary perspectives on attention and the development of self-regulation. *Progress in Neurobiology, 82*(5), 256–286.

Biederman, J., Monuteaux, M. C., Doyle, A. E., Seidman, L. J., Wilens, T. E., Ferrero, F., et al. (2004). Impact of executive function deficits and attention-deficit/hyperactivity disorder (ADHD) on academic outcomes in children. *Journal of Consulting and Clinical Psychology, 72*(5), 757–766.

Bishop, S. R., Lau, M., Shapiro, S., Carlson, L., Anderson, N. D., Carmody, J., et al. (2004). Mindfulness: A proposed operational definition. *Clinical Psychology Science and Practice, 11*(3), 230–241.

Blomqvist, M., Holmberg, K., Lindblad, F., Fernell, E., Ek, U., & Dahllof, G. (2007). Salivary cortisol levels and dental anxiety in children with attention deficit hyperactivity disorder. *European Journal of Oral Sciences, 115*(1), 1–6.

Bohus, M., Haaf, B., Simms, T., Limberger, M. F., Schmahl, C., Unckel, C., et al. (2004). Effectiveness of inpatient dialectical behavioral therapy for borderline personality disorder: a controlled trial. *Behaviour Research and Therapy, 42*(5), 487–499.

Braaten, E. B., & Rosen, L. A. (2000). Self-regulation of affect in attention deficit-hyperactivity disorder (ADHD) and non-ADHD boys: Differences in empathic responding. *Journal of Consulting and Clinical Psychology, 68*(2), 313–321.

Broderick, P. C. (2005). Mindfulness and coping with dysphoric mood: Contrasts with rumination and distraction. *Cognitive Therapy and Research, 29*, 501-510.

Brown, K. W., & Ryan, R. M. (2003). The benefits of being present: mindfulness and its role in psychological well-being. *Journal of Personality and Social Psychology, 84*(4), 822-848.

Brown, K. W., Ryan, R. M., & Creswell, J. D. (2007). Mindfulness: theoretical foundations and evidence for its salutary effects. *Psychological Inquiry, 18*, 211-237.

Bush, G., Valera, E. M., & Seidman, L. J. (2005). Functional neuroimaging of attention-deficit/hyperactivity disorder: A review and suggested future directions. *Biological Psychiatry, 57*(11), 1273-1284.

Cahn, B. R., & Polich, J. (2006). Meditation states and traits: EEG, ERP, and neuroimaging studies. *Psychological Bulletin, 132*(2), 180-211.

Cantwell, D. P. (1996). Attention deficit disorder: a review of the past 10 years. *Journal of the American Academy of Child and Adolescent Psychiatry, 35*(8), 978-987.

Cardinal, R. N., Winstanley, C. A., Robbins, T. W., & Everitt, B. J. (2004). Limbic corticostriatal systems and delayed reinforcement. *Annals of the New York Academy of Sciences, 1021*, 33-50.

Clark, T., Feehan, C., Tinline, C., & Vostanis, P. (1999). Autistic symptoms in children with attention deficit-hyperactivity disorder. *European Child and Adolescent Psychiatry, 8*(1), 50-55.

Creswell, J. D., Way, B. M., Eisenberger, N. I., & Lieberman, M. D. (2007). Neural correlates of dispositional mindfulness during affect labeling. *Psychosomatic Medicine, 69*(6), 560-565.

Davidson, M. C., Amso, D., Anderson, L. C., & Diamond, A. (2006). Development of cognitive control and executive functions from 4 to 13 years: evidence from manipulations of memory, inhibition, and task switching. *Neuropsychologia, 44*(11), 2037-2078.

Diamond, A. (2002). *Normal development of prefrontal cortex from birth to young adulthood: Cognitive functions, anatomy, and biochemistry.* London, UK: Oxford University Press.

Dodson, W. W. (2005). Pharmacotherapy of adult ADHD. *Journal of Clinical Psychology, 61*(5), 589-606.

Draganski, B., Gaser, C., Busch, V., Schuierer, G., Bogdahn, U., & May, A. (2004). Neuroplasticity: Changes in grey matter induced by training. *Nature, 427*(6972), 311-312.

Draganski, B., Gaser, C., Kempermann, G., Kuhn, H. G., Winkler, J., Buchel, C., et al. (2006). Temporal and spatial dynamics of brain structure changes during extensive learning. *Journal of Neuroscience, 26*(23), 6314-6317.

Escobar, R., Soutullo, C. A., Hervas, A., Gastaminza, X., Polavieja, P., & Gilaberte, I. (2005). Worse quality of life for children with newly diagnosed attention-deficit/hyperactivity disorder, compared with asthmatic and healthy children. *Pediatrics, 116*(3), e364-369.

Fan, J., McCandliss, B. D., Sommer, T., Raz, A., & Posner, M. I. (2002). Testing the efficiency and independence of attentional networks. *Journal of Cognitive Neuroscience, 14*(3), 340-347.

Faraone, S. V., Biederman, J., & Mick, E. (2006). The age-dependent decline of attention deficit hyperactivity disorder: a meta-analysis of follow-up studies. *Psychological Medicine, 36*(2), 159-165.

Faraone, S. V., Perlis, R. H., Doyle, A. E., Smoller, J. W., Goralnick, J. J., Holmgren, M. A., et al. (2005). Molecular genetics of attention-deficit/hyperactivity disorder. *Biological Psychiatry, 57*(11), 1313-1323.

Graybiel, A. M. (1998). The basal ganglia and chunking of action repertoires. *Neurobiology of Learning and Memory, 70*(1-2), 119-136.

Hariri, A. R., Bookheimer, S. Y., & Mazziotta, J. C. (2000). Modulating emotional responses: Effects of a neocortical network on the limbic system. *Neuroreport, 11*(1), 43-48.

Hayes, S. C., Follette, V. M., & Linehan, M. M. (2004). *Mindfulness and acceptance: Expanding the cognitive-behavioral tradition.* New York: Guilford Press.

Hayes, S. C., & Shenk, C. (2004). Operationalizing mindfulness without unnecessary attachments. *Clinical Psychology Science and Practice, 11*(3), 249-254.

Hesslinger, B., Tebartz van Elst, L., Nyberg, E., Dykierek, P., Richter, H., Berner, M., et al. (2002). Psychotherapy of attention deficit hyperactivity disorder in adults – a pilot study using a structured skills training program. *European Archives of Psychiatry and Clinical Neuroscience, 252*(4), 177-184.

James W., *Principles of Psychology*, Volume I page 424 of original 1890 edition (page 401 of Harvard University Press edition, ISBN 0-674-70625-0)

Jensen, P. S., Arnold, L. E., Swanson, J. M., Vitiello, B., Abikoff, H. B., Greenhill, L. L., et al. (2007). 3-year follow-up of the NIMH MTA study. *Journal of the American Academy of Child and Adolescent Psychiatry, 46*(8), 989-1002.

Jensen, P. S., Mrazek, D., Knapp, P. K., Steinberg, L., Pfeffer, C., Schowalter, J., et al. (1997). Evolution and revolution in child psychiatry: ADHD as a disorder of adaptation. *Journal of the American Academy of Child and Adolescent Psychiatry, 36*(12), 1672-1679; discussion 1679-1681.

Jha, A. P., Krompinger, J., & Baime, M. J. (2007). Mindfulness training modifies subsystems of attention. *Cognitive, Affective, & Behavioral Neuroscience, 7*(2), 109-119.

Kabat-Zinn, J. (1990). *Full catastrophe living: Using the wisdom of your body and mind to face stress, pain, and illness.* New York: Delacorte Press.

Kaneko, M., Hoshino, Y., Hashimoto, S., Okano, T., & Kumashiro, H. (1993). Hypothalamic-pituitary-adrenal axis function in children with attention-deficit hyperactivity disorder. *Journal of Autism and Developmental Disorders, 23*(1), 59-65.

Kessler, R. C., Adler, L., Barkley, R., Biederman, J., Conners, C. K., Demler, O., et al. (2006). The prevalence and correlates of adult ADHD in the United States: results from the National Comorbidity Survey Replication. *American Journal of Psychiatry, 163*(4), 716-723.

Kessler, R. C., Adler, L. A., Barkley, R., Biederman, J., Conners, C. K., Faraone, S. V., et al. (2005). Patterns and predictors of attention-deficit/hyperactivity disorder persistence into adulthood: results from the national comorbidity survey replication. *Biological Psychiatry, 57*(11), 1442-1451.

King, J. A., Barkley, R. A., & Barrett, S. (1998). Attention-deficit hyperactivity disorder and the stress response. *Biological Psychiatry, 44*(1), 72-74.

Klingberg, T., Fernell, E., Olesen, P. J., Johnson, M., Gustafsson, P., Dahlstrom, K., et al. (2005). Computerized training of working memory in children with ADHD – a randomized, controlled trial. *Journal of the American Academy of Child and Adolescent Psychiatry, 44*(2), 177-186.

Konrad, K., Neufang, S., Hanisch, C., Fink, G. R., & Herpertz-Dahlmann, B. (2006). Dysfunctional attentional networks in children with attention deficit/hyperactivity disorder: evidence from an event-related functional magnetic resonance imaging study. *Biological Psychiatry, 59*(7), 643-651.

Kratter, J. (1983). The use of meditation in the treatment of attention deficit disorder with hyperactivity. *Dissertation Abstracts International, 44*(1965).

Lazar, S. W., Kerr, C. E., Wasserman, R. H., Gray, J. R., Greve, D. N., Treadway, M. T., et al. (2005). Meditation experience is associated with increased cortical thickness. *Neuroreport, 16*(17), 1893-1897.

Leary, M. R., Tate, E. B., Adams, C. E., Allen, A. B., & Hancock, J. (2007a). Self-compassion and reactions to unpleasant self-relevant events: the implications of treating oneself kindly. *Journal of Personality and Social Psychology, 92*(5), 887–904.

Leary, M. R., Tate, E. B., Adams, C. E., Allen, A. B., & Hancock, J. (2007b). Self-compassion and reactions to unpleasant self-relevant events: the implications of treating oneself kindly. *Journal of Personality and Social Psychology, 92*(5), 887–904.

Lieberman, M. D., Eisenberger, N. I., Crockett, M. J., Tom, S. M., Pfeifer, J. H., & Way, B. M. (2007). Putting feelings into words: affect labeling disrupts amygdala activity in response to affective stimuli. *Psychological Science, 18*(5), 421–428.

Loo, S. K., Humphrey, L. A., Tapio, T., Moilanen, I. K., McGough, J. J., McCracken, J. T., et al. (2008). Executive Functioning Among Finnish Adolescents With Attention-Deficit/Hyperactivity Disorder. *Journal of the American Academy of Child and Adolescent Psychiatry, 46(12)*, 1594–1604.

Lu, A. T., Ogdie, M. N., Jarvelin, M. R., Moilenan, I. K., Loo, S. K., McCracken, J., et al. (2008). Association of the cannabinoid receptor gene (CNR1) with ADHD and post-traumatic stess disorder. *AM J Hum Genet: Part B Neuropsychiatric Genet.*

Lynn, D. E., Lubke, G., Yang, M., McCracken, J. T., McGough, J. J., Ishii, J., et al. (2005). Temperament and character profiles and the dopamine D4 receptor gene in ADHD. *American Journal of Psychiatry, 162*(5), 906–913.

Maguire, E. A., Gadian, D. G., Johnsrude, I. S., Good, C. D., Ashburner, J., Frackowiak, R. S., et al. (2000). Navigation-related structural change in the hippocampi of taxi drivers. *Proceedings of the National Academy of Sciences of the United States of America, 97*(8), 4398–4403.

Marlatt, G. A., Witkiewitz, K., Dillworth, T. M., Bowen, S. W., Parks, G. A., MacPherson, L. M., et al. (2004). Vipassana Meditation as a Treatment for Alcohol and Drug Use Disorders. In S. C. Hayes, V. M. Follette & M. M. Linehan (Eds.), *Mindfulness and acceptance: Expanding the cognitive-behavioral tradition*. New York: The Guilford Press.

Mauss, I. B., Cook, C. L., Cheng, J. Y., & Gross, J. J. (2007). Individual differences in cognitive reappraisal: Experiential and physiological responses to an anger provocation. *International Journal of Psychophysiology, 66(2)*, 116–24.

McGough, J. J., Smalley, S. L., McCracken, J. T., Yang, M., Del'Homme, M., Lynn, D. E., et al. (2005). Psychiatric comorbidity in adult attention deficit hyperactivity disorder: findings from multiplex families. *American Journal of Psychiatry, 162*(9), 1621–1627.

Mechelli, A., Crinion, J. T., Noppeney, U., O'Doherty, J., Ashburner, J., Frackowiak, R. S., et al. (2004). Neurolinguistics: structural plasticity in the bilingual brain. *Nature, 431*(7010), 757.

Moretti-Altuna, G. (1987). The effects of meditation versus medication in the treatment of attention deficit disorder with hyperactivity. *Dissertation Abstracts International 47*(4658).

Nigg, J. (2003). ADHD: Guides for the perplexed reflect the state of the field. *Journal of Clinical Child and Adolescent Psychology, 32*(2), 302–308.

Nigg, J. T., Blaskey, L. G., Stawicki, J. A., & Sachek, J. (2004). Evaluating the endophenotype model of ADHD neuropsychological deficit: results for parents and siblings of children with ADHD combined and inattentive subtypes. *Journal of Abnormal Psychology, 113*(4), 614–625.

Nigg, J. T., & Casey, B. J. (2005). An integrative theory of attention-deficit/hyperactivity disorder based on the cognitive and affective neurosciences. *Development and Psychopathology, 17*(3), 785–806.

Nudo, R. J., Milliken, G. W., Jenkins, W. M., & Merzenich, M. M. (1996). Use-dependent alterations of movement representations in primary motor cortex of adult squirrel monkeys. *Journal of Neuroscience, 16*(2), 785–807.

Ochsner, K. N., & Gross, J. J. (2005). The cognitive control of emotion. *Trends in Cognitive Sciences, 9*(5), 242-249.

Olesen, P. J., Westerberg, H., & Klingberg, T. (2004). Increased prefrontal and parietal activity after training of working memory. *Nature Neuroscience, 7*(1), 75-79.

Pagnoni, G., & Cekic, M. (2007). Age effects on gray matter volume and attentional performance in Zen meditation. *Neurobiology of Aging, 28*(10), 1623-1627.

Panzer, A., & Viljoen, M. (2005). Supportive neurodevelopmental evidence for ADHD as a developmental disorder. *Medical Hypotheses, 64*(4), 755-758.

Pelc, K., Kornreich, C., Foisy, M. L., & Dan, B. (2006). Recognition of emotional facial expressions in attention-deficit hyperactivity disorder. *Pediatric Neurology, 35*(2), 93-97.

Plessen, K. J., Bansal, R., Zhu, H., Whiteman, R., Amat, J., Quackenbush, G. A., et al. (2006). Hippocampus and amygdala morphology in attention-deficit/hyperactivity disorder. *Archives of General Psychiatry, 63*(7), 795-807.

Pressman, L. J., Loo, S. K., Carpenter, E. M., Asarnow, J. R., Lynn, D., McCracken, J. T., et al. (2006). Relationship of family environment and parental psychiatric diagnosis to impairment in ADHD. *Journal of the American Academy of Child and Adolescent Psychiatry, 45*(3), 346-354.

Rapport, L. J., Friedman, S. R., Tzelepis, A., & Van Voorhis, A. (2002). Experienced emotion and affect recognition in adult attention-deficit hyperactivity disorder. *Neuropsychology, 16*(1), 102-110.

Roemer, L., & Orsillo, S. M. (2007). An open trial of an acceptance-based behavior therapy for generalized anxiety disorder. *Behavior Therapy, 38*(1), 72-85.

Rostain, A. L., & Ramsay, J. R. (2006). A combined treatment approach for adults with ADHD - results of an open study of 43 patients. *Journal of Attention Disorders, 10*(2), 150-159.

Safren, S. A. (2006). Cognitive-behavioral approaches to ADHD treatment in adulthood. *Journal of Clinical Psychiatry, 67 Suppl 8*, 46-50.

Safren, S. A., Otto, M. W., Sprich, S., Winett, C. L., Wilens, T. E., & Biederman, J. (2005). Cognitive-behavioral therapy for ADHD in medication-treated adults with continued symptoms. *Behaviour Research and Therapy, 43*(7), 831-842.

Schwartz, J., & Begley, S. (2002). *The mind and the brain: Neuroplasticity and the power of mental force* (1st ed.). New York: Regan Books.

Schwartz, J., Gullifor, E. Z., Stier, J., & Thienemann, M. (2005a). *Mindful awareness and self directed neuroplasticity: Integrating psychospiritual and biological approach to mental health with focus on obsessive compulsive disorder.* Haworth Press.

Schwartz, J. M., & Beyette, B. (1997). *Brain lock: Free yourself from obsessive-compulsive behavior.* New York: Harper Collins.

Schwartz, J. M., Stapp, H. P., & Beauregard, M. (2005b). Quantum physics in neuroscience and psychology: a neurophysical model of mind-brain interaction. *Philosophical Transactions of the Royal Society of London. Series B: Biological Sciences, 360*(1458), 1309-1327.

Segal, Z. V., Williams, J. M. G., & Teasdale, J. D. (2002). *Mindfulness-based cognitive therapy for depression: A new approach for preventing relapse.* New York: Guilford Press.

Seidman, L. J. (2006). Neuropsychological functioning in people with ADHD across the lifespan. *Clinical Psychology Review, 26*(4), 466-485.

Seidman, L. J., Biederman, J., Faraone, S. V., Weber, W., & Ouellette, C. (1997). Toward defining a neuropsychology of attention deficit-hyperactivity disorder: performance of children and adolescents from a large clinically referred sample. *Journal of Consulting and Clinical Psychology, 65*(1), 150-160.

Shapiro, D. H. (1982). Clinical and physiological comparison of meditation and other self-control strategies. *Am Journal Psychiatry, 139*, 267-274.

Shekim, W. O., Asarnow, R. F., Hess, E., Zaucha, K., & Wheeler, N. (1990). A clinical and demographic profile of a sample of adults with attention deficit hyperactivity disorder, residual state. *Comprehensive Psychiatry, 31*(5), 416-425.

Singh, N., Lancioni, G. E., Joy, S. D. S., Winton, A. S. W., Sabaawi, M., Wahler, R. G., et al. (2007). Adolescents with Conduct Disorder Can be Mindful of Their Aggressive Behavior. *Journal of Emotional and Behavioral Disorders, 15*(1), 56-63.

Skounti, M., Philalithis, A., & Galanakis, E. (2007). Variations in prevalence of attention deficit hyperactivity disorder worldwide. *European Journal of Pediatrics, 166*(2), 117-123.

Slagter, H. A., Lutz, A., Greischar, L. L., Francis, A. D., Nieuwenhuis, S., Davis, J. M., et al. (2007). Mental Training Affects Distribution of Limited Brain Resources. *PLoS Biology, 5*(6), e138.

Smalley, S. L. (2008). Reframing ADHD in the Genomic Era. *Psychiatric Times, 25(7).*

Smalley, S. L., McGough, J. J., Moilanen, I. K., Loo, S. K., Taanila, A., Ebeling, H., et al. (2007). Prevalence and Psychiatric Comorbidity of Attention Deficit Hyperactivity Disorder in Adolescent Finnish Population. *Journal of the American Academy of Child and Adolescent Psychiatry, 46(12)*, 1572-1583.

Sondeijker, F. E., Ferdinand, R. F., Oldehinkel, A. J., Veenstra, R., Tiemeier, H., Ormel, J., et al. (2007). Disruptive behaviors and HPA-axis activity in young adolescent boys and girls from the general population. *Journal of Psychiatric Research, 41*(7), 570-578.

Stadler, C., Sterzer, P., Schmeck, K., Krebs, A., Kleinschmidt, A., Poustka, F. (2007). Reduced anterior cingulate activation in aggressive children and adolescents during affective stimulation: Association with temperament Traits. *Journal of Psychiatry Research, 41*(5), 410-417.

Stevenson, C. S., Whitmont, S., Bornholt, L., Livesey, D., & Stevenson, R. J. (2002). A cognitive remediation programme for adults with Attention Deficit Hyperactivity Disorder. *Australian and New Zealand Journal of Psychiatry, 36*(5), 610-616.

Strayhorn, J. M., Jr. (2002). Self-control: toward systematic training programs. *Journal of the American Academy of Child and Adolescent Psychiatry, 41*(1), 17-27.

Swanson, J. M., Schuck, S., Mann, M., Carlson, C. L., Hartman, C. A., Sergeant, J. A., et al. (2001). Categorical and dimensional definitions and evaluations of symptoms of ADHD: The SNAP and SWAN ratings scales. Retrieved June 6, 2006., from http://adhd.net

Talge, N. M., Neale, C., & Glover, V. (2007). Early Stress, Translational Research and Prevention Science Network: Fetal and Neonatal Experience on Child and Adolescent Mental Health. *Journal of Child and Psychology and Psychiatry, 48*(3-4), 245-261.

Teasdale, J. D., Scott, J., Moore, R. G., Hayhurst, H., Pope, M., & Paykel, E. S. (2001). How does cognitive therapy prevent relapse in residual depression? Evidence from a controlled trial. *Journal of Consulting and Clinical Psychology, 69*(3), 347-357.

Teasdale, J. D., Segal, Z. V., Williams, J. M., Ridgeway, V. A., Soulsby, J. M., & Lau, M. A. (2000). Prevention of relapse/recurrence in major depression by mindfulness-based cognitive therapy. *Journal of Consulting and Clinical Psychology, 68*(4), 615-623.

Teasdale, J. D., Segal, Z. V., & Williams, J. M. G. (2003). Mindfulness training and problem formulation. *Clinical Psychology Science and Practice, 10*(2), 157-160.

Tyrka, A. R., Mello, A.F., Mello, M.F., Gagne, G.G., Grover, K.E., Anderson, G.M., Price, L.H., Carpenter, L.L. (2006). Temperament and hypothalamic-pituitary-adrenal axis function in healthy adults. *Psychoneuroendocrinology, 31*(9), 1036-1045.

Urry, H. L., van Reekum, C. M., Johnstone, T., Kalin, N. H., Thurow, M. E., Schaefer, H. S., et al. (2006). Amygdala and ventromedial prefrontal cortex are inversely coupled during regulation of negative affect and predict the diurnal pattern of cortisol secretion among older adults. *Journal of Neuroscience, 26*(16), 4415-4425.

Verte, S., Geurts, H. M., Roeyers, H., Oosterlaan, J., & Sergeant, J. A. (2006). The relationship of working memory, inhibition, and response variability in child psychopathology. *Journal of Neuroscience Methods, 151*(1), 5-14.

Wasserstein, J., & Lynn, A. (2001). Metacognitive remediation in adult ADHD. Treating executive function deficits via executive functions. *Annals of the New York Academy of Sciences, 931*, 376-384.

Wender, P. H. (1998). Pharmacotherapy of attention-deficit/hyperactivity disorder in adults. *Journal of Clinical Psychiatry, 59 Suppl* 7, 76-79.

Wilens, T. E., Biederman, J., & Spencer, T. J. (2002). Attention deficit/hyperactivity disorder across the lifespan. *Annual Review of Medicine, 53*, 113-131.

Winston, D. (2003). *Wide Awake: A Buddhist Guide for Teens*: Perigee Trade.

Yuill, N., & Lyon, J. (2007). Selective difficulty in recognising facial expressions of emotion in boys with ADHD: General performance impairments or specific problems in social cognition? *European Child and Adolescent Psychiatry, 16*(6), 398-404.

Zuddas, A., Ancilletta, B., Muglia, P., & Cianchetti, C. (2000). Attention-deficit/hyperactivity disorder: A neuropsychiatric disorder with childhood onset. *European Journal of Paediatric Neurology, 4*(2), 53-62.

Zylowska, L., Ackerman, D. L., Yang, M. H., Futrell, J. L., Horton, N. L., Hale, T. S., et al. (2008). Behavioral and cognitive changes in Attention Deficit Hyperactivity Disorder using a mindfulness meditation approach. *Journal of Attention Disorders, 11*(6), 737-746.

18

Mindfulness and Psychosis

Antonio Pinto

Homo sum. Humani nihil a me alienum puto (Heautonti-moroumenos) (163 A.C.) I am human. Nothing human can be alien to me.

Terentius

Introduction

In the last years, mindfulness significantly contributed to promote the ultimate goal of all medical and psychological treatments: easing patients' suffering (Segal, Williams, & Teasdale, 2002).

Indeed, patients with disorders of whatever cause or nature all raise the same desperate and hopeful cry: "help me feel better, help me live better," which all the while points out the intolerability of their material condition of being ill, as well as the existential one of being sufferers.

Thus, all psychotherapies are called upon to deal with the issue and causes of suffering.

There are no doubt innumerable causes of suffering, such as stress, illnesses, people, one's own feelings, goals and wishes. Yet most of the times we suffer occur when different factors combine in a non-harmonious way.

While psychotherapies help people solve, work on, remove or better cope with what causes their suffering, mindfulness introduces a new important element: helping its practitioners and patients change their attitude towards suffering itself. It helps develop the necessary skills to be less reactive to what is occurring at the moment, allowing us to deal with different types of experiences in a way that lowers our levels of suffering, while a sense of well-being is enhanced (Germer, 2005).

Mindfulness also involves gaining greater acceptance and awareness. Acceptance of things as they are, without immediately judging and/or rejecting them; acceptance of one's self and others' selves, which means greater benevolence towards one's nature, limits, feelings and thoughts (Kabat-Zinn, 2005).

It is possible to practice mindfulness with varying degrees of intensity: from everyday practice in our habitual environment, allowing us to experience mindful moments, to the more intense and continuous one of the monks or practitioners of meditation who live in extraordinary contexts. Whatever the level and degree of intensity of our practice, mindfulness allows us to reach a higher level of awareness of thought, feeling, emotion, wishes and actions, as well as suffering itself (Kabat-Zinn, 1990).

As mentioned before, suffering is a constant in the human condition and the more it is approached as nonsensical and meaningless, the more unbearable it is, for the possibility to communicate and share it becomes lower, which slowly and inevitably leads sufferers to shut themselves away in a desperate attempt to find possible causes and solutions. Experiencing suffering merely as an inner private dimension shifts people away from their possibility to be comforted and open to a relational dialogue that is based most of all on mutual sharing and understanding (Bowlby, 1969).

Severe Patients

This is the typical inner experience of life of many severe patients who, besides their great suffering, present a series of issues that thwart treatment effectiveness, such as poor or absent illness insight, mood instability, withering emotional intensity, bizarre and hardly understandable behaviours (eventually violent towards themselves and others) and a tendency to bring rejection and to become an outcast. Furthermore, such patients often live within family environments with predominating high levels of expressed emotions (EE), which together with criticism and communication problems cause the pathology to worsen or relapse (Falloon I. et al., 1985). These patients' ascertained deficits make it hard for them to use some metacognitive functions that are necessary for their therapy to be successful, such as decentralization, distancing, mastery and other skills (Linehan, 1993). Traditional psychotherapies have proved to be scarcely effective in these cases, as shown by the high dropout or clinical ineffectiveness levels. Even the widely validated cognitive-behavioural therapy (CBT) is not enough with patients of this kind and adjustments in the standard protocol become necessary. The first change to make is surely the introduction of a monitoring of the therapeutic relationship and the therapist's relational stance towards that particular type of patient, as a source for learning and changing within the psychotherapy.

Creating a quiet, safe and validating therapeutic environment, in order to make patients feel safe and trustful towards the therapist, is therefore a crucial step for achieving clinical changes (Bowlby, 1988).

What we have said so far explains and motivates what, in our opinion, the difficulties are in treating and trying to help these particular patients return to a living path that is characterized by lower levels of suffering. In order to achieve this, we believe mindfulness might be a helpful additional tool that could integrate those kinds of therapies that have already been shown to be effective.

In fact, owing to what has already been explained, not all psychotic patients might be eligible for or able to bear mindfulness protocols in the forms that are validly structured for other pathologies (i.e. depression, anxiety and so on). It is therefore necessary to briefly overview the main features of psychosis, in order to better understand its intrinsic nature and identify which strategies can be used to adapt the basic principles of mindfulness in a way that better suits the needs and characteristics of patients, in order to achieve the best possible outcomes.

General Characteristics of Psychosis

Psychoses and schizophrenia, in particular, are no doubt in a position of prominence among the above-mentioned highly complex pathologies. They are a series of severe psychiatric disorders, characterized mainly by an altered perception of reality, up to a profound loss of contact with the surrounding world and lack of illness insight, which in severe cases can even be total. Through the years, there have been several attempts to identify the basic diagnostic criteria of schizophrenia. Today, despite these attempts, various controversial points remain. However, it is generally accepted that disorders of thought form and content, loss of functional abilities and a particular course over time are psychopathological aspects common to various forms of psychosis.

Schizophrenia is characterized by a series of symptoms, such as hallucinations, delusions, disorganized thinking, affective flattening and catatonic behaviour. Symptoms must persist for at least 6 months. Moreover, cognitive functions may deteriorate over time (American Psychiatric Association, 2000).

We, however, emphasize the importance of considering the extreme variability of phenotypic manifestations of schizophrenia for diagnosis and therapy purpose.

Indeed, if it is true that this disease has a negative course in the long run, psychic deterioration should be lower at an early stage, which means higher possibilities for intervention. On the other hand, patients with a long history of illness should be likely to have more severe cognitive and social/functional impairment (McGorry P.D., 1999). Moreover, as suggested earlier, the level of illness insight can vary greatly from patient to patient and, even complex delusions do not necessarily prevent communicating and sharing at least some aspects of reality. Finally, we should not forget the great variety of clinical pictures among the forms of schizophrenia with prevailing positive/negative symptoms or with alterations in the formal organization of cognitive architecture, rather than in the contents of thought, which causes extremely disorganized and confused cognitive and behavioural manifestations (Andreasen, Arndt, Alliger, Miller, & Flaum, 1995).

Today it is widely accepted that schizophrenia is a mental disorder or a series of diseases transmitted genetically and/or caused by perinatal or prenatal traumas (Weinberger D.R., 1987; Roberts G.W., 1991).

For many years, the idea of schizophrenia has been affected by Kraepelin's approach, which found its basis on a pejorative course that would culminate in a dementia-like picture (Kraepelin, 1919).

It was therefore seen as a disease that would basically have a chronic course.

The dogma of a progressive devolution of the pathology has contributed to a climate of mistrust and pessimism among both therapists and patients' families. Such approaches have resulted in orienting therapeutic choices towards the isolation of the subject from his/her social environment (especially before neuroleptics were used) or in the attempt of containing the patients' disabilities, seen as obstacles to their return to the community and to their possibility to reach normal levels of autonomy and social functioning.

Later studies on the course of schizophrenia (Liddle P.F. 1999) were determining for a "crisis of the concept of chronicity and presumption of incurability" (Ciompi & Müller, 1976; Huber G., 1979), both widely related to the emphasis given by Kraepelin on deterioration in "Dementia Praecox" (Kraepelin, 1919). The two main studies conducted by the World Health Organization (WHO) on the epidemiology of schizophrenia revealed a wide range of variations in the course and outcome of this disorder. The International Pilot Study on Schizophrenia (IPSS) in particular (WHO, 1973) documented how, in a two-year follow-up, only 37 per cent of the sample evaluated at the beginning was still in a psychotic state, the remaining two-thirds of the sample could either still present some non-psychotic or be totally recovered.

Furthermore, today we know how the course and outcome of an apparently universal phenomenon such as schizophrenia is in fact widely influenced by factors that do not depend on the intrinsic features of the pathology. Bleuler himself would say, "...what is determined is only the *direction* of the course and not the course itself. The outcome is not a feature of the disorder, but it depends on *actual internal and external factors*" (Bleuler, 1911). In support of this, WHO data reveal a better prognosis of schizophrenia in those developing countries with a substantially more supportive family and social environment playing an important role against isolation and stigma (WHO, 1973, 1979; Jablensky, 1987, 1989, 1992; Sartorius et al., 1986).

Currently indisputable data shows that the illness course is basically influenced by environmental events and that patient's environmental modification can lead to important effects (Bellack Mueser et al., 1997).

Traditionally, schizophrenia has been the purview of psychiatric treatment, with *antipsychotic medication* as primary intervention and *psychosocial rehabilitation* as secondary (Bellack & Mueser, 1993; Penn & Mueser, 1996).

Recently, the perception of the nature of psychotic syndromes and the possibility to positively influence their course has gradually yet firmly changed, although, for the following reasons, psychotic patients are hardly considered eligible for radical structured psychotherapy.

Difficulties in Structuring a Setting for Psychotic Patients

- **The first concerns a presumption of incurability**. Generated by the concept of chronicity. Such an assumption has long represented fundamental scientific bias, affecting motivation to engage in serious clinical research, aiming to identify adequate strategies: it would not be worthwhile to undertake a complex therapeutic treatment, to determine substantial changes in the patient's way to interpret reality and deal with it, in case of a genetically determined pathology that's inexorably condemned to evolve (or rather devolve) into a chronic degenerative and defective process.
- **Excessively protective attitude of mental health centres**. After asylums, mental health centres, in their several divisions, appeared to be a possible solution to try and contain and possibly uncover some of the complex issues underlying the structure of the schizophrenic phenomenon.

Mental health service structures found a solid and innovative epistemological reference point in the vulnerability model, renewing their impulse towards the care of schizophrenic patients. This shook off psychiatrists' sense of resigned impotence towards planning a therapeutic intervention programme, so common in the last decades. Mental health service would thus try its best to protect patients from the risk of a crisis caused by exposure to a stress they could not cope with, as this would appear coherent with its reference model; in other words mental health service and its staff would act as a defensive barrier, preserving patients from suffering and offering them adequate medical and social support. Yet, the concrete risk of following the theoretical vulnerability model literally is to create a sort of "protective belt" around vulnerability, rather than patients, paradoxically fostering the "*chronicization of vulnerability*" itself. Indeed, interventions through standardized and predetermined programmes, aiming mainly at the remission of symptoms and "normalizing" of behaviours, show psychiatrists as "*gardeners of madness*," whose task is "*pruning*" anything that appears pointless and potentially dangerous (smothering) for a "better" growth of the individual (Lazslo & Stanghellini, 1993). Although in a particular historical moment such an attitude might no doubt have been useful, following the latest scientific achievements in the psychological and pharmacological field (not least the advent of atypical antipsychotics), it does not seem to meet the needs of those who rather believe in the possibility to apply, with schizophrenic patients as well, the general principles underlying psychopharmacological and psychotherapeutic treatments used for other psychiatric pathologies.

- **Difficulties in establishing good relational attunement and building a solid therapeutic alliance**. Schizophrenic patients very often appear scarcely willing to be helped, having a suspicious and distrustful attitude, even displaying outright hostility to the therapist. Furthermore, while attempting to structure a stable setting for therapy there may often be a lack of attunement between the therapist and the patient's needs, with no apparent possibility for reasonable mediation. At times therapists and patients seem to be engaged in a rational struggle in which therapists try to encourage patients' critical sense in order to increase their sense of reality, while they are intent on defending at any cost their ideas and own interpretation of events and surrounding reality. This often causes a gap between therapist and patient.

More issues compromising the therapeutic alliance are:

Lack of clarity on the goals to be achieved. Through the years, different types and models of therapeutic intervention with schizophrenic subjects have been developed, aiming mainly at a remission of the symptoms and at a better management of the patient's dysfunctional behaviours (Burti, 1993; Hogarty, 1998). Such interventions are part of the so-called biopsychosocial approach (Penn & Mueser, 1996) and range from a hospital treatment model for crisis management, to the so-called psychosocial rehabilitation, mainly implemented within community-based structures. In our opinion, such models have not always considered the subjects' subjective perception of well-being as the main purpose of therapy, nor as one of the outcome indicators that usually trace the specific purposes of a psychotherapy treatment (psychological independence, tolerance to frustration, mental flexibility, etc.) (Paltrinieri & De Girolamo, 1996).

Moreover, as long as therapists consider patients' main psychopathological symptoms (delusions, hallucinations and bizarre behaviours), as nonsensical. Hard to investigate and therefore hindrances to therapy, they will inevitably convey to patients, intentionally or not, the idea that they will not actually improve until they come around to the fact that delusions and hallucinations are the core issues of their disease. Patients are indeed likely to make a stand against this, further complicating the formation of a therapeutic alliance.

Another aspect to take into account when trying to understand the reasons for the difficulties in starting psychotherapy with schizophrenic patients is the

- **little attention given to patients' personal history and dysfunctional assumptions underlying their cognitive structure**, which might contribute, whether uncovered and investigated, to achieve a better understanding of patients.

Examples of dysfunctional assumptions may be: constantly being in danger; being a bad person; not deserving esteem and love; having committed some sins; being condemned to social isolation or eternal damnation; not being capable; risking to lose control of their own actions; having to be the best, never making mistakes; having to pursue perfection at all costs; associating making mistakes with total failure and so on.

Patients seldom spontaneously express such assumptions, on the contrary, the fact that delusions and hallucinations drink in all their energies (as well as those of therapists) may hold them back from achieving greater awareness of their origin and relationship with the causes of their problems. Indeed, these patients have severe communication issues, owing both to their disorganized structure of verbalization and the presence of thought contents that are apparently meaningless or have a complex and obscure meaning that is hardly understandable for therapists.

Last but not least,

- **the general feeling of non-acceptance and foreignness to schizophrenic people's way of being**, which concurred in creating a social stigma affecting and holding back clinical research, and has been playing a definitely negative role in the attempt to engage in a psychotherapeutic process with these patients.

Although in the past this state of things has actually been impeding the care of schizophrenic patients, we now believe that a possible alternative may be in the reminding of psychiatrists about their existential responsibility for taking care of others, not just curing them.

Taking care in the sense of attending to someone, avoidance of forcing them to adapt to an everyday pace that does not belong to them or prevent them from planning their own existential development path. As Bruno Callieri said, such responsibility consists in *"feeling the inward duty to recover a dimension of otherness to the alienus..., not quieting our conscience*

*like the Pharisee in front of the troublesome and demanding dimension
of an intersubjective relationship."*

In this view, acceptance, compassion and a non-judgmental mindful attitude are inescapable not only in handling disturbing thoughts and emotions, but first of all in dealing with such severe patients, who owing to
their unfathomable manifestations are also likely to have received throughout their existence continuous signs of non-acceptance, rejection and deser-
tion, which fed further on their constitutively strong sense of non-belonging.
A compassionate attitude will increase therapists' awareness of the importance of the suspension of judgment (epoché), strengthening their wish to
cultivate listening instead; not as a skill to learn, but rather as a dimension
of intersubjective responsibility (Callieri, 1984a) where the other-from-self
can be understood. Listening to who is asking for help paves the way to
understanding their message, which is rich in contents, plans and interconnected truths that, though often tangled, do reveal another way to "be-in-the-
world"; saying it Mundt's way a disturbed wilfulness, revealing great difficulty
in developing the self, the object world and processes of social reciprocity
(Mundt, 1985).

When analyzing the key components of a relationship from this point of
view, particular notice should be given to the *state of mind and attitude
of a therapist* the moment he/she *meets* a mentally ill person, particularly
a schizophrenic, as the moment of the encounter has extraordinary human,
clinical and therapeutic implications.

Running into certain psychotic manifestations for the first time can no
doubt give a feeling of foreignness, as they are alien to the usual categories
for relating to others and the world. The symbolic meaning of delusions,
certain absurd behaviours, the intrusion of the far-fetched, the reporting
of sensory experiences that are actually hallucinations, the contact with an
apparently far away inner world are dismaying experiences for psychiatrists,
who instinctively take an objectifying attitude, characterized by an aseptic
neutrality, justified by their necessity to observe and explain (Callieri, 1985,
1993a, 1984b). Enduring such an attitude would prevent the development of
a genuine dialogue and affect the therapist's possibility to see the one in front
of him/her as an *alter*, rather than an *alienus*; another who is constitutionally
similar to us, with whom a process can begin, leading to being together like
fellow-men (socii), rather than one in front of the other, which is a typical
stance for studying or observing.

Let us think of *Weltuntergangserlebnis*: the extraordinary and upsetting
schizophrenic experience of the end of the world, admirably described by
Bruno Callieri, where an attempt to establish an order through epitomiza-
tions will end up in an ego-world relationship melting away and total loss of
contact with logic, as well as any other element commonly characterized by
a continuity value. In a kaleidoscopic series of images, the patient will prove
to be radically out of any structures of meaning the therapist might ever share
(Callieri, 1993b).

In front of such an experience, the only alternative to reifying and taking cognizance of alienity is asserting that person's *presence*. Being with the
other *(mitsein)* can convey the sense of sharing of an experience that may
not be understood in its components and symbols, yet is happening in that
particular moment that can therefore be shared *(hic et nunc)*, as long as such

experience is not considered as a private dimension. This would allow recognition of the other person's suffering in the same existential matrix as one's own. *Being there* can thus be a sign of shared *Humanitas* but also a *therapeutic element*: the presence of the other, a fellow-person, can help bridge that broken *ego-world relationship* and allow the conveyance of structures of meaning to be connected to symbols and contents that would otherwise be incomprehensible. In this way *Lebenswelt* (lifesworld) is given back the existence of an individual put away by the social world *(Mitwelt)*, offering his/her *willingness*, which until then was "frozen" owing to psychotic rigidity, the possibility to unfold and tend to the object *(protensio)* again.

Cognitive-Behavioural Therapy as an Adjunct to Standard Care

The use of CBT as an adjunct treatment for psychotic patients seems to have provided, in recent years, the necessary tools for shifting what we described in theory in the previous paragraph to a clinical framework. Indeed, CBT for psychotic patients seems to have seized and overcome some of the issues that had been thwarting attempts to structure therapy interventions that could give adequate consideration both to the characteristics of this kind of patient and to the need for types of interventions that could be standardized and, therefore, reproduced.

CBT (opportunely revisited and adapted to these patients' specific needs) starts from a fundamental premise: all kinds of patients, regardless of presented symptoms, can to some extent improve their subjective perception of well-being and, as a consequence, the quality of their lives (Perris and Skagerlind, 1994). This can only be possible if the achievement of a strong and solid therapeutic alliance is identified as a core factor to therapy success and is therefore set as a high-priority goal. Taking advantage of their role, therapists can try to get to represent a "safe base" for patients, structuring an acceptance-oriented relationship (Bowlby J., 1988). Only afterward will therapists try to develop, along with patients, a programme for achieving specific shared goals.

Collaborative empiricism, as well as giving importance to patients as thinking beings who are able to express sensical and meaningful ideas, are the ingredients that make it possible to access a wide range of both cognitive and behavioural techniques, allowing therapist-patient pairs to reduce current symptoms or at least prevent them from thwarting an acceptable and satisfying standard of living.

Let us outline two different CBT based approaches to this matter:

a)   The first one is based on the idea of discontinuity between normal and abnormal functions and involves an important psychoeducational component. Its main purposes are: strengthening coping strategies, distancing from and correcting psychotic symptoms, training in a wide variety of social skills and psychosocial rehabilitation techniques (Tarrier et al., 1990).

b)   The most normalizing one is based on the idea of continuity between normal and abnormal functions and sees psychotic symptoms as the extreme end of an experiential continuum (both delusions and hallucinations). It aims at doing the greater job "within delusions," in order to seize the existential issues in them, the personal meaning underlying delusional ideas and hallucinations and re-enact the history of patients' development to help them go back to their living path (Kingdon and Turkington, 1994).

Recently, there has been substantial evidence for the effectiveness of CBT for psychosis. Since the end of the 90 s, several randomized controlled trials have been conducted (Kingdon & Turkington, 2005). Some data from these findings are summarized below:

The London-East Anglia group published positive findings (Kuipers et al., 1997). They showed benefits for CBT over usual treatment in the treatment of people with stable psychotic symptoms. Tarrier et al. (1998) in a well-designed methodologically robust study tested CBT against supportive counselling and routine care. Their results showed that both CBT and supportive counselling (SC) were significantly better than standard treatment as at 3 months. CBT had a significant effect on positive symptoms whereas SC did not. Significantly more people who received CBT showed an improvement of greater than fifty per cent in positive symptoms. Relapse rate and time spent in hospital were significantly worse for the treatment as the standard group. However, it was found, after one year, that the results from this brief, intensive therapy of this study were not significantly different from supportive therapy after discontinuation of therapy. In Italy, Pinto et al. (1999) carried out a randomized study of CBT in people who were beginning treatment with Clozapine. The CBT group showed a significant effect in terms of overall symptoms. Sensky et al. (2000) compared nine months of CBT with befriending (designed to be a control for "non-specific" therapy factors including time spent with subjects) in an RCT. At the end of therapy, both groups had made substantial improvements in depressive, positive and negative symptoms. In the CBT group, further gains were made in the subsequent nine months, whilst the befriending group scores began to return to their previous levels. Durham et al. (2003) have found positive but modest results using a group of CBT trained therapists who had limited training and supervision in CBT for psychosis. Gumley, O'Grady, and McNay (2003) have also shown positive benefits on relapse.

In summary (we refer the reader to specialized literature on this subject), many studies have shown therapeutic effectiveness resulting from an integrated pharmacological and psychotherapeutic treatment on outcome and relapse prevention of psychotic symptoms. Meta-analyses (Zimmermann et al., 2005) and more than twenty randomized controlled trials confirmed the effectiveness of CBT in reducing persistent positive symptoms in schizophrenia (Turkington, Kingdon, & Weiden, 2006).

Creating a Mindful Atmosphere to Overcome the "Loss of Intersubjectivity"

One of the first things to take into account is that this particular type of patients lacks an intersubjective dimension, that is the event of encounter and communication (Binswanger,1928). This is considered to be one of the main obstacles to understanding and taking care of these people: corollary of such structural limit is the issue of therapeutic alliance, for example, the difficulty in establishing a stable therapeutic relationship, which is necessary for any structured programme to be started.

This issue has long been considered as one of the main hindrances to the cure of these patients.

On the contrary, we believe that the therapeutic alliance should be considered as a high-priority goal to be achieved with specific tailored strategies, rather than as a requirement for treatment; an initial lack of compliance, which may often be a characteristic of the pathology itself, cannot therefore be a sufficient reason not to try adequate strategies.

A Therapist's Role

Thus, therapists have a key role, as they themselves are required to become tools for therapy. Indeed, as mentioned before, a mindful and compassionate attitude towards the patient can indirectly contribute to convey the essence of a mindfulness-based approach from the very beginning of a treatment, before explicitly goal-oriented psychoeducational phases can begin.

From the first crucial phases of the encounter, therapists must help their patients to perceive how they can be and look at their being without judging or criticizing it; without classifying or measuring it, or worrying whether others' approval of them depends on how many right or wrong things they do; without having to ask themselves if they can get to be loved, accepted only if they behave correctly, only in so far as they meet the expectations of others.

Therapists will try to create a setting allowing much time for patients to introduce themselves, tell about their stories of fears, wishes, feelings and irrational thoughts, which are leitmotifs of an existence interrupted in its evolution by the outbreak of an illness, yet whose framework is perhaps held together by those core contents that are indecipherable to most people, but represent patients' only bridge between a shareable reality and what appears to be total chaos.

In order to actualize a relational atmosphere that is grounded on this sort of philosophy of acceptance of the other, it will be appropriate to allow very flexible time limits to the patient. It will be up to the therapist to show patients attention, care and therefore importance, besides giving proper credit to their existential value, starting from adapting to and respecting their timing and modalities (let us not forget their difficulties with communication and abstract thinking).

Indeed, more than any other type of patients, psychotic people come from a history of alienation, sense of not belonging and marginalization from the rest of humanity, as a reaction to the contents of their thoughts and related behaviours. Furthermore, as their behaviours would be considered as nonsensical, their whole existence would end up being devalued.

This would be enough to determine, or at least affect those typical attitudes in the schizophrenic experience, such as shutting oneself away and withdrawing from the world.

If instead patients experience feeling safe within the atmosphere of a neighbourly, non-judgmental therapy setting and are helped by the therapist hold the same attitude towards themselves, their permanent state of alarm, triggering delusions and hallucinations, is likely to have no more reason to exist.

Indeed, decentred awareness of automatic thoughts of self-reproach and self-criticism contributes to loosen patients' defensive stance deriving from ascribing to others' thoughts their own negative self-beliefs. Such a metacognitive deficit can easily generate delusional ideas of reference, as well as a sense of danger and threat. Criticism can be so destructuring and destructive for the subject that it may come to be perceived as a genuine threat to his/her physical integrity (Mills, 2001) and hetero-aggressive acting out would not then be an unlikely possibility.

On the other hand, establishing a climate of acceptance and abstention from judgment in a therapy setting will allow patients to experience a new way to relate with others, finally being able to exchange their views with someone who is not focused on making them change their minds and showing them how weird and abnormal their way of thinking is. They will find someone who is interested in their ideas, feelings, ways of living and thoughts about themselves; someone who will even be interested in talking about personal and private aspects such as their body (their physical sensations, their way of breathing, etc.) or their life-plan with its values, purposes and goals.

This attitude, grounded on compassion and understanding, is one of the necessary requirements for patients to find, later on, interest and motivation in putting their ruminations aside for a while, in order to focus their attention on relating to someone else, starting from the therapist, who will show them (rather than teach them) how to deal with themselves and their actions in a different way from what they are used to (Allen & Knight, 2005).

The "*loss of intersubjectivity*" is often fed by the fear of others, who will judge and rate them. On the contrary, a more compassionate attitude towards themselves is likely to affect their state of mind towards people around them, experienced as threatening and dangerous until then. Greater openness towards others, meaning less distrust and greater concern about their needs and difficulties, starts a virtuous circle leading patients to also receive positive feedback (Allen & Knight, 2005). Their sense of personal worth and mastery can increase as they begin to develop decentring skills and attention to others, since in this way they can experience being able to feel compassion for someone who is other-from-self, as well as feeling attending and caring, therefore able to take an interest in and worry about someone else.

In this kind of setting, the gap between patients and people around them should narrow, making it easier to create an existential bridge between them, as people who encounter one another to share an experience, who do not, at the time, construct hypotheses or evaluate actions and behaviours. An "*encounter*" is a clear example of a shared experience, representing both the starting point and the goal of this first phase of therapy. The encountered is an *alter* not an *alienus*; an alter with whom harmony and synchrony of intents is possible, an alter who breathes and walks with us so we can recognize him/her as similar and trust him/her, instead of being afraid. In other words, patients are helped broaden their sense of sharing and belonging.

If this emotional state is reached, it will allow us to proceed with less difficulties and "resistance" towards a phase that involves more actively addressing sensory experiences and ideative ruminations in a "defused" way, up to the use of cognitive restructuring techniques and/or learning new social and behavioural skills through the integration of other structured treatment approaches, CBT firstly.

Accepting Patients' Ideas

One of the goals of a mindfulness-based therapy is having patients see how their suffering and discomfort do not come from the symptoms themselves, but from how they react to them and what they decide to do (or not) in order to try and overcome or suppress them.

Patients should for instance be explained that *thoughts are just thoughts* and *voices are just voices*, therefore they don't have any power to harm (Pankey & Hayes, 2003). Similarly to the already validated mindfulness programmes for depression (Segal et al., 2002), patients are expected to slowly manage, through practice, to defuse from ruminations and unpleasant feelings, stop automatically making negative assumptions about themselves and their own discomfort, as well as having reactive behaviours which, in turn, increase their discomfort or end up being its main cause.

On the contrary, we believe that in the first phases of therapy, therapists cannot and should not try to get across the message that (delusional) thoughts are only thoughts, and what makes them suffer is just how they react to them, for such a message might be misunderstood by these patients. They indeed do not always have those cognitive and metacognitive skills that allow understanding of what is being explained to them, experiencing it in a defused way. Any patients adhering to the content of a delusional idea and initially showing no insight are likely to find it illogical and nonsensical to consider that thoughts are not troublesome. In our opinion, this would undermine the therapeutic alliance, so fragile at first, since the theoretical stance of the therapist would appear to be the same as that of the rest of the world, which seems to say "your ideas do not deserve to be considered, as they are just nonsense."

We indeed know that psychotic patients can be totally absorbed in their world, both from a sensory and ideative point of view, structuring and performing their own way to interpret reality, come into contact with other people, their own categories of meaning and their ideas about self-evaluation.

It is important to take adequate precautions to ward off the risk that patients doubt that the therapist's attempt to help them distance themselves from behaviours and ways of thinking that cause them to suffer is in fact a polite way to invalidate their core mental constructions (i.e. "*it is not me who is an inept, they want me to make mistakes*").

One of my first patients suffered from paranoid psychosis, having strong feelings of persecution; when I tried to use "standard" mindfulness procedures with him, after a few sessions he would say: "*There is something wrong with this place, doctor ... I don't feel safe ... they must have managed to locate me ... they are powerful ... I think they're influencing you too*" ... I realized that he was going into a state of alarm that was not apparently justified by what we were actually doing, but in fact I had been going too fast. My patient was not ready to start relating to someone in a way that was not known to him. He would not trust that someone might want to help him, but most of all he would not trust himself. My attitude, so finely focused on finding out what was underneath his delusion, would only reinforce his already strong sense of inefficiency and his low self-esteem, layered during the long years of a tormented existence, along with its emotional and relational failures.

We must take into account that these patients are structured in a way that necessarily leads them to continuously deal with concepts (automatic thoughts and cognitive schemas), which are represented (also as metaphors) within delusions and which they are closely tied to. Thus, we should extend, at least at the beginning, our attitude of acceptance and acquisition of awareness without judgment to the contents of the psychotic experience itself, showing patients that we believe they are worth listening to, being believed and taken seriously for what they think and believe to be correct, as we would do with any other human being.

If for instance we assume (or notice) that the voices patients hear or their delusional thinking represent ideas of low self-esteem or personal value (i.e. insulting voices), we will try to highlight these aspects and prepare patients to change their attitudes, developing greater tolerance and compassion towards themselves. In this case, as shown by CBT, attention will not be focused on symptoms like voices or delusional ideas, but rather on what they represent. Learning to have a more compassionate attitude means helping patients develop greater tolerance towards those aspects of themselves they consider as negative and responsible for their own condition of life. Even people with such characteristics can learn to love themselves more just the way they are and, once they do, they will experience a more peaceful and quiet, less stressful inner condition.

In order to prevent relational deadlocks during therapy, especially when it is still to be consolidated, it is appropriate to pay maximum attention to patients' history, having them perceive our willingness to try and understand together what happened or what is happening with them, placing their (psychotic) experience within their walk of life, whose key stages should also be re-enacted together, if possible, assuming that they would lead to some useful elements for a better understanding of present issues.

This will of course be done in an atmosphere of compassion, empathy and sincere interest for patients' feelings and the suffering caused by their situation.

The analysis of delusional contents, performed with the patient, may allow the therapist to identify problematic areas showing the existence of specific dysfunctional assumptions patients have made about themselves, others and the world (Beck, 1970).

Therapists can help patients focus their attention on themselves in order to find the significant past life events in which certain ideas emerged for the first time, as well as other events contributing to maintain and reinforce those ideas (Beck, 1976).

It will be therefore crucial to begin such exploration starting from the subject's early childhood, studying: (a) the attachment style within the early relationship with parents ("parenting"); (b) the creation of "internal working models" (Liotti, 1995); (c) the presence of deficits in several metacognitive activities (Guidano & Liotti, 1983).

The themes to be explored will perhaps not yet be totally clear to patients: what they think about themselves, of their personal worth, their ability to be loved and accepted, their difficulties in interpersonal relations; of others' behaviour towards them and of others and their behaviours in general.

It will also be important to get more information on patients' opinion on their own disorder, (making sure to focus on "problems" rather than symptoms), their reaction towards it and their symptoms.

Discussing these matters may cause specific dysfunctional assumptions to emerge and, if identified, they would no doubt help decode and better understand the content of certain delusions and hallucinations, besides explaining the reason for the patient's apparently inexplicable behaviours (Fowler, Garety, & Kuipers, 1995; Bedrosian & Beck, 1980).

Furthermore, since clients' negative experiences and convictions about themselves often produce issues of stigma and consequences for personal and social adjustment, such as isolation and lack of social skills, therapists encourage them to identify their negative schemas and more effective assumptions and behaviours will be gradually discussed and introduced later on (Perris, 1989).

This work of exploration and understanding can be done harmoniously integrating mindfulness within a cognitive-behavioural approach. Coherently with the extensively validated CBT procedures for psychosis, initial work shall be done (at least with some patients) exclusively' "within delusions," while any cognitive defusing techniques shall be put aside. Whereas it will be possible to give attention to what comes after delusional ideas, that is, their emotional and behavioural consequences on patients.

Another possible step is highlighting the subtle, yet fundamental difference between ruminations (which cannot lead to solving a problem and are therefore a source for ongoing and self-feeding stress and anxiety) and a problem-solving oriented thinking, providing that patients are shown attention and interest in the ideas and issues that cause them suffering, as well as in their private truths (Lorenzini & Sassaroli, 1992), making sure to never make them feel judged or ridiculed. They shall also be shown a willingness to accept and share the troublesome situations they find themselves in (no matter how plausible they are), trying to find together a sense that can be reconnected to significant moments of their evolution.

Here is an example of what can be said to patients:

> *I understand that the things you told me about represent a problem for you. Though if at the moment there does not seem to be a way to solve them, although having tried to find one, it is pointless to ceaselessly think about them, or you would feel even more worried, distressed and anxious. It would be more useful to learn how to distract yourself, letting all those troublesome thoughts go. Then, when you feel ready and want to, we can go back to them. I know it is not easy, if I had the same problem myself I would as well think about it all the time but, in all fairness, I know it would be useless. Mindfulness can be of help here.*

A delusion can contain a patient's whole life and all its issues, thus, delusional thinking might be the patients' only way to find explanations about how the world works, while at the same time preventing the deepest cores of their identity to collapse into fragments. It is therefore crucial not to run the risk of leaving them destitute of the importance of what they believe in, until they have developed some new interpretation key (Lorenzini & Sassaroli, 1998).

A non-judgmental, mindful attitude shall be shown towards patients' states of mind and actions, which will nurture their self-esteem and sense of personal worth.

Patients can be very tense and anxious owing to the great discomfort originated by their delusional ideas and, since stressful situations may in turn trigger relapses or reinforce symptoms (Morrison, 1998), they will be helped not by being overwhelmed by ruminations and problems that cannot be solved straight away, but by taking advantage of the practice of keeping anxiety at a minimum and of an increased ability to accept and tolerate it for what it is (Williams, 2002).

We believe that, at this stage, patients will be more willing to temporarily set certain thoughts aside, becoming more aware that if they are not overwhelmed by them but allow them smaller space and time during the day, their suffering can be reduced.

In this way we address the following purposes:

- narrowing the existential gap between patients and the rest of humanity, caused by feeling alone, not being understood and/or being negatively judged for their way of thinking
- sharing their "private truths," creating an opportunity to work together on them
- nurturing their hope for an actual solution of the problem they have been long been going through
- increasing their willingness to accept the idea of cognitive defusion, as it does not require them to give up any of those parts of themselves and their history that lay beyond delusions and represent the centrepiece of their existence itself.

Proposing a Change

As soon as a therapeutic relationship is well-established and a patient can feel the closeness of his/her therapist, as well as his/her sincere willingness to help, he/she can be guided to the possibility to detach from disturbing thoughts and emotional states.

As we mentioned in the previous paragraph, patients are not required to be more or less aware of being ill. In fact, from a therapy viewpoint, it can be seen as a success, or at least a good outcome if they just accept to freely talk about their delusional ideas and hallucinations without hesitating or being afraid. Indeed, patients are often afraid to lay themselves bare; they may in fact worry about being negatively judged because of their "strange" thoughts or the unusual sensory phenomena they experience. They can also feel ashamed or embarrassed about being eventually called crazy. Their lives have taught them that their thoughts can make others become distrustful and hostile, insomuch that they can be threatened and verbally or even physically assaulted. In fact, forced hospitalizations have often occurred as a consequence of patients' behaving coherently with their view of the world or of their attempt to find confirmation of or share the existence of the voices. Their weird and bizarre, sometimes restless behaviours indeed scare and puzzle people around them, who in turn feel threatened.

Thus, the first step with these patients is get to persuade them that they can freely talk to us, since we will consider their thoughts equally valid as those of any other person. Perris has already talked about conveying to patients and their families the importance of an approach based on learning how "*to substitute symptoms to treat with problem to solve*" (Perris, 1989).

The normalizing approach of CBT for psychosis represents the conceptual basis to start from: delusional beliefs and hallucinations differ only quantitatively from processes that are common among all individuals (Kingdon & Turkington, 1991, 2005). Hence, delusional thoughts can trigger emotional and behavioural responses, just like any other kind of thoughts, becoming in turn an actual source of discomfort.

It is though commonly acknowledged that many problems cannot be solved immediately, nor in the desired way, yet it is possible to find adequate strategies to keep stress derived from a persisting unresolved issue at a minimum.

There is no doubt that delusions and hallucinations, as well as their emotional and behavioural consequences, represent the biggest issues for psychotic patients, who, with time, developed their own personal ways to react to or avoid them. Indeed, both pharmacological and psychosocial interventions in general have often been programmed in an attempt to extinguish, or at least dramatically reduce symptoms but, paradoxically, in certain cases symptoms ended up being exacerbated (Morrison, 1994; Morrison, Haddock, & Tarrier, 1995) and in others, little or no result was reached, while, on the other hand, new maladaptive behaviours and unpleasant sensations arose. Thus, it would be very useful if patients could learn how to deal with such material in a new way, if it were suggested to them that, very often, the most stressful and disturbing consequences they experience are not triggered by symptoms, but rather by their response to them.

A typical example is the so feared and fought hospitalization, which on most occasions is not executed due to a relapse, but because of the way patients behave as a reaction to the voices (bothering others, hurting themselves/others and so on) (Rogers, Anthony, Toole, & Brown, 1991).

For this reason, it shall be explained to patients that the core of their issue is not a symptom but the way they choose to respond to it: *voices* or *thoughts* do not have the power to autonomously operate on reality, so they cannot harm them, nor anyone else.

We ask patients to perform an accurate description of their symptoms, feelings and sensations in general, paying attention to any subsequent reactions. They will surely notice how some of their behaviours respond to certain phenomena and aim at exercising some sort of control over them. Drug, alcohol or medication abuse, for instance, reflect their need to lower the high levels of tension and anxiety that are triggered by troublesome situations, while obeying the voices may make patients feel safe from eventual frightful consequences (Birchwood & Chadwick, 1997).

In other words, patients can gradually gain greater awareness of their own responses to the voices or to stressful thoughts, yet they will be invited not to oppose, but rather just notice them, as they will flow away themselves, gradually becoming less intense and eventually disappearing, just like any other feeling. It would indeed be impossible to hold feelings back, even if we wanted to, yet patients might have never had the chance to experience this.

Mindfulness needs to be explained to patients, what it is for and how it can represent a new possibility for them to deal with stressful experiences. The practice of mindfulness can help them to not be overwhelmed by the images, unusual thoughts and unpleasant feelings they continuously run into. There is in fact no way to prevent anything from getting into our minds, so the real challenge is to learn not to try and hold feelings back (they are doomed to pass away) but relate to them in a different way: attentively addressing feelings and sensations, even the unpleasant ones, being curious about them instead of fighting against or avoiding them or trying to make them disappear (Chadwick, 2006). Encouraging patients to carefully and curiously observe their feelings and sensations will lead them to see how they continuously change; indeed, as an example, voices will seldom be found to persist for a consistent length of time.

After mindfulness has been explained, patients shall be invited to spend some time focusing on their breath and body, with no lessons, but just being guided towards an increase of their level of awareness. Then, their attention shall be gently brought to whatever comes up, not opposing any kind of sensation, be it pleasant or not. We shall remind them that as they address sensations or anything else that may come up, simply noticing them without judging, their stress decreases. Practically, patients are able to awarely accept the experience of hallucination for what it is, without adhering to its content but instead keeping sufficiently detached from it; bearing in mind their project of life and plans and stay focused on their sources of well-being and satisfaction, and they will gradually realize that they can achieve their life goals, regardless of their unusual sensory experiences.

We highlight the importance of staying anchored to their values and core life purposes, as this can be an effective tool not to be entangled in ruminations or chain reactions. Patients who bear in mind what is important to them (interpersonal relations, achieving and maintaining some degree of autonomy, economical independence and so on) feel more motivated to keep focused on the behaviours that are useful for achieving their goals, rather than letting their choices and behaviours follow the urge of delusional beliefs (Pankey & Hayes, 2003). Hence, any patients not having clear ideas on this matter must be helped identify possible goals to be achieved.

We emphasize once again the importance of integrating goal-oriented CBT programmes, as patients' lives can often be unsatisfactory because of their difficulties in achieving goals (Kendall, 1984).

Training in *problem solving* can be of great help for patients to give up adopting avoidance strategies with any issues they consider to be unsolvable. They will in fact experience the necessary skills to do what people normally do, as soon as they learn how to better tolerate initial feelings of anxiety and discomfort, being then able to use adequate strategies to tackle one obstacle at a time. This will nurture their self-esteem and sense of personal worth, further motivating them to continue therapy. In this view, even simple *social skills training*, opportunely revised, can be a valid tool (Bellack, Mueser, Gingerich, & Agresta, 1997).

Moreover, in theory, an increased sense of personal worth and mastery may in turn determine an increase in self-esteem and, therefore, reduce patients' sense of isolation and non-belonging, which is also fed by the lack of sharing of even the most common aspects of everyday life.

In order to achieve this goal, patients can be trained to first identify and then give up those strategies that merely aim at controlling their emotional states and, subsequently, recognize and accept any thoughts and troublesome feelings, simply by becoming aware of them in a decentred way, not having to strive to suppress them. This will help patients to notice how having been long focused on symptoms had interfered with their life projects (Hayes, Kirk, & Wilson, 1999).

Patients are though not only absorbed in their own unpleasant feelings but also chastise themselves for feeling something they should not be feeling. Non-acceptance is the cause for an exponential increase of suffering, which in turn is fed by patients' conviction that symptoms have some obscure power and therefore have to be suppressed at any cost. This triggers an inner struggling, fostering isolation and loss of common sense, which leads to a spiral of increasing separation from reality, becoming the theme of patients' unshareable malaise.

A therapy that involves offering patients the described relational experience is a means for promoting the idea that self-acceptance is the missing ring in their search for sense and meaning. There may though be hindrances to accepting unpleasant feelings and unusual sensory experiences; patients might indeed find it hard to "*let everything go*" (that is stop giving serious consideration to the content of "thoughts" and "voices"), as they might expect negative consequences from giving up their fight, or, they may be so used to staying anchored to such perceptions that they are afraid to lose some fundamental element of their life (Chadwick, 2006).

Therapists will have to discuss with patients the fact that acceptance does not mean avoidance of an issue or passive resignation about what they identify as a cause for their suffering. On the contrary, they will be encouraged to stick to reality for what it is. Accepting everything that happens within their sensory range means "*this is my experience and my reality, now*" and this inescapable fact can be a good basis for developing non-judgmental thinking. *Self-acceptance* is, indeed, obviously thwarted by our negative self-beliefs. Mindfulness can also help increase awareness of our own reactive judgments, which, just as emotional responses, can be addressed as understandable and transitory: they can be seen as a part of the self that comes and goes but is actually not the self.

Thus, having "bad thoughts" does not mean being a bad person, but just that "*in this particular moment, for some reason, I am having these thoughts*" and they will pass away and will be replaced by others. They do not determine my way of being or my actions, but I can turn away from them if I want.

The fact is that some patients find it very difficult to maintain a mindful attitude towards psychotic experiences.

What can we do with them?

Chadwick suggests that they should be reminded that everything they feel or sense is doomed to pass away; at the same time their decentred awareness of any feeling, sensation or reaction should be validated and, moreover, they should be encouraged to keep connected to their body and to breathing in particular (Chadwick, 2006).

Yet, it will still be likely that patients feel they have failed once again and that their inadequacy makes it impossible for them to follow the programme. This may in turn feed their tendency to ceaselessly make negative self-judgments. Therefore, great emphasis must be given on the fact that trying to achieve a condition of acceptance of unpleasant feelings, as well as subsequent physical sensations, is in fact a process to follow, rather than a goal to achieve.

Patients will slowly and gradually be guided along the path to awareness and their constancy and perseverance will continuously be encouraged in order not to let them feel discouraged. Any difficulties, i.e. being distracted by intrusive thoughts or voices will be normalized and shared.

We might as well invite patients to deliberately expose themselves to their bizarre thoughts or disturbing sensory experiences, obviously trying not to transform, control or understand them, but just awarely noticing them.

Later on, it will also be possible to help patients release the literal content of thoughts, through a process of cognitive defusion (Luoma & Hayes, 2003). They will be once again reminded that thoughts do not have any power to directly transform reality or determine our behaviours.

Thoughts are in fact just thoughts. The essence of defusing techniques is getting accustomed to seeing thoughts and feelings for what they are (just experiences), rather than what they seem to mean (structured realities) (Bach & Hayes, 2002).

A Sense of Bodily Fragmentation

Another common issue among these patients is their sense of fragmentation and destructuration, mainly located in their body in the form of an altered coenaesthesia. An altered perception of the body scheme has been reported in highly stressful interpersonal contexts, such as families with high levels of expressed emotion where communication is extremely disturbed and confused, characterized by high hostility and criticism that are conveyed through improper use of verbal language tones and contents. This causes patients to constantly feel in danger or even physically threatened and, in psychological and/or physical trauma patients, such clinical manifestations take the structure and defensive meaning of dissociative states. (Falloon, 1988; Kuipers & Bebbington, 1988).

Furthermore, these patients' cognitive deficits often prejudice their ability to quickly and properly decode words (McKenna & Oh, 2005), so their only way to find a meaning in what happens around them is by holding on to what comes from their body sensations and emotional states: feeling scared or terrorized, besides having intense physical sensations they cannot account for and which, in turn, become causes of further fear and concern. In this way, their initial state of alarm will be amplified.

It is thus likely that patients construct multiple, not integrated mental representations of self, so their sense of bodily fragmentation may be intended as a metaphor for something that would otherwise be impossible to communicate.

Indeed, in this search for sense and meaning, it will be useful to set body as a starting point, in order to help patients develop a more mindful relationship with it (Mills, 2001).

Once patients learn to relate with their bodies in a different way, becoming more aware of their common sensations, including the pleasant ones, they more easily manage to also transform their relationship with stressful and unpleasant sensory experiences.

Case Report

A patient we can call "John" suffered from severe paranoid schizophrenia. He would live in a condition of significant social isolation and relational impairment. The only activity he could engage in was bodybuilding, of which he had become an eager practitioner. His father, who wanted to try and encourage him to broaden his interests, would oppose this only passion and this triggered violent family fights with bitter criticism. Immediately after these high-pitched arguments, John would feel deep anxiety and anguish, as well as a strong sense of danger and threat. He would also bring up an increasing sense of bodily disaggregation, "as if my body would break into pieces." He could not feel it anymore, nor he could tell which was its position in space; he would feel his blood disappearing from his veins, "as if someone had been sucking it out." After a while he would see his father "turning into a monster... a sort of vampire." At that point, he could not do anything but run away, making them lose track of him, and would usually be found after a few days in confusional state.

In fact, when under stress, John could not decode his own high levels of tension and anxiety and, as a consequence, he would construct mental representations of a physical identity, based on a misinterpretation of physical sensations connected to fear and to feeling threatened. His psychotic structure would then lead him to make up a world, as well as intrinsically coherent meanings, that could provide the necessary explanations for him to choose which behavioural steps to take.

Managing to keep their attention focused on their body and on catching and enhancing every sensation coming from any specific district of it; being fully aware of their senses, moment after moment, can distract them from feeling overawed and devastated by terrifying and disaggregating thoughts and feelings that hamper their full and fluent relationship with reality.

This kind of concentration is not a mere exercise of the mind, but a renewed ability to develop a new sense of the self. Patients with a weak ego unity and stability will take advantage of the practice of "*body scan*" or "*mindful walking*" (Kabat-Zinn, 1990; see also Appendix A of this volume). They will be invited to notice everything that happens, everything they perceive and every body sensation; they will be asked to notice what comes up and concentrate on their mental representation of what they are perceiving, just noticing, without commenting.

This will help the process of "*embodiment*" and regaining of patients' sense of corporeity, threatened by their feelings of fragmentation, and will foster a more competent and stable sense of the self, protecting them from a disaggregation and dissolution of their ego, otherwise they would find in delusions the only way to give events a meaning.

Being in motion, as a unitary organism, held together by the ability to perceive all sensations, elicits the impression that different parts of the body are connected to each other and communicate with each other. The fragmentation these patients report is not simply an abstract idea, but an actual physical sensation. Experimenting a new, more aware way to be in motion, feeling more centred and relate to the surrounding world in a new way, can help transform one's "being-in-the-world" (Mills, 2001).

Indeed, everything concerning corporeity can by right combine to bring about self awareness or, in other words, *presence*; yet not for its own sake, within the boundaries of a more or less defined body scheme: body can be a means for connecting with others: *the body I am*, a subject-body, makes encounters with other subjects bodies possible and is opposed to *the body I have* (Callieri, 1989), an object-body that, according to the constrained and petrified psychotic meanings is object of spells of violence and is anyway passive towards anything coming from who is other-from-self. See the enlightening pages by Merleau-Ponty (1945) on this subject.

Being able to experience areas of well-being, as well as a different way to perceive oneself, one's corporeity and sensations through an aware and intentional use of the described practice can therefore help increase self-esteem, as well as a sense of empowering connected to having developed a focused awareness as an alternative to being swept away by the ceaseless torrent of thoughts. In other words, focusing on one's self and one's own corporeity can be an opposite experience to fragmentation, providing a sense of safeness and integrity to be used as a resource when coping with every-day stressful events. Becoming aware of one's emotions and sensations is also identifying them as what they are (just feelings), not having to resort to alternative interpretations such as delusions, in order not to dissolve once again into the inexplicable and the unspeakable.

> *After clinical stabilization, John willingly got involved in a CBT programme for psychotic patients, which of course included some mindfulness sessions. Because of his taste for physical activity, he showed particular interest in the importance that was given to corporeity. Focusing on his breathing and body through "body scan," and on his body-environment interactions through "mindful walking," he slowly developed a new perception of himself and the functioning of his body. Being aware of an underlying physical integrity, despite any changes in his physical sensations, due to variations in his emotional state, provided the patient with a new cognitive scheme allowing him to go on with psychotherapy with more confidence and peace of mind.*

Some Practical Variations of the Protocol

Mindfulness-based strategies for treatment of psychotic patients have already been implemented (Chadwick, 2006; Garcìa Montes et al., 2004).

Chadwick highlights some examples of the use of a modified mindfulness protocol, stressing in particular the effectiveness of mindfulness in coping with the voices *"rather than getting rid of them*:

From the very outset I clarify that mindfulness will not get rid of voices, thoughts, images, and so on. It involves practicing a different way of responding to them. It is about learning to accept and live with these experiences without feeling preoccupied, ruled, dominated and overwhelmed by them" (Chadwick, 2006).

We fully share his adjustments to the standard protocol as necessary to adapt it to the specific characteristics of this kind of patient.

They indeed seem hardly able to tolerate the usual 20–45 minute meditation sessions, since in that length of time it is reasonable to expect their attention to come and go, as they tend to be distracted by external stimuli (especially auditory) and internal ruminations. One of the cognitive deficits often found in these patients concerns in fact the ability to keep their attention focused on an internal or external object (Wykes & Reeder, 2005). This would thus increase the risk of patients' exposure to the "voices" that, not yet understood and adequately dealt with, may in turn cause anxiety, determining, as already proved (Birchwood & Tarrier, 1992), a condition of stress that might trigger delusions and hallucinations. Meditation itself might then be experienced as extremely hard and stressful, discouraging patients from engaging in it again in the following sessions.

During the first experimental phases with a group of ten patients, I remember one of them saying, after a session of about 25 minutes:

> *Doctor, everything is so strange: during the first few minutes I was feeling calm and could follow your instructions, then I heard a voice (external?) telling me not to do that..., saying you were deceiving me and if I had kept breathing that way I would have activated the device I have in my head...I was scared.*

This example shows how, if all necessary precautions are not taken, even the experience of meditation may be encompassed in a patient's delusional world, so it should be introduced and offered considering everything that was said about the use of CBT with psychotic patients (Chadwick, Birchwood, & Trower, 1996).

Another very useful variation Chadwick introduced is to *avoid prolonged silence* during sessions. Therapists will indeed give short instructions to patients during practice, in order to continuously stimulate their attention, preventing them from going astray in their (delusional) inferences and/or ruminations, which might increase, rather than lower, their sense of alienation, not belonging and detachment from the real world.

For the same reason, continued practice at home will not be recommended to all patients, especially at the beginning of therapy, especially in the case of someone is thought not to have sufficient metacognitive, decentring and self-mastery skills. Another good reason to share this experience with a therapist is that its relational component can be seen as a means and a chance for patients to increase their sense of sharing and belonging to the human assembly, while alone in their homes, in a family environment where tranquillity and understanding are not always guaranteed, they would be exposed to the risk of being pointed out and judged as "*the ones who do strange, unfathomable things*" and are again different.

Hence, we believe that getting involved with a group practice is the best way to start out, yet not until a therapeutic relationship has been consolidated in an individual therapy setting, where the therapist has gained reasonable knowledge of the patient's possibilities and, most of all, not before the patient is able to fully trust his/her interlocutor and his/her level of clinical stability is acceptable.

Therapists will have to take care not to proceed too fast when offering this new type of experience and only after having provided sufficient explanations of its nature and of the intended outcomes.

This psychoeducational approach will be further extended to family members, should patients be encouraged to do some short practice sessions at home.

In the fullness of time, patients who seem to be in good contact with reality, but find it difficult to concentrate on their breathing (as too much of an abstract task), can be invited to focus on what they do for themselves. They can be asked to perform a few everyday actions with greater awareness and especially those tasks that are more gratifying and make them feel somehow enriched and satisfied. For example, it can be suggested that they pay more aware attention to what they do:

> "*Now I am walking,*" "*Now I am touching the door handle,*" "*Now I am bringing the toothbrush close to my mouth,*" and so on.

This has a double effect: helping them learn how to recognize themselves and to focus their attention, where they want it, with little effort, as too hard tasks may, in case of failure, further weaken their sense of personal worth and self-esteem; and it also leads them to find out how they can take care of themselves in a simple way, giving importance to their small everyday actions and contributing in this way to form a new, more positive image of themselves ("*I am able to do something for myself and feel satisfied from it*"), not having to say to themselves they have to change or do something different, but just noticing and revaluing what they already do spontaneously.

In other words, learning to accept themselves for who they are and what they do, no matter what it is and how it is done.

As for defusing from the voices, we find the hints provided during the fourth MBCT session extremely useful (Segal et al. 2002).

The protocol involves a "mindfulness of sounds" moment, designed to increase awareness of sounds through the practice of mindfulness (see also Appendix A of this volume). In order to keep patients from getting stuck on the contents of voices, which are known to trigger emotional and behavioural responses, we invite them to pay attention to some of their formal components, such as tonality, timbre, pitch and length, as well as the rhythm they make as they come one after the other. This encourages patients to do the opposite of what they would normally do, that is avoiding or being afraid of the voices. In fact the aim is to arouse their curiosity to observe them in a different way, to catch some details and finding out particular aspects they had never noticed before, living in the present moment and refraining from any evaluation; just noticing them and, in case they find themselves lingering on their possible meaning, they should gently drive their attention back to their sensory features, trying not to blame or come down on themselves for not doing the exercise the right way.

In this way, patients are helped to change the way in which they deal with misperceptions. They will realize that they do not just have to suffer them, but can decide whether to amplify them or not, or whether to observe or ignore them.

Moreover, this occasion shall be used to reinforce the idea that what is important is the process, not the outcome, and that managing to give up the idea of *having to do things well*, while pointing out that of *just doing them*, will be a further step towards moving from *doing mode* to *being mode* which is itself an object of focused awareness.

The Heterogeneousness of Clinical Pictures

As already mentioned before, the extreme heterogeneousness of symptoms and phenotypic pictures has to be taken into consideration when planning a therapy. Patients with structured delusions, but no formal thought disorder or hallucinations present different issues from those with a prevalent hallucinatory component or with low social functioning and/or high levels of cognitive impairment.

In our opinion, group therapy should always aim at improving clinical conditions, groups should never be uneven, as this makes mutual acceptance and sharing much harder to learn and may instead increase patients' sense of otherness and non-belonging, as well as their fear of being criticized or judged.

After a session of group practice, a patient asked if he could talk to me in private:

> Doctor, as I was trying to concentrate on my body and on my breath, trying to release every unpleasant sensation related to the voices, I felt embarrassed and anxious thinking that my experience was totally unknown and not very understandable for the others...so I thought that if this makes me so tense, maybe it is not good for me.

Another one told me "*he could not understand why I was considering him similar to those mad people hearing things that were not there and how he could possibly trust them...*"

If on the one hand we try to help patients develop a habit to relate mindfully to all experiences, including the psychotic one in general, it is also true that this is a goal, not a requirement, and patients must be placed in a condition in which they can achieve it.

In this view the grouping of patients with similar symptoms can be useful, as this will make them feel less exposed to criticism and embarrassment.

If all group members share the same kind of sensory experiences or the same issues, i.e. relational (let us think, as an example, of the tendency to relate to others through the lenses of persecutory ideas), it is more likely that they will reach acceptance of their present experience without judging it.

We shall not forget that, even in the best-case scenario, these patients have a labile illness insight, so it is not always possible to count on their acceptance of explanations for the origin and nature of their thoughts and experiences.

In other words, what we consider a psychotic experience is, for many patients, the ordinary, self-evident, irrefutable one and the only way to perceive reality and interpret facts.

A further issue that shall not be neglected is that these patients may lose their sense of time and space and, eventually, even of their own physical boundaries.

Hence, it is important to evaluate if a patient should or should not be asked to close his/her eyes during practice. An alternative to closing their eyes can be the focusing on a point on their chest and/or keeping one hand either on their chest or abdomen, in order to help them feel their body and follow their breath.

Finally, it can be suggested to patients who easily fall into a delusional state or who are noticed to have an increased sense of otherness after even very short sessions, that they concentrate their attention on the movements of the chest of who is in front of them and try to be in tune with their breathing (Chadwick, 2006).

DV-SA Questionnaire

We invited our patients to perform a self-administered questionnaire on subjective opinion about delusions and voices (*DV-SA questionnaire*: delusion and voices self-assessment questionnaire, Pinto, Gigantesco, Morosini, & La Pia, 2007), developed and validated in collaboration with the Italian National Institute of Health. Our purpose was not to get a quantitative psychopathological score (assessing the eventual presence of delusions and/or hallucinations), but rather to have patients focus their attention on their own responses to voices and/or other (delusional) beliefs.

Patients are in fact asked to answer questions about a certain (delusional) idea, which was previously identified:

> *How often do you think about this idea?, how does this idea make you feel?, to what extent does this idea affect your relationship with others or interfere with your everyday actions?*
> *About the voices*:
> *How often do you hear the voices?, do you think they are other people's voices?, do they make you feel stressed and nervous? or do they make you feel good?, do they ordain you? And do you obey?, to what extent do they interfere with your relationship with others and your everyday activities?*
> and so on.

In order to check the extent to which their answers and those of patients overlap DV-SA can also be completed by therapists The goal is knowing patients better, in order to improve therapist-patient attunement and make the most of therapy: not everything that therapists assume to know about their patients matches with what they actually feel or think, especially if patients have communication issues or fear to lay themselves bare. This can thwart relational attunement and prevent therapists from grasping everything that makes a patient's inner world.

DV-SA questionnaire can be useful both as a diagnostic and therapy tool, assuring patients an initial distancing from triggering factors, which is an important step towards dis-identification and experiential practice of decentred awareness (Segal et al., 2002).

Conclusion

Therapists attempts to make "strange" signs and symptoms disappear at any cost has too long been the core of a therapeutic relationship with psychosis patients and this has led to clinicians feeling impotent and frustrated. Inexorably, this state of things has affected the course of the pathology itself, which was thereby relegated among incurable illnesses.

Whereas, the core of CBT and mindfulness is people, and getting to know and understand all of their manifestations rather than finding an explanation of them.

Perhaps, this increases the possibility to establish a therapeutic relationship that is first of all human; a relationship that is based on comparing lives and experiences that are often very hard, be they real or imaginary. Regardless of the extent to which suffering characterizes and permeates every aspect of our life, it is still authentic, natural and therefore shareable.

Clinical evidence for our research has still to be provided, yet, perhaps, if we manage to encourage patients to learn to accept things for what they are, without judging them, this message might soon translate into acceptance of themselves and others and we would have helped another human being leave loneliness and otherness behind, coming through a private, unapproachable dimension that is relentlessly doomed to be out of space and time.

References

Allen, N., & Knight, W. E. J. (2005). Mindfulness, compassion for self, and compassion for others. In P. Gilbert (Ed.). *Compassion*. London and New York: Routledge.

American Psychiatric Association (2000). *Diagnostic and Statistical Manual of Mental Disorders (DSM IV TR)*. Washington, DC: American Psychiatric Association.

Andreasen, N. C., Arndt, S., Alliger, R., Miller, D., Flaum, M. (1995). Symptoms of Schizophrenia. Methods, meanings, and mechanisms. *Archives of General Psychiatry, 52*, 341-351

Bach, P., & Hayes, S. C., (2002). The use of acceptance and commitment therapy to prevent the rehospitalization of psychotic patients: A randomized controlled trial. *Journal of Consulting and Clinical Psychology, 70*(5), 1129-1139.

Beck, A. T. (1970). *Cognitive therapy: Nature and relation to Behavior therapy. Behavior Therapy 1*, 184.

Beck, A. T. (1976). *Cognitive therapy and emotional disorders*. New York: International Universities Press.

Bedrosian, R. C., & Beck, A. T. (1980). Principles of cognitive therapy. In M. J.Mahoney (Ed.) *"Psychotherapy process"*: New York: Plenum Press.

Bellack, A. S., & Mueser, K. (1993). Psychosocial treatment for schizophrenia. *Schizophreni Bulletin, 19*, 317-336

Bellack, A. S., Mueser, K., Gingerich, S., Agresta, J. (1997). *Social skills training for schizophrenia. A step by step guide. New York*: The Guilford Press.

Binswanger,L. (1928). Lebensfunktion und innere Lebensgeschichte. *Monatsschrift für Psychiatrie und Neurologie, 68*.

Birchwood, M. & Chadwick, P. (1997). The omnipotence of voices: Testing the validity of a cognitive model. *Psychological Medicine, 27*,1345-1353.

Birchwood, M., & Tarrier, N. (1992) (Eds.), *Innovations in the psychological management of schizophrenia*. Chichester: Wiley

Bleuler, E. (1911). *Dementia Praecox oder gruppe der Schizophrenien*. Deutick, Leipzig.

Bowlby, J., (1969) *Attachment and loss*. London: Hogarth Press.

Bowlby J. (1988). *A secure base*. London: Routledge.

Burti, L. (1993). Commentary. In L. Burti *L.* (Ed.), Forum: Models of psychosocial rehabilitation for chronic psychiatric patients. *Italian Journal of Psychiatry Behavioral Science, 3*, 147.

Callieri, B. (1984a). La Clinica come demitizzazione della psichiatria. *Psyche*, pag. 69, Abano, Piovan.

Callieri, B. (1984b). La fenomenologia antropologica dell'incontro: il "noi" tra l'homo natura e l'homo cultura. In C. L. Cazzullo, & C. Sini (Eds.), *Fenomenologia: Filosofia e psichiatria* (pp. 53-62). Milano: Masson.

Callieri, B. (1985). Antropologia e psichiatria Clinica. *Quaderni Italiani di Psichiatria*, IV, 3, pp.207-223.

Callieri, B. (1989). Dimensioni antropologiche della psicopatologia della "corporeità". *Psyche*, 3.4., pp 213-223,

Callieri, B. (1993a). Aspetti antropofenomenologici dell'incontro con la persona delirante. - *Riv. di psichiatria*, vol. 28, n. 6, novembre dicembre.

Callieri, B. (1993b). Contributo allo studio psicopatologico dell'esperienza schizofrenica di fine del mondo. In "*Percorsi di uno Psichiatra*". Roma: Edizioni Universitarie Romane, pp. 15-42.

Chadwick, P. (2006). *Person-based cognitive therapy for distressing psychosis*. Chichester: Wiley & Sons.

Chadwick, P., Birchwood, M., & Trower, P.(1996) C*ognitive therapy of voices delusions and paranoia*. Chicester, UK: Wiley

Ciompi, L., & Müller, C. (1976) Labenslauf und Alter der Schizophrenen: eine katamneische Lagzeitstudie bis ins Senium. Berlin: Springer.

Durham, R. C., Guthrie, M., R. V., et al. (2003). Taysyde-Fife clinical trial of cognitive-behavioural therapy for medication-resistant psychotic symptoms: Results to 3-month follow-up. *British Journal of Psychiatry*, 182,303-311.

Falloon, I. (1988). Expressed emotion: Current status. *Psychological Medicine, 18*, 269-274

Falloon, I., et al. (1985) Family management in the prevention of morbidity of schizophrenia: clinical outcome of a two-year longitudinal study. *Archives of General Psychiatry, 42*, 887-896.

Fowler, D., Garety, P., Kuipers, E. (1995). *Cognitive behaviour therapy for psychosis: theory and practice*. Chichester:Wiley.

Garcia Montes, J. M., Soriano, C. L., et al. (2004). Aplicacion de la terapia de aceptacion y Compromiso (ACT) a sintomatologia delirante: un estudio de caso. *Psichothema, 16* (1), 117-124.

Germer, K. C. (2005). Mindfulness, what is it? What does it matter? In C. K. Germer, R. Siegel, P. R. Fulton (Eds.), *Mindfulness and psychotherapy*. New York: The Guilford Press.

Guidano, V. F., & Liotti, G., (1983). *Cognitive processes and emotional disorders*. New York: Guilford.

Gumley, A., O'Grady, M., & McNay, L. (2003). Early Intervention for relapse in schizophrenia: Results of a 12-month randomized controlled trial of cognitive behavioural therapy. *Psychological Medicine, 33*, 419-431.

Hayes, S. C., Kirk, D. S., & Wilson, K. G. (1999). *Acceptance and commitment therapy*. New York: The Guilford Press.

Hogarty, G. E. (1998). L'integrazione degli interventi. In C. L.Cazzullo, M. Clerici, & P., Bertrando. (Eds.), "*Schizofrenia ed ambiente. Modelli della malattia e tecniche di intervento*" (pp. 163-177). Milano: Franco Angeli.

Huber, G., & Schüttler R (1979). *Schizophrenie*. Berlin: Springer.

Jablensky, A. (1987) Multicultural studies and the nature of schizophrenia: A review. *Journal of Rojal Social Medicine, 80*, 162-167

Jablensky, A. (1989). An Overview of the World Helath Organization Multi-Centre Studies of Schizophrenia. In P. Williams, G. Wilkinson, & K. Rawnsley (Eds.), *The scope of epidemiological psychiatry: Essays in honour of michael sheperd*, (pp. 225-239). Esat sussex: Routledge.

Jablensky, A. (1992). Schizophrenia: Manifestations, incidence and course in different cultures. A world Health Organization ten-country study. *Psychological Medicine.* Suppl.20.

Kabat-Zinn, J. (1990) *Full catastrophe living: using the wisdom of your body and mind to face stress, pain, and illness.* New York: Dell.

Kabat-Zinn, J. (2005). *Coming to our senses: Healing ourselves and the word through mindfulness.* New York. Hyperion

Kendall, P. C. (1984). Cognitive processes and procedures in behavior therapy. In C. M. Franks, G. T. Wilson, P. C. Kendall, & K. D. Brownell. *Annual review of behavior therapy; theory and practice*, (Vol. 10, pp. 123-163). New York: Guilford Press.

Kingdon, D. G., & Turkington, D. (1991). The use of cognitive behavior therapy with a normalizing rationale in schizophrenia. Preliminary report. *Journal of Nervous and Mental Disease, 179*(4), 207-211.

Kingdon, D. G., & Turkington, D. (1994). *Cognitive behavior therapy of schizophrenia.* New York: Guilford Press

Kingdon, D. G., & Turkington D. (2005). *Cognitive therapy of schizophrenia.* New York: Guilford Press.

Kuipers, L., & Bebbington, P. (1988). Expressed Emotion research in schizophrenia: theoretical and clinical implications. *Psychological Medicine, 18*, 893-909

Kuipers, E., Garety, P., Fowler,D., et al. (1997). London-East Anglia randomised controlled trial of cognitive-behavioural therapy for psychosis: 1. Effects of the treatment phase. *British Journal Psychiatry, 173*, 319-327.

Kraepelin E. (1919). *Dementia praecox and paraphrenia.* Livingstone, Edinbourgh.

Laszlo P., & Stanghellini G. (1993). La vulnerabilità e il suo impatto sui Servizi. In A. Ballerini, F. Asioli, & G. Ceroni, (Eds.), *Psichiatria nella Comunità*, (pp. 70-94). Bollati Boringhieri, Torino.

Liddle P. F. Diagnosis and Pathophysiology of Schizophrenia (1999) In M. May, & N. Sartorius (Eds.) *Schizofrenia* 1.4; 45-47

Linehan, M. (1993) *Cognitive Behavioural treatment of borderline personality disorder.* New York: Guilford Press.

Liotti, G. (1995). *La dimensione interpersonale della coscienza.* Roma: NIS.

Lorenzini, R., & Sassaroli, S. (1992). Perchè si delira. In R. Lorenzini, & S. Sassaroli (Eds.). "La *verità privata. Il delirio e i deliranti* (pp. 39-49). – Roma: La Nuova Italia Scientifica.

Lorenzini, R., & Sassaroli, S. (1998). Patogenesi e Terapia Cognitiva del disturbo delirante. In C. Perris & P. D. McGorry (Eds.), *Cognitive Psychotherapy of Psychotic and Personality Disorders.* Chichester: Wiley

Luoma, J. B. & Hayes, S. C. (2003). Cognitive defusion. In W. O'Donohue, J. Fisher, & S. C. Hayes (Eds.), *Cognitive behaviour therapy: Applying empirically supported techniques in your practice.* New Jersey: John Wiley & sons

McKenna, P., & Oh, T.,(2005). *Schizophrenic speech.* Cambridge: Cambridge University Press.

Merleau-Ponty M. (1945) *Phénoménologie de la perception.* Paris: Gallimar.

Mills, N. (2001). The experience of fragmentation in psychosis: Can mindfulness help?. In I. Clarke (Ed.), *Psychosis and spirituality.* London and Philadelphia: Whurr Publishers.

Morrison, A. P. (1994). Cognitive behaviour therapy for auditory hallucinations without concurrent medication: A single case. *Behavioural & Cognitive Psychotherapy, 22*, 259-264.

Morrison, A. P. (1998). A cognitive analysis of the maintenance of auditory hallucinations: Are voices to schizophrenia what bodily sensations are to panic? *Behavioural and Cognitive Psychotherapy, 26*, 289–302.

Morrison, A. P., Haddock, G. & Tarrier, N. (1995). Intrusive thoughts and auditory hallucinations: A cognitive approach. *Behavioural & Cognitive Psychotherapy, 23*, 265–280.

Mundt, C. (1985) *Das Apathiesyndrom der Schizophrenen.* Berlin, Heidelberg, New York: Springer.

Paltrinieri, E., & De Girolamo, G. (1996) La riabilitazione psichiatrica oggi: Verso una pratica "evidence-based". *Noos, 3*(1), 201.

Pankey, J., & Hayes S. C. (2003). Acceptance and Commitment therapy for psychosis. *International Journal of Psychology and Psychological Therapy, 3*(2), 311–328.

Penn D. L., & Mueser K. T. (1996). Research update on the psychosocial treatment of Schizophrenia. *American Journal of Psychiatry, 153*(5), 607.

Perris, C. (1989) *Cognitive therapy with schizophrenic patients.* New York: The Guilford Press.

Perris, C., & Skagerlind, L., (1994). Cognitive therapy with schizophrenic patients. *Acta Psychiatrica Scandinavica*, 89(382), 65–70.

Pinto, A., Gigantesco, A., Morosini, P., & La Pia, S. (2007). Development, reliability and validity of a self-administered questionnaire on subjective opinion about delusions and voices. *Psychopathology, 40*(5), 312–320.

Pinto, A., Kingdon, D., Turkington, D., (In press). Cognitive Behaviour Therapy for Psychosis: Enhancing the therapeutic relationship to improve the quality of life. In G. Simos (Ed.), *CBT -A guide for the Practicing Clinician-Vol. II.* East Sussex: Routledge, 1–17.

Pinto, A., La Pia, S., Mennella, R., et al. (1999). Cognitive Behavioral therapy and clozapine for clients with treatment refractory schizophrenia. *Psychiatric Services, 50*, 901–904.

Roberts, G. W. (1991) Schizophrenia a neuropathological perspective. British Journal of Psychiatry, 158, 8–17, January.

Rogers, E., Anthony, W. A., Toole, J., & Brown, M. A. (1991). Vocational outcomes following psychosocial rehabilitation: A longitudinal study of three programs. Journal of Vocational *Rehabilitation, 1*, 21–29

Sartorius N., Jablensky A., Korten A., Ernberg G., Anker M., Cooper J., et al. (1986). Early manifestations and first-contact incidence of schizophrenia in different culture. *Psychological Medicine, 16*, 909–928.

Segal, Z. V., Williams, J. M., & Teasdale, J. D. (2002) *Mindfulness-based cognitive therapy for depression.* New York: Guilford Press.

Sensky, T., Turkington, D., Kingdon, D., et al. (2000). A randomized controlled trial of cognitive-behavioural therapy for persistent symptoms in schizophrenia resistant to medication. *Archives of General Psychiatry, 57*, 165–172.

Tarrier, N., Harwood, S., Yusupoff, L., et al. (1990). Coping Strategy Enhancement (CSE): a method of treating residual schizophrenic symptoms. *Behavioural Psychotherapy, 18*, 283.

Tarrier, N., Yusupoff, L., Kinney, C., et al. (1998). Randomised controlled trial of intensive cognitive behaviour therapy for patients with chronic schizophrenia. *British Medical Journal, 317*, 303–307.

Turkington, D., Kingdon, D., & Weiden, P. J. (2006). Cognitive behavior therapy for schizophrenia. *American Journal of Psychiatry, 163*, 365–373.

Weinberger D. (1987). Implications of normal brain development for the pathogenesis of schizophrenia. *Archives of General Psychiatry, 44*(7), 660–669, July.

Williams, S., (2002). Anxiety, associated physiological sensations, and delusional catastrophic misinterpretation: Variations on a theme? In A. P. Morrison (Ed.), *A casebook of cognitive therapy for psychosis.* New York: Brunner-Routledge.

Word Health Organization. (1973) *The International Pilot Study of Schizophrenia*, Chapter 11. World Health Organization, Geneva.

World Health Organization (1979). *Schizophrenia: An international follow-up study*. Chichester, UK: Wiley.

Wykes, T., & Reeder, C. (2005) *Cognitive remediation in therapy*. East Sussex: Routledge.

Zimmermann, G., Favrof, J., Trieu V. H. et al. (2005). The effect of cognitive behavioural treatment on the positive symptoms of schizophrenia spectrum disorders: A Meta-Analysys. *Schizophrenia Research, 77*, 1-9.

19

Mindfulness-Based Stress Reduction for Chronic Pain Management

Jacqueline Gardner-Nix

"Pain is not just a 'body problem', it is a whole-systems problem."
Jon Kabat-Zinn

It is time the medical community acknowledged the other half of the system
Jackie Gardner-Nix

Introduction

Pain is a common complaint in primary care, with chronic pain reported in 20% of visits to general practitioners (McCaffrey et al., 2003). Twenty percent of adults suffer from chronic pain, rising to half of those of the older age population (Cousins et al., 2004). Chronic pain, defined as "intermittent or continuous pain persisting longer than six months or beyond the regular healing time for a given injury" can impact on patients' physical and emotional well-being (Siddall et al., 2004) and may be associated with disability disproportionate to degree of injury, as well as with depression and anxiety (Bair et al., 2003). Despite analgesics, surgeries and procedures, pain is poorly controlled by traditional Western medicine (Cousins et al., 2004, Furrow, 2001). Opioids are sometimes prescribed for chronic pain, but the undesirable side-effects of these drugs and their ability to lose their effects over time are well-documented (Gardner-Nix, 2003). Consequently, many patients have turned to alternative modalities to control their suffering.

Psychological factors such as mood changes and anxiety have been shown to alter pain perception (Jensen et al., 1994; Villemure and Bushnell, 2002). A meta-analysis of psychological interventions for chronic low back pain (Hoffman et al., 2007) provided support for the efficacy of psychological interventions in reducing self-reported pain, pain-related interference, depression, and disability in sufferers of low back pain. The study also demonstrated that multidisciplinary programs that included psychological interventions were superior to other active treatment programs at improving work-related outcomes at both short and long-term follow-up.

The workings of the mind in appreciating pain (Seminowicz and Davis, 2007) and even in permitting or clearing painful responses such as inflammation, nerve irritation and muscle spasm at painful body sites are especially interesting in view of studies showing no correlations between pain perception and imaging studies of painful areas such as with CAT scans. Boos et al. (1995) showed no correlation between pathological findings and back pain symptoms, and that disk herniation was just as common amongst patients with no back pain as patients with back pain. Boden et al. (1990) showed abnormal MRI scans of the lumbar spines in individuals with no back pain. Adding to the mystery of why some suffer for years with chronic pain is the discovery of a genetic predisposition to feel and suffer more pain in certain people inheriting a variant of the catechol-O-methyltransferase (COMT) gene versus others considered more stoical to pain (Zubieta et al., 2003), and the discovery that past experiences of abuse, such as in childhood, in susceptible individuals might predispose to poor healing and chronic pain in later adulthood (Schofferman and associates 1993; Grzesiak, 2003).

In trying to understand what influences susceptibility to developing chronic pain, work in other areas of illness connecting psychosocial factors to predisposition to illness may shed light. Kobasa (1979) posed the question: what distinguishes those who are exposed to stressful life events and do not get sick from those who do? She studied middle and upper level executives and in a sample of 161, she found that those not getting sick in general show more hardiness, having a stronger commitment to self, an attitude of vigor toward the environment, a sense of meaningfulness, and an internal locus of control. The work of Rosengren et al. (2004) found stress, anxiety and depression increased the risk of heart attacks as much as obesity, cholesterol, and hypertension, also increasing understanding of psychological influences on health, which might shed further light on why psychological interventions are so important in illnesses involving chronic pain.

Bruehl et al. (2002, 2003) found correlations between trait anger and anger style (anger in versus anger out) and sensitivity to acute and chronic pain stimuli, and response to opioids. Carson et al. (2005) reported lack of forgiveness correlated with an increased likelihood of life being affected by chronic low back pain. Carson et al. (2006) reported an eight week loving-kindness meditation program pilot study on 43 chronic low back pain patients randomly assigned to study group or usual care controls; they showed significant decreases in pain and psychological distress in the study group.

Baliki et al. (2006) have also shown that long term back pain on functional MRI imaging shows activity in the prefrontal cortex as an imprinted memory and fear of pain, and that the longer the person has suffered from the pain the higher the activity in that part of the brain: described as cumulative memory. Millecamps et al. (2007) showed that erasing the emotional pain in that area of the brain with a drug: D-cycloserine in rats, appeared to cause them to no longer be bothered by the pain even though the physical pain, as experienced in the thalamus where the sensation is registered, had only partly reduced. Erasing the emotional pain also reduced the physical sensitivity at the site of injury in the animal model. D-cycloserine has been used to treat phobias in humans.

The above studies suggest that treatments targeting the higher cognitive centers which are involved in the chronic pain experience might be more fruitful than targeting pain sensation or pain vigilance and attention. These reports give some insights into the ways in which Mindfulness and Meditation may influence the experience of chronic pain.

Mindfulness-Based Stress Reduction (MBSR) and Pain

Kabat-Zinn (1982) reported on the outcomes of MBSR in a sample of 51 individuals afflicted with chronic pain. Dominant pain categories were back, neck, shoulder and headache. Sixty-five percent of the participants showed a reduction of ≥33% in pain ratings and 50% showed a reduction of ≥50%. In addition, 76% of participants reported a reduction in mood disturbance of ≥33 and 62% of participants reported a reduction of ≥50%. A limitation of the study was that there was no control group.

A follow-up study (Kabat-Zinn et al., 1985) compared chronic pain sufferers who participated in a 10 week mindfulness program with a group receiving traditional treatment protocols including nerve blocks and medication. The results in the control group demonstrated no improvement in parameters that were found to significantly improve in the mindfulness group: anxiety, depression, present moment pain, negative body image and inhibition of activity by pain. Pain-related drug utilization reduced in the mindfulness group and activity levels and self-esteem increased. This remained the same at 15-month follow-up for both groups, except for present moment pain which returned to pre-intervention levels in the treatment group.

Kabat-Zinn et al. (1987) later reported significant reductions in medical and psychological symptoms continuing up to four years after the completion of the course in 225 participants. Response rates to questionnaires ranged from 53 to 70%. Twenty percent cited that they had developed a "new outlook on life" while 40% stated that they had the ability to control, understand, or cope better with their pain and stress. A weakness of the study is inherent in the likelihood that responders to the questionnaires might have been more likely to be those who did benefit.

Mindfulness meditation has been found to facilitate significant improvements in the mental as well as the physical aspects of chronic pain. A study by Sephton et al. (2007) investigating 91 women diagnosed with fibromyalgia showed that the mindfulness meditation intervention group experienced a significant decrease in depressive symptoms when compared to a waitlist control group, and these effects remained stable two months after the end of the study. When depressive symptoms were broken down into the subtypes of cognitive and somatic symptoms, it was found that MBSR significantly decreased the occurrence of both types in patients in the intervention group.

Sagula and Rice (2004) investigated the effects of MBSR on the bereavement process for their losses in chronic pain sufferers. They compared 39 participants with 18 in their control group who were on a waiting list or receiving other therapies. The Mindfulness group advanced significantly more quickly through the initial stages of grieving than the control group, and demonstrated significant reductions in depression and state anxiety, though did not differ from the control group in the final stages of grieving and trait anxiety. Pain outcomes were not measured.

Ott et al. (2006) surveyed the literature for the effectiveness of Mindfulness courses for cancer patients for many parameters including depression, fatigue, sleep, and physical parameters, but found only one conference abstract measuring influences on pain. This was in 10 patients undergoing stem cell/autologous bone marrow transplants undergoing lengthy hospitalization. They found a significant decrease in pain from the intervention, as well as increases in happiness, relaxation and comfort, and found that most were still using mindfulness up to three months post-discharge.

Plews-Ogan et al. (2005) reported on a pilot study of a comparison of 8 weekly sessions of MBSR with once a week massage, and standard care (seen every 3 months with medication adjustments) in 30 chronic musculoskeletal pain sufferers (23 female), randomized to the intervention. The numeric pain scale (Farrar et al., 2001) and the SF 12 (brief quality of life questionnaire) were used in assessment. In the MBSR group there were three dropouts before the start of the eight week course, only five completing seven of eight sessions and one attending only three sessions, though completing all the questionnaires. There was only one drop out in the massage group and two in the standard care group. Although there was a trend toward pain decrease in all groups the only drop in pain scale score to reach significance was in the massage group at week eight, reducing by a mean of almost three points on the numeric pain scale, but by week 12 it was not maintained or statistically significant. For the quality of life scores there was a significant increase in mental health scores in both the massage and MBSR group by week 8, but not in the standard care group, an increase which was only sustained in the MBSR group by week 12 when the interventions had been stopped for 4 weeks.

Pradham et al. (2007) reported significant improvements in psychological distress (35% reduction) in 31 women suffering from rheumatoid arthritis up to 6 months after completing an MBSR program which was followed by a 4-month maintenance program, compared to a randomized wait-list control group, but there was no significant change in disease parameters and pain changes were not reported.

Morone et al. (2008a) reported on the effect of the MBSR course on 37 older adults, 65 years and older, suffering pain, randomized to wait list control or active intervention, and also tested them three months after taking the course. Meditation occurred on an average of 4.3 days a week, for an average of 31.6 minutes a day. Their outcomes suggested significantly improved acceptance of their limits, increased activity, and improved physical function. In another paper Morone et al. (2008b) used grounded theory and content analysis to do a qualitative study on diary entries of 27 MBSR older adult participants, with pain, demonstrating that they had been able to achieve pain reduction by mindfully focusing on tasks and mindfully pacing activities which had been causing pain increases, and had greater insight into their emotional processing which worsened pain.

However, psychological interventions such as mindfulness and meditation have been demonstrated to have physiological effects, which likely mediate the improvements experienced by the participants in these programs. Studies which included looking at immune system parameters showed improvements associated with Mindfulness program participation in breast and prostate cancer (Carlson et al., 2003), in T cell counts in HIV positive men receiving instruction on relaxation, hypnosis and meditation (Taylor, 1995), in flu vaccine response in normal workers (Davidson et al., 2003) and that meditation increased the rate of clearing of psoriasis lesions compared to controls (Kabat-Zinn et al., 1998). It is possible that inflammation and neural instability at the site of damage in chronic pain patients might change in participants of these courses leading to reduced pain and enhanced healing.

Mindfulness-Based Chronic Pain Management Courses

We have explored the effectiveness of a mindfulness-based chronic pain management (MBCPM) program which we developed based on MBSR. The program was modified to increase accessibility to those who had been referred to the pain management clinics of two Toronto teaching hospitals (Gardner-Nix et al., 2008).

A concern for most of the Mindfulness research in the literature has been the lack of randomized controlled studies. We felt that to randomize would bias the study in the direction of those who were of lower acuity and higher motivation to do the course and who would therefore be prepared to agree to a delay of possibly several months. Pre-course start drop out rates were high as patients with severe pain (our population's "usual" pain was scored around 6/10 where 10 is excruciating), tended not to agree to wait long for an intervention, which was not going to be a fast fix. We therefore used non-randomized wait-list controls.

Classes are once a week for two hours for ten weeks, at two Toronto teaching hospitals, or at the patients' local hospitals linking by telemedicine. Some classes involve mixing the onsite patients with distant site, while other classes are conducted separately. The use of telemedicine (IP transmission at 384 kbit/s; Gardner-Nix et al., 2008) for inclusion of those living in rural areas has proven very important as traveling long distances increases the pain, which is also increased by stress.

Mindfulness for Chronic Pain: Course Outline

At the initial classes participants are taught about mindfulness and the concept of meditation versus relaxation, using initially the breath as a focus. They are started on meditations of five minute durations only, and encouraged to participate in the class from any position: they may lie on the floor or stand for the entire class if their physical pain requires that. Classes also involved teaching on lifestyle habits: diet, exercise, sleep, and relationships, as well as on the attitudes described in Kabat-Zinn's "Full Catastrophe Living" (p. 33–41). Large group and small group discussions on the topic of the week are conducted in each class. Meditation tracks are provided on CDs narrated by the class facilitator (JGN) and include a 30 minute body scan (started in the third week) which is quite anatomical and highly relevant to pain sufferers. During the body scan they are encouraged to watch what happens emotionally and to their pain intensity and quality when scanning the part(s) of the body that hurts, and see if there is a tendency to mentally amputate or ignore it/them. This tends to improve over time, though some report having to return to the scan later after using other meditations, to note that they have now "taken back" those parts of their body.

Patients are asked to meditate daily at home to a selection of CD meditation tracks varying from 5 to 30 minutes in length and encouraged to use meditative positions which are comfortable given their pain condition. Jon Kabat-Zinn's lake and mountain meditation tracks are also used. Some meditations involve visualization of their pain with guidance to decrease it For example, they may see their pain as like a block of ice, and bring their attention fully to it and start to observe it melt. Meditations longer than 30 minutes are thought not to be as acceptable for those in chronic pain and might reduce compliance after course end.

Yoga is replaced by mindful movements, most of which are based on hatha yoga, which can all be done from a standing position, with some being done from a sitting position. Participants are encouraged to trust their judgment about which they can or cannot do. Walking meditation is usually assigned as homework to see if that becomes a preferred meditation. It is suggested that consideration be given to transforming the walking meditation into swimming if the patients move with less pain in water, and mindful movements can also be done in water rather than on dry land. Where there is agitation, anxiety, panic attacks, flashbacks, an increase in stress or a tendency to always fall asleep, movement or walking meditation is usually preferred.

Homework includes: watching their tendency to judge, rather than just note and evaluate; determining what exacerbated their pain and what helped it, paying attention to emotional factors as well as physical ones; doing simple or mundane tasks mindfully (showering, cleaning out a cupboard, watching a teabag diffuse), which they then described in small group work, and mindfully preparing and eating a meal, also discussed in small group work. Artwork or collage is requested in the latter part of the course to commit their idea of their pain to paper, or to a 3D structure. The symbolism of the artwork is discussed in class if the class member wishes to share it. Some prefer to journal rather than draw. Homework also includes readings from Jon Kabat-Zinn's book "Full Catastrophe Living," specifically on attitudes, stress, pain, and chapters pertaining to the different types of meditation.

There is no silent day-long retreat introduced between later classes in the course due to poor attendance at that day, apparently due to fear, during the first year the course was offered. Participants are allowed to repeat the courses, and frequently do. There is approximately a 33% drop out rate from the course defined as those attending 4 of 10 classes or less, with a higher rate of drop outs in onsite classes versus distant site.

Case Scenario 1

A 39-year-old male factory worker, was referred for pain control. He had had four back surgeries after injuring his back at work in 1989, was on Worker's Compensation, and was reporting pain scores of 8 to 9/10. He was initially optimized in the pain clinic on transdermal fentanyl 100 mcg/hr every 2 days, methadone 9 mg every 12 hours, gabapentin 900 mg 3 x a day, and acetaminophen 325 mg/oxycodone 5 mg, 4 tablets a day for rescue analgesia. He was referred for the MBCPM course, driving 11/2 hours weekly to attend the initial course, and repeating the course from a distant site once we were able to link through telemedicine to his community. Towards the end of the first course he found he was able to deal with extended family relationships, which he had found quite troublesome throughout his life. He began to reduce his medications. During the second course he was able to wean himself off the rest of his medications, and start a running program. Three years later, he is currently working in a non manual job, and reports he continues to meditate daily, sometimes several times a day, for 10 to 40 minutes at a time.

Case Scenario 2

A 38-year-old female auto assembly line worker was referred to the pain clinic with a continuous severe headache 1 month after surgical removal of two cavernous hemangiomas from her cervical spine, reporting pain scores of 8-9/10 (zero = no pain, 10 = excruciating pain). She had sensory loss below T4 after her surgery but was being retrained to walk. CT/MRI studies were negative. Tricyclic antidepressants and anticonvulsants were unhelpful, and she was tried on all opioids sequentially, including methadone. Over next 2 years her opioid dose increased to 400 mg CR-oxycodone every 8 hours, with hydromorphone 72 mg every 4 hours for rescue analgesia. She was ambulating with a walker, was prone to pneumonia, was on oxygen, used a continuous positive airway pressure (CPAP) machine at night, and received attendant care at home.

Pain scores on her medications were usually 7/10. She completed two courses of the MBCPM, connected by telemedicine from a distant site, separating the two courses by four months. She stabilized her medication requirements during the first course, unusual for her as she reported tolerance to her opioid medications approximately every 2 months. Six months after the start of the second course she had been able to reduce her CR-oxycodone dosage to 40 mg every 12 hours, her hydromorphone rescue analgesic to 24 mg 3 times a day, and she was off oxygen and walking without a walker. She no longer needed attendant care, and her "usual" pain scores were around 3-4/10. She would have returned to work except for the sensory loss below T4. She reported she was meditating 30 minutes a day, and if she missed for a few days her pain scores rose and she experienced reduced function.

In the next year she separated from her husband and became a single mother of two teens. She reported her pain scores rose when in the presence of her ex-husband.

Two years later she has been able to convince her employers to allow her to return to work. She was retrained for a job in her car plant which would be safe given her sensory loss. She continues to meditate, using the body scan, daily.

Outcomes

We hypothesized that participants in the treatment group would experience an overall decrease in pain ratings (Numeric pain rating scale, Farrar et al. 2001), pain catastrophizing (Sullivan et al., 1995), and suffering (Pictorial Representation of Illness and Self Measure: PRISM test, Büchi et al., 2002), and an increase in their quality of life (SF 36 v2, Ware, 2000) when compared to those in the waiting list control group by class 10. We also looked at response by gender, hypothesizing that females in the treatment group would show greater improvement in these areas than males, as this is the trend that has been observed in the previous literature. Women made up 70% of the population presenting to our pain clinics and classes, an observation in line with reports that men are less willing to report pain than women (Robinson et al., 2001) and those men who seek pain management report greater levels of mood disturbance than women (Fow and Smith-Seemiller, 2001).

Finally as we were offering the course through telemedicine to outlying areas in Ontario, Canada, we compared outcomes between the course participants taught in person and those taught through telemedicine (Gardner-Nix et al., 2008).

Two hundred and thirty three chronic noncancer pain patients were studied, and included 178 females and 55 males, participating onsite ($N = 95$), by telemedicine from a distant site ($N = 79$) and fifty nine wait-list controls.

Health conditions included back pain, headache and facial pain, arthritis, fibromyalgia, and "other." Eighty seven patients with chronic back or neck pain were also analyzed separately from the total treatment group.

Previous research has found that pain catastrophizing, defined as "an exaggerated negative orientation toward pain stimuli and pain experience" is a significant predictor of suffering and disability (Sullivan et al., 1995, 1998). These scores seemed the most sensitive measure to change during MBCPM. Overall pain catastrophizing showed significant improvement over time, for both distant and onsite groups. Both onsite and distant groups experienced less pain magnification and helplessness over time than the control group, and the distant group also ruminated less over time than controls. Highly significant reductions which occurred in patients' pain catastrophizing scores over time did not differ between males and females, or patients with back pain versus other pain.

Treatment with mindfulness and meditation did significantly improve patients' quality of life in terms of role physical, general health, vitality, social functioning, and mental health scores, results consistent with those found by Sephton et al. (2007) who studied fibromyalgia sufferers. Treatment was less successful in the physical domains of the SF-36v2 than in the mental health domains, suggesting that ten weeks is not a long enough time period in which to observe significant changes in the physical aspects of quality of life in prolonged pain sufferers. Distant site participants benefited as much as onsite participants, though they started the course with significantly lower physical quality of life scores than onsite participants (Gardner-Nix et al., 2008). It was speculated that participants onsite had to cope with big city traffic and parking and were less likely to sign up for the course if too disabled to manage such challenges. There were no significant differences in effectiveness due to gender or pain type (back pain versus other pain).

It has been reported that a drop of 2 points on the numeric zero to ten pain scale should be considered clinically significant but the authors did not analyze the influence of this drop on disability, mood, and perceived suffering (Farrar et al. 2001). Patients have reported a "reframing" of their pain with mindfulness, and we have observed anecdotally reduced disability levels in the presence of only slightly changing pain scale scores. In this study "usual" pain scores differed between groups: the "usual" pain of the onsite patients improved significantly by the end of the course, though by an average of only 1 point on the pain scale, compared to controls, but not the distant site. Males in the treatment group had lower usual pain ratings than females at weeks 1 and 10. Significant differences were also seen between patients with back pain versus patients with other pain conditions: initially, the back pain patients rated their usual pain as significantly higher than patients with other conditions, and when measured again at Week 10, this difference was still present, though "usual" pain levels did decrease over the course.

The PRISM test is a visual/tactile tool thought to assess the burden of suffering due to illness and the intrusiveness and controllability of the illness or its symptoms, and has been validated for Rheumatoid Arthritis (Büchi et al., 2002), and Lupus (Buchi et al., 2000). We recently validated this tool for use in the chronic pain population (Kassardjian et al., in press). Patients are presented with an $8.5'' \times 11''$ paper with a yellow disk (7 cm diameter) in the bottom left-hand corner representing "self," and handed five additional disks (5 cm diameter) representing pain, work, partner, family, and recreation. Patients are asked to place the disks relative to the self-disk to describe the intrusiveness or importance of each of these influences on their lives. Disks that are placed in close proximity to the self-disk are considered prominent features in the patient's life. The distances (in centimeters) between the center of the self-disk and the centers of the other disks provide quantitative parameters. If treatment has been effective in reducing suffering due to pain, the distance between the "pain" disk and the "self" disk will increase, while the other disks might move closer to the self, provided they represent positive aspects of the individual's life. Interpretations of the non-pain disks can only be made in the context of the patients' lives.

It was found that overall, there was a significant difference in PRISM pain scores for both onsite and distant site groups relative to controls. Males' and females' pain suffering was shown to differ significantly. The males' mean distances between the pain and self-disks were greater than those of females at week 1, suggesting that males experienced less pain suffering before treatment began. This is contrary to observations by Fow and Seemiller (2001) if mood disturbance is correlated with suffering. At week 10, males and females distances between pain and self-disks showed similar significant improvements. Patients with back pain were also found to differ in terms of pain suffering when compared to those with other pain conditions, who appeared to suffer less as a result of their pain than those with back pain at week 1. Though both groups improved significantly the difference between them was observed again at Week 10, suggesting that the patients with chronic back pain indicated greater suffering than patients experiencing other types of chronic pain.

An interesting effect of the mindfulness course appeared in validating the PRISM test for the chronic pain population using the parallel data being collected to study the effectiveness of the MBCPM course. In assessing convergent validity, better correlations were found at class 10 than class 1. This suggested the patients were either more familiar with the concept of this test at class 10, or they were more mindful of the influences of the parameters being studied on "self."

The Future of Mindfulness in Chronic Pain Management

A major part of the training on mindfulness involves arriving at acceptance of the pain and disability in the present moment and a letting go of the struggle to return to pre morbid status. McCracken (McCracken et al., 2004a, b; McCracken and Eccleston, 2005; McCracken and Yang, 2006; McCracken et al., 2007; McCracken, 2007; McCracken and Vowles, 2007) has written extensively on the role of acceptance in chronic pain and a refocusing of participating in valued actions in life irrespective of the pain. Hayes (2004) has published on the effectiveness of acceptance and commitment therapy, which incorporates mindfulness to train patients to engage in valued activities regardless of pain. McCracken and Eccleston (2005) reported that pain intensity and functioning were unrelated, but those reporting greater acceptance of their pain were better in terms of emotional social and physical functioning when assessed 3.9 months after first evaluation, using less medication and report a better work status. Their work is questioning the cognitive-behavioral beliefs, which follow the assumption that if attention and awareness of pain are lessened, the physical and emotional effects of pain will reduce. Acceptance correlated with better functional and emotional outcomes than reduction in awareness of and vigilance to pain.

Along with acceptance it seems likely that a predisposition to a heightened stress response and slower recovery which is cumulative due to past stressful events (McEwen, 2007) might accompany the perpetuation of pain, and Goleman and Swartz (1976) described, 31 years ago, that recovery from the stress response was hastened by meditation practice.

These findings may question the drive of pain management programs to work with decreasing pain perception such as on numeric scales and correlating the degree of decrease with clinical improvement. The acceptance literature also suggests that data on pain intensity reductions due to standard interventions (such as procedures, medication) should be followed prospectively to monitor whether emotional and functional improvements result, are maintained, and continue to improve, or whether they return to pre-intervention levels in a few months. Pain scales may prove less useful in the future and tools such as the chronic pain acceptance questionnaire (CPAQ) (McCracken et al., 2004b), chronic pain values inventory (CPVI) (McCracken et al., 2006), and the PRISM test (Buchi and Sensky, 1999) may have more relevance.

Acute physical pain is a warning that something in the body is malfunctioning and damaged. Chronic pain may be a warning that the body/mind has been challenged for too long or too intensely in some way, and is not able to remain well, heal or cope beyond a certain level of physical or emotional stress, which may be cumulative. Although in the US this is the decade dedicated to the elimination of pain, even chronic pain should be seen as a symptom: a warning that something needs to change more globally in the patient's life. Mindfulness, and acceptance and commitment therapy are interventions which may increasingly offer that opportunity in the future of pain management.

References

Bair M. J., Robinson R. L., Katon W., Kroenke K. (2003). Depression and pain comorbidity: A literature review. Archives of Internal Medicine, *163*, 2433–2445.

Baliki M. N., Chialvo D. R., Geha P. Y., Levy R. M., Harden N., Parrish T. B., Apkarian A. V., (2006). Chronic pain and the emotional brain: Specific brain activity associated with spontaneous fluctuations of intensity of chronic back pain. *The Journal of Neuroscience, 26*(47), 12165–12173.

Boden S., Davis D., Dina T., Patronas N., Wiesel S., (1990). Abnormal magnetic resonance scans of the lumbar spine in asymptomatic subjects. Journal of Bone Joint Surgery, *72*, 403-408.

Boos N., Reider R., Schade V., Spratt K., Semmer N., Aebi M., (1995). The diagnostic accuracy of magnetic resonance imaging, work perception and psychosocial factors in identifying symptomatic disc herniation. *Spine, 20*, 2613-2625.

Bruehl S., Burns J. W., Chung O. Y., Ward P., Johnson B., (2002). Anger and pain sensitivity in chronic low back pain patients and pain-free controls: The role of endogenous opioids. *Pain, 99*(1-2), 223-233.

Bruehl S., Chung O. Y., Burns J. W., Biridepalli S., (2003). The association between anger expression and chronic pain intensity: Evidence for partial mediation by endogenous opioid dysfunction. *Pain, 106*(3), 317-324.

Büchi S., Buddeberg C., Klaghofer R., Russi E. W., Bandli O., Schlosser C., Stoll T., Villiger P. M., Sensky T. (2002). Preliminary validation of PRISM (Pictorial Representation of Illness and Self Measure) - A brief method to assess suffering. *Psychother Psychosom, 71*(6): 333-341.

Buchi S., Sensky T. (1999). PRISM: Pictorial representation of illness and self measure: A brief nonverbal measure of illness impact and therapeutic aid in psychosomatic medicine. *Psychocsomatics, 40*, 314-320.

Buchi S., Villiger P., Kauer Y., Klaghofer R., Sensky T., Stoll T. (2000). PRISM (Pictorial Representation of Illness and Self Measure)-A novel visual method to assess the global burden of illness in patients with systemic lupus erythamatosis. *Lupus, 9*, 368-373.

Carlson L. E., Speca M., Patel K. D., Goodey E. (2003). Mindfulness-based stress reduction in relation to quality of life, mood, symptoms of stress, and immune parameters in breast and prostate cancer outpatients. *Psychosomatic Medicine, 65*, 571-581.

Carson J. W., Keefe F. J., Goli V., Fras A. M., Lynch T. R., Thorp S. R., Buechler J. L. (2005). Forgiveness and chronic low back pain: A preliminary study examining the relationship of forgiveness to pain, anger, and psychological distress. *Journal of Pain, 6*, 84-91.

Carson J. W., Keefe F. J., Lynch T. R., Carson K. M., Goli V., Fras A. M., Thorp S. R., (2006). Loving-kindness meditation for chronic low back pain: Results from a pilot trial. *Pain, 124*, 287-294.

Cousins M. J., Brennan F., Carr D. B. (2004). Pain relief: A universal human right. Pain, *112*, 1-4.

Davidson R. J., Kabat-Zinn J., Schumacher J., Rosenkranz M., Muller D., Santorelli S. F., Urbanowski F., Harrington A., Bonus K., Sheridan J. F. (2003). Alterations in brain and immune function produced by mindfulness meditation. *Psychotherapy and Psychosomatic Medicine, 65*, 564-570.

Farrar J. T., Young J. P., LaMoreaux L., Werth J. L., Poole R. M. (2001). Clinical importance of changes in chronic pain intensity measured on an 11- point numeric pain rating scale. *Pain, 94*, 149-158.

Fow R. N., Smith-Seemiller L. (2001). Impact of gender, compensation status and chronicity on treatment response in chronic pain patients. *Journal of Applied Rehabilitation Counseling, 2*, 32.

Furrow B. (2001). Pain management and provider liability: No more excuses. *Journal of Law Medicine and Ethics, 29*, 28-51.

Gardner-Nix J. (2003). Principles of opioid use in chronic noncancer pain. *CMAJ, 169*, 38-43.

Gardner-Nix, J., Backman, S., Barbati, J. Grummitt, J. (2008) Evaluating Distance Education of a Mindfulness-based Meditation Programme for Chronic Pain Management. *Journal of Telemed. and Telecare, 14*, 88-92.

Goleman D. J., Schwartz G. E. (1979). Meditation as an intervention in stress reactivity. *Journal of Consulting and Clinical Psychology, 44(3)*, 456-466.

Grzesiak R. C. (2003). Revisiting pain-prone personalities: Combining psychodynamics with the neurobiological sequelae of trauma. *American Journal of Pain Management, 13*, 6-15.

Hayes S. C., (2004). Acceptance and commitment therapy, relational frame theory, and the third wave of behaviour therapy. *Behaviou Therapy, 35*, 639-665.

Hoffman B. M., Papas, R. K., Chatkoff, D. K., Kerns, R. D. (2007). Meta-analysis of psychological intervention for chronic low back pain. *Health Psychology, 26*(1), 1-9.

Jensen M. P., Turner J. A., Romano J. M. (1994). Correlates of improvement in multidisciplinary treatment of chronic pain. *J Consult Clin Psychol 62*, 172-9.

Kabat-Zinn J. (1982). An outpatient program in behavioral medicine for chronic pain patients based on the practice of mindfulness meditation: Theoretical considerations and preliminary results. *General Hospital Psychiatry, 4*, 33-47.

Kabat-Zinn J., Lipworth L., Burney R. (1985). The clinical use of mindfulness meditation for the self-regulation of chronic pain. *Journal of Behavioral Medicine, 8*, 163-190.

Kabat-Zinn J., Lipworth L., Burney R., Sellers W. (1987). Four-year follow-up of a meditation-based program for the self-regulation of chronic pain: Treatment outcomes and compliance. *Clinical Journal of Pain, 2*, 159-173.

Kabat-Zinn J., Wheeler E., Light T., Skillings A., Scharf M. J., Cropley T. G., Hosmer D., Bernhard J. D., (1998). Influence of a mindfulness meditation-based stress reduction intervention on rates of skin clearing in patients with moderate to severe psoriasis undergoing phototherapy (UVB) and photochemotherapy (PUVA). *Psychosomatic Medicine, 60*, 625-632.

Kassardjian C, Gardner-Nix J. S., Dupak K, Barbati J, Lam-Mc Culloch J. "Validation of PRISM method of assessing global burden of illness and self measure in non cancer pain patients". *Journal of Pain*. (In press).

Kobasa S. (1979). Stressful life events, personality, and health: An inquiry into hardiness. *Journal of Personality and Social Psychology, 37*, 1.

McCaffrey R., Frock T. L., Garguilo H. (2003). Understanding chronic pain and the mind-body connection. *Holistic Nursing Practice, 17*, 281-287(quiz):288-289.

McCracken L. M. (2007). Contextual analysis of attention to chronic pain: What the patient does with their pain might be more important than their awareness pr vigilance alone. *Journal of Pain, 8*, 230-236.

McCracken L. M., Carson J. W., Eccleston C., Keefe F. J. (2004a). Acceptance and change in the context of chronic pain. *Pain, 109*, 4-7.

McCracken L. M., Eccleston C. (2005). A Prospective study of acceptance of pain and patient functioning with chronic pain. *Pain, 118*, 164-169.

McCracken L. M., Gauntlett-Gilbert J., Vowles K. E. (2007). The role of mindfulness in a contextual cognitive-behavioral analysis of chronic pain-related suffering and disability. *Pain, 131*, 63-69.

McCracken L. M., Vowles E. K. (2007). Psychological flexibility and traditional pain management strategies in relation to patient functioning with chronic pain: An examination of a revised instrument. *Journal of Pain, 8*, 700-707.

McCracken L. M., Vowles K. E., Eccleston C., (2004b). Acceptance of chronic pain: component analysis and a revised assessment method. *Pain, 107*, 159-166.

McCracken L. M., Yang, S. (2006). The role of values in a contextual cognitive-behavioral approach to chronic pain. *Pain, 123*, 137-145.

McEwen B. S. (2007). Physiology and neurobiology of stress and adaptation: central role of the brain. *Physiological Reviews, 87*, 873-904

Millecamps M., Centeno M. V., Berra, H. H., Rudick, C. N., Lavarello S., Tkatch T., Apkarian, A. V. (2007). D-cycloserine reduces neuropathic pain behaviour through limbic NMDA-mediated circuitry. *Pain, 132*, 1-2.

Morone N. E., Lynch C. S., Greco C. M., Tindle H. A., Weiner D. K. (2008a). "I Feel Like a New Person". The Effects of Mindfulness Meditation on Older Adults with Chronic Pain: A Qualitative Narrative Analysis of Diary Entries. *Journal of Pain, 9*, 841-848.

Morone N. E., Greco C. M., Weiner D. K. (2008b). Mindfulness meditation for the treatment of chronic low back pain in older adults: A randomized controlled pilot study. *Pain, 134*, 310-319.

Osman A., Barrios F., Gutierrez P., Kopper B., Merrifield T., Grittmann, L. (2000). The pain catastrophizing scale: Further psychometric evaluation with adult samples. *Journal of Behavioral Medicine, 23*, 351-365.

Ott M. J., Norris R., Bauer-Wu, S. (2006). Mindfulness meditation for oncology patients: A discussion and critical review. *Integrative Cancer Therapies, 5*, 98-108.

Plews-Ogan M., Owens J., Goodman M., Wolfe P., Schorling J. (2005). Brief report: A pilot study evaluating mindfulness-based stress reduction and massage for the management of chronic pain. *Journal of General Internal Medicine, 20*, 1136-1138.

Pradham E. K., Baumgarten M., Langenberg P., Handwerger B. Gilpin A. K., Magyari, T., Hochberg M. C., Berman B. M. (2007). Effect of mindfulness-based stress reduction in rheumatoid arthritis patients. *Arthritis and Rheumatism, 57*(7), 1134-1142.

Robinson M. E., Riley J. L. III, Myers C. D., Papas R. K., Wise E. A., Waxenberg L. B., Fillingim R. B. (2001). Gender role expectations of pain: Relationship to sex differences in pain. *Journal of Pain 2*, 251-257.

Rosengren A., Hawken S., Ôunpuu S., Sliwa K., Zubaid M., Almahmeed W., Ngu Blackett K., Sitthi-amorn C., Sato H., Yusuf S. (2004). Association of psychosocial risk factors with risk acute myocardial infarction in 11 119 cases and 13 648 controls from 52 countries (the INTERHEART study): case-control study. *Lancet, 364*, 953-962.

Sagula D., Rice K. G. (2004). The effectiveness of mindfulness training on the grieving process and emotional well-being of chronic pain patients. *Journal of Clinical Psychology in Medical Settings, 11*, 333-342.

Schofferman J., Anderson D., Hines R., Smith G., Keane G., (1993). Childhood psychological trauma and chronic refractory low-back pain. *Clinical Journal of Pain, 4*, 260-265.

Seminowicz D. A., Davis K. D. (2007). A re-examination of pain-cognition interactions: Implications for neuroimaging. *Pain, 130*, 8-13.

Sephton S. E., Salmon P., Weissbecker I., et al. (2007). Mindfulness meditation alleviates depressive symptoms in women with fibromyalgia: Results of a randomized clinical trial. *Arthritis Rheum, 57*, 77-85.

Sherbourne J. W. C. (1992). The MOS 36-item short-form health survey (SF-36). *Medical Care, 30*, 473-483.

Siddall P. J., Cousins, M. J. (2004). Persistent pain as a disease entity: Implications for clinical management. *Anesthesia and Analgesia, 99*, 510-520.

Sullivan M. J. L., Bishop S. R., Pivik J. (1995). The Pain Catastrophizing Scale. *Psychological Assessment, 7*, 524-532.

Sullivan M. J. L., Bishop S. R., Pivik J. (2005). The pain catastrophizing scale: Development and validation. *Psychological Assessment, 7*, 524-532.

Sullivan, M. J., Stanish, W., Waite, H., Sullivan, M. Tripp, D.A. (1998). Catastrophizing, pain, and disability in patients with soft-tissue injuries. *Pain, 77*, 253-260.

Taylor D. N. (1995). Effects of a behavioral stress management program on anxiety, mood, self-esteem and T-cell count in HIV positive men. *Psychological Reports, 76*, 451-457

Telemed J., & Telecare. Goleman D and Schwartz G.E., (1976). Meditation as an intervention in stress reactivity. *Journal of Consulting and Clinical Psychology, 44*, 456-466.

Villemure C., Bushnell M. C. (2002). Cognitive modulation of pain: how do attention and emotion influence pain processing? *Pain, 95*, 195-199.

Ware J. E. Jr. (2000). SF-36 health survey update. *Spine, 25*, 3130-3139.

Zubieta J. -K., Heitzeg M. M., Smith Y. R., Bueller J. A., Xu K., Xu Y., Koeppe R. A., Stohler C. S., Goldman D. (2003). COMT genotype affects u-opioid neurotransmitter responses to a pain stressor. *Science, 299*, 1240-1243.

20

Mindfulness-Based Interventions in Oncology

Linda E. Carlson, Laura E. Labelle, Sheila N. Garland, Marion L. Hutchins, and Kathryn Birnie

"I realized that you can't do anything about the cancer, but you can do something about how you feel about it and how you react to it."
Sylvia (cancer patient)

The Impact of Cancer Diagnosis and Treatment

Negative Effects

Cancer is a leading cause of death worldwide, accounting for 7.6 million (or 13%) of all deaths in 2005 (World Health Organization, 2005). According to cancer prevalence statistics, as of January 1, 2004, it was estimated that there were 10.7 million cancer survivors in the United States alone, which represents approximately 3.6% of the country's population (Surveillance, Epidemiology, and End Results (SEER) Program, 2007). These numbers will only grow as treatments for cancer become more successful and a larger cohort of patients survive long-term. Regardless of increasingly promising survival statistics (up to 65% of all patients now survive beyond 5 years in North America (National Cancer Institute of Canada, 2007; Ries et al., 2007)), receiving a diagnosis of cancer and undergoing cancer treatment continues to be a source of dread and fear for many.

Indeed, cancer diagnosis and treatment is routinely associated with high levels of emotional distress (Strain, 1998; Zabora, BrintzenhofeSzoc, Curbow, Hooker, & Piantadosi, 2001). Despite recent development of targeted therapies and biologic treatments offering effective treatment with fewer side effects (Baselga & Hammond, 2002; van der Poel, 2004), cancer and its treatment are associated with a host of physical symptoms (e.g., nausea, fatigue, pain, hair loss), and both temporary and permanent changes in physical appearance. Emotional reactions of fear, confusion, anxiety and anger are common given the prospect of debilitating and lengthy treatment protocols and disruption of normal life trajectories (Burgess et al., 2005; Epping-Jordan et al., 1999; Hughes, 1982; Shapiro, 2001). Hardship often extends beyond the patient, emotionally impacting family members and friends (Compas et al., 1994; Donnelly et al., 2000; Pitceathly & Maguire 2003). Unfortunately, this increase in stress occurs at a time when there may be an urgent need for emotional and physical resources to help cope with the illness.

After completing primary treatments many patients continue to have high levels of distress requiring psychosocial care (Carlson, Speca, Patel, & Goodey, 2004). Anxiety, depression (Kissane et al., 2004; Strain, 1998), fatigue (Carlson et al., 2004), and sleep problems (Fortner, Stepanski, Wang, Kasprowicz, & Durrence, 2002) are common among cancer survivors. Fear of recurrence, sexual problems, and concerns about body image are reported by a large proportion of survivors (Kornblith & Ligibel, 2003). Threat of disease recurrence and alterations in future life plans can create considerable psychological stress (Northouse, Laten, & Reddy, 1995). Adjustment to cancer-related stress involves psychological and behavioral coping responses (e.g., cognitive and emotional responses to receiving a diagnosis) that may influence psychological functioning (e.g., Walker, Zona, & Fisher, 2006) and the severity of cancer-related symptoms (e.g., Roscoe et al., 2002). It follows that the potential benefits of psychosocial interventions designed to enhance coping with stress and improve quality of life are substantial for cancer patients and survivors.

Positive Effects

Clinicians and researchers in the field of psycho-oncology have often prioritized the importance of identifying and reducing negative psychological reactions following a cancer diagnosis. This is understandable as the focus of effort has been to reduce the suffering of patients and families. However, there has been a recent surge of interest in the perceived benefits of the cancer experience. Being diagnosed with cancer can lead one to renegotiate life priorities and search for purpose and meaning of one's diagnosis and in one's life more generally. Research findings suggest that despite decreased physical health and functioning, some cancer patients indicate positive psychosocial change, including increased spirituality, a deeper appreciation of life, and more positive perceptions of significant others (Andrykowski, Brady, & Hunt, 1993; Cordova, Cunningham, Carlson, & Andrykowski, 2001).

The experience of discovering or actively searching for benefits, or positive implications, of the cancer diagnosis and the life changes that follow is termed posttraumatic growth (PTG). Research on PTG, while still in early stages, indicates greater levels of PTG among cancer patients when compared with age and education matched healthy controls (Cordova et al., 2001). Patients have reported more compassion for others and a willingness to express feelings more openly (Katz, Flasher, Cacciapaglia, & Nelson, 2001). Moreover, both patients and their partners report an increased sense of personal strengths and new possibilities for life (Manne et al., 2004).

Spirituality may also play a significant role in the context of fighting a life-threatening illness (Cotton, Levine, Fitzpatrick, Dold, & Targ, 1999). Despite lack of current consensus, definitions of spirituality generally highlight the importance of providing a context in which people feel whole, at peace and hopeful amid life's most serious challenges (Brady, Peterman, Fitchett, & Cella, 1999). Definitions of religiosity are typically narrower and less inclusive, and emphasize adherence to institutionally sanctioned beliefs and practices associated with a particular faith group. Alternatively, the notion of spirituality refers more generally to the feelings and experiences associated with the search for connection with a transcendent power (Peterman, Fitchett, Brady, Hernandez, & Cella, 2002). Research has confirmed the importance of spirituality to both patients and caregivers (Murray, Kendall, Boyd, Worth, & Benton, 2004; Taylor, 2003).

Spirituality and PTG have been linked with other positive outcomes, such as increased quality of life, psychological adjustment, and positive affect, as well as decreased physical discomfort and dysfunction following cancer diagnosis (Carver & Antoni, 2004; Cotton et al., 1999; Katz et al., 2001; Krupski et al., 2006). Moreover, a need has been identified to provide interventions that may encourage the development of spirituality and posttraumatic growth (Lechner & Antoni, 2004; Linley & Joseph, 2004). Psychosocial interventions which increase perceived benefits among cancer patients may help individuals adapt and adjust to the disease and its consequences.

Hence, the need has been identified to focus both on alleviating some of the more distressing negative symptoms associated with cancer diagnosis and treatment, as well as working to enhance the ability of patients and families to use the transition of the cancer experience as a catalyst to enhance personal growth and spirituality. The Mindfulness-Based Stress Reduction (MBSR) program has the potential to create an opportunity for both of these aspects in cancer patients and families.

Mindfulness-Based Stress Reduction

General Description

Mindfulness meditation, a technique involving moment-to-moment nonjudgmental awareness of internal and external experience, including thoughts, emotions, and body sensations, has become an increasingly popular stress reduction tool used to improve symptoms associated with several clinical illnesses, including cancer (Baer, 2003). Recent interest in the potential health benefits of mindfulness meditation has risen from the development of treatment programs modeled after the MBSR program of Jon Kabat-Zinn and colleagues (1990) at the Stress Reduction Clinic of the University of Massachusetts Medical Center. MBSR is a group intervention consisting of mindfulness meditation and gentle yoga that is designed to have applications for stress, pain, and illness (Kabat-Zinn, 1990). The program is perceived as qualitatively distinct from other forms of meditation (e.g., mantra based), and is not aimed at achieving a state of relaxation, but more at the cultivation of insight and understanding of self and self-in-relationship via the practice of mindfulness (Kabat-Zinn, 2003). Within a framework of nonjudging, acceptance and patience, the individual is taught to focus attention on the breath, body sensations, and eventually any objects (e.g., thoughts, feelings) that enter his or her field of awareness. Although mindfulness meditation is formally practiced while seated, walking or lying down with eyes closed, individuals may also practice mindfulness "informally" when engaged in everyday activities. MBSR programs are being implemented and evaluated in health-care settings across the globe to help address a need for effective psychosocial care.

General Efficacy

Studies suggest that MBSR may be efficacious for treating some of the symptoms associated with a broad range of chronic medical and psychiatric problems. In a meta-analysis of the health benefits of MBSR, Grossman, Niemann, Schmidt, and Walach (2004) identified 20 studies that met the criteria of acceptable quality or relevance to be included in their analyses. Ten of the 20 studies had randomized controlled designs, while six investigations employed forms of active control intervention to account for general or non-specific effects of treatment. Overall, both controlled and uncontrolled studies assessing mental and/or physical health variables showed similar effect sizes of approximately $d = 0.5$. This indicates a relatively strong effect of mindfulness interventions for improving physical symptoms (e.g., chronic pain), and participants' ability to cope with everyday distress and disability, and with serious disorders or stress (Grossman et al., 2004). In general, treatment effects of one-half of a standard deviation ($d = 0.5$) are considered to represent clinically meaningful improvements in symptomatology (Norman, Sloan, Wyrwich, & Norman, 2003). Grossman et al. (2004) conclude that although as a whole the current quality of evidence for the efficacy of MBSR on physical correlates of disease suffers from serious methodological flaws including a lack of randomized controlled studies, findings are generally supportive for the hypothesis that mindfulness training has beneficial effects on psychological and physical well-being.

Two other conceptual and empirical reviews of the general MBSR literature have been conducted independently (Baer, 2003; Bishop, 2002), each examining mindfulness training as a clinical intervention and discussing conceptual and methodological issues relevant to the research. The authors of each review conclude that mindfulness-based interventions may be useful in the treatment of several disorders. However, Baer (2003) emphasizes the need for methodologically sound investigations to clarify the utility of these interventions, while Bishop (2002) expresses "cautious optimism" with his conclusion that there exists some preliminary evidence that supports the need for further evaluation of the mindfulness-based approach.

Description of the Tom Baker Cancer Centre MBSR Program

Given the high level of emotional distress experienced following a cancer diagnosis (Carlson et al., 2004), and accumulating evidence of the efficacy of MBSR in other patient populations (Baer, 2003; Bishop, 2002), this intervention seemed well-suited for implementation at the Tom Baker Cancer Centre (TBCC). The TBCC's MBSR program was modeled on the work of Jon Kabat-Zinn and colleagues (1990), and is adapted and standardized to the clinical context of the TBCC. As described by Speca, Carlson, Goodey, and Angen (2000), the MBSR program offered through the TBCC aims to provide an opportunity to become aware of one's personal responses to stress and to learn and practice meditation techniques that will bring about healthier stress responses. The core of the program consists of the practice of mindfulness meditation. Attitudes of nonjudging of personal experience, seeing and accepting situations as they are, patience during the practice and in daily life, non-striving and loosening of goal-oriented stances, and letting go of uncontrollable outcomes are suggested and modeled by group leaders (Speca et al., 2000). Group members are encouraged to take an active role in their healing process, and are taught options for self-care that promote feelings of competence in terms of managing stress. The core of the program consists of the practice of mindfulness meditation. The two instructors provide a safe and supportive group environment in which self-disclosure regarding the experience of cancer can serve to enhance skill acquisition (Speca et al., 2000).

The intervention is provided over the course of eight weekly, 90-minute group sessions, as well as one 6-hour intensive session on a Saturday between weeks six and seven. The program consists of three components: didactic instruction, experiential practice, and group process. Topic areas covered didactically in-session and in a participant manual are: (a) the impact of stress on one's physical and psychological health, including the psychological and physical symptoms of stress, (b) emotional, cognitive, and behavioral patterns and how they may influence our stress responses, and (c) concepts fundamental to mindfulness meditation and mindful living. Participants learn to apply the principles taught didactically, through experiential practice of mindfulness meditation at home and during group sessions. In group sessions, instructors guide participants through experiential activities including various types of mindfulness meditation (e.g., sitting, walking) and gentle hatha yoga. When the yoga component is taught, it is framed as a modality for practicing mindfulness (moving meditation), rather than a physical exercise. Participants are encouraged to practice the prescribed meditation and yoga techniques daily, for 45 minutes. Guided meditation CDs are provided to support home practice. During each session, group discussions are facilitated to encourage self-disclosure regarding experiences and challenges encountered through the practice of mindfulness meditation. Instructors and other program participants offer constructive feedback and support to help problem solve when there are impediments to effective practice. Supportive interaction between group members is encouraged.

Several specific issues involved in therapy for cancer patients are considered in the delivery of MBSR at the TBCC. Sensitivity to the physical and mental implications associated with the various types and stages of disease, and medical treatments received, is critical. It follows that the timing of a cancer patient's enrollment is an important factor to consider. The program's format and scheduling requirements are discussed with patients at a pre-intervention interview, at which time concerns regarding pain, fatigue, nausea, immobility and other factors influencing motivation to participate are discussed. Patients are encouraged to discuss any concerns regarding participating in MBSR with their treating physician. Some patients find that participating in MBSR during the course of a demanding treatment regime is difficult or impossible, while other patients find they can engage fully in the program while undergoing treatment. Appropriate management of expectations and concern for safety often permits debilitated patients to fully engage in the program. For example, consideration of physical limitations is emphasized with regards to the yoga component of the program; instructors provide modifications of standard yoga *asanas* (i.e., postures) as necessary, to ensure individual comfort and safety. Many patients find the program useful for coping with day-to-day demands of treatment such as waiting for appointments, tolerating venipuncture and chemotherapy or radiation therapy administration and coping with uncomfortable tests and scans. Others find that the program is particularly helpful after treatment completion when they sometimes feel "abandoned" by the treatment team and are often struggling with fears of recurrence and issues around how to live a genuine and authentic life moving forward, but still re-integrate into mainstream society.

Review of Empirical Support for MBSR in Oncology Settings

Quantitative Findings – Symptom Reduction Outcomes

MBSR is gaining credibility and interest for use in oncology settings (Ott, Norris, & Bauer-Wu, 2006). Several independent reviews of the literature of MBSR in oncology settings indicate that although the research is still at an early stage, MBSR may be efficacious as an adjunct treatment for improving psychological functioning of cancer patients (Lamanque & Daneault, 2006; Mackenzie, Carlson, & Speca, 2005; Matchim & Armer, 2007; Ott et al., 2006; Smith, Richardson, Hoffman, & Pilkington, 2005). The first published study in this area was our randomized controlled trial of the effects of MBSR on symptoms of stress and mood disturbance in a diverse population of cancer outpatients (Speca et al., 2000). When compared to a waitlist control group, MBSR participants indicated significantly less total mood disturbance, tension, depression, anger, and more vigor following the intervention. Program participants also reported reduced symptoms of stress, including peripheral manifestations of stress, cardiopulmonary symptoms of arousal, central neurological symptoms, gastrointestinal symptoms, habitual stress behavioral patterns, anxiety/fear, and emotional instability, when compared with controls. In addition, more home meditation practice over the course of the program was associated with fewer reported stress symptoms and decreased total mood disturbance. Results of a 6-month follow-up study which included intervention and control group participants together revealed that psychological benefits were maintained at the follow-up assessment (Carlson, Ursuliak, Goodey, Angen, & Speca, 2001). The largest improvements were seen on subscales of anxiety, depression, anger and irritability.

Evaluations of the efficacy of MBSR for improving sleep quality among cancer outpatients also offer promising results. Sleep disturbance in cancer patients has been found to range from 40 to 85% across studies, clearly indicating that sleep is a problem for this clinical population (Carlson et al., 2004; Engstrom, Strohl, Rose, Lewandowski, & Stefanek, 1999; Koopman et al., 2002; Savard & Morin, 2001). In a study of the effects of an MBSR program on sleep quality in a heterogeneous cancer patient population, results indicated significant reductions in overall sleep disturbance and improved subjective sleep quality, as assessed by the Pittsburgh Sleep Quality Index (Carlson & Garland, 2005). When using a conservative cutoff on this measure, sleep disturbance was reduced in the entire sample by 11%. After the program, participants reported they were sleeping a mean of 1 hour more per night, which is considered clinically significant. Reductions in symptoms of stress, mood disturbance, and fatigue were also observed; changes in symptoms of stress and fatigue correlated in expected ways with improvement in sleep quality.

In an earlier study of the effects of MBSR on sleep, Shapiro, Bootzin, Figueredo, Lopez, & Schwartz (2003) compared an MBSR and a "free choice" active control condition on sleep complaints in a group of breast cancer patients. Both MBSR and control participants demonstrated significant improvement on daily diary sleep quality measures. Participants in the MBSR group who reported greater mindfulness practice improved significantly more on the sleep quality measure most strongly associated with distress (i.e., feeling rested after sleep) (Shapiro et al., 2003).

Observations of other research groups who are applying modifications of MBSR in oncology settings complement the above-described findings. Monti et al. (2006) conducted a randomized waitlist-controlled trial to evaluate the efficacy of a mindfulness-based art therapy (MBAT) program designed for cancer patients. MBAT incorporates mindfulness meditation and art therapy with the goal of decreasing distress and improving quality of life. Participants in the study were women with a variety of cancer diagnoses. MBAT participants demonstrated significant decreases in emotional distress, and improvements in general health, mental health, vitality, and social functioning, when compared with waitlist controls. Gains associated with MBAT participation were maintained at a 2-month follow-up assessment (Monti et al., 2006). Another research group has presented pilot qualitative data attesting to the potential benefits of integrating mindfulness techniques into psychoeducational programs for sexual problems subsequent to gynecological cancer (Brotto & Heiman, 2007). Finally, studies evaluating modifications of MBSR have been presented at scientific meetings, representing ongoing clinical application of MBSR in oncology populations (e.g., Bauer-Wu & Rosenbaum, 2004; Baum & Gessert, 2004; Lengacher et al., 2007; Moscoso, Reheiser, & Hann, 2004).

Quantitative Findings – Biological Outcomes

In addition to improving psychological functioning, MBSR is hypothesized to impact biological systems in cancer patients, who may exhibit dysregulation of these systems (Abercrombie et al., 2004; Sephton, Sapolsky, Kraemer, & Spiegel, 2000; Touitou, Bogdan, Levi, Benavides, & Auzeby, 1996; van der Pompe, Antoni, & Heijnen, 1996). Our group evaluated the effects of MBSR on immune, neuroendocrine, and autonomic function in early stage breast and prostate cancer patients who were at least 3 months posttreatment (Carlson, Speca, Patel, & Goodey, 2003; Carlson et al., 2004). Participants completed self-report measures to assess quality of life, mood states, and stress symptoms, and provided blood samples to measure immune cell numbers and function. Salivary cortisol (assessed three times/day), plasma dehydroepiandrosterone sulfate (DHEAS, a steroid product of the adrenal glands), and salivary melatonin were also measured pre- and post-intervention (Carlson et al., 2004). Significant improvements were observed in overall quality of life, symptoms of stress, and sleep quality. Although there were no significant changes in the overall number of lymphocytes or cell subsets, T cell production of cytokines interleukin (IL)-4 increased and interferon gamma decreased, whereas natural killer cell production of IL-10 decreased. These changes in patients' immune profiles were behaviorally associated with a shift away from a depressive pattern to one more consistent with healthy immune function. In addition, approximately 40% of patients shifted from an abnormal "inverted V-shaped" pattern of diurnal cortisol secretion, to a healthier "V-shaped" pattern. This change was driven by a decrease in afternoon and evening cortisol levels in some participants. Improvements in quality of life were associated with decreases in afternoon cortisol levels. In sum, although the lack of a control group limits interpretation, findings suggest that the MBSR program alters immunological and neuroendocrine profiles of cancer patients in a direction more consistent with healthy functioning (Carlson et al., 2003, 2004).

More recently a 1-year follow-up paper of this same group of breast and prostate cancer patients has been published (Carlson, Speca, Patel, & Faris, 2007). We found that improvements in stress symptoms and quality of life were maintained over the full year of follow-up. In addition, cortisol levels continued to drop over the year, and salivary cortisol levels at 1-year follow-up were associated with stress symptoms, such that those patients with less stress also had lower cortisol values. Continued regulation in immune system values, particularly pro-inflammatory cytokines, was also seen. This is usually interpreted as a sign of stabilization of the immune system, which may have been producing a maladaptive inflammatory response to the cancer. Finally, systolic blood pressure values decreased over the course of the MBSR program. Any decreases in blood pressure are desirable, as elevated blood pressure is the best predictor of subsequent heart disease (Carlson et al., 2007).

Confirming this last finding in a much more methodologically rigorous manner, preliminary results from a waitlist controlled trial conducted by our group indicate a beneficial impact of MBSR on resting blood pressure in women with cancer (Van Wielingen, Carlson, & Campbell, 2007). Twenty-nine women with a diagnosis of cancer (mostly breast) who had completed treatment at least 1 month prior to study entry were either registered for immediate MBSR participation, or were waiting for the next program. Resting blood pressure was assessed weekly at home over the 8-week study period in both groups. For participants with relatively high levels of baseline systolic blood pressure at entry to the study, participation in the MBSR program was associated with a significant decrease in resting systolic blood pressure over the 8 weeks relative to the control group. In addition, MBSR participation was associated with decreased self-reported symptoms of stress, depression, rumination, and increased mindful attention awareness. This study confirms our previous findings that the MBSR program may be efficacious in reducing resting blood pressure. The decrease in systolic blood pressure observed (15.5 mmHg) is clinically meaningful, and is comparable to the drop seen for antihypertensive medication or a 10 kg drop in body weight (The Trials of Hypertension Prevention Collaborative Research Group, 1997; Wua et al., 2005). In the same study, when compared with waitlist controls, preliminary data suggests that MBSR participants appear to demonstrate greater systolic blood pressure recovery following a public speaking stressor at post-intervention (Van Wielingen, Carlson, & Campbell, 2006). It remains to be seen whether preliminary results from this ongoing trial hold up at study completion. As blood pressure levels are predictive of the development of cardiovascular morbidity and mortality, MBSR may have the potential to improve health outcomes for cancer patients, many of who are already at increased risk due to heart-related side effects of cancer treatments.

In another study which included biological outcomes, Saxe et al. (2001) evaluated the effects of combining a dietary intervention with MBSR on levels of prostate specific antigen (PSA), an indicator of the level of tumor activity in men with prostate cancer. Results suggested this 4-month combined program resulted in a slowing of the rate of PSA increase in a pilot sample of 10 men (Saxe et al., 2001). Findings from the larger RCT may confirm whether this combined dietary and mindfulness-based intervention alters PSA levels in prostate cancer patients.

Quantitative Findings – Positive Psychology Outcomes

The effects of the MBSR program on positive outcomes such as spirituality and PTG are in the early stages of investigation. Garland, Carlson, Cook, Lansdell, & Speca (2007), compared the effects of an MBSR intervention and a creative arts-based ("Healing Arts") program for facilitating PTG and spirituality in cancer outpatients. Participants in the MBSR group demonstrated significant increases in PTG and spirituality over the course of the program; increases in spirituality as well as decreases in anger and overall stress symptoms were significantly greater for MBSR versus Healing Arts program participants (Garland et al., 2007). This preliminary study indicates future research into the effects of MBSR on positive psychological outcomes in cancer patients is warranted.

Quantitative Findings Summary

In general, MBSR is thought to have potential as a clinically valuable intervention for cancer patients (Mackenzie et al., 2005; Ott et al., 2006; Smith et al., 2005). However, there is a need for replication of randomized controlled trials that include active control groups and long-term follow-up. In the future, incorporating both positive (e.g., things we want to enhance such as PTG) and negative (e.g., things we want to decrease such as depression) psychological outcomes alongside biological indices may foster greater breadth and depth of understanding of changes incurred through the program. Studies comparing MBSR to other psychosocial interventions developed for cancer patients (e.g., supportive-expressive therapy) and dismantling studies will enable identification of the program's key ingredients. Brown and Ryan (Brown & Ryan, 2003) reported that increased mindfulness over the course of the MBSR intervention predicted decreases in symptoms of stress and mood disturbance, alluding to emerging research on the mediating role of mindfulness in cancer-related outcomes (Brown & Ryan, 2003; Ott et al., 2006). According to Ott et al. (2006), "further work is needed to explicate the mediating factors and better understand the unique benefits of mindfulness meditation and MBSR (p. 107)."

Qualitative Findings and Case Conceptualization

A qualitative understanding of participants' experiences may be used to tailor MBSR programs to better assist patients during cancer diagnosis, treatment and recovery. Findings from a recent qualitative study support and inform quantitative findings indicating that the MBSR program has a positive impact on psychological and emotional dimensions in cancer patients (Mackenzie, Carlson, Munoz, & Speca, 2007). Nine cancer patients who had participated in an 8-week TBCC MBSR program and who continued to attend weekly drop-in MBSR sessions were interviewed for this study. Using a grounded theory analytic approach, data from semi-structured interviews and a focus group were analyzed to identify themes concerning the effects patients experienced by adding meditation to their lives. Five major themes emerged from the data: (1) opening to change; (2) self-control; (3) shared experience; (4) personal growth; (5) spirituality. This information was used to develop a theory regarding mechanisms through which MBSR effects change for cancer patients (Mackenzie et al., 2007).

Case Study

The following case study was developed as part of a larger qualitative research investigation conducted at the TBCC in Calgary, Alberta. Individual semi-structured interviews were conducted with cancer patients who had recently completed an 8-week MBSR program. The aim of the interviews was to explore items of interest that had been previously identified in questionnaires assessing positive and negative aspects of psychological functioning, which were administered before and after an MBSR program. Questionnaires included the Functional Assessment of Chronic Illness Therapy – Spiritual Well-Being Scale (FACIT-Sp), Posttraumatic Growth Inventory – revised (PTGI-r), Symptoms of Stress Inventory (SOSI), and the Profile of Mood States (POMS). Items that changed significantly for the sample as a whole on the questionnaires were chosen as the focus for the interviews, and representative patients who demonstrated a change on those items were selected. All participants provided informed consent, and the study was approved by the Conjoint Health Research Ethics Board of the University of Calgary Faculty of Medicine and Alberta Cancer Board. The case of Sylvia was chosen for presentation because it illustrates emerging themes common to the application of MBSR in the context of cancer treatment and recovery.

Personal Background and Disease Context

Sylvia is a 50-year-old woman who lives with her common-law partner and has no children. She has 13 years of education and has been employed as a middle manager for 31 years. Sylvia was diagnosed with Stage I breast cancer in February 2006. She had two surgeries to remove affected tissue of the left breast. She then received 25 radiation therapy treatments daily (M-F) for a period of 5 weeks, beginning in August 2006. Radiation therapy, or radiotherapy, is the use of ionizing radiation to control malignant cells. Radiotherapy itself is painless, but can cause various acute and long-term side effects, including skin reactions (e.g., redness, soreness) and reduced skin elasticity due to scarring. Following surgery and radiation, Sylvia began a 5-year course of Tamoxifen, an adjuvant therapy, which interferes with the activity of the hormone estrogen, reducing the chance of recurrence of the disease. Tamoxifen is commonly administered following primary treatment for early-stage breast cancer. The side effects of Tamoxifen are similar to the symptoms commonly associated with menopause, such as hot flashes and irregular menstrual periods; the nature and degree of side effects varies across patients.

Sylvia began the 8-week MBSR program shortly after she finished radiation in October 2006. When she began the program, she considered herself to be very familiar with cancer-related stress, and hoped the program would help her cope with the cancer experience. Sylvia described herself as "needy" for support and stated she sought out the program because she did not know where else to find help.

Findings

Common themes that emerged from the qualitative interviews related to reduced symptoms of stress, improved mood, increased feelings of spiritual connectedness, and perceived benefits from the cancer experience. These themes that emerged included the importance of present-focused awareness for identifying and dealing with stress, the development of self-efficacy for coping with challenges, the importance of accepting things as they are, and learning to let go of unknowable or uncontrollable outcomes.

In particular, participating in the MBSR program appeared to increase Sylvia's present-focused attention/awareness, influencing how she fets about herself.

> I never knew that we always thought about the past and the future. I just had no idea that that was where our mind always went and it's so true. I mean, it's kind of embarrassing to say that you didn't know that before. But, you know, we kept hearing that and it was when you are in the present you feel so much different about yourself than when you think about the past, if you think about the future. The present is a really good place to be.

It appeared that Sylvia developed greater *self-efficacy* with regard to coping with stress.

> I learned that when you react to things when you're under stress, you're only hurting yourself really. You know, because, I remember when I used to react to things, you know, it would still fester and boil up in me. And now, when I sort of let it go, when I have a stressful situation and I breathe and I think about it [. . .] and then I deal with it, it's not so bad.

Sylvia acknowledged that she had felt depressed for some time and felt that the program was integral in *improving her mood*.

> I think that I am better. I stand at better peace with myself. And it's because of the meditation by all means I know that. I know that because without that I think I would've had the time, but nothing would have changed. It's still minus a body part and you still don't know, you [are] still unsure. . . .I think you can be depressed though for a long time. So, the fact that I had this [program] for a couple of months and I feel a change. So, again I feel that I have to attribute it to the meditation because I could still be the way I was going for so many months.

She expressed a *reduction in fear* surrounding cancer recurrence, feeling that if the cancer recurred she would be able to cope with it.

> I was always thinking about [the cancer] and I was depressed. . .And I'm not anymore. . .And if it recurs, I think I'm prepared for that. I sure wasn't before [the program]. [. . .] I realized that you can't do anything about the cancer but

you can do something about how you feel about it and how you react to it. I do much better.

In particular, Sylvia described her change in attitude from needing to know what caused her cancer to an attitude of *acceptance* of the cancer experience after participation in the program. She finally felt able to *let go* of trying to determine why she got cancer.

> When I had cancer…what I questioned all the time was, "ok, what am I going to learn from this"?…there's a reason why I got this…I needed to know that because I thought I could deal with things differently and I was adamant to know….And for the longest time I thought that's the only way I could deal with it, so I was always thinking about that and I was depressed…And then it just kind of didn't matter. It didn't matter where I got it from.

Sylvia described increased *acceptance* of what is occurring in the present moment.

> So, I learned how to be in the present and I use that a lot on a daily basis – when I'm stressed out, you know even in traffic. You say, "I'm here now. This is where I'm going to be. I'll worry about the grocery store later." I just accept things a lot easier now than I did before.

Issues around *spirituality*, encompassing feelings of hope, peace, and understanding, surfaced and resonated strongly with Sylvia despite that the focus of the MBSR program is secular and does not specifically address spirituality.

> After the [full-day meditation] retreat I said that I was at such peace and it was so spiritual…

The increased feelings of spirituality and peace expressed by Sylvia had particular implications related to her own experience of cancer.

> I'm at peace. I understand it [the cancer] a lot better. I understand it. And if it recurs, I think I'm prepared for that. […] I know things happened for a reason, always. Always."

This comment is congruent with the definition of spirituality as an ability to see the divinity, or greater organization in life, and to use this understanding to deal with life challenges.

Significant increases in *PTG* were also evident in Sylvia's interview. She described experiencing positive changes related to the cancer experience after participation in the program, and linked specific skill acquisition in dealing with the cancer experience to her participation in the MBSR course.

> I always knew that there was something that I had to learn from this and I never knew what it was - I never knew. And I think now what I've learned (and probably from the course) is, what I've learned is to appreciate things, to take time for things, which I think before I was always so busy and always so controlling, and you know, quite bossy. I realized that you can't do anything about the cancer but you can do something about how you feel about it and how you react to it.

It is clear from this interview that many of the themes of the program resonated with Sylvia's experience of learning MBSR, particularly around issues of feeling a need to know and have some certainty about why cancer occurred, and whether it was coming back. This inherent uncertainty in the illness experience is often one of the most difficult issues for cancer survivors to live with. Sylvia's comments provide some insight into how the program can help patients find peace even within this vast inability to know the future with any degree of certainty. Somehow through the practice she learned to tolerate uncertainty and uncontrollability much better than before her cancer experience.

Sylvia's responses during this qualitative interview represent only one patient's perception of the effects of MBSR on positive and negative outcomes, but do resonate well with what other patients have articulated. The interviews in general reveal a broad range of improvements related to a greater appreciation for life and improved coping self-efficacy. Encouragement of the adoption of attitudes such as acceptance and letting go appear to have contributed to patients' increased feelings of spirituality and PTG, and decreased stress and mood disturbance. Based on qualitative analyses, there appears to be a strong link between mindfulness practice and a healthier view of the cancer experience and its impact on daily functioning.

Summary and Conclusions

Distress and other negative reactions to a cancer diagnosis and all that it entails are common and expected experiences for cancer patients and their families. Fears of premature death and of the pain and indignities of cancer treatment are natural and well founded in many cases. Despite the hurdles such experiences present, patients are often able not only to adjust to such a massive life stress, but even to thrive and grow as a result. We have reviewed the rational suggesting MBSR may be helpful for cancer patients and families, and provided an overview of the clinical research detailing its efficacy for alleviating a wide range of negative outcomes including stress symptoms, anxiety, anger, fear, sleep disturbance and depression. We have also shown evidence of enhancement in overall quality of life, improved ability to find benefit in the situation and grow through trauma, including enhancement of a sense of spirituality and meaning and purpose in life, as well as enhanced ability to tolerate uncertainty. In addition to these psychological benefits, patients often show improved biological regulation of a variety of circadian systems that are essential to promote health and homeostasis, such as cytokine expression, cortisol secretion, and blood pressure. We have attempted to integrate methods of inquiry including both qualitative and quantitative approaches in the hopes of better understanding not only the outcomes of MBSR in people living with cancer, but also the potential mechanisms that may help to explain how and why MBSR is effective in this group. Future research efforts of our group and others should help to lend further understanding not only to the full range of effects of MBSR, but also some insight into these intriguing questions of how and why.

Acknowledgements: Dr. Linda E. Carlson holds the Enbridge Endowed Research Chair in Psychosocial Oncology, co-funded by Enbridge Inc., the

Canadian Cancer Society, and the Alberta Cancer Foundation. Laura E. Labella is funded by an Alberta Heritage Foundation Medical Research PhD Scholarship and a Social Sciences and Humanities Research Counsel of Canada PhD Fellowship, and Sheila Garland is funded by the Social Sciences and Humanities Research Counsel of Canada PhD Fellowship. The research described in this chapter has been funded by the Canadian Institutes of Health Research, National Cancer Institute of Canada, Canadian Breast Cancer Research Alliance, and Calgary Health Region through grants awarded to Dr. Linda E. Carlson. None of this work would be possible without the cooperation and dedication of the patients who have given generously of their time to participate in our research programs – heartfelt thanks are extended to them all.

Appendix: Description of Specific Didactic Learning and Experiential Exercises

Following group discussion and problem solving about home practice, the didactic components of Week 3 ("Mind-body Wisdom and Healing") and

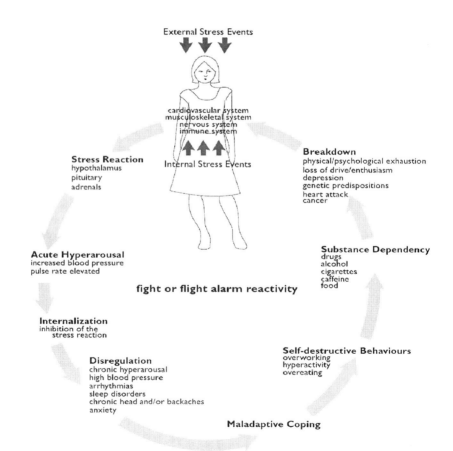

Figure. 20.1. The stress reaction.

Week 4 ("Balance in the Autonomic Nervous System") in our MBSR program include a description of the automatic physical, emotional and behavioral reaction to stress, compared with the response when we choose to attend mindfully to our experience. Short and long-term emotional, cognitive, behavioral, and physiological aspects of these two different responses are illustrated and discussed (Figures 20.1 and 20.2; adapted from Kabat-Zinn, 1990). In addition, participants complete a self-assessment checklist of symptoms of stress, in order to develop awareness of the ways in which stress may influence emotions, sensations, and behaviors (Figure 20.3).

In Weeks 3 and 4, following didactic instruction, participants are guided through a series of experiential exercises involving bringing awareness to

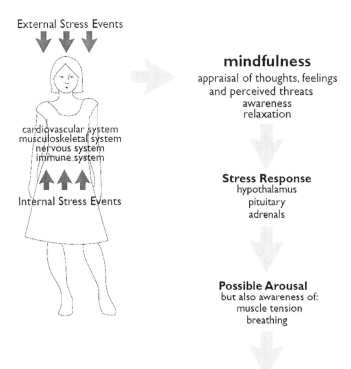

Figure. 20.2. The stress response.

SYMPTOMS OF STRESS – SELF ASSESSMENT

Check off any of the following symptoms of stress that you have experienced in the last week:

Physical Symptoms

❑ Headaches	❑ Sleep difficulties	❑ Racing heart
❑ Indigestion	❑ Dizziness	❑ Restlessness
❑ Stomach aches	❑ Back pain	❑ Tiredness
❑ Sweaty palms	❑ Tight neck, shoulders	❑Ringing in ears

Behavioural Symptoms

❑ Smoking	❑ Grinding teeth at night
❑ Bossiness	❑ Overuse of alcohol
❑ Compulsive gum chewing	❑ Compulsive eating
❑ Critical attitude	❑ Inability to get things done

Emotional Symptoms

❑ Crying	❑ Overwhelming feeling of pressure
❑ Nervousness, anxiety	❑ Anger
❑ Boredom, no meaning to things	❑ Loneliness
❑ Edginess, ready to explode	❑ Unhappiness for no reason
❑ Feeling powerless to change things	❑ Easily upset

Cognitive Symptoms

❑ Trouble thinking clearly	❑ Indecisiveness
❑ Forgetfulness	❑ Thoughts of running away
❑ Lack of creativity	❑ Constant worry
❑ Memory loss	❑ Loss of sense of humor

Spiritual Symptoms

❑ Emptiness	❑ Martyrdom	❑ Cynicism
❑ Loss of meaning	❑ Looking for magic	❑ Apathy
❑ Doubt	❑Loss of direction	❑ Need to prove self
❑ Unforgiving		

Relational Symptoms

❑ Isolation	❑ Hiding	❑ Lack of intimacy
❑ Intolerance	❑ Clamming up	❑ Using people
❑ Resentment	❑ Lowered sex drive	❑ Fewer contacts with friends
❑ Loneliness	❑ Nagging	❑ Lashing out
❑ Distrust		

Figure. 20.3. Symptoms of stress self-assessment.

the breath. These are taught in conjunction with the basic sitting meditation and yoga postures that occur during each weekly class. These exercises are referred to as "mini" mindfulness exercises. "Minis" are focused breathing techniques that are practiced to help reduce anxiety and tension in any place, at any time, and can be engaged in without others taking notice. For example, "minis" can be performed when stuck in traffic, when feeling overwhelmed, when waiting in the doctor's office, waiting in line or when experiencing pain. Participants are guided through the experience of mindful slow, deep diaphragmatic breathing then use the various techniques to focus breath patterns and awareness (Figures 20.4–20.8).

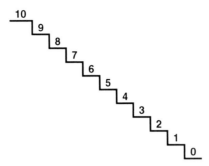

Figure. 20.4. Balanced mini breathing exercise with counting. (BALANCED MINI 1: Count from ten down to zero – one number for each in and out breath, like walking down a set of stairs. With the first diaphragmatic breath say "ten" to yourself; with the next breath say "nine"; -8-7-6-5-4-3-2-1-0).

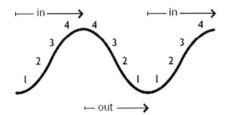

Figure. 20.5. Balanced mini breathing exercise with counting 2. (BALANCED MINI 2: As you inhale, count very slowly up to four. As you exhale, count slowly back down to one. Do this several times).

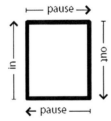

Figure. 20.6. Balanced mini breathing exercise with holding. (BALANCED MINI 3: After each inhalation pause for a few seconds. After you exhale, pause again for a few seconds. Do this for several breaths).

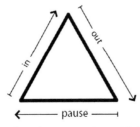

Figure. 20.7. Relaxing mini breathing exercise with holding after the outbreath. (RELAXING MINI: Triangular breath. Breathe in fully, then out fully. Pause and hold after the out breath.)

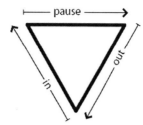

Figure. 20.8. Arousing mini exercise with holding after the inbreath. (AROUSING MINI: Inverted triangular breath. Breathe out fully, then in fully. Pause and hold after the in breath).

References

Abercrombie, H. C., Giese-Davis, J., Sephton, S., Epel, E. S., Turner-Cobb, J. M., & Spiegel, D. (2004). Flattened cortisol rhythms in metastatic breast cancer patients. *Psychoneuroendocrinology, 29,* 1082–1092.

Andrykowski, M. A., Brady, M. J., & Hunt, J. W. (1993). Positive psychosocial adjustment in potential bone marrow transplant recipients: Cancer as a psychological transition. *Psycho-oncology, 2,* 261–276.

Baer, R. A. (2003). Mindfulness training as clinical intervention: A conceptual and empirical review. *Clinical Psychology: Science and Practice, 10,* 125–143.

Baselga, J., & Hammond, L. A. (2002). HER-targeted tyrosine-kinase inhibitors. *Oncology, 63,* 6–16.

Bauer-Wu, S. M., & Rosenbaum, E. (2004). Facing the challenges of stem cell/bone marrow transplantation with mindfulness meditation: A pilot study. *Psycho-oncology, 13,* S10–S11.

Baum, C., & Gessert, A. (2004). Mindfulness-based stress reduction (MBSR) classes as a tool to decrease the anxiety of cancer patients. *Psycho-oncology, 13,* S13.

Bishop, S. R. (2002). What do we really know about mindfulness-based stress reduction? *Psychosomatic Medicine, 64,* 71–83.

Brady, M. J., Peterman, A. H., Fitchett, G., Mo, M., & Cella, D. (1999). A case for including spirituality in quality of life measurement in oncology. *Psycho-oncology, 8,* 417–428.

Brotto, L. A., & Heiman, J. R. (2007). Mindfulness in sex therapy: Applications for women with sexual difficulties following gynecologic cancer. *Sexual and Relationship Therapy, 22*(1), 3–11.

Brown, K. W., & Ryan, R. M. (2003). The benefits of being present: Mindfulness and its role in psychological well-being. *Journal of personality and social psychology, 84,* 822–848.

Burgess, C., Cornelius, V., Love, S., Graham, J., Richards, M., & Ramirez, A. (2005). Depression and anxiety in women with early breast cancer: Five year observational cohort study. *BMJ, 330,* 702–705.

Carlson, L. E., Angen, M., Cullum, J., Goodey, E., Koopmans, J., Lamont, L., et al. (2004). High levels of untreated distress and fatigue in cancer patients. *British Journal of Cancer, 90*(12), 2297–2304.

Carlson, L. E., & Garland, S. N. (2005). Impact of mindfulness-based stress reduction (MBSR) on sleep, mood, stress and fatigue symptoms in cancer outpatients. *International Journal of Behavioral Medicine, 12,* 278–285.

Carlson, L. E., Speca, M., Patel, K. D., & Faris, P. (2007). One year pre-post intervention follow-up of psychological, immune, endocrine and blood pressure outcomes of mindfulness-based stress reduction (MBSR) in breast and prostate cancer outpatients. *Brain, behavior, and immunity,* Online view DOI: 10.1016/j.bbi.2007.04.002

Carlson, L. E., Speca, M., Patel, K. D., & Goodey, E. (2003). Mindfulness-based stress reduction in relation to quality of life, mood, symptoms of stress, and immune parameters in breast and prostate cancer outpatients. *Psychosomatic Medicine, 65*(4), 571–581.

Carlson, L. E., Speca, M., Patel, K. D., & Goodey, E. (2004). Mindfulness-based stress reduction in relation to quality of life, mood, symptoms of stress and levels of cortisol, dehydroepiandrosterone-sulfate (DHEAS) and melatonin in breast and prostate cancer outpatients. *Psychoneuroendocrinology, 29*, 448–474.

Carlson, L. E., Ursuliak, Z., Goodey, E., Angen, M., & Speca, M. (2001). The effects of a mindfulness meditation based stress reduction program on mood and symptoms of stress in cancer outpatients: Six month follow-up. *Supportive Care in Cancer, 9*, 112–123.

Carver, C. S., & Antoni, M. H. (2004). Finding benefit in breast cancer during the year after diagnosis predicts better adjustment 5–8 years after diagnosis. *Health Psychology, 23*, 595–598.

Compas, B. E., Worsham, N. L., Epping-Jordan, J. E., Grant, K. E., Mireault, G., Howell, D. C., et al. (1994). When mom or dad has cancer: Markers of psychological distress in cancer patients, spouse and children. *Health Psychology, 13*, 507–515.

Cordova, M. J., Cunningham, L. L., Carlson, C. R., & Andrykowski, M. A. (2001). Posttraumatic growth following breast cancer: A controlled comparison study. *Health Psychology, 20*, 176–185.

Cotton, S. P., Levine, E. G., Fitzpatrick, C. M., Dold, K. H., & Targ, E. (1999). Exploring the relationships among spiritual well-being, quality of life, and psychological adjustment in women with breast cancer. *Psycho-oncology, 8*, 429–438.

Donnelly, J. M., Kornblith, A. B., Fleishman, S., Zuckerman, E., Raptis, G., Hudis, C. A., et al. (2000). A pilot study of interpersonal psychotherapy by telephone with cancer patients and their partners. *Psycho-oncology, 9*, 44–56.

Engstrom, C. A., Strohl, R. A., Rose, L., Lewandowski, L., & Stefanek, M. E. (1999). Sleep alterations in cancer patients. *Cancer Nursing, 22*, 143–148.

Epping-Jordan, J. E., Compas, B. E., Osowiecki, D. M., Oppedisano, G., Gerhardt, C., Primo, K., et al. (1999). Psychological adjustment in breast cancer: Processes of emotional distress. *Health Psychology, 18*(4), 315–326.

Fortner, B. V., Stepanski, E. J., Wang, S. C., Kasprowicz, S., & Durrence, H. H. (2002). Sleep and quality of life in breast cancer patients. *Journal of Pain & Symptom Management, 24*(5), 471–480.

Garland, S. N., Carlson, L. E., Cook, S., Lansdell, L., & Speca, M. (2007). A non-randomized comparison of mindfulness-based stress reduction and healing arts programs for facilitating post-traumatic growth and spirituality in cancer outpatients. *Supportive care in cancer: official journal of the Multinational Association of Supportive Care in Cancer*, Online view DOI: 10.1007/s00520-007-0280-5

Grossman, P., Niemann, L., Schmidt, S., & Walach, H. (2004). Mindfulness-based stress reduction and health benefits. A meta-analysis. *Journal of Psychosomatic Research, 57*(1), 35–43.

Hughes, J. (1982). Emotional reactions to the diagnosis and treatment of early breast cancer. *Journal of Psychosomatic Research, 26*(2), 277–283.

Kabat-Zinn, J. (1990). *Full catastrophe living: Using the wisdom of your body and mind to face stress, pain and illness*. New York: Delacourt.

Kabat-Zinn, J. (2003). Mindfulness-based interventions in context: Past, present, and future. *Clinical Psychology: Science and Practice, 10*, 144–156.

Katz, R. C., Flasher, L., Cacciapaglia, H., & Nelson, S. (2001). The psychosocial impact of cancer and lupus: A cross validation study that extends the generality of "benefit-finding" in patients with chronic disease. *Journal of Behavioral Medicine, 24*, 561–571.

Kissane, D. W., Grabsch, B., Love, A., Clarke, D. M., Bloch, S., & Smith, G. C. (2004). Psychiatric disorder in women with early stage and advanced breast cancer: A comparative analysis. *Australian and New Zealand Journal of Psychiatry, 38*, 320–326.

Koopman, C., Nouriani, B., Erickson, V., Anupindi, R., Butler, L. D., Bachmann, M. H., et al. (2002). Sleep disturbances in women with metastatic breast cancer. *The Breast Journal, 8*, 362–370.

Kornblith, A. B., & Ligibel, J. (2003). Psychosocial and sexual functioning of survivors of breast cancer. *Seminars in Oncology, 30*(6), 799–813.

Krupski, T. L., Kwan, L., Fink, A., Sonn, G. A., Maliski, S., & Litwin, M. S. (2006). Spirituality influences health related quality of life in men with prostate cancer. *Psycho-oncology, 15*, 121–131.

Lamanque, P., & Daneault, S. (2006). Does meditation improve the quality of life for patients living with cancer? *Canadian Family Physician, 52*, 474–475.

Lechner, S. C., & Antoni, M. H. (2004). Posttraumatic growth and group-based interventions for persons dealing with cancer: What have we learned so far? *Psychological Inquiry, 15*, 35–41.

Lengacher, C. A., Kip, K. E., Moscoso, M., Johnson-Mallard, V., Molinari, M., Gaurkee, D., et al. (2007). Mindfulness-based stress reduction (MBSR) improves physical and psychological symptoms, and general health status among breast cancer survivors. *Poster Presented at the Center for Mindfulness in Medicine, Health Care, and Society*, Worcester, MA.

Linley, P. A., & Joseph, S. (2004). Positive change following trauma and adversity: A review. *Journal of Traumatic Stress, 17*, 11–21.

Mackenzie, M. J., Carlson, L. E., Munoz, M., & Speca, M. (2007). A qualitative study of self-perceived effects of mindfulness-based stress reduction (MBSR) in a psychosocial oncology setting. *Stress and Health: Journal of the International Society for the Investigation of Stress, 23*(1), 59–69.

Mackenzie, M. J., Carlson, L. E., & Speca, M. (2005). Mindfulness-based stress reduction (MBSR) in oncology: Rationale and review. *Evidence Based Integrative Medicine, 2*, 139–145.

Manne, S., Ostroff, J., Winkel, G., Goldstein, L., Fox, K., & Grana, G. (2004). Posttraumatic growth after breast cancer: Patient, partner, and couple perspectives. *Psychosomatic Medicine, 66*, 442–454.

Matchim, Y., & Armer, J. M. (2007). Measuring the psychological impact of mindfulness meditation on health among patients with cancer: A literature review. *Oncology Nursing Forum, 34*(5), 1059–1066.

Monti, D. A., Peterson, C., Kunkel, E. J., Hauck, W. W., Pequignot, E., Rhodes, L., et al. (2006). A randomized, controlled trial of mindfulness-based art therapy (MBAT) for women with cancer. *Psycho-oncology, 15*(5), 363–373.

Moscoso, M., Reheiser, E. C., & Hann, D. (2004). Effects of a brief mindfulness-based stress reduction intervention on cancer patients. *Psycho-oncology, 13*, S12.

Murray, S. A., Kendall, M., Boyd, K., Worth, A., & Benton, T. F. (2004). Exploring the spiritual needs of people dying of lung cancer or heart failure: A prospective qualitative interview study of patients and their carers. *Palliative Medicine, 18*, 39–45.

National Cancer Institute of Canada. (2007). *Canadian cancer statistics*. Canadian Cancer Society.

Norman, G. R., Sloan, J. A., Wyrwich, K. W., & Norman, G. R. (2003). Interpretation of changes in health-related quality of life: The remarkable universality of half a standard deviation. *Medical Care, 41*, 582–592.

Northouse, L. L., Laten, D., & Reddy, P. (1995). Adjustment of women and their husbands to recurrent breast cancer. *Research in Nursing and Health, 18*, 515–524.

Ott, M. J., Norris, R. L., & Bauer-Wu, S. M. (2006). Mindfulness meditation for oncology patients. *Integrative Cancer Therapies, 5*, 98-108.

Peterman, A. H., Fitchett, G., Brady, M. J., Hernandez, L., & Cella, D. (2002). Measuring spiritual well-being in people with cancer: The functional assessment of chronic illness therapy–spiritual well-being scale (FACIT-sp). *Annals of Behavioral Medicine: A Publication of the Society of Behavioral Medicine, 24*(1), 49-58.

Pitceathly, C., & Maguire, P. (2003). The psychological impact of cancer on patients' partners and other key relatives: A review. *European Journal of Cancer, 39*(11), 1517-1524.

Ries, L. A. G., Melbert, D., Krapcho, M., Mariotto, A., Miller, B. A., Feuer, E. J., et al. (2007). *SEER cancer statistics review, 1975-2004.* Bethesda, MD: National Cancer Institute.

Roscoe, J. A., Morrow, G. R., Hickok, J. T., Bushunow, P., Matteson, S., Rakita, D., et al. (2002). Temporal interrelationships among fatigue, circadian rhythm and depression in breast cancer patients undergoing chemotherapy treatment. *Supportive Care in Cancer, 10*, 329-336.

Savard, J., & Morin, C. M. (2001). Insomnia in the context of cancer: A review of a neglected problem. *Journal of clinical oncology: Official journal of the American Society of Clinical Oncology, 19*, 895-908.

Saxe, G. A., Hebert, J. R., Carmody, J. F., Kabat-Zinn, J., Rosenzweig, P. H., Jarzobski, D., et al. (2001). Can diet in conjunction with stress reduction affect the rate of increase in prostate specific antigen after biochemical recurrence of prostate cancer? *Journal of Urology, 166*, 2202-2207.

Sephton, S. E., Sapolsky, R. M., Kraemer, H. C., & Spiegel, D. (2000). Diurnal cortisol rhythm as a predictor of breast cancer survival. *Journal of the National Cancer Institute, 92*(12), 994-1000.

Shapiro, S. L. (2001). Quality of life and breast cancer: Relationship to psychosocial variables. *Journal of Clinical Psychology, 57*, 501-519.

Shapiro, S. L., Bootzin, R. R., Figueredo, A. J., Lopez, A. M., & Schwartz, G. E. (2003). The efficacy of mindfulness-based stress reduction in the treatment of sleep disturbance in women with breast cancer: An exploratory study. *Journal of Psychosomatic Research, 54*, 85-91.

Smith, J. E., Richardson, J., Hoffman, C., & Pilkington, K. (2005). Mindfulness-based stress reduction as supportive therapy in cancer care: Systematic review. *Journal of Advanced Nursing, 52*, 315-327.

Speca, M., Carlson, L. E., Goodey, E., & Angen, M. (2000). A randomized, wait-list controlled clinical trial: The effect of a mindfulness meditation-based stress reduction program on mood and symptoms of stress in cancer outpatients. *Psychosomatic Medicien, 62*(5), 613-622.

Strain, J. J. (1998). Adjustment disorders. In J. F. Holland (Ed.), *Psycho-oncology* (pp. 509-517). New York: Oxford University Press.

Surveillance, Epidemiology, and End Results (SEER) Program. (2007). *Prevalence database: "US estimated complete prevalence counts on 1/1/2004"*National Cancer Institute.

Taylor, E. J. (2003). Spiritual needs of patients with cancer and family caregivers. *Cancer Nursing, 26*, 260-266.

The Trials of Hypertension Prevention Collaborative Research Group. (1997). Effects of weight loss and sodium reduction intervention on blood pressure and hypertension incidence in overweight people with high normal blood pressure. *Archives of Internal Medicine, 157*, 657-667.

Touitou, Y., Bogdan, A., Levi, F., Benavides, M., & Auzeby, A. (1996). Disruption of the circadian patterns of serum cortisol in breast and ovarian cancer patients: Relationships with tumour marker antigens. *British Journal of Cancer, 74*, 1248-1252.

van der Poel, H. G. (2004). Smart drugs in prostate cancer. *European Urology, 45*(1), 1-17.

van der Pompe, G., Antoni, M. H., & Heijnen, C. J. (1996). Elevated basal cortisol levels and attenuated ACTH and cortisol responses to a behavioral challenge in women with metastatic breast cancer. *Psychoneuroendocrinology, 21,* 361-374.

Van Wielingen, L. E., Carlson, L. E., & Campbell, T. S. (2006). Mindfulness-based stress reduction and acute stress responses in women with cancer., *15* S42.

Van Wielingen, L. E., Carlson, L. E., & Campbell, T. S. (2007). Mindfulness-based stress reduction (MBSR), blood pressure, and psychological functioning in women with cancer. *Psychosomatic Medicine, 69*(Meeting Abstracts), A43.

Walker, M. S., Zona, D. M., & Fisher, E. B. (2006). Depressive symptoms after lung cancer surgery: Their relation to coping style and social support. *Psycho-oncology, 15*(8), 684-693.

World Health Organization. (2005). *WHO cancer control programme.*

Wua, J., Kraja, A. T., Oberman, A., Lewis, C. E., Ellison, R. C., & Arnett, D. K. (2005). A summary of the effects of antihypertensive medications on measured blood pressure. *American Journal of Hypertension, 18,* 935-942.

Zabora, J., BrintzenhofeSzoc, K., Curbow, B., Hooker, C., & Piantadosi, S. (2001). The prevalence of psychological distress by cancer site. *Psycho-oncology, 10*(1), 19-28.

Part 4

Mindfulness-Based Interventions for Specific Settings and Populations

21

Mindfulness-Based Intervention in an Individual Clinical Setting: What Difference Mindfulness Makes Behind Closed Doors

Paul R. Fulton

I would like to beg you to have patience with everything unresolved in your heart and try to love the questions themselves as if they were locked rooms or books written in a very foreign language. Don't search for the answers, which could not be given to you now, because you would not be able to live them. And the point is, to live everything. Live the questions now. Perhaps then, someday far in the future, you will gradually, without even noticing it, live your way into the answer.

– Rainer Maria Rilke (1875–1926), Letters to a Young Poet

Introduction

In my teens, when I began my study of Buddhist and Western clinical psychology, few resources were available. Most published materials were general and theoretical, such as Erich Fromm's *Zen Buddhism and Psychoanalysis* (Fromm, Suzuki, & DeMartino, 1960), or Hubert Benoit's (1955) *The Supreme Doctrine*. There was no practical literature, and like many others, I was left to explore the territory without a map. When a group of like-minded individuals formed a study group in the early 1980s, the idea of the integration of psychotherapy with meditation remained mildly disreputable. Meditation was associated with New Age self-help and exotic spirituality, and we lingered quietly at the margins of the mainstream.

In these early efforts to integrate these two disciplines, most of the influence of mindfulness was through the therapist's own practice, remaining unnamed and invisible to the patient, a potent but transparent background to the encounter. However, with the growing popularity of mindfulness, patients are more receptive to its use (Psychotherapy Networker, 2007). In my own practice it is common for people already interested or deeply grounded in meditation to seek me out because of it. While it is relatively rare for me to recommend meditation, if I feel it is appropriate, I now do so without the squeamishness I felt early in my clinical career. The issue of how one introduces meditation to patients has all but disappeared.

Mindfulness has gained respectability due to the recent explosion of published literature, much of it providing empirical support of its clinical efficacy. Excellent guidance is increasingly available to new generations of clinicians. To make such research possible, the concept of mindfulness, derived from Buddhist practice and literature, has required refinement and definition. For meaningful clinical trials to be conducted, it has been necessary to define consistent treatment conditions, to try to isolate the "active ingredients" in mindfulness, and control for extraneous variables. Consequently, much of the available literature focuses on protocol-driven use of mindfulness, applied in a structured manner with well-defined populations.

What is determined to be effective in a protocol-driven research trial may not translate naturally to the individual treatment setting. What actually happens in the face to face encounter between patient and therapist in the use these concepts and techniques? This volume provides a number of responses to this question. In this chapter I take up the issue through case examples, from a first-person real world perspective, learned by doing, informed by study and (periodically inconsistent) meditation practice of nearly 35 years, to illustrate some relatively unformulaic ways mindfulness informs the treatment process.

Please note that in this chapter, my use of the term "mindfulness" lacks a certain precision, and is offered as a kind of abbreviation for a range of practices, perspectives, or observations gained through mindfulness practice and study that are broader than redirection of attention or mental training.

The Continuum

As I ended a day-long program teaching about mindfulness to mental health professionals, an elderly psychiatrist and former colleague came up to me and asked with genuine puzzlement, "So, what *is* a mindfulness-based intervention?" I was embarrassed that the answer remained unclear. The problem, I decided, is that for all the efforts to arrive at a consistent and concise definition of mindfulness, it remains elusive for the breadth of its application. In the clinical setting, the concept of mindfulness quickly loses precision because its influence can be seen at a variety of levels. Describing these levels provides a kind of map to locate what we mean when discussing mindfulness.

The intersection of mindfulness and psychotherapy can be described as occurring along a continuum. One pole of this continuum might be called the "implicit" end, where mindfulness is practiced by the therapist, but is otherwise invisible to the patient. Elsewhere I have written about the "implicit" end of the continuum, describing the contribution mindfulness practice makes to the mind of the therapist, and through it, to the therapy (2005). Mindfulness, I argued, helps the therapist to cultivate mental capacities and qualities such as attention, affect tolerance, acceptance, empathy, equanimity, tolerance of uncertainty, insight into narcissistic tendencies, and perspective on the possibility of happiness. The degree to which the therapist's own mindfulness practice influences treatment outcome is just beginning to receive empirical attention.

Moving along the continuum, the use of mindfulness becomes more explicit, incorporating concepts informed by mindfulness, to psychotherapy overtly incorporating specific mindfulness techniques. Some of the stations along this continuum are described by Germer (2005) as a mindfulness-practicing psychotherapist, mindfulness-informed psychotherapy, and mindfulness-based psychotherapy. The explicit end of this continuum, however, does not stop there, as many patients will take up meditation per se, perhaps first as preparation to enable themselves to enter therapy, as an adjunct to therapy, or as a parallel activity conducted as a spiritual practice of awakening quite apart from the therapy's original presenting problem.

Of course, no unidimensional continuum can adequately describe the many ways psychotherapy and mindfulness come together in life, as the clinical examples below attest. This chapter will focus on a variety of ways mindfulness practice informs what actually occurs in the individual clinical setting at different levels of this implicit-explicit continuum.

In addition to the continuum, we can also imagine a Venn diagram in which the domains of psychotherapy and meditation are each described by circles. While each has its own original purpose and range of effectiveness, the circles overlap in mindfulness-oriented psychotherapy (Figure 21.1).

However, when the therapist is a meditator, *all* activities, whether the conduct of psychoanalysis, mindfulness-based cognitive therapy, or doing the laundry, are all informed by mindfulness. This might be depicted by drawing a third circle encompassing both of the other two (Figure 21.2).

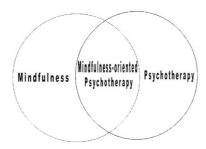

Figure. 21.1. Mindfulness-oriented psychotherapy as the area of overlap between mindfulness and psychotherapy

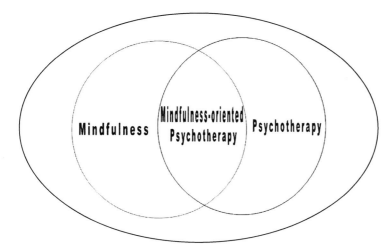

Figure. 21.2. Psychotherapy when the clinician practices mindfulness.

General Considerations

One begins to see the difficulty establishing distinctions about what constitutes mindfulness-based psychotherapy. This integration may be most simple when we craft techniques clearly inspired by mindfulness. For example, one can teach exercises such as the "Three Minute Breathing Space," (Segal, Williams, & Teasdale, 2002), visualizations conducive to acceptance (Hahn, 1976; Kabat-Zinn, 1994), or prescribe techniques intended to use emotions as objects of mindfulness (Brach, 2003).

But mindfulness is not reducible to a class of interventions or techniques, and must be understood in a much broader context. It originates as the methodological cornerstone of a system of understanding, focused on the nature of suffering and the nature of happiness. It is an understanding that, with time and practice, we *become*. When practiced wholeheartedly, it becomes inseparable from all we do, including our clinical work. It is manifest as a quality of attention, a way to hold experience, a commitment to ethical conduct, and an understanding of a path to be traversed. The common denominator of all applications of mindfulness is the turning toward experience; the common therapeutic factor is a changed relationship to experience.

A fundamental contribution of mindfulness is its formulation of the nature of suffering and its relief, which differs from the way distress is often formulated in traditional clinical terms. In the medical model, suffering is regarded as symptom of an underlying disorder, a developmental arrest, learned errors in thought, perception, or conduct, or psychological injury. Treatment is often based on identifying and treating the underlying disorder to relieve the symptomatic distress. By contrast, the Buddhist formulation, upon which mindfulness rests, holds that suffering is inevitable and arises due to a misdirected effort to manipulate our experience to our liking. That is, in our actions large and imperceptibly small, we are constantly trying to hold on to what is pleasurable, and rid ourselves of the unpleasant. In Buddhist terms this is often described in shorthand as grasping. As most experience is tinged by these valences, the effort to control is nearly ceaseless. In this respect, suffering is universal, its operation identical irrespective of this or that putative underlying disorder, or the particular conditions to which we react. It may manifest in overt misery, or it may be extremely subtle in its expression as a sense of unease or dissatisfaction, even in the face of abundance. Grasping is also seen in a tendency to identify with our thoughts and mental constructions, investing them with greater reality and durability than they possess. Suffering arises when we cling to that which is unreliable for being changing and ultimately empty. Understanding this formulation of suffering as originating in our effort to control or grasp offers an opportunity to radically reframe the problem of our patients' suffering.

Mindfulness and Its Influence on the Practice of Psychotherapy

Inevitably, patients arrive with their own hypotheses, or in many cases, convictions, about what is wrong, what must be changed, lost, or gained before their distress can be lifted. Often the formulation is itself an obstacle. This is illustrated by the case of Lydia.

A former therapist herself, Lydia came to treatment after her previous therapist of 10 years moved away. She was recently divorced by her choice, and was now working to rebuild her life and a career in her chosen field. For years she was beset by the fear that she would be alone, left out, and isolated, a fate she concluded was evidence that something was wrong with her. Her previous therapies had focused on identifying and fixing what was wrong, but she still was susceptible to downward spirals of self doubt and despair, driven by her harsh self inquiry conducted with the emotional tone of an inquisition. When I asked if she had established what was wrong with her, she said she had not; her previous therapy had yet to get to the bottom of it. I asked what she really wanted, and she was clear that it was to be happier. When I asked how it felt when she tried to analyze her problems, she said she felt truly terrible. I suggested that given that her desire was to be happy, and this inquiry made her miserable, had she considered setting it aside? Lydia was appalled. After all, this picking away at her wounds was the only method she could imagine, and she believed (against all evidence) that it was the lifeline that would ultimately be her rescue. I suggested that in light of her experience to date, the next time she noticed she was engaged in this spiral, she consider how she felt, and if so inclined, stop as best she could, redirect her attention, and see how she felt as a result. She was threatened by this idea, and the next several sessions were given to understanding the nature of her doubt. Some of this doubt came from her own early professional training in analytic psychotherapy. Lydia conceded that her efforts had been counterproductive, and she might consider an alternative. This experiment became the shared working formulation between us, and she was able to notice when she started down this steep and painful slope, and arrest her fall. Together we began to apply the same approach to other facets of her life, and she became more adept at identifying mental habits relatively quickly after appearing in experience, and exercise a choice in how to proceed. For example, when she found herself grumbling about having to file a stack of papers, she noticed her irritability, and spontaneously saw how it was not the filing itself, but her mind, that was causing her torment. She remained introspective, but what she sought to understand shifted away from the diagnosis of a deficit and toward consideration of the impact of her current mental activity on her sense of well-being. The issue of whether redirecting her attention constituted an abandonment of some truth-seeking became irrelevant; she was freeing herself, and that was rewarding enough.

There are several elements of this reframe that owe a debt to mindfulness. The first is that it offered an alternative to the vestigial impulse, inherent in the medical model, to fix or rid oneself of something. Rather than analyzing or interpreting the underlying meaning of distress, the focus shifted to a pragmatic investigation of what brings relief and what brings more distress, as judged with genuine open-mindedness. In the process, Lydia turned her attention to her here-and-now experience, rather than invest her energy in the unproductive rehearsal of familiar stories.

This touches on another element of formulations derived from mindfulness. That is, what we do is effectively being practiced and strengthened, exactly as a pianist's skills are honed by rehearsal. Conversely, what we cease to do is gradually weakened, and perhaps ultimately extinguished. When we point out to our patients that what they do (whether in thought, speech, or action) is being practiced and strengthened, it offers a new basis to evaluate the impact of those actions on their well-being.

This is illustrated by Andrew, a genuinely caring man who was concerned over his tendency to become impatient or angry, which he took to be signs of failure and moral weakness. In any angry encounter, he suffered both the inherently unpleasant anger itself, as well as the self-judgment he leveled for his loss of control. Even when he thought his anger was justified, he felt bad and helpless to change his reactions. These angry events stuck with him. I asked if he found relief in revisiting these episodes, or if they perpetuated the feelings of anger and shame. Andrew said it made him feel worse. I introduced the idea of practice as strengthening these pathways of anger and judgment, and some neurophysiological evidence behind it (which appealed to his scientific background). I pointed out the way that his lingering over the offending event and his own reactions amounted to a sustained rehearsal. Andrew understood, and immediately brightened at the idea that each new episode offered an opportunity to relate to his anger differently, as a chance to practice something different. I suggested that he practice directing his attention to the subjective mental and physical experience of anger before responding. In this way, he gradually became a student of his own experience and a trained observer of how his anger is triggered in real time. In the process, he gained access a broader palate of responses. The emphasis on practicing took his anger out of the domain of moral weakness, which only tended to cause him to add fuel to his shame, and recast it as something workable in the moment of its arising, something one *does*, rather than evidence of a relatively immutable character flaw or statement about "what kind of person" he was.

The role of practice and learning is not unique to mindfulness, of course. What mindfulness contributes to this commonsense observation is an expanded range of mental qualities that are amenable to simple cultivation. Qualities we often consider to be relatively fixed and trait-like, such as generosity, compassion, anger, impatience, or even interest in our reactions, are all legitimate subjects for on-the-job training. Such observations serve as an antidote to the tendency to see ourselves as relatively static, and to define ourselves in fixed, often uncharitable ways. They invite us to try to become what we value in a practical way. In practice, attending to "what one does" is more workable than fixating on "what one is." The liberating benefit of learning to limit our tendency to form and attach to any fixed perception of ourselves is one benefit of a nuanced mindful understanding of our mental activity.

Often, our patients' habits of mind are harsh and self-punitive. This was true of both Lydia and Andrew. I asked them to attend to the quality of their minds when, for instance, Lydia engaged in her well-practiced self-analysis, or Andrew resided in familiar guilt. In both cases the feeling was unpleasant, regardless of how hygienic they felt these activities to be. When I pointed out that, despite their positive intentions, these habits appeared unkind, both got the message. They had permission to consider their conduct in the light of compassion, as a form of granting or denying self-care. Redefining their own mental habits along the axis of "kind and conducive of happiness," rather than along dimensions of health or morality, offered them more freedom to experiment. How could each be different with themselves in the moment of difficulty? Framing actions in terms of compassion, toward oneself as much as toward others, in practice rather than as an abstract ideal, is both method and fruit of mindfulness.

Note that none of the examples cited above depended on meditation or formal mental training, nor is mindfulness invoked to the patient. They are "interventions" that rest on the therapist's understanding and personal experience, communicated in the language of commonsense to the patient. Nor does the role of mindfulness necessarily lead to a turning away from one's history, in flight to the here and now. This is seen in the case of Carol.

Carol was an experienced meditator, but a novice to therapy, having kept her difficult emotional life from her friends and her kind but unattuned husband. None knew the sort of emotional torment she carried for most of her 50 years. Carol's mother had been an indifferent parent, entirely uninterested in babies or children, a fact made clear in her failure to mirror her gifted daughter's efforts to be seen and accepted. Carol was desperate not to disappoint her mother, but inevitably failed, as her mother wanted only to be the center of attention and the life of the party. Her father was loving, but intolerant and angered by any expression of dissent by Carol. She felt as though she did not exist, and as a young girl would rock on her bed, repeating "I *do* exist." Though she was academically gifted and later, professionally successful, she received no recognition from her parents, nor nourishment for herself, for her accomplishments. She felt counterfeit, learning to hide beneath an exterior of competence to mask a deep sense of illegitimacy. In adulthood she earned a doctorate, but every step was an enormous challenge, as she felt she lacked the right to the self-assertion implied by creating works of original scholarship. What seemed like a natural expression of competence required Herculean effort to overcome a commensurate inner resistance. It was as though she had one foot fully on the gas pedal and another on the brake. Carol was in a helping profession, and though socially competent, being with others was deeply fraught and exhausting. She avoided unnecessary contact for measured periods of time.

Carol chose me as her therapist because she knew of my interest in meditation, though we rarely discussed – and never used – meditation or mindfulness. However, her meditation experience was crucial to the therapy. She had developed some capacity to tolerate her difficult emotional experience, enabling her to endure the overwhelming early months of the therapy. The fear and shame of speaking her formerly disavowed and unspoken thoughts left her trembling and tearful, and she had to sit in her car for a long spell after our sessions. She dreaded the sessions, but was surprised to feel relief as well. Together we learned to pace the therapy to keep it manageable. I was deeply impressed with her courage.

By contrast with Lydia who needed assistance dislodging her attention from the personal archeological investigation that characterized her previous therapies, Carol needed to open to her history and difficult emotional content, to enter and reclaim her story. In this movement she was honoring the truth of her experience, which she had formerly sought to deny. This is the work of conventional therapy, though it felt as if conducted on a high wire. At one point I asked Carol if she felt there was anything authentic in her experience. She thought a moment, and said that the direct experience of the breath, encountered in moments of silent meditation, felt authentic. While Buddhist meditation is often described in terms of seeking to illuminate the illusory nature of the self, in meditation Carol had found a way to locate herself, to herself. She was familiar with the Buddhist doctrine of no-self, but said clearly, "That's not what this was about." We both understood that the self she was in need of inhabiting was something different from the illusory self described by Buddhist psychology, and we understood that both activities were real and valid.

Carol's journey was perilous, and I am convinced that she would have been unable to undertake it were it not for the qualities of courage and fortitude cultivated in her years of meditation practice. It enabled her to become more real to herself as a counterbalance to her sense of inauthenticity. This sort of contribution can never be reduced to a set of techniques, a formulation, or a perspective. Nor was her meditation a substitute for psychotherapy, addressing difficulties that could only be fully summoned in relationship. In meditation she had skillfully found a form of self-care and a source of emotional survival. Though not an explicitly applied technique in the therapy, as part of her own background it was an essential ingredient in her treatment and her life.

Becoming More Explicit

Some uses of mindfulness and its underlying principles are nearer the explicit end of the spectrum. I have often shared specific suggestions lifted more or less directly from Buddhist lore, to good effect.

Leonard was a regional vice president of sales for a large national furniture company. He lived in terror of his semiannual sales presentations at his company's national office, and would over prepare with reams of overhead slides and notes. I had referred him to a MBSR program, from which he had received some benefit, but his fear of these meetings kept him awake at night. I told Leonard of a sermon given by a Zen master, which, in its entirety, was two words long: "Soon dead." Leonard was delighted, and was excited to tell me, after his return from the sales meeting, that the only notes he brought with him were these same two words written large on a legal pad. Leonard knew his material cold, and paradoxically, his voluminous notes only added to his anxiety. The reminder of the proper place of a sales presentation in his life was freeing, and he gave his best presentation ever. Rather than heighten his anxiety, the reflection on life's transience allowed him to loosen his frightened grip on how his sales performance would define him. He saw this event from a larger perspective.

Andrew often wondered when it was appropriate to correct a subordinate, and how to distinguish when he was acting skillfully from when he was speaking from anger.

I suggested that when faced with this uncertainty, he could apply three questions, which I had lifted directly (without full attribution) from one of the Buddha's own discourses (the Abhaya Sutta). First, is what he wants to say true? If not, then don't say it. If it is true, he might then ask if it is beneficial to say it. If it is both true and beneficial, then ask if it is the correct time and place to say it. Besides requiring a moment to reflect (which already helps curtail an impulsive response), posing these practical questions to oneself provides a way to practice non-harm, thereby avoiding escalation of one's own anger and aggression.

The Buddhist formulation for working skillfully with emotions differs from the clinical notions of "abreaction," "getting it out," or catharsis. Anger or hostility are seen as harmful, whether directed toward others or, through judgment and self-rejection, toward oneself. While knowing difficult emotions in the fullness of mindful awareness is essential, expressing them in speech or action requires great care to avoid fueling the anger. This practice of full present-moment awareness of a difficult emotion delicately balanced against and verbal/behavioral restraint is a well developed practice in Buddhist psychology.

Consider this dynamic in the case of Margaret, formerly a teacher but now disabled by the cumulative debilitating effects sadistic childhood abuse. She had repeatedly asked her neighbor not to walk her dog in Margaret's tiny yard. One day, called to the yard by the nearby sound of a fire truck's siren, she found herself standing in the midst of voluminous dog manure. Enraged, she smeared the neighbor's porch, door, and outdoor children's toys with the manure. Then, terrified of what she had done, she called the clinic where I was providing backup coverage for her vacationing therapist, for an emergency appointment. The "expression" of anger had shaken her badly, and she was frightened. In the course of our meeting I asked her if there was someone about whom she felt kindly, even in the midst of this storm. She was able to locate feelings of kindness toward an elderly shut-in neighbor. I suggested to Margaret that she consider doing something for this neighbor. We made a follow-up appointment for the next day. When Margaret returned, she told me how she had brought ice cream to her elderly neighbor, in the process breaking the spell of her rage. She asked me, "How did you know?" She was later able to speak to the neighbor who owned the dog about what each of them had done, and resolved it amicably in a way that had seemed impossible in the heat of her fear.

The Buddha purportedly said that hatred is never appeased by hatred, but only by non-hatred (Dhammapada 5). More than an elevated shibboleth, this expresses a pragmatic approach to difficult emotions that does not deserve to be segregated in spiritual literature and admired from a distance. It offers a practical way to work with inner experience in the interest of cultivating inner and outer peace. Resisting actions rooted in anger, in speech or behavior, toward oneself or toward others, is the practice of compassion, not one of avoidance, isolation, or repression. As with most practices offered by the Buddha, the encouragement is to see for oneself if they work to bring mental peace.

In each case cited above is the invitation to patients to turn toward their experience *as it is*, in full acceptance, not because of their like or dislike of it, but because it is "true" for being present. In this movement is the subtle suggestion that we need not be cured, fixed, or rid of anything as a precondition for healing. Relief from suffering may be difficult to win, but it is nearer at hand than the notion of cure would suggest. When suffering is divested of being regarded as evidence of failure, weakness, or illness, it may become an opportunity to embrace more of life. This startling reframing points the way suffering may gradually loses its sting.

Conclusion

These few case examples do not suggest the application of interventions cribbed from treatment handbooks, but neither are they esoteric or mysterious in nature. They arise from an understanding of the universal underlying dynamic of human suffering. Books can provide invaluable guidance, but mindfulness interventions and formulations arise naturally when, as therapists, we have tested their utility for ourselves in the crucible of our own experience. The sustained idiographic study of our own minds becomes the seat of creative discovery, and the potential contributions of mindfulness to therapy become as countless as the moments we spend with our patients. When we have come to see how we entrap ourselves and how we might cease such harming activity, we learn to see how others, too, fall into cycles of suffering despite their deepest wishes for relief. We are better equipped to provide guidance to our patients in this movement to well-being when we have experiential understanding of this path, whether the use of mindfulness remains unspoken or becomes an explicit part of the therapeutic contract between ourselves and our patients. Then all that we do as therapists become mindfulness-based interventions.

References

Benoit, H. (1955). *The supreme doctrine*. Pantheon Books.

Brach, T. (2003). *Radical acceptance: Embracing your life with the heart of a Buddha*. New York: Bantam Dell.

Dhammapada 5, The Pairs: Heedfulness. (1985). Acharya Buddharakkhita (Trans.) Kandy: Buddhist Publication Society.

Fromm, E., Suzuki, D. T., & DeMartino, R. (1960). *Zen Buddhism and Psychoanalysis*. New York: Harper.

Fulton, P., Anatta: Self, non-self, and the therapist, (2008). In S. Hicks, & T. Bien, (Eds.), *Mindfulness and the therapeutic relationship*. New York: Guilford.

Fulton, P. (2005). Mindfulness as Clinical Training, In C. Germer, R. Siegel, & P. Fulton (Eds.), *Mindfulness and Psychotherapy* (pp. 55–72). New York: Guilford.

Germer, C. (2005). What is mindfulness? In C. Germer, R. Siegel, & P. Fulton (Eds.), *Mindfulness and psychotherapy* (pp. 3–27). New York: Guilford.

Hanh, T. N. (1976). *The miracle of mindfulness*. Boston: Beacon Press.

Kabat-Zinn, J. (1994). *Wherever you go there you are: Mindfulness meditation in everyday life*. New York: Hyperion.

Majjhima Nikaya 58, Abhaya Sutta.

The Most Influential Therapists of the Past Quarter-Century. (2007, April/March) *Psychotherapy Networker*. Retrieved June 28, 2007 from http://www.psychotherapynetworker.org/index.php?category=magazine&sub_cat=march_april_2007

Rilke, Rainer Maria. (1984). *Letters to a Young Poet*. (S. Mitchell, Trans.). New York: Random House. (Original work published 1929)

Segal, Z., Williams, J., & Teasdale, J. (2002). *Mindfulness-based cognitive therapy for depression: A new approach to preventing relapse*. New York: Guilford Press.

22

Mindfulness with Children: Working with Difficult Emotions

Trudy A. Goodman and Susan Kaiser Greenland

"Then it is only kindness that makes sense anymore, only kindness that ties your shoes. . .only kindness that raises its head from the crowd of the world to say it is I you have been looking for, and then goes with you everywhere like a shadow or a friend."

– Naomi Shehab Nye

Introduction

In Buddhist psychology, difficult emotions are defined as forces that visit the mind. Imagine that your mind is like water in a pot and your emotions are the wind. When the wind blows, the water ripples on the surface and the still water below is hidden from view. If you were to gaze at the water's surface your reflection would be obscured by ripples. Damaging emotions make it especially difficult to see the water's surface clearly; they make waves, and in the ensuing turbulence you may feel upset and confused. Mindfulness practice helps you see and calm the emotional turbulence, allowing your mind to be clearly reflected on the surface of the water. This is one way we talk to children about their feelings.

In this chapter we discuss mindfulness as a way to help children understand their emotional pain. We present a method that we dub *scram* to help children loosen the grip of their difficult emotions and respond more mindfully to them. We choose this acronym because children and mentors (therapists, teachers, parents, and others working with children) often want to scram – or quickly leave – when faced with difficult emotions. *scram* is a step-by-step approach toward a mindful resolution of a painful emotion or experience: *Stop* or slow down; *Calm* your body; *Remember* to look at what is happening both inside and out; and only after completing the first three steps, take mindful *Action* with kindness or *Metta*.[1]

This chapter is a collaboration between two writers with different perspectives. Trudy Goodman (Trudy) co-founded the Institute for Meditation and Psychotherapy in 1995, and founded InsightLA in 2002, a not-for-profit organization for the teaching of mindfulness. Trudy, a psychotherapist for 25 years, has worked with children and mindfulness in

---

[1] Metta – Pali for friendly.

a variety of therapeutic settings and family mindfulness programs. Susan Kaiser Greenland (Susan) co-founded *InnerKids* in 2000, which brings mindful awareness practices to children in pre-kindergarten through high school. In collaboration with educators and therapists, she adapts traditional mindfulness practices so that they are developmentally appropriate for children/teens and suitable for use in a secular setting. We hope that by bringing together insight from mindfulness, psychotherapy and classroom experience, this article will contribute to the emerging body of knowledge regarding the secular practice of mindful awareness with children.

Background

The traditional objective of mindfulness is both practical and therapeutic; by viewing experience with clarity and discernment at the moment it occurs, it is possible to free the mind from emotional suffering. This process, in and of itself, trains attention, promotes emotional balance, and cultivates compassion[2]. It is well suited to children because the approach can be playful, experimental and is always experiential; we invite children to "come and see, to try this for yourself."

"What is unique about mindfulness-oriented child therapy (or education) is the enhanced ability to return to the present moment again and again, with openhearted, nonjudgmental attention to both the experience of the child and to one's own experience." (Goodman, 2005.). The objective of practicing mindfulness with children is to develop and strengthen their ability "to pay attention to their inner and outer experience, with curiosity and kindness"(Kaiser-Greenland, In Press) in a variety of ways consistent with their level of development. Through this process children are encouraged to become gently introspective, to look a little closer at life experience as it is happening. As a result, they learn to objectively see: (a) internal processes, how they tend to act and react; (b) external interactions, how they interact with others including setting boundaries and managing conflict; and (c) connections between themselves, others and the environment. (Kaiser-Greenland, In Press.) This letter from Eliot, one of Susan's fifth grade students, illustrates this process:

> "I get mad easily and [mindfulness] helped me calm down. On the test, I got mad at some questions and got out of concentration. [Focusing on my breath] got me back on track. I just let the monkeys go." (Monkeys refer to the colloquial Buddhist term "monkey mind," where thoughts and emotions swing through the mind like monkeys in a jungle, swinging through the trees.)

Through the practice of mindfulness, Eliot observed his internal processes (he gets mad easily), external interactions (he lost his concentration on the test), then made a connection between his inner experience, outer experience and mindfulness (breath awareness got him back on track by helping him calm down and focus).

---

[2] *InnerKids* programs refer to attention, balance, and compassion as the *New ABCs* of learning.

Attention

Mindfulness is a word that has come to mean many different things to many different people, but in Buddhism mindfulness, or bare attention, is in the very first perception – a fleeting moment of open awareness, before the conceptual, thinking mind takes over. From Sarah Doering: "Mindfulness is the observing power of the mind, the active aspect of awareness. It is present in a moment of seeing that's nonverbal, pre-verbal. It's seeing with very great clarity and no thought. The object noticed is not yet separated out, but is simply part of the whole flow of the process of life." (Sarah Doering, 2003.) This is the realm of mindfulness. Whatever is happening is accurately reflected, as if in a clear mirror. It simply reflects, without passion or prejudice, what is here.

There is overlap between the quality of attention fundamental to mindfulness and executive function (the mental capacity to control and purposefully apply one's own mental skills). In what may seem to be a tautology, mindfulness strengthens executive function while executive function strengthens mindfulness. Pilot studies suggest that this may be true for teens and children as young as four years old. The Mindful Awareness Research Center at UCLA recently completed two pilot programs studying the effect of mindfulness on attention in teens and pre-school children. A small pilot study in ADHD teens, found improved performance on selected executive function tests (specifically, tests measuring inhibition or conflict attention) and reduced self-report symptoms of ADHD (Zylowska et al., 2006). In a larger randomized and controlled study conducted at UCLA's Early Childcare Center, pilot data shows that pre-school children's participation in an InnerKids mindfulness program that Susan developed, was associated with improvements in executive function specifically working memory, planning and organization, global executive functioning and emergent metacognition (thinking about thinking). (Smalley and colleagues, 2007.) While this data is preliminary and requires further investigation, the results are promising.

Robust executive function in and of itself does not constitute mindfulness, however. The quality of attention, or one's perspective, is critical. Susan describes this mindset to children as one of curiosity and kindness. Dr. Jeffrey Schwartz has adopted the more formal term "impartial spectator" to describe this stance: "the part of your mind that has the ability to become aware of the difference between "me" (the watcher/observer) and "my brain" (the thought or feeling)" (Schwartz, 1998). When practicing mindfulness with children Susan refers to this perspective as one of a *friendly and impartial spectator*, combining both the concepts of kindness and of impartiality into a single phrase. This view helps children differentiate between identifying with an emotion ("I am angry") and observing the emotion ("I know this angry feeling"). By making a clear distinction between identification and observation, a child can begin to understand that an emotion does not necessarily reflect who she is, it only reflects how she's feeling right *now* about what's happening right *now*. Viewing emotions as a from the perspective of a *friendly and* impartial spectator is not meant to take children out of their experience, nor does it mean becoming dissociated. Rather, it is a way to help them develop confidence in their capacity to stand fully in their experience and observe it for what it is, seeing it clearly and as completely as possible given their developmental stage.

A child in the grip of frightening or overwhelming emotions is frequently unable to attend to the task at hand. An example of this emerged from Susan's work with one of her students, Sara. Here is the way Susan's work in the classroom unfolds:

In mindfulness class we use secular and age appropriate exercises and games to promote awareness of inner experience (thoughts, emotions and physical sensations), outer experience (other people's thoughts, emotions and physical sensations) and both together without blending the two. The program consists of 8–12 consecutive weekly sessions with each session broken down into three standard sequences: the first and last sequences contain introspective practices and the middle sequence contains activities and games that promote each week's learning objective. The program is designed to expose children to progressively longer periods of introspective practices each week. This is accomplished by gradually extending the duration of the first sequence (which includes a brief period of sitting introspection) and the third sequence (which includes a modified body scan or concentration practice while lying down). As the duration of the first and last sequences increase, the duration of the second sequence containing more goal directed (as opposed to introspective) practices decreases. This dynamic course structure permits the length of time students engage in introspective practice to increase gradually and organically, through the course of the program.

Recently Susan taught an *InnerKids* mindful awareness program in a public school (pre-k through middle) located in a shelter for moms and children who are victims of domestic violence. Sara is a 10-year-old student who was enrolled in one of Susan's classes.

Quiet and studious, Sara was always one of the first to participate in class discussions and enthusiastically engage in mindfulness activities and games. Sara was a leader within the shelter and frequently helped younger students on the playground and at home. It was hard to imagine she was the victim of extreme physical and sexual abuse.

Sara was not able to participate in the last sequence of mindfulness class because she was too frightened to lie on the floor in the presence of other people. Her understandable fear of lying down in public paralyzed her so that she was unable to focus on anything else. Sara's experience is not uncommon in this setting and demonstrates clearly how painful emotions can interfere with even the most basic activities.

The first challenge when working with Sara was to help her identify her fear and view it – even for a fleeting moment – from the perspective of a *friendly and impartial spectator*. Over a period of several weeks Susan integrated the mindful process scram into her work with Sara. First, Susan encouraged Sara to simply notice the fear when it occurred by *stopping* doing whatever she was doing when it happened. Period. There was no expectation that She lie down or engage in another, less frightening, introspective practice. It was enough for Sara to make the connection that her fear was triggered by lying on the classroom floor.

Eventually Sara made that connection and was able to *calm* her body and quiet her mind with breath awareness practices. Once she felt calmer, she could *remember* that these emotions occurred every time the class practiced introspection while lying down. By the end of the 12-week course,

Sara was able to *act* mindfully and cautiously lie down with the rest of the class with *metta* or kindness toward herself by understanding her feelings. Sara was never able to close her eyes during the body scan, nor was she able to physically relax. But she overcame her fear and lay on the floor with her peers. Sara discovered the courage to do so by practicing mindfulness and *metta*.

The case of Sara illustrates an important caveat about working with children suffering from posttraumatic stress disorder. The potential for flooding, especially in classroom situations, must be taken seriously and mentors must be trained in recognizing signs that flooding may be immanent. Safety and flexibility are most important in clinical settings, as well. When attention is destabilized by traumatic memories and strong emotions, the mentor can support a child by helping turn their attention *away* from awareness of inner feelings and toward awareness of the outer world.

Emotions Are Viewed as Visitors

To a child, a difficult emotion sometimes feels strong and solid, particularly in the early years when children are concrete thinkers. Children can get stuck in painful emotional states because they believe them to be permanent and an inherent aspect of who they are. Children often become so caught up in a feeling that they immediately act on it, unable to imagine that there could be a more objective perspective. We have found the Buddhist teaching of impermanence, that everything changes and nothing stays the same, an extremely useful concept that children can easily recognize and understand when embodied by their mentors. Mentors with a visceral understanding of impermanence will model how to relate to emotions as impermanent states, inside and out. Practicing mindfulness, children and their mentors see together how emotions arise with each moment of experience, in a continuously flowing, changing stream. Through relationship with a mentor who sees through the lens of impermanence, children can learn to experience difficult emotions as transient and situational, rather than a permanent condition intrinsic to them.

One way that emotions are described in Buddhist psychology is as passing, or adventitious, visitors to the heart. Emotions are viewed as healthy (leading to wise actions and happiness) or unhealthy (leading to unwise expressions that bring unhappiness in their wake). We recognize that this view of emotions is a simplification and propose it only as a practical and therapeutic way of approaching complex emotional processes with children who often find it easier to view psychological pain more clearly if they personify the emotion.

Negative emotions that naturally accompany the inevitable painful aspects of relational life can get blown out of proportion and become damaging when children are left alone with them, or if their mentors get frightened or angry when they don't know how to help. Then both children and mentor naturally try to avoid the emotions (to *scram*); thus giving them an authority they don't have. From the perspective of *scram*, it doesn't matter whether emotions are positive or negative, we work with both in the same mindful way as. Simply the integrative, dynamic activity of the mind, an expression of being alive. But when emotions are blown out of proportion, they obscure awareness of both clear mind and its objects.

Personifying difficult emotions and the problems they cause as visitors, albeit unwelcome ones, allows children and their mentors to consider many aspects of mood, emotion and the possibility of their transformation by:

- Talking about emotions as impermanent, like guests who visit and then leave. We cannot overemphasize the compassionate role of the mindful mentor in helping children gently slow into their experience so they can begin to identify their emotions, to stop themselves from acting them out, and to see how they change.
- Experimenting with purposeful attention in the company of a mentor, children may see that it is possible to have some control over how they respond to their emotions. While children cannot choose their feelings, with guidance and support, they can learn and practice new ways of responding to them.
- Acknowledging we have a choice about how to entertain our visitors; a child may not be able to prevent them from arriving, but with help, she may choose whether to invite them to stay. This may open new possibilities. Together with her mentor, a child can reflect about how long she is willing to stay with this particular guest. For the time of a play date? A sleepover? Does she let them move in, take over and cause problems? Or even get in the way of growing up?
- Recognizing times when she is not bothered by unwelcome guests, where she is able to relax and be herself. Acknowledging those times with her mentor, even celebrating them together. These moments when nothing else seems to be happening can be an opportunity for quiet non-verbal sharing of attention and connection.

The quiet nonverbal sharing mentioned above describes an important way of teaching mindfulness, without necessarily saying a word. Through attentive, quiet presence, a mentor can *embody* mindfulness and model how *scram* can be used in real-life relationships. Embodied mindfulness may also be an effective means by which a mentor becomes better attuned with (or "felt by") a child. From Dan Siegel, "As this joining evolves, we begin to resonate with each other's states and become changed by our connection. Attunement can be seen as the heart of therapeutic change." Attunement is expressed in the safety, comfort, and relief a child may feel when seen through a mentor's eyes, as being whole and complete just as she is. By accompanying, by staying with the child as all the child's "visitors" come and go, the mentor embodies trust in the child's underlying, inherent clarity and wisdom. As trust and attunement with the mentor deepen, a child may be better able to integrate the mentor's positive view and make it her own.

In the following example, Trudy models mindfulness in her response to a boy's provocative actions.

A 7-year-old boy, Xavier, was referred to psychotherapy for being oppositional with teachers and fighting at school. Xavier was a perfectionist who would angrily destroy his work if he made the slightest mistake. He came to therapy clutching his after-school snack, a big box of Fruity Pebbles cereal. He was bright and presented himself as friendly and playful. But the fun play immediately broke down when he couldn't have his way. He would regress and become furious, expressing intense self-hatred. Inevitably, Xavier would lose control and the cereal would suddenly fly all over the room. The first time it happened, he and Trudy both stopped, stunned. They looked at the rug covered in multi-colored tiny pieces of cereal. Xavier was visibly frightened by the aggression in his act of flinging the cereal around Trudy office. He became defiant and hostile, daring her to get mad.

Just stopping and looking at the therapeutic space bedecked in colorful fruity pebbles, Trudy understood why this tightly controlled little boy, an only child who lived in an environment where no misstep went unnoticed or unpunished, needed to let his precious snack fly all over the space. Suddenly it was funny, the office was a mess! It became a *scram* practice when the cereal flew; they *stopped*, saw what was happening at the moment it happened, and *calmed* down to *remember* that the mess was not a big deal. After taking these first three steps, Xavier was able to *act* mindfully as they swept up the cereal together with an attitude of kindness, understanding why Xavier acted as he did.

Trudy's stance of mindfulness and kindness allowed Xavier to feel safe enough to talk about the beatings he received when he was "bad." Trudy and his school counselor found help for his mother and a therapy group for Xavier, where he could work on improving relationships with peers and develop self-regulating behaviors. This was a case where a mentor's compassion, mindfulness and humor allowed a frightened, angry boy to express his truth.

We understand that limits may need to be set for children to keep them and their peers safe. By embodying mindfulness the mentor can both establish boundaries, and convey empathic attunement of a child just the way she is, without needing to fix, rescue or change her. Together mentor and child can use *scram* to help build the child's capacity for self-compassion and understanding.

Because children are deeply embedded in a *family system*, it is not surprising that the degree to which a child benefits from mindfulness-based therapy is highly associated with the amount of parental involvement. (Semple et al., 2006.) A parent's capacity to reflect on her inner life, and the inner life of her child, can also be a significant predictor of the child's security of attachment to the parent (Fonagy & Target, 1977). Thus it is important to look at practicing mindfulness with children from a systems perspective and, whenever possible, involve parents from the outset. In keeping with this approach a pilot pediatric obesity study currently underway at University of California, San Francisco, is delivered to the child through the adult caregiver (whether overweight or not). The pilot intervention extends MB-EAT[3] (Kristeller & Hallett, 1999) to children and parents, using *MB-EAT* and *InnerKids* programs adapted for this population. It is deliberately focused on preadolescent children who are embedded in the family unit. Michele Meitrus-Snyder, lead investigator of the study, is persuaded from limited pilot experience that the mutual understanding gleaned through the shared mindfulness experience, fosters improved connections between parent and child that may be as important as any other facet of the intervention. (Mietus-Snyder et al., 2007).

---

[3] MB-EAT is a mindfulness-based intervention for adults with binge eating disorders. It was developed by Jean L. Kristeller, Department of Psychology, Indiana State University, Ruth Quillian-Wolever, Center for Integrative Medicine, Duke University and their colleagues.

While the application of *scram* is simple and can be taught to the entire family, the embodiment of this steady, gentle way of being is not easy. From Buddhist meditation teacher and psychologist Jack Kornfield: "An important part of mindfulness practice is being conscious of and taking responsibility for *embodying* mindfulness through our own thoughts, feelings and actions" (Kornfield, 2007). Taking responsibility for your own mindfulness, learning to walk-the-walk, is the most effective way to transmit compassionate mindfulness skills to children.

If you are not already a practitioner, we recommend you gently introduce yourself to mindfulness practice in order to get a felt sense of the experience. Dr. Jon Kabat-Zinn, who first taught and researched clinical applications of mindfulness, says:

> First, we become receptive to actually feeling the subtly changing sensations in our bodies, so often overlooked in our daily lives. We become aware of our physical location and movements, thereby bringing the mind and body to the same place at the same time. It can be surprising to see how rarely the mind is where the body is, here, in the present, instead of thinking about something or somewhere else. Literally *embodying* mindfulness, we observe direct sensory experience, opening all the senses – "sensing" – the non-verbal world of touch, sound, sensation, smell, sight etc."
>
> (Kabat-Zinn, 2005)

These techniques that enhance sensory awareness, build the skills of mindfulness through actually being mindful. As mentioned earlier, mindfulness is both the means and the end of our practice; what strengthens mindfulness the most is the practice of mindfulness itself! For those new to this way of working, here are some guidelines:

- Recognize that there is a learning curve. Mindfulness takes practice; insight and compassion are experiences that cannot be forced.
- Your credibility comes from knowing first-hand the clarity and gentleness that come from doing this practice patiently, over and over again.
- As you continue in your own practice of mindfulness meditation, insights about the children with whom you work will likely occur quite spontaneously. You may find that your intuition becomes sharper and you become more willing to trust it.
- The more you become acquainted with this process, the more you may be able to creatively introduce it in appropriate ways to the children with whom you work.
- Learn as much as you can from others who have done pioneering work in the field.

Using *Scram* in Psychotherapy

A 12-year-old girl named Manouj was suffering from constant anxiety and panic. Manouj's family had emigrated to the USA shortly after her father was released from prison, three years before. He was a political prisoner for months, taken at gunpoint from their home while Manouj was at school. Shortly before entering therapy with Trudy she had been visiting cousins in the Middle East, and the war between northern Israel and Hezbollah broke out. This triggered intense terror in Manouj.

Manouj, told Trudy in tears, that she's afraid to fall asleep because there might be spiders in her bed, she's afraid to eat lunch with her friends because the taco might be poisonous, she can't eat outside because an insect might fall into her food. Salad reminds her of a poisonous plant and she might die if she touches it. Even the food her mother has cooked for her might be bad. The little spot on her T-shirt could be dangerous. . . She is sobbing as she tells all this, in Arabic, with her mother as interpreter.

Trudy enters her world through mindful attunement to her feelings of fear and sadness. Trudy names fear as a visitor who got its foot in the door when her father was taken to prison.

Together, they practice *scram* when fear arrives: *Stop* and slow down, calmly breathe through the fear, and remember fear is visiting. Wordlessly, through her willingness to just come and be open, Manouj can attune to her therapist and begin to act mindfully to change her relationship to fear.

Trudy shifts into an active internal practice of mindfulness and metta: her attention is attuned to her experience and Manouj's simultaneously. Trudy deliberately suffuses the atmosphere with kindness, "holding" Manouj in her stable presence. A mindful mentor can lend the strength of her ability to be present with experience to the child; Manouj can begin to see how fear can be there, she can feel anxious, without losing her own capacity to be mindful. Fear doesn't have to be in charge of her thoughts, feelings, and choices. *Calmly* she can recover her balance and confidence.

As we sit and talk, Trudy checks in with Manouj; she reflects, in English now: "The more I talk about it, the more fear goes away and the better I feel." Her voice is calmer, lower, and she is not crying anymore. Manouj is relaxed now, body draped across her mom's lap, her head resting on the arm of the couch. Her mother, a sensitive meditator and attuned parent, is quietly holding her. The room is peaceful and still. Trudy encourages her mother to act with metta by holding Manouj and being silent, "as if you are meditating." Sitting still, they are all quiet together. Manouj seems to be soaking up the peace that is palpable in the room. The session ends this way.

A tear-stained and angry Manouj arrives at the next meeting, reluctant to come in, hiding behind her mother. Manouj is upset, afraid that coming to talk about her fears will make then come back, when she's actually been feeling less scared this past week. She despairs that it would happen again from seeing Trudy and is angry with her mother for bringing her.

Fear was not around for much of her weekend. When it came back, her mother remembered *scram* and brought Manouj on to her lap while she sat quietly. Manouj feel asleep, held in the arms of her mother's mindfulness meditation, and, the next morning woke up free of fear again.

Trudy *reflects* aloud if fear might be trying to protect her from present dangers – could fear be trying to protect her from growing up too fast? She nods. From having to go to high school? From having her body change and mature? Manouj tells her mother that she wishes she could just stop the world, go somewhere for a while and then get back on.

Trudy teaches Manouj mindfulness meditation at this point, as a way to stop and be very grounded in the present moment, able to observe fear's comings and goings. Manouj learns to be aware of her body sitting, of her breath flowing rhythmically, in and out. When thoughts go through her mind, Manouj can bring her attention gently back to the movement of the breath.

They sit together for 8 minutes, and Manouj gives a thumbs-up when finished. She was able to notice when her mind wandered away from what she was doing, and to relax and feel peaceful as she practiced being mindful of her breathing. Smiling and rosy, Manouj looks genuinely happy for the first time.

Manouj arrives at our next meeting, glad to see Trudy and asks her mother to go out for a walk, so they can be alone together. This is new. Being held in her mother's attuned mindfulness, with the guidance of her mentor, Manouj is learning to hold and calm herself, too.

In the next session, Manouj imagines empathetically how difficult it must have been for her parents when she was in so much emotional pain. She describes how she is healing the past terror and loss of her childhood home. "Moving to Los Angeles was a big shock for me. The story behind it and the story after it makes me realize how strong I have become. If you get hurt, you will heal,. . .as you realize what's here and what's there, your mind will be strong, and become healthy, that alone will heal the wound. That is how I got through (my fears), back to my real world."

At the end of the session, Manouj acts mindfully! She stands on her head, using her arms for support. It's a wonderful metaphor for learning how to handle her world being turned upside down with balance, self-efficacy and confidence.

For over a year, Manouj was free from fear and anxiety. After around 18 months, Manouj became mildly anxious and Trudy saw her again. Her parents felt Manouj's anxiety was an internal problem of her own. They are not yet willing to acknowledge how much their family's past trauma and losses still affect their relationships, to one another and to their new life. Until they find a way to do this, Manouj may continue to be vulnerable to fear.

Guidelines for Working with Children

- *Mentoring and Embodiment*

  ○ Children learn to build their own mindfulness skills more effectively when the adult *embodies* mindfulness. Having and maintaining an established mindfulness practice is a prerequisite for this work.
  ○ It is critical that the mentor has experience with the specific mindfulness practices that are being taught. Many have blown on a pinwheel to teach children breath awareness, but to use the practice effectively you must know how to apply it to different learning objectives – how do you use the pinwheel to train focused attention? wide-open awareness? to soothe the body? When used skillfully this one practices can be used to help a child feel the experience of each of these qualities – concentration, awareness, and calming.
  ○ Mindfulness is relational, attuned, and connected. Sharing attention and caring may strengthen both mentor and child's capacity to access a calm and clear state-of-mind.
  ○ The benefits of practicing mindfulness take time and are not always obvious. Patience is the heart of the process and developed by focusing on the practice itself rather than a specific goal or end point. From Lonnie Zeltzer: "It is precisely the moving away from the need to have

results that often contributes to a lessening of the child's suffering"
(Zeltzer, 2005).

- *Practices*

  o Mindfulness teaches children to note and label emotions. Noting is an
  effective tool for becoming aware of emotions and being able to see
  them as occasional visitors.

  o Mindfulness games and activities can be framed in ways that are appropriate to various ages and developmental abilities, from pre-school
  through adulthood.

  o Because children often have relatively short attention spans and,
  depending on their age, their memory may not be completely developed, we engage in reflective practices for periods of short duration
  and repeat them frequently.

  o *Fun* is a key concept when practicing mindfulness with children. If the
  activities are not fun and playful young children will resist them.

  o Practicing mindful awareness may not be for everyone and it is not skillful to insist that a child engage in introspective practices if she is not
  comfortable doing so.

  o Breath awareness alone is an extremely valuable tool for all ages, and if
  taught correctly, it is in and of itself a practice of mindfulness.

  o In a classroom setting it is virtually never appropriate for children to
  drop into deep states of meditation or introspection. The mentor must
  take care to monitor the students. If it appears that a child is having a
  difficult time sitting still or is becoming sad, it is appropriate to gently
  ease out of a reflective practice into a more active one.

- *Metta*

  o The use of mindfulness techniques to train children in attention is com-
  plemented by training in kindness and caring (*metta*), and learning how
  to include both oneself and others in a circle of compassion.

  o Through compassion for self and others *embodied* by the mentor, a
  child is show a process through which she can develop a new relationship to her difficult emotions, built upon insight and courage.

- *Family Systems*

  o It is important that parents are informed about every aspect of your
  work and are integrated as much as possible. We recommend a parent
  meeting before and after mindfulness skills are taught to children. We
  often give children prompts (or homework) at the end of a session and
  it is helpful if parents participate in the home practice.

Conclusion

The playful acronym *scram* takes breath awareness further than calming the
body and mind. It charts a step-by-step mindfulness-based process to help
children free themselves from the often complex webs of tangled and difficult emotions that are a natural part of growing up. *Scram* invites children to
stop, calm their bodies/quiet their minds, and *remember* to be mindful when

a painful emotion arises. Using this process, children *act* only after taking a moment to *reflect* on and viscerally sense their inner and outer experience. *Scram* reminds them to do so with kindness or *metta*.

Scram is most effectively taught through a combination of verbal and non-verbal methods; with one's own mindfulness practice as a fundamental prerequisite of this work. How long must one practice mindfulness before being qualified to teach children? This is the subject of vigorous debate in the field and there is no definitive answer. We know, however, that in order to *embody* or model *scram* one must viscerally understand how the work is rooted in mindfulness, and that the intention of mindfulness-oriented work with children is education, healing and service. In the drawing of the *InnerKids* tree, with roots deep in awareness practice, service is represented by the trunk of the tree, which underlies and quietly supports the work with children in families, schools and clinical or community settings. For the work to be authentically transmitted, it must remain connected to its trunk and roots – connected to the intention of service with deep roots in the practice of mindfulness.

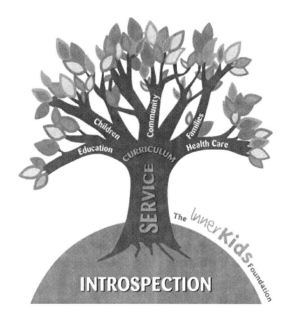

The Sanskrit root of the word *sati*, mindfulness (in Pali), means "to remember." In our work we remind children "remember! – Remember to notice, to pay attention to what's happening within you and around you, from moment to moment to moment." It's easy to overlook the first moments of mindful awareness, which can be so fleeting. By teaching children to remember to notice, we are helping them value and extend moments of pre-verbal attention that come naturally, but so often are unnoticed or forgotten.

Remembering to practice mindfulness over and over again can be as transformative for the mentor as for the child, by giving, the mentor an opportunity to viscerally understand the child's experience and the child an opportunity to feel deeply seen and understood. This nonconceptual way of knowing has a profound effect on all those who experience it, inherent in which is Mindful the potential to change the way that children and mentors relate to their emotions, their relationships, and their world.

We do not have a magic bullet to alleviate the suffering of children faced with painful emotional experiences, but we've seen even the most basic mindfulness practice have a remarkable impact on the life of a child. As with many things, this is best summed up by a child:

> I learned one thing about mindfulness. I learned that when you don't feel so well, maybe you can breathe, In-then-out, that is what I learned.
>
> *InnerKids' Second Grade Student, Lucy*

References

Doering, S. (2003). Insight Journal Archives; The Five Spiritual Powers, Barre Center for Buddhist Studies.

Fonagy, P. & Target, M. (1977). Attachment and Reflective Function: Their role in self organization. Development and Psychopathology, 9(4) 679–700.

Goodman (2005). Trudy Working with Children: Beginner's Mind. In: Germer, C., Siegel, R. & Fulton, P. (Eds.), Mindfulness and Psychotherapy (p. 198). New York: Guilford Press.

Kabat-Zinn, Jon (2005). Guided Mindfulness Meditation Practice CDS Series 3, in conjunction with Coming to Our Senses: Healing Ourselves and the World through Mindfulness. New York: Hyperion.

Kaiser Greenland, S (In Press), The Mindful Child, New York: Free Press.

Kornfield, J. (2007) personal communication

Kristeller, Jean L., & Hallett, C. Brendan, (1999). An Exploratory Study of a Meditation-Based Intervention for Binge Eating Disorder, Journal of Health and Psychology, 4(3) 357–363.

Mietus-Snyder et al., (2007). paper in preparation.

Schwartz, Jeffrey M., (1998). Dear Patrick, Life is tough – Here's some good advice (p. 122). New York: HarperCollins.

Semple R. J., Lee J., & Miller J. L. (2006). Mindfulness-based cognitive therapy for children. In: Baer R. A., (Ed.) Mindfulness-Based Treatment Approaches (pp. 143–166). New York: Academic Press.

Siegel, Daniel J., (2007). The Mindful Brain; Reflection and Attunement in the Cultivation of Well-Being (p. 290), New York: W. H. Norton & Company, Inc.

Smalley, S. (2007) Personal correspondence.

Zeltzer, Lonnie K., & Blackett Schlank, Christina (2005). Conquering Your Child's Chronic Pain, A Pediatrician's Guide for Reclaiming a Normal Childhood (p. 231). New York: HarperCollins.

Zylowska L., Ackerman D. L., Yang M. H., et al. (2006). Mindfulness meditation training in adults and adolescents with Attention Deficit Hyperactivity Disorder—A feasibility study. J Atten Disord.

23

Mindfulness-Based Elder Care: Communicating Mindfulness to Frail Elders and Their Caregivers

Lucia Mc Bee

"The most important intervention we can offer is ourselves, who we are in each moment, being present with the other, feeling our connection, and verbally and non-verbally conveying this felt sense."

Introduction

Since its inception in 1979, mindfulness-based stress reduction Mindfulness-Based Stress Reduction (MBSR) has been introduced into many community and institutional settings with a variety of populations. There is an understood caveat that the participants are able to understand and follow instructions, have a good attention span, are able to commit to the experience, and to participate in some form of exercise. In this chapter, I discuss group and individual interventions offered to populations who often are not able to meet the above criteria.

While MBSR has prescribed interventions and tools, the core of these interventions lies in the skillful application and intentions of the teacher. The "heart of mindfulness" or the basic elements are not the tools, which could be described as a finger that points to the moon, not to be confused with the moon itself. The skill of the teacher arises from a personal practice of mindfulness that allows resourcefulness and flexibility. With a physically or cognitively frail population, the key is in the adaptation of the skills and the teacher's embodiment of mindfulness.

Since 1995, I have been offering mindfulness-based elder care (MBEC) groups to frail elders and their caregivers, most frequently in the nursing home setting. I have made moderate to significant adaptations to the MBSR model while maintaining the core intention of mindfulness. In MBEC groups, participants learn the techniques of meditation, gentle yoga, and mindfulness, and discuss ways to integrate these techniques into their day-to-day lives. MBEC groups and mindfulness practice foster an awareness of life, moment by moment, allowing them to face illness, pain, and loss with increased presence and equanimity. My hope is that readers of this chapter will be encouraged to conduct their own work with frail elders and their caregivers, and also consider additional adaptations of mindfulness to younger populations with significant cognitive and physical disabilities.

Rationale

In 2001, Kinsella and Velkoff reported that the world's population of people 65 and older was growing by almost 800,000 a month. Lower infant mortality, increased birth rates and declining death rates lead to estimates that this trend will continue. In addition, the fastest growing segment of the 65-plus population belongs to people over 80 years old (Kinsella & Velkoff, 2001). Increasing the quantity of our lives may not increase the quality of our lives. Elders disproportionately suffer from chronic illness and multiple losses. In the United States, 80% of the over 65 population is living with at least one chronic condition and 50% have two (Centers for Disease Control and Prevention, 2003). Cognitive, as well as physical health can have a profound impact on elders' quality of life. International studies document that dementia affects 1 in 20 people over the age of 65 and 1 in 5 over the age of 80. Worldwide, there are an estimated 24 million people with dementia. By 2040 the number will have risen to 81 million (Hebert et al., 2003).

Pain and stress affect the quality of life of older adults (Ferrell, 1991; Landi et al., 2001). Frail nursing home residents are even more frequently at risk for pain. In a study of one nursing home, 71% of the residents were found to experience at least one pain complaint, and 34% reported constant pain (Ferrell, Ferrell, & Osterweil, 1990). In a review of studies from 14 nursing homes, residents were found to have prevalence of pain from 27 to 83% (Fox, Raina & Jadad, 1999). In addition, the multiple losses of friends, family, home, and health can lead to despair and other emotional problems (Cohen-Mansfield & Marx, 1993; Parmelee, Katz, & Lawton, 1991). Recent US statistics have found major depression in 1–5% of community dwelling elders, but over 13.5% in elders who require home health care and 11.5% in elder hospital patients (Hybels & Blazer, 2003).

The impact of illness and disability on a nation's finances, health care services, and caregiving needs are significant. Some predict that "health expectancy" will become as important a measure as life expectancy is today (Kinsella & Velkoff, 2001). The growth in the aging population also has implications for both formal and informal caregiving. Research increasingly demonstrates the impact of caregiving on the caregivers' emotional and physical well-being (Schulz & Martire, 2003). These populations will need multiple tools and interventions to enjoy the quality as well as the quantity of their lives.

Theoretical Framework

Interventions that focus on curing are not always realistic or appropriate, especially for elders. Patients are learning that chronic conditions may not be cured, but may be managed, and lives lived fully despite ailments. Elders often have complex, multiple, physical and cognitive disabilities, requiring a multifaceted approach. Pharmacological treatment alone often does not resolve pain and distress and may have unwanted side effects. For elders and their caregivers, mindfulness practices can offer holistic relief from the multiple losses of aging. Elders and caregivers often feel disempowered by conventional treatment models. Mindfulness practices provide a model for inclusion and specific skills to promote increased well-being. Older adults are constantly reminded of their losses and their disability. In mindfulness practice, they are reminded of their inner strengths and resources. Daily, elders and their caregivers face the profound spiritual issues of loss, pain and death. Mindfulness practices can provide a format for reconnecting with individual spiritual practices and forming new meaning and understanding. Moreover, mindfulness practice has a demonstrated acceptability with elders and their caregivers (McBee, 2008; McBee, 2003; McBee, Westreich, & Likourezos, 2004; Smith, 2004, 2006).

Caregiving staff for the frail elderly are often at risk for stress and stress-related problems. Direct caregiving for the confused and, at times, combative older adult is among the most physically demanding and emotionally taxing of jobs. Nursing home residents, whether demented or cognitively intact, easily discern the physical and emotional state of caregiving staff. Furthermore, stressed out staff tend to be less satisfied with their jobs and to have secondary health problems (Pekkarinen, Sinervo, Perala, & Elovainio, 2005; Zimmerman, Williams, Reed, Boustani, Preisser, Heck et al., 2005). For professionals who are trained to cure, the chronic illness, pain, and disability associated with aging may lead to feelings of helplessness and frustration.

Families and other informal, unpaid caregivers also experience stress related to the caregiving role. They may not feel they have the time or skills to cope with their own distress (Schultz and Matire, 2004). Formal and informal caregivers must face their own feelings about aging, illness and death. The time-limited groups and skill training offered in mindfulness stress reduction can provide crucial tools for coping with caregiving stress.

Empirical Evidence

MBSR has been studied in multiple settings and with a variety of populations. Few studies, however, solely target mindfulness training for adults over age 65, or populations with significant communication, cognitive or physical disabilities. In 1978, Garrison reported that a stress-management training including relaxation skills, meditation practice and homework was found helpful in reducing tension and anxiety in elders. In 1996, Moye and Hanlon reported that introducing nursing home residents to relaxation training enhanced morale and decreased pain. Results for residents with cognitive impairment suggested the most helpful interventions were focused, frequent, and simple in structure. A six-month, weekly yoga class for healthy elders 65–85 demonstrated improvement in quality-of-life measures of well-being, energy and fatigue as well as balance and flexibility compared to exercise and wait-list control groups (Oken et al., 2006). Similar to mindfulness training, the experimental yoga groups included not only yoga poses or asanas, but also meditation and encouragement of practice outside the class.

In 1996, I co-led a group based on the principles of MBSR and adapted for residents on a dementia unit of a nursing home. Following the program, staff perceived a reduction in agitation and behavioral problems (Lantz, Buchalter, & McBee, 1997). Shalek and Doyle (1997) found that distressed and agitated residents on a dementia unit appeared "peaceful and smiling" after their relaxation group. In research published in 2004, I described modified

MBSR groups offered to nursing home residents with cognitive and physical frailties. Following each of 10 groups, residents reported feeling less sad and a trend toward feeling less pain as compared to a recreational activity program (McBee, Westreich, & Likourezos, 2004). In qualitative interviews, 41% of the participants reported increased sense of relaxation and mentioned benefits from the "sense of community."

Smith (2004, 2006) has offered MBSR classes slightly modified in length to community dwelling elders with mild cognitive and physical impairments. Anecdotal findings of six groups were mixed – some participants (and their health care workers) reported benefits while others reported no benefits. Further research may discern the commonalities among those who report benefits, as well as those who do not. Smith also studied three mindfulness-based cognitive therapy groups for adults over age 65 with at least three episodes of unipolar depression but without significant cognitive impairment. Yoga stretches were modified. One year after this class, 62% of the participants reported global as well as specific improvements that were "Extremely useful." Lynch, Morese, Mendelson, and Robins (2003) found that a group of 34 depressed elders (60 and over) treated with dialectical behavior therapy (DBT; the core practice in DBT is mindfulness) experienced a statistically significant remission of depression as compared to a group treated with medication only. In 2005, Lindberg published a review of research conducted in the previous 25 years about elders, meditation and spirituality. She found reported evidence of physical and emotional benefits, and also that elders, even those in the nursing home, could be taught meditative practices.

Mindfulness training targeting caregivers can also benefit care receivers (Singh, Lancioni, Winton, Wahler, Singh, & Sage 2004). Informal caregivers of frail elders in Spain were offered a stress-management program that included cognitive restructuring, diaphragmatic breathing and the homework of increasing pleasant events (Lopez, Crespo, & Zarit, 2007). Stress management was offered as a traditional group and in a minimal therapist contact (MTC) format. The MTC format provides skill training and support via phone contact, brief meetings, manuals and audiovisual material. A control group was wait-listed. The traditional group experienced higher reductions in anxiety and depression than both the MTC and wait-listed control groups.

To date, no empirical studies have been published that demonstrate the effectiveness of mindfulness training for informal or formal caregivers of frail elders. Waelde, Thompson, and Gallagher-Thompson (2004) described a six-session yoga and (mantra focused) meditation intervention offered to 12 dementia caregivers. Participants were significantly less depressed and anxious following the series.

In 2005, I led an eight-week MBSR class for informal caregivers of nursing home residents and found a moderate effect size for reduction in stress and burden after the intervention and again four weeks following the end of the group (Epstein-Lubow, McBee, & Miller, 2007). Several published studies report positive outcomes post mindfulness training for formal and informal caregivers of multiple populations with chronic and end-of-life conditions (Bruce & Davies, 2005; Minor, Carlson, Mackenzie, Zernicke, 2006; Schenström, Rönnberg, & Bodlund, 2006).

Mindfulness-Based Elder Care in the Nursing Home

Elders in the nursing home cope with trauma, loss, disability, pain, and life-threatening illness. While traditional MBSR programs might prove unfeasible for those with these physical and cognitive limitations, adaptations to the model can offer it in an acceptable format. I have found older adults and their caregivers generally to be receptive to mindfulness groups and interventions, and many report benefits. Key to adapting mindfulness teaching for those with cognitive and physical disabilities was my own mindfulness practice. I also found it helpful to be flexible and creative in communicating mindfulness both verbally and non-verbally (McBee, 2008).

Nursing Home Resident Groups

MBEC groups in the nursing home are quite feasible when knowledge about working with elders is integrated into the teaching practices. Adaptations consider the possibility of poor hearing or eyesight, physical limitations, longer processing times, and cognitive impairments. Shorter sessions (approximately one hour) and ongoing, rather than time-limited, groups prove to be more effective. I adopt the gentle yoga exercises for participants in wheelchairs, and with significant disabilities. I am more directive and less open-ended in groups with frail elders. The skills I teach include: diaphragmatic breathing, meditation, gentle yoga, and informal mindfulness practice. I also use guided imagery.

Environmental challenges of running groups in an institution should also be considered. My groups are taught in busy dining areas or the nursing home units. I use aromatherapy and gentle music, at times, to create a calming milieu. Group discussion and mutual support are an important component for this population. Finding poor compliance with homework assignments, I nevertheless encourage participants to use the techniques of deep breathing and mindfulness outside of the group. The underlying focus on ability, not disability proved to be quite appropriate and successful. Nursing home residents often struggle with dependency issues; MBEC practices remind participants of what is still under their control.

Mindfulness on a Dementia Unit

Elders with dementia often manifest physical and verbal agitation, and behavior problems. Current thinking attributes these behaviors to an attempt to communicate. While traditional communication skills may be diminished by dementia, feelings remain. MBEC for those with dementia provides solace and skills in a supportive environment. Classes I offer on a dementia unit follow a simple, repeated structure, but have the flexibility to allow for unpredictable events. I often begin with breath awareness, followed by deep, belly breathing. Aromatherapy and music help create a sacred space in the midst of a noisy hospital dining room where confused residents often wander in and out. I explain simple chair stretches verbally as well as physically demonstrate, and assist hands-on when needed. I usually end the group with a guided meditation- either the body scan or imagery – using simple, concrete language. I focus on non-verbally communicating mindfulness practices using body language, voice tone and pacing, and facial expression to convey acceptance and presence. When I am centered and calm, even residents who cannot follow instructions or respond cognitively to the class practices usually respond positively.

Isolated Elders

Elders are often isolated in the nursing home or the community, adding to their distress. In the nursing home, some elders are in their rooms for medical conditions, or are unable to participate in groups due to communication or cognitive problems. In those cases, I offer individualized meditation, mindfulness, and instruction in gentle stretches. Yoga stretches may be adapted for those in wheelchairs or bedbound. Participants who are physically disabled are especially receptive to adapted poses. These poses offer a powerful message that, as stated by Kabat-Zinn (1990), there is more right with us than wrong with us.

Persons at the end of life also are often isolated. Concerned caregivers may feel helpless at times. MBEC creates a supportive environment in which the patient and the caregiver can fully experience sadness and yet appreciate each available moment. I have found that aromatherapy and hand massage can be a mindful experience that benefits both the care receiver and the caregiver. Breath work can also allow for communication. By observing the breath's rhythm, it is possible to connect to patients who are no longer communicative otherwise. A connection may be established by synchronizing one's breath to the patient's, and breathing in harmony (Mindell, 1989).

Homebound Elders

The Telephone Mindfulness Group

Many elders are confined to their homes. While for some, it is preferable to nursing home placement, it can be isolating. I offered a series of five, 50-minute stress-reduction classes to eight homebound participants over a conferenced telephone call. The class received pre-mailed handouts and cassette tapes for homework practice, visually demonstrating and supporting the classwork. I verbally gave instructions on the mindfulness skills, and group members shared questions and feedback. Following the group, class members reported continued use of the skills, especially the deep breathing. One participant, Ms. C, states that during the past 6 years, the mindfulness "guidance and your wonderful tape kept me alive and helped me to become the real person I am today. Without your help I never would have reached my 90th birthday, and had the courage to go to Florida after my dear son passed."

Use of CDs and Tapes

In a long-term, home health care program, CDs and tapes of meditation, a body scan exercise, and other mindfulness practices help homebound elders and their caregivers. Social work or nursing staff provide initial guidance on tape and CD use. Following this introduction, the homebound elder and the caregiver can follow instructions on the CD or tape. Both benefit by the shared experience of listening to the CDs together and practicing the mindfulness exercises.

Formal and Informal Caregivers

Staff Caregivers

Stress-reduction classes and mindfulness training for caregivers can benefit both the caregiver and the elder. A one-hour class for interdisciplinary staff can provide a basic introduction to stress and stress management. I include an introduction to stress and to the mind–body connection; simple deep breathing; a brief experience of mindfulness with chair and standing yoga; and a guided meditation. I find it is helpful to offer practical tips on coping with the real job stress that staff experience daily, and to provide a resource list for those who wish to pursue further options.

A more substantial commitment is required for a traditional MBSR class, although it, too, can be slightly altered to enable increased participation. I offered a seven-week, one-hour, traditional MBSR class to approximately 100 staff members. Staff were encouraged to participate in all sessions and asked to do practice homework. Following the group, staff retention on the units that participated in the class was 100%, and nursing staff satisfaction showed improvement.

I have also adapted mindfulness and stress reduction for the nursing units. I have found that the most successful programs offered "mini-breaks" at the times we knew staff were more available. These mini-breaks take place in the dining area and last around 15 minutes. Smaller numbers of staff sit in, and some come and go, as they are able to make time. While the practices of meditation and yoga were foreign to many, there was a broad acceptance and enthusiasm for them in all of the above formats. Direct care workers often reported practicing the skills outside of groups and even sharing them with their families. Anecdotal reports included the following quotes: "The deep breathing was so soul searching and relaxing. It makes me more aware of myself." "I appreciate taking the time during the day when it's stressful, to learn ways to come back to a state of equilibrium." and "I know how to control myself when I feel nervous and angry." This continued popularity in the face of job demands underscores the importance to both caregivers and care receivers of creating ongoing opportunities within the work schedule and environment to engage in stress-reduction programs.

Informal Caregivers

Mindfulness groups offered to family and friend caregivers can also provide skills and support. Informal caregivers frequently report stress and stress-related illness, and yet informal caregivers often find it hard to care for themselves. Mindfulness groups encourage self-care in the context of care provision. The groups are one and one-half hours long and generally in the early evening at the facility providing care for the institutionalized elders.

Many group members reported a decrease in somatic complaints and an increased satisfaction in the caregiving role. Caregivers can be "in the moment" with their loved one, rather than worrying about the past or future. As one group member responded: "I feel less anxious about stresses than I formerly did. I think about 'riding the waves' instead of getting anxious about them or 'fighting' the waves. I feel less responsible for my husband's well-being."

Group members also reported learning new ways to cope with stress, such as using deep breathing when feeling upset. Experiencing the "groupness" was also important, as shared by this member: "I think what was most helpful was the energy you received from the group. Everyone seemed to want to be there and wanted to participate and learn."

Practical Issues

Teacher Requirements

MBSR teaches informal and formal practices that, if employed regularly, can lead to profound life changes. Below are listed some of the practices taught and the adaptations made for frail elders and their caregivers. Clinicians desirous of initiating mindfulness training with older adults and their care-givers should have an established mindfulness practice, MBSR instructor training, and geriatric experience. Practitioners may also consider partner-ing with persons who have complementary expertise. It is not possible in the span of this chapter to detail the varied accommodations to the interven-tions based on the individual or group needs and abilities. What cannot be substituted is the mindfulness practice of the teacher. The most important intervention we can offer is ourselves, who we are in each moment, being present with the other, feeling our connection, and verbally and non-verbally conveying this felt sense.

Mindful Eating

Mindfulness in daily living is frequently taught initially by an eating aware-ness. Group members are given a few raisins and asked to slowly eat them while observing physical sensations, thoughts and feelings. They observe the raisins, without judgment. Participants may find an increased awareness of sensations, just by slowing down and paying attention. There may be elders who are not able, for a variety of reasons, to follow all of your instructions. They may have swallowing difficulties or medical conditions that prohibit certain foods. Consider different foods, or even different activities, in order to include as many residents as possible in the experience. Elana Rosenbaum, who has worked with cancer patients in the hospital, describes using ice chips for a mindful experience (Rosenbaum, 2005).

Group Discussion

Group discussion with residents in the nursing home will have a natural focus on the very real and immediate pain and distress of medical conditions and institutional living. Residents may feel disempowered and unable to control any aspect of their lives. In MBEC groups, we discuss and learn new ways of being with pain and distress. Residents find that they still have abilities, con-trol over their perceptions, and increased choices in how they respond to situations. Group discussion often starts with a resident complaining about having to wait for care provision, or other residents, or the food, or pain. Rather than focus on resolving these issues, we discuss how what we practice and learn in the group might apply to these situations. If a resident is upset because he had to wait to get a glass of water, for example, we might discuss what he could do while he waited. He could take a deep breath, or practice meditation or stretches. This shift in focus enables residents to feel increased control over situations where they previously felt victimized and dependent. In qualitative reports, the group experience was reported to be the most valued aspect by group members. They reported: "I've always liked this [group] since I started... being quiet, relaxed... a special feeling." And, "I feel uplifted. I realize we all have pain. We talk about how we are getting along. It is important to be with other people."

Caregivers also, report the group experience to be helpful. Sharing common stressors is often an initial theme. As the group progresses, however, caregivers begin to share how they use mindfulness skills to cope with these stressors. In addition, caregivers who work together provide support and reminders to practice on the job.

Diaphragmatic Breathing and Breath Awareness

I often tell group members that anyone can participate in the group as long as they are breathing. In a setting where the focus is on disability, it is helpful for residents to remember what they still can do. Mindful meditation often begins with an awareness of the breath, not trying to change the breath, just noticing if it is fast or slow, even or ragged, deep or shallow. A deep, belly breath is intentional and directed. With a soft belly, participants are encouraged to deeply fill the belly, ribs and upper chest with air, and then, very slowly release it. Both residents and caregivers report that the deep belly breath is the intervention most utilized. It only takes a few moments and can be utilized anytime, anywhere. The deep belly breath can also provide the space we need to respond thoughtfully in moments of intensity.

Deep breathing can be challenging for nursing home residents with breathing problems. I use it as an opportunity to talk about expanding our boundaries. Mindfulness classes encourage participants to explore their limits, knowing when we can expand them and when we need to respect them. I use deep breathing as an example of how we can stretch a little further each day, with regular practice.

Meditation

Seated meditation practice may initially appear foreign to an elder and caregiver population. The instructor can offer guidance and encouragement. Shorter practice times are also important, and yet, participants should be encouraged to gradually expand their practice. I have found that residents with cognitive and physical limitations are able to participate in the experience of meditation. On the dementia unit, many group members sat quietly, with their eyes closed, for periods of time following a simple explanation and demonstration.

Rose was an 84-year-old nursing home resident who was physically frail, with minimal family involvement and a life-long psychiatric history. Her

*fixed paranoid delusions often kept her from sleeping as she was convinced
there was a network of people plotting to harm her. I knew Rose well, and
during the group closely monitored her for potential negative impact. She
attended the group faithfully and reported that the chairs in the group
were more comfortable than other chairs. (In fact, they were the same
chairs she sat in for eating and other activities.) Rose often fell asleep in
group and declared that it was the only place she found peace. She also
said the meditation practice reminded her of her Jewish roots, when she
used to light candles on Friday night.*

Gentle Yoga and Mindful Movement

Despite significant physical disability, elders report enjoying simple yoga
stretches. Chair and bed adaptations can include the basics of yoga stretches
and poses. Instruction for the poses can be given verbally, demonstrated by
the instructor and hands-on assistance given as needed. In addition, staff caregivers are often out of shape and do not care for their own bodies. For residents and staff with limited physical experience, yoga provides wonderful
opportunities to experience their bodies in a new way.

I adapt the poses to bed and chair, and focus on the groups' abilities, not
disabilities. For example, when stretching our arms, I might say that those
who cannot use one or both arms, to just stretch the arm that is available
to them. If they cannot move their arms at all, I ask them to focus on their
breathing and imagine they are stretching with us. Residents never express
any distress that they cannot participate in all the exercises; to the contrary,
they are pleased to be included.

Standing and walking meditation may not be an option for nursing home
residents in wheelchairs. A "wheeling" meditation can be suggested for these
residents. I often use mindful movement with elders on the dementia unit,
combining movement, music, imagery, and play. While seated, we imagine
we are walking, moving our feet up and down in a walking motion. I ask
people where they would like to go. Some might say Central Park, or Broadway, or the beach. I ask what we would see, smell, feel, and hear there. We
might swing our arms and turn our heads. Music may ease the movements.
For residents who are rarely able to leave a facility, this experience provides
some release and remembrance.

Guided Imagery

When introduced skillfully, this practice does not serve to escape the present
moment, but provides a powerful metaphor to illuminate the process of
shifting to a mindful awareness. I found that many elders responded to the
use of imagery, especially of nature, or to address pain. Guided imagery
tapes calmed even some residents on the dementia unit. While not able to
understand all of the words, these residents understood the tone, pacing
and simple, concrete language. An exercise as easy as breathing into the
pain, and gently releasing it with the out breath, may offer relief. On the
other hand, it may not. What is important is to accept whatever arises with
equanimity.

Body Scan

The body scan uses guided imagery to observe the body without judgment. Elders with disabilities may be acutely aware of their body's limitations. The body scan allows us to observe our bodies as they are, without needing to change anything. Again, a lack of comprehension of all the instructions does not prevent those with dementia from participating. Caregivers may also have unpleasant feelings about their bodies, and this exercise can increase their self-acceptance and compassion.

Homework

Nursing home residents in my groups rarely participated in the homework assignments of a formal practice. They did, however, report using the skills of deep breathing and reframing outside of class. Some residents had difficulty operating CD or tape players. Staff would set up the equipment and encourage residents. Staff also were not able to consistently practice formal skills. Many held two jobs or provided caregiving at home for family after work. In caregiver classes, I emphasized in class skills that could be practiced while waiting in line, driving, or on the bus or subway. Formal and informal caregiver classes also discussed specific stresses of caregiving and strategized ways to cope with them.

Other Considerations

There are logistical and practical problems that you may want to consider as you plan your group. The following are some of the issues that came up as I developed and led groups over the past 13 years (McBee, 2008).

Environment

Mindfulness groups in institutional environments can present environmental difficulties. Often, there are no quiet or secluded spots to hold meditation groups. In the nursing home, I hold groups in one corner of a large dining/recreation room. We hear loudspeakers and alarms; confused residents may wander into the group; and once, a doctor even entered the group and pulled a resident's wheelchair out while the group was in progress! When I find it especially challenging, I remind myself that this is the environment that many residents are in 24 hours a day, seven days a week. If they can experience some restoration and skill building during the group, it may help them when they are not in the group. Staff groups, also, are often held in the dining area. I use aromatherapy and music for some groups to create a milieu that may support the mindfulness practice.

Exclusionary Criteria

Given the broad adaptations of mindfulness skills, there is no reason to exclude anyone who can safely participate from MBEC. MBSR classes often screen out persons with a history of trauma or abuse. Psychosocial history of frail elders may be limited, and they may not be able to supply information themselves. Therefore, teachers should be aware of participant's verbal and non-verbal response to the interventions and make adjustments accordingly.

Nursing home residents may have cognitive or physical impairments, or both. Unless a resident is unable to get to the group, physical impairments should not prevent participation in appropriate exercises. Residents with cognitive impairments can also be included in groups unless their behavior is too unsafe or disruptive to other participants. I usually allow for some interruptions, encouraging the participant to settle in. If the disruptive behavior continues, I will ask staff to take the resident to the other end of, or out of, the room. Encouraging acceptance of others in the group can be part of the group's practice.

When I first thought about offering such groups to our population, I wondered if the elders would be open to new experiences. What I found is that most residents are surprisingly open and receptive. There are also some residents who are clearly not interested. One resident, discussing her pain, said, "Just give me a pill."

I also consider the language I use to describe the group and the practices: Meditation can be sitting quietly, yoga can be gentle stretches, and the groups can be stress-reduction groups or relaxation groups. During the course of the group, I integrate language that might be less familiar to them, including meditation and mindfulness.

Communicating

One of the most difficult losses for elders is the loss of ease in communication. Some elders are vision impaired. Others may be hard of hearing. Others may speak very softly due physical problems. The group is a wonderful opportunity to focus on strengths! For example, I will sit next to a resident who is hard of hearing so that I can speak directly into his or her good ear. I move around a lot in groups so that I can make sure that I am communicating with each resident. I often repeat what one resident said so that the entire group will hear. I find hands-on and touch are also helpful in guiding residents.

Ongoing Groups or Time Limited

A key component of traditional MBSR groups is that they are time-limited. For nursing home residents, however, I found that ongoing groups are more beneficial. Residents face many daily challenges in the nursing home and carryover, the ability to maintain the practices and learning, is difficult. As previously discussed, residents did utilize some of the practices, like deep breathing, but were not able to practice other skills outside of class. Concrete reminders like handouts can help participants recall the mindfulness practices. Long-term effectiveness for caregivers may reflect the results documented in multiple studies on MBSR. Given the stress of caregiving, however, refresher groups may be helpful.

Conclusion

The explosive growth of the older adult population with the concurring projected growth in chronic conditions cries out for modalities that address these conditions. Complementary and alternative medicine (CAM) use is increasingly accepted and utilized. In 2000, approximately 1000 United States citizens over 52 were interviewed about their use of CAM and 31% of those over 65 utilized meditation (Ness, Cirillo, Weir, Nisly, & Wallace, 2005). Tilden et al. (2004) interviewed 423 caregivers about the use of CAM during end of life care. Decedents median age was 57 and 50% of the caregivers reported the decendent's use of relaxation techniques. Another US study reported that of 2055 adults interviewed in 1997–1998, one in five used at least one mind-body therapy in the last year. Meditation, imagery and yoga were the most commonly reported (Wolsko, Eisenberg, Davis, & Phillips, 2004).

Mindfulness training adaptations benefit frail elders holistically offering skills to address physical, spiritual and emotional needs. In addition, training caregivers in mindfulness practices impacts both those who give care and those who receive it. Future research will dictate and refine the differential use of mindfulness interventions for cognitively and physically impaired populations and their caregivers. The difficulty in quantifying results in a population often unable to communicate, and with results related to quality of life and difficult to quantify, should not deter further investigation into the benefits of their profound practice for this compellingly needy population.

Acknowledgements: The author wishes to thank Victoria Weill-Hagai for her editorial assistance, and Sue Young and Dr. Gary Epstein Lubow for their comments.

References

Bruce, A. & Davies, B. (2005). Mindfulness in hospice care: Practicing meditation-in-action. *Qualitative Health Research, 15*(10), 1329–1344.

Centers for Disease Control and Prevention. (2003). Public health and aging: trends in aging- United States and worldwide. *Morbidity and Mortality Weekly Report, 52*(06), 101–106.

Cohen-Mansfield, J., & Marx, M. S. (1993). Pain and depression in the nursing home: corroborating results. *Journal of Gerontology: Psychological Sciences, 48*(2), 96–97.

Epstein-Lubow, G. P., McBee, L., & Miller, I. W. (2007, March). *Mindful caregiving: a pilot study of mindfulness training for family members of frail elderly*. Poster session at the 5th annual conference of the Center for Mindfulness in Medicine, Healthcare and Society. Worcester, MA, US.

Ferrell, B. A. (1991). Pain management in elderly people. *Journal of the American Geriatric Society, 39*, 64–73.

Ferrell, B. A., Ferrell, B. R., & Osterweil, D. (1990). Pain in the nursing home. *Journal of the American Geriatrics Society, 38*, 409–414.

Fox, P. L., Raina, P. & Jadad, A. R. (1999). Prevalence and treatment of pain in older adults in nursing homes and other long-term care institutions: A systemic review. *Canadian Medical Association Journal, 160(3)*, 329–333.

Garrison, J. E. (1978) Stress management training for the elderly: A psychoeducational approach. *Journal of the American Geriatrics Society, 26*(9), 397-403.

Hebert, L. E., Scherr, P. A., Bienias, J. L., Bennett, D. A., & Evans, D. A. (2003) Alzheimer's disease in the US population: Prevalence estimates using the 2000 census. *Archives of Neurology, 60*(8), 1119-1122.

Hybels, C. F. & Blazer, D. G. (2003). Epidemiology of late-life mental disorders. *Clinics in Geriatric Medicine, 19*, 663-696.

Kabat-Zinn, J. (1990). *Full catastrophe living: Using the wisdom of your body and mind to face stress, pain and illness.* New York: Dell Publishing.

Kinsella, K. & Velkoff, V. A. (2001). *An aging World: 2001.* (U.S. Census Bureau, Series P95/01-1). Washington, DC.: U.S. Government Printing Office.

Landi, F., Onder, G., Cesari, M., Gambassi, G., Steel, K., Russo, A., et al. (2001). Pain management in frail, community-living elderly patients. *Archives of Internal Medicine, 181*(22), 2721-2724.

Lantz, M. S., Buchalter, E. N., & McBee, L. (1997). The Wellness Group: A novel intervention for coping with disruptive behavior in elderly nursing home residents. *The Gerontologist, 37*(4), 551-555.

Lindberg, D. A. (2005). Integrative review of research related to meditation, spirituality, and the elderly. *Geriatric Nursing, 26*(6), 372-377.

Lopez, J.; Crespo, M.; & Zarit, S. H. (2007). Assessment of the efficacy of a stress management program for informal caregivers of dependent older adults. *The Gerontologist, 47*(2), 205-214.

Lynch, T. R., Morese, J., Mendelson, T., & Robins, C. (2003). Dialectical behavior therapy for depressed older adults: a randomized pilot study. *American Journal of Geriatric Psychiatry. 11*, 33-45

McBee, L. (2008). *Mindfulness based elder care.* New York: Springer Publishing Company.

McBee, L. (2003). Mindfulness practice with the frail elderly and their caregivers: changing the practitioner-patient relationship. *Topics in Geriatric Rehabilitation, 19*(4), 257-264.

McBee, L., Westreich, L., & Likourezos, A. (2004). A psychoeducational relaxation group for pain and stress in the nursing home. *Journal of Social Work in Long-Term Care, 3*(1), 15-28.

Mindell, A. (1989). *Coma: The dreambody near death.* London: Penguin Books.

Minor, H. G., Carlson, L. E., Mackenzie, M. J., & Zernicke, K. (2006). Evaluation or a Mindfulness Based Stress reduction (MBSR) program for caregivers of children with chronic conditions. *Social Work in Health Care, 43*(1), 91-109.

Moye, J. & Hanlon, S. (1996). Relaxation training for nursing home patients: Suggestions for simplifying and individualizing treatment. *Clinical Gerontologist, 16*(3), 37-48.

Ness, J., Cirillo, D. J., Weir, D. R., Nisly, N. L., & Wallace, R. B. (2005). Use of complementary medicine in older Americans: Results from the Health and Retirement Study. *The Gerontologist, 45*(4), 516-524.

Oken, B. S., Zajdel, D., Kishiyama, S., Flegal, K., Dehen, C., Haas, M. et al. (2006). Randomized, controlled, six-month trial of yoga in healthy seniors: effects on cognition and quality of life. *Alternative Therapies in Health Medicine, 12*(1), 40-47.

Parmelee, P. A., Katz, I. R., & Lawton, M. P. (1991). The relation of pain to depression among institutionalized aged. *Journal of Gerontology: Psychological Sciences, 46*, 15-21.

Pekkarinen, L., Sinervo, T., Perala, M-L. & Elovainio, M. (2005). Work stressors and the quality of life in long-term care units. *The Gerontologist, 44*, 633-643.

Rosenbaum, E. (2005). *Here for now: Living well with cancer through mindfulness.* Hardwick, MA: Satya House Publications.

Shalek, M., & Doyle, S. (1997). Relaxation revisited: an adaptation of a relaxation group geared toward geriatrics with behavior problems. *Alternative Therapies in Clinical Practice*, November/December, *215-220*.

Schenström, A., Rönnberg, S. & Bodlund, O. (2006). Mindfulness-based cognitive attitude training for primary care staff: a pilot study. *Complementary Health Practice Review, 11*(3), *144-152*.

Schulz, R., & Martire, L. M. (2003). Family caregiving of persons with dementia: prevalence, health effects, and support strategies. *American Journal of Geriatric Psychiatry 12*, 240-249.

Singh, N. N., Lancioni, G. E., Winton, A. S. W., Wahler, R. G., Singh, J., & Sage, M. (2004). Mindful caregiving increases happiness among individuals with profound multiple disabilities. *Research in Developmental Disabilities: A Multidisciplinary Journal, 25*(2), 207-218.

Smith, A. (2004). Clinical uses of mindfulness training for older people. *Behavioral and Cognitive Psychotherapy, 32*, 423-430.

Smith, A. (2006). Like waking up from a dream: mindfulness training for older people with anxiety and depression. In R. Baer (Ed.), *Mindfulness based treatment approaches* (pp. 191-215). Burlington, MA: Elsevier.

Tilden, V. P., Drach, L. L., & Tolle, S. W. (2004). Complementary and alternative therapy use at end-of-life in community settings. *The Journal of Alternative and Complementary Medicine, 10*(5), *811-817*.

Waelde, L. C., Thompson, L., & Gallagher-Thompson, D. (2004). A pilot study of a yoga and meditation intervention for dementia caregiver stress. *Journal of Clinical Psychology, 60*(6), 677-687.

Wolsko, P. M., Eisenberg, D. M., Davis, R. B., & Phillips, R. S. (2004). Use of mind-body medical therapies. *Journal of General Internal Medicine, 19*, 43-50

Zimmerman, S., Williams, C. S., Reed, P. S., Boustani, M., Preisser, J. S., Heck, E., & Sloane, P. D. (2005). Attitudes, stress, and satisfaction of staff who care for residents with dementia. *The Gerontologist, 45*, 96-105.

24

Mindfulness-Based Interventions in an Inpatient Setting

Fabrizio Didonna

Only in quiet waters things mirror themselves undistorted.
Only in a quiet mind is adequate perception of the world.
                                                    – Hans Margolius.

Introduction

In the past two decades the use of mindfulness-based interventions in clinical settings has quickly become more and more common especially in outpatient treatment and above all with patients whose problems are not extremely serious and who are not in the acute phase of the disease (Baer, 2003). There has been debate about whether or not it is possible and useful to use mindfulness therapy with serious, chronic psychiatric pathologies in the acute phase (Baer, 2003; Segal, Williams, Teasdale, 2002, see also Chapter 18 of this volume). There is, however, some evidence that acceptance and mindfulness-based treatment programs can be usefully adopted in clinical inpatient settings and for challenging problems, especially for suicidal adolescent inpatients (Katz, Gunasekara, & Miller, 2002; Katz et al., 2000) patients with borderline personality disorder (BPD) (Barley et al., 1993; Bohus et al., 2000), psychotic patients (Bach, P., & Hayes, S. C., 2002; York, 2007; Gaudiano & Herbert, 2006), and to enhance treatment team process (Singh, Singh, Sabaawi, Myers, & Wahler, 2006).

Keeping in mind that mindfulness approaches (e.g., MBSR, MBCT, ACT) easily lend themselves to applications in a group-therapy setting and on account of an excellent cost-efficient ratio resulting from this sort of application, these kinds of interventions are particularly suitable in psychiatric inpatient settings and especially in units specialised in the treatment of specific forms of psychopathology. This form of treatment seems to obtain good compliance and appears to be well tolerated even by patients with high levels of distress or disturbance (Mason & Hargreaves, 2001). As will be detailed later in this chapter, mindfulness-based intervention has many attributes that make it highly suitable for use in short-term inpatient treatment. Nevertheless, there are some difficulties and obstacles involved in using mindfulness treatment in an inpatient setting. These challenges are mostly non-existent in outpatient treatment so mindfulness-based interventions must be re-organized and follow a specific format when used for hospital patients and environments.

Based on the personal experience of the author in implementing and planning mindfulness-based treatments for hospital programs for psychiatric patients, this chapter aims to show how it is possible to successfully implement mindfulness interventions within an inpatient unit in a Mental Health Service for severe and challenging problems by rationally integrating them with established inpatient treatments and protocols. More specifically, the chapter will clearly outline the obstacles and challenges related to these inpatient mindfulness-based protocols and propose some guidelines to overcome them.

Why Should a Mindfulness-Based Program Be Implemented in an Inpatient Setting?

There are several reasons that make mindfulness-based training a cost-efficient intervention in the context of an inpatient treatment program. First of all, clinical experience and empirical observation suggest that, in general, the more serious the problems of patients admitted to inpatient units, the greater the need to provide an environment that promotes mindfulness practice. These patients require a more intense degree of practice than that which characterizes outpatient settings, for example, at least on a daily basis, and more help in learning how to carry out the exercises and in understanding how they relate to and can be useful in helping them learn to manage their problems. During hospitalization, if all the treatment staff share a mindfulness-based model, patients can live in a *mindful therapeutic setting*: patients can feel a sense of calm in an environment that is free from judgements and pressure and that demonstrates tolerance, emotional validation and empathy. The style of communication and messages from therapeutic team, therefore, need to be consistent with mindfulness-based principles (acceptance, presence, here and now, non-judgement, etc.).

Normally in an inpatient setting, the ward milieu can be considered a "safe place" in which patients feel safe, accepted, protected and cared for. Indeed, very often patients begin to improve shortly after admission even before they start any sort of treatment. This atmosphere is needed in order to allow severely disturbed patients to become familiar with and effectively use mindfulness practices, often for the first time in their lives. In this setting they can do regular mindfulness practice without being disturbed by the factors that they often can find in their own personal environment (e.g., family conflicts, expressed emotion, feeling of loneliness, psychological or physical violence, etc.).

Unlike outpatient mindfulness training, in which participants may often have difficulty finding the time, spaces and willingness to do meditation practice on a regular basis, especially individuals with challenging problems (e.g., BPD, depression, OCD), during hospitalization patients can be assisted in doing intensive and regular practice. Because of the specificity of the program, planned inpatient treatment involves daily practice, which is assisted by the nursing staff and psychological professionals. Furthermore, in an inpatient setting, patients have more opportunities to find moments and spaces for mindfulness practice because most of their time during inpatient treatment is to be used for therapeutic reasons.

Another advantage of this kind of treatment in an inpatient setting is the chance to use mindfulness-based interventions in vivo with the patients' problems when they arise, explaining and showing the effects and importance of acceptance, non-judgement, and decentering attitudes when anxiety, sadness, anger or any other emotion or problematic states arise.

As is the case for all group therapeutic interventions in inpatient programs mindfulness-based group therapy is a cost-efficient intervention in that it can make optimal use of the staff and maximize the often limited resources of the mental health units. It has also been noticed that inpatients, during the sessions together with individuals suffering from different disorders (heterogeneous group), can share a sense of *common human suffering* with each other regardless of the diagnosis), and this is one of basic principles of mindfulness. Patients in group therapy can realize that suffering is an impermanent normal condition that can be present in people with different ages, cultures, and social status and that the suffering has a common origin (e.g., the three causes of suffering, see Introduction, Chapters 1 and 2 of this volume). This understanding can be reached by sharing of a mindfulness-based problem formulation, which offers a simple and uniform approach across diagnoses and gives the individual a clear and non-accusatory way of understanding how their breakdown has occurred.

There is also some evidence that when mindfulness-based mentoring is provided to professionals involved in inpatient programs, it can be an efficient and effective intervention for enhancing and maintaining the performance of treatment teams in adult psychiatric hospitals. Singh et al. (2006) investigated changes in treatment team functioning in an adult inpatient psychiatric hospital after the implementation of a mindfulness-based mentoring intervention. Their results showed that with the introduction of mindfulness-based mentoring, treatment team performance was enhanced, patients' attendance at therapeutic groups and individual therapy sessions was maximized, and patient and staff satisfaction with treatment team functioning increased substantially, with patient satisfaction showing greater gains than staff satisfaction.

Another important point is that hospital units and wards are normally staffed by multidisciplinary teams characterized by very different orientations. A mindfulness-based approach is a trans-epistemological perspective, which can be easily used by professionals from different therapeutic orientations (psychodynamic, cognitive-behavioral, existentialist, etc.). What is important is that all the professionals in the treatment team share the same mindfulness view of suffering and of mind functioning and, if possible, have a regular meditation practice. For this reason, in order to implement an effective mindfulness-based program in an inpatient treatment, it is important to highlight the fact that all therapeutic staff need to be trained in mindfulness and that supervision is required on a regular basis.

Features and Difficulties of an Inpatient Mindfulness-Based Group

Providing mindfulness training for severe and acute disorders is not an easy task and, compared with outpatient treatment, it requires that first those providing the training clearly understand the obstacles and challenges that characterize inpatient units. First of all, the disorders of hospitalized patients are much more severe, comorbid, and chronic than those of outpatients, and inpatients are often in an acute phase, especially at the beginning of the inpatient treatment. They may also have a seriously disturbed relationship with the body (often because of traumatic experiences or psychotic problems), which is usually an important focus in mindfulness exercises, and feel extreme fear of loosing control during the mindfulness exercises. Furthermore, during hospitalization patients are usually on medication. This can often create some problems with patients during group sessions because of the side effects of the medication. Thus, during the exercises they may fall asleep or have several physical symptoms that can make concentration or participation during sessions difficult or even impede it.

Another important point is that in inpatient treatment, because of the intensity and the relatively limited duration of the stay, there is a rapid turnover of patients. This fact can make it difficult to provide group interventions in which participants start with a group of people and finish with the same one, as is, on the other hand, more so the case in outpatient groups. There is an ongoing change in the makeup of the group and this can lead to lack of homogeneity in each meeting with regards to the level of learning and understanding of the participants. Indeed, each session can be the first session for some patients and this often makes it difficult to provide more advanced exercises to the patients who have been in the hospital and in the group for longer periods of time.

These problems mean that the standard mindfulness-based group format must be adapted to the specificity of the severe mental health problems of patients admitted to the unit and to the features of an inpatient treatment program.

Features and Advantages of Heterogeneity in Mindfulness Groups

Another typical feature that we normally find in inpatient mindfulness groups, and which is often considered an obstacle for the process and outcome of treatments, is *heterogeneity*. This is related in particular to the kind of the disease, level of severity, age, and socio-cultural level. The author's clinical experience with hundreds inpatients suggests that heterogeneity can actually be turned into a resource if we are able to understand and exploit some of the advantages of heterogeneous groups.

Heterogeneity and the atmosphere of mindfulness-based groups tend to deactivate the "agonic/competitive modes" (which activate anger, shame, etc.) are normally activated in other more homogeneous settings (e.g., skills training groups for borderline patients). For many patients, participating in a group with people of different ages, status and kinds of disorder allow them to de-identify themselves from the *"pathological role and identity"* that they often have. In groups this discourages the expression of typical pathological modes and behaviors (anger, acting-out, expressing emotions or avoidance), which are often connected to the identification of the patients with their own disorder. This phenomena is often observed, for example, in BPD or depressed patients, who show some behaviors during mindfulness groups that are totally different from the ones they have in all other conditions and environments.

Heterogeneity during the sessions can also allow patients to feel a sense of "normality" of the experience of suffering (human condition implies/includes suffering) regardless age, diagnosis, symptoms, and so on. This is especially true because during mindfulness group sessions, the instructor never talks about the specificity of the disorders, but always explains that each person has different ways of manifesting suffering all of which have a common origin (attachment, aversion, delusions and distortions, automatic pilot, judgement, etc.) and that each individual's own form of suffering is probably only quantitatively different, and not necessarily qualitatively different, from that of people with different disorders and of people without clinical problems.

The Importance of Regular Practice

Developing mindfulness skills is not easy and requires the regular practice of meditation. When working with severe disorders, it is important to bear in mind that these patients are generally not used to doing meditation and often they don't even know what meditation is. It is important to explain to patients that mindfulness can be considered a therapeutic skill, connected in various ways to their problems, and that as is the case all new abilities, regular practice is required in order to learn the new skill. A useful analogy for patients is that of athletes: when a person wants to learn a new sport, they have to train regularly, with the help of a coach or trainer in order to face the challenges that the competition (life) will present them with.

One of the basic strategies for dealing with the chronic difficulties inpatients have with doing meditation is to provide them with guided regular practice of mindfulness on a daily basis. This is particularly important with challenging patients because they find it hard to feel motivated and willing to practice alone. This is important because empirical observation and clinical experience show that the more patients do formal and informal meditation, the more stable and beneficial the effects of the meditation practice. One way to help inpatients learn to practice meditation regularly (if possible even after discharge) is to provide them with a half hour of guided mindfulness practice early in the morning and another half hour late in the afternoon. This allows patients to understand that mindfulness is not just a simple technique, but rather that it could become a regular way of being which can affect/condition their emotional states and give them a sense of calm and balance all day long.

This kind of daily practice should be guided, if possible, by a healthcare professional (psychologist, psychiatrist, nurse, social worker), but in the absence of professional resources even by an intern or practitioner who can use a recorded mindfulness exercise (audio tape, audio CD) and just coordinate and check the state of patients during the practice. Daily practice can be a powerful and helpful complement to the weekly mindfulness sessions with the instructor.

Problem Formulation in Inpatient Treatment

Other chapters in this book (see Chapters 5 and 11) have already highlighted the importance in clinical application of mindfulness of sharing a clear conceptualization of the patient's problem as well as a clear understanding of the clinical mechanisms of change of mindfulness that can help modify the activating and maintaining factors that are highlighted in the problem formulation. This becomes even more important during inpatient treatment in which patients are receiving several different kinds of therapeutic intervention and may have difficulties understanding the meaning and rationale of each one and their coherence and integration. Problem formulation is also a helpful tool for developing and enhancing motivation for mindfulness practice inside and outside group sessions.

Problem formulation can be shared during individual sessions before starting the mindfulness training and also by using special sheets and verbal descriptions or explanations during group sessions.

An example of mindfulness-based problem formulation is that done with patients suffering from BPD, which is one of the most frequent diseases found in inpatient treatment, often in comorbidity with other problems. In order to allow borderline patients to understand the power, potential and relevance of mindfulness intervention, it is helpful to share a cognitive-behavioral conceptualization of the borderline crises with patients (Figure 24.1). After the occurrence of an impulsive crisis characterized by different maladaptive behaviors (such as self-injury, substance abuse, suicidal attempts), in time patients experience a stage of remission from the symptoms, which is here called "*temporary calmness.*" Then, at a certain moment some specific events (such as invalidating experiences or messages, abandonment or exclusion behaviors on the part of others, traumatic memories, etc.) can arise and consequently the patients activate and perceive several inner changes at emotive (guilt, anger, disgust, feeling of emptiness shame), cognitive (flashes, rumination) or physical bodily sensations connected to past abuse, hyper-arousal levels. These perceived changes are eval-

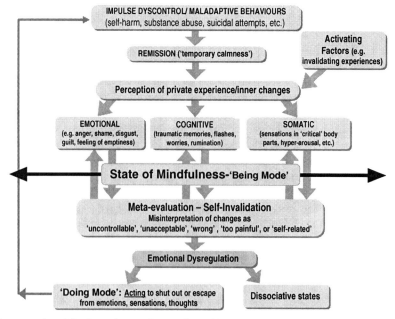

Figure. 24.1. The hypothesized role of mindfulness-based interventions with respect to the process of crisis activation in borderline personality disorder.

uated (meta-cognition) in terms of *"uncontrollable, intolerable, unaccept-able, very painful* or *self-related* (which means that patients identify them-selves with those contents)" experiences and they may also self-invalidate their own inner states. This misinterpretation and/or self-invalidation acti-vate *emotional dysregulation* (Linehan, 1993), a psychological state char-acterized by chaotic and uncontrollable feelings and confusion. This state normally leads patients *to react* (and not to 'respond') by activating a "doing mode" in which they (differently from depressed patients who are generally unable to act) tend to act in order to shut out or escape from the intolera-ble emotions, sensations, or thoughts. The only way that borderline patients know how to act in order to deal with this experience is by escaping from the subjectively terrifying and unacceptable reality through dissociative states or by activating maladaptive behaviors, thus leading them into a new *borderline crises*, and the vicious circle is maintained.

The Author hypothesizes that mindfulness-based interventions can help these patients on a first level by helping them prevent or stop each meta-evaluation that they tend to activate regarding the distressful private experience (emotions, thoughts, sensations) that arises. On a second level, indirectly, mindfulness states help patients to prevent or neutralize the con-sequent emotional dysregulation also because they are trained to not react immediately to a negative experience when one occurs but rather to *observe, describe and stay in touch with it, accepting it as it arises without judging.* Doing so they can learn to avoid starting the vicious circle that leads to fur-ther impulsive crises or avoidant behaviors (e.g., dissociation). They can do this using decentering, defusion and disidentification as cognitive styles and modes and using acceptance as well, learned through mindfulness training.

Clinical observation during group sessions shows that mindfulness-based interventions, in particular in inpatient treatment, can help patients with impulse dyscontrol problems (e.g., BPD) to learn a different *mental style and metacognitive attitude* toward problematic and emotional states, sensations and cognitions which are incompatible with the impulsive and maladaptive behaviors (self-harm, binge eating, substance abuse, etc.) that patients use to deal with these states. Other important effects have been highlighted by Linehan (1993; Linehan, Armstrong, Suarez, Allmonn, & Heard, 1991), who included in her cognitive-behavioral model for borderline patients – dialectical-behavior therapy – an important component of mindfulness-based intervention (see also Chapter 13 of this volume). This kind of training can increase attention control, improve awareness of self and others, reduce emotional reactivity, provide a foundation for self-validation, and reduce feel-ings of emptiness and self and cognitive dysregulation.

The use of metaphors in the context of mindfulness groups (such as *thoughts like clouds in the sky* or *seeing emotions or cognitions like a waterfall*) could also be helpful in helping patients stay in touch, decenter and overcome the distressful private experience.

It has been observed that in order to help borderline patients, especially those with severe problems, to learn mindfulness skills, it is useful to pro-vide specific inpatient mindfulness-based groups in which individuals can find a setting that better allows them to overcome, step-by-step, the unavoid-able difficulties that they would normally find in practicing formal meditation exercises in outpatient settings.

Clinical Goals in a Mindfulness-Based Inpatient Program

Within inpatient psychiatric units where there are patients suffering from mood disorders, anxiety disorders and problems related to impulsivity (e.g., BPD, bulimia nervosa) the goals of mindfulness training are:

— to help individuals diagnosed with *major depression* (during partial remission or a moderate/not acute symptomatic phase) to learn the skills that will help them to deal effectively with dysphoria and changes in their mental states and to stop and prevent rumination and possible subsequent relapse;

— to train patients who have problems *controlling impulses* (e.g., BPD) adopt a different *mental style and metacognitive attitude* toward problematic emotional states, sensations and cognitions, incompatible with impulsive and maladaptive behavior (self-harm, binge eating, substance abuse, etc.) or experiential avoidance (flight, dissociation, etc.) that patients use to deal with these states;

— to help patients with *anxiety disorders* (panic, generalized anxiety disorder, obsessive-compulsive disorder) to develop a new and more functional mental attitude (observation, acceptance and decentering) toward their own physical symptoms and, in general, toward their inner experience.

In general, all inpatients, regardless of the diagnosis, are trained to observe and intentionally become aware at all times of their thoughts, body sensations and emotions, being and remaining in the present time, developing a different way of relating to their private experience. More specifically, they are trained to acquire and develop the capacity to *recognize* and *consciously accept* without judging (not "turning away" and not "attachment") undesired emotions and thoughts as an alternative to activating their customary, automatic, pre-programmed modes, which tend to perpetuate their psychiatric problems. Furthermore, patients learn how to acquire the capacity to choose the most effective response to any unpleasant thought, sensation and situation that they may encounter (i.e., responding vs. reacting, shifting from a "doing" mode to a "being" mode, etc.). Some other skills and attitudes taught in mindfulness groups are not being guided during mindfulness exercises by an objective, not striving to attain a particular state (e.g., relaxation, happiness, peace, etc.) and developing awareness of how a problem can manifest itself in and through the body.

An Example of a Mindfulness-Based Program in Inpatient Treatment (M-BPIT)

Setting

An example of the application of a meditation approach for hospitalized patients can be found in the mindfulness-based therapy program in inpatient treatment (M-BPIT) provided by the Department of Psychiatry of the *Villa Margherita* clinic in Vicenza (Italy), where an adapted version of mindfulness-based cognitive therapy (MBCT) (Segal, Williams & Teasdale, 2002) forms the most important part of an integrated treatment program primarily based on the cognitive-behavioral approach. More specifically, this department offers mindfulness training for the inpatients of its Unit for Mood and Anxiety Disorders and for the Unit for BPD.

In this program the duration of hospitalization is four weeks; the frequency of the mindfulness training is two weekly sessions (2 h/session) plus two daily practice sessions of a half-hour each (*morning and evening mindfulness sessions*). The number of participants varies significantly and ranges from six to eighteen because it depends on the physical and psychological condition of the patients each day.

Material provided during the sessions includes handout sheets containing the rationale behind the session and usefulness of the group, explanations and instructions on how to carry out the exercises, problem formulation, quotes, stories and an audio tape or CD ROM with guided mindfulness exercises for daily practice. For BPD patients, mindfulness training is integrated with a skills training group (Linehan, 1993), body/expressive group therapy and individual cognitive-behavioral therapy (CBT). For patients suffering from anxiety or mood disorders (in particular major depression and severe obsessive-compulsive disorder), mindfulness training is integrated with cognitive group-therapy sessions, body/expressive group therapy and individual CBT.

The mindfulness groups are always led by two professionals, an instructor and an assistant.

Adapted Form of MBCT

Within the inpatient unit program, the treatment team has found it useful to provide and implement an adapted form of MBCT, (Segal et al., 2002) which differs from the original approach in the duration of some of the exercises, the introduction to new meditation exercises, the format of the sessions and the frequency of the meetings (twice a week). As is the case in all mindfulness-based training, participants are trained to practice both *formal* (mindfulness meditation) and *informal* (the application of mindfulness attitudes and skills in everyday life) exercises (see also Chapter 1 of this volume). The *formal meditation exercises* include "mindful walking," "mindful eating" (the raisin exercise), "sitting meditation" (mindfulness of breathbody/sounds/thoughts; see also Appendix A of this volume), "mindfulness of the body" (body scan, see also Appendix A of this volume), "mindful movements, stretching/yoga," "the secure place" (guided imagery exercise), *practice of the morning* (mindful breathing), and *practice of the evening* (mountain meditation, lake meditation, sea meditation, etc.), exercises outdoors, and relational mindfulness (in couples). The *informal meditation exercises* include mindfulness during everyday activities, mindfulness when experiencing pleasant/unpleasant events, mindful breathing (breathing as an "anchor"), the *three-minute breathing space* and the "thoughts-are-not-facts" exercises (Segal et al., 2002), free mindful walking, mindfulness of sight and sound (see Appendix A), and eating meditation during meals.

Typical Format of an Inpatient Mindfulness-Based Group Session

The duration of a mindfulness group session is one and a half hours, in a large room in which patients are provided with cushions, mats and chairs. They are free to choose whether they prefer to sit on a chair or a mat, but most of them choose the mats.

In each session the following steps are normally used.

— After patients have settled down in the room and on their mats or chairs and after the roll call (only the patients considered to be ready for treatment by the team of professionals are admitted to the session), the instructor starts to explain and illustrate the aims of the group, the general meaning and rationale of mindfulness for the patients' problems (problem formulation, acceptance, non-judgemental attitude, exposure), and the consistence and integration of the group with the other therapies in the treatment program.

— Explanation of the first mindfulness exercise, normally chosen depending on the group composition of the given session, evaluating the possible problems of the patients present.

— Formal mindfulness exercise (20–40 min).

— Practice review and sharing comments on the exercise.

— Understanding the meaning and rationale of the exercise for the patients' problems using comments, suggestions, questions, difficulties and benefits that arose during the exercise.

— Break (10 min).

— Final meditation (10–15 min).

— Sharing comments on the exercise.

— Homework and handing out of material for participants (sheets, descriptions of exercises, quotations, CD for practice).

Exercises and themes of the group would be run in continuing cycles.

Obstacles and Difficulties in Inpatient Groups

As has already been stated, during inpatient mindfulness groups we have to deal with several problems that are usually not as frequent in outpatient groups.

— *Emotional activation*: Several mindfulness exercises, in particular the ones in which patients are asked to stay deeply in touch with their body and physical sensations, can activate intense emotions, especially anxiety. Patients can often feel a sense of lack of control during a long sitting or meditation exercise done lying down because of the relaxation feelings and because they don't want to be in touch with an often hated body (usually in sexually abused and traumatized patients) that they have avoided or harmed or punished in the past. For these reasons some patients may activate intense feelings of shame, guilt, disgust and anxiety and might be frequently and easily distracted, and may ask for a break or even suddenly abandon the group.

— *Dissociative crisis*: Dissociation can be considered a more extreme form of avoidance from undesired and painful feelings. This symptom is normally found in patients suffering from posttraumatic stress disorder (see also Chapter 16 of this book) or BPD. It can be an important and disabling problem during a group, but not as frequent as might be imagined. In the author's clinical experience, there have only been four or five severe dissociative crises during mindfulness group sessions in several years of trainings with hundreds of inpatients with traumatic experiences and BPD.

— *Patients that fall asleep*: Patients may fall asleep as a result of medication, excessive relaxation or even as a form of avoidance.

— *Disturbing background noises*: Inpatient settings and mental health services are usually not designed to be "meditation centers." Therefore, noises that are normal in these contexts but intrusive for the session may disturb patients during the meditation exercises. Patients are always invited to consider noises as particular sounds and impermanent events that become the object of awareness in the here and now and to turn them into opportunities to develop a non-judgemental acceptance toward difficulties.

— *Late comers*: It is not uncommon for inpatients to arrive late to group sessions. This can disturb the mindfulness exercises, which require silence. This happens because of the difficulties many patients have following rules either because of their psychological problems or because they have inadequate priorities during their stay in the inpatient setting.

— *Physical problems or malaise*: Some patients, especially older ones (see also Chapter 23 of this book), may associate to psychological disease with physical problems; this can create several difficulties when trying to practice some specific mindfulness exercises (e.g., sitting meditation or mindful walking).

Coping Strategies to Deal with Difficulties

In order to deal with the problems and obstacles that severe inpatients can have during the group, the following strategies, which have been developed through clinical experience, may prove to be helpful.

— *Ensuring daily practice*: One of the most important strategies to effectively deal with challenging problems during an inpatient mindfulness group is ensure that patients are practicing mindfulness in a consistent and regular way on a daily basis with the guidance of instructors who have extensive experience and competence regarding the problems the inpatients suffer from.

— *Providing two therapists for each session*: It is very important that mindfulness groups for severe inpatients are guided and conducted by two leaders: a leader (instructor) and an observer (assistant). This is important so that should a patient have any difficulty, the observer, or co-leader, can intervene in order to try and help the patient to overcome the problem or resist until the end of the exercise, while the leader can continue to provide the instructions of the exercise for the rest of the group.

— *Providing individual help*: Difficult patients need to be provided with individual help between group sessions to optimize and allow their participation in the group. In order to prevent counter-productive experiential avoidance, it is important to help patients

who are ready to be in the group but who either are hesitant to participate for the first time or have had difficult or frightening experiences
in a session and are hesitant to return to the group.

— *Avoiding, if possible, large groups* with severe patients (max 8–10
participants). Large groups increase the risk of significant and difficult
problems that have to managed during the sessions. This is especially
a problem if the leaders do not have extensive experience in leading
mindfulness groups for psychiatric problems.

— *Selection of patients*: Not all patients admitted to the ward may be
ready to participate in the mindfulness group because of various clinical and personality features (see next section).

— *Giving/providing more instructions during exercises than what is
done in outpatient groups*: Inpatients normally need to be frequently
guided during the process of meditation because they tend to get distracted more easily than outpatients, their minds easily tend to wander off or ruminate, and they easily loose the contact with the here
and now.

— *Keeping the more difficult patients close to the group leader*: In
order to provide patients that may easily have problems (e.g., anxiety,
dissociation, pain) during a session prompt help, it might be useful
to ask them to sit or lay down close to the leaders. This often gives
patients a sense of protection and safety that allows them to get and
stay in touch with difficult inner states.

— *Providing support and encouraging patients in difficulty*. If necessary or appropriate, the leaders can hold the hands of patients who
are nervous, anxious or at risk of dissociation.

— *Accompanying patients having difficulty coping back to their ward*:
If necessary, patients who find it very difficult to cope with their problems should be accompanied back to their ward in order to prevent
intense crises (e.g., dissociation, panic, etc.) that could compromise
the continuity of the entire session.

— *Not allowing late arrivals to enter*: Once a group has already begun,
late arrivals should not be allowed to enter the group because they
may disturb participants during a meditation exercise. Furthermore,
it is important to set rules and discipline in order to transmit and
share a sense of priority and respect toward each other.

— *Using background music*: In order to allow inpatients to stay in
touch with their private experience in the here and now for a long
time, it is often useful to use soft background music that can gently accompany patients during the difficult process of the exploration of challenging and disturbing internal experiencing. Normally
background music is not experienced as a source of distraction and
it helps allow patients to maintain concentration in the present
moment.

— *Gradual progress in implementing exercises*: As the difficulty of
exercises increases, inpatients with challenging patients must be
introduced to the exercises in a more gradual way than with outpatients. This can be done by passing from exteroceptive (external sensory awareness; e.g., mindfulness of sight and sounds) to interoceptive (inner mindfulness; e.g., body scan, sitting meditation) exercises,

from shorter (5–10 min) to longer exercises (30–40 min) and from informal (mindfulness of daily life) to formal meditation.

— *Selecting the exercises of the session depending on the makeup of the group*: If there are many new, inexpert or disturbed patients in a group, leaders should consciously choose exercises that are not too activating.

— *Encouraging patients to use difficulties as opportunities*: During group sessions, patients should be encouraged to use difficulties (e.g., stressful emotions and thoughts, self-discomfort or malaise, backward noises, disturbing behaviors from participants, etc.) during session *as opportunities* to promote and develop acceptance and non-judgmental attitudes rather than as problems or obstacles.

— *Patients who fall asleep during the session should be woken up*: Mindfulness means being present moment by moment. When people fall asleep they simply are not aware in the present moment and they loose an opportunity to learn this attitude.

Criteria for Exclusion from an Inpatient Mindfulness-Based Group

Clinical experience suggests that mindfulness-based groups are not suitable for severe inpatients that show certain stable or temporary clinical conditions and features. Therefore, patients should be carefully selected for participation in each group session. The conditions which would determine the unsuitability of certain patients are:

— *patients in an acute depressive phase and too severely affected to be able to establish a rapport with the instructor and the group*;

— *patients with active severe psychotic symptoms or with an extensive delusional system*;

— *bipolar patients in an euphoric/manic state*;

— *patients with severe risk of dissociative crisis*;

— *patients with severe cognitive deficit/impairment and gross retardation or agitation, and who present poor insight*;

— *poorly-motivated or hypercritical patients with an opposing attitude, or who are unwilling or unable to collaborate with a group*;

— *patients under the effects of drugs or substances (alcohol, opioids, cannabis, etc.)*

When the above-mentioned conditions are no longer stable and patients begin to improve during hospitalization, they can be admitted to the mindfulness group.

Useful Messages for Dealing with Difficulties in Groups

During mindfulness group sessions, the instructor can help participants deal with any difficulties that might arise using specific messages that are consistent with mindfulness attitudes and principles toward suffering. Some examples are given below.

— "Stay in touch with your experience" (emotion, thought, sensation, feeling); "You can do it"; "Yes, you can"; "Allow it to be..."; "Don't avoid it..."; "Don't fight it"; "Do not try to escape from it"; "Accept it"; "Don't judge it" (Acceptance, allowing the inner experience);

— "Take a breath"; "Stay in touch with your breath"; "Breathe together with me" (Breath as an anchor, decentering and defusion);

— "It's OK to feel like this, it is not wrong"; "Whatever it is, it's OK"; "It is just what it is right in this moment (non-judgement);

— "Feel this emotion"; "Don't escape from it"; "It doesn't hurt" (going toward and trough private experience);

— "Thoughts are only thoughts, transient and impermanent mental events"; "This thought is not 'you' or reality"; "Thoughts are not facts" (relating in a different way to thoughts, disidentification);

The aim of all these statements and phrases is to help patients to overcome, during the session, the point in which they would tend to activate experiential avoidance or maladaptive reactions (e.g., self-harm, rumination, etc.) as difficulties and problems related to the private experiences that arise. Very often patients report that over time they were able to embody and interiorize these messages and use them autonomously to deal with difficulties in non-therapeutic situations.

Summary

Acceptance and mindfulness-based treatment programs can be effectively adopted in clinical inpatient settings, especially in specialized units for specific disorders, and they are interventions that can optimize the resources of the staff. These kinds of approaches offer a cost-efficient way to generically teach useful skills for disengaging patients from the dysfunctional cognitive processing modes that characterize severe and acute disorders. Furthermore, this form of treatment seems to obtain a good compliance and appears to be well tolerated even by patients with high levels of discomfort or disturbance.

Unlike outpatient treatment, in an inpatient setting the environment and the ward milieu, can play an important role in the implementation and effects of mindfulness-based interventions. Inpatient settings may offer patients the opportunity to follow an intensive program with more frequent mindfulness sessions and meditation practice on a daily basis.

Nevertheless, providing mindfulness training for severe and acute disorders in an inpatient setting is not an easy task and requires practitioners and professionals understand the many obstacles and challenges that characterize inpatient units, and which are basically inexistent in outpatient treatment. These difficulties mean that specific formats and organization must be used when implementing mindfulness-based interventions in an inpatient setting, that is, the structure of the interventions must be adapted to the hospitalized population and environment. Furthermore, several specific and general coping strategies that are useful for dealing with patients' difficulties during mindfulness groups must be used. However, as was explained above, mindfulness intervention is not suitable for all inpatients and the selection of who is fit or unfit can be made using some criteria of exclusion from mindfulness groups which come from the author's clinical experience.

In order to implement an effective mindfulness-based program in inpatient treatment, it is important to point out that all therapeutic staff need to be trained in mindfulness and it is important to try and keep the approach of different members of staff as consistent as possible. Supervision is also required on a regular basis.

In all the treatment interventions and for the entire duration of the patients' stay, the emphasis must be on the principles of *acceptance* and the *here and now*. It is also important that both patients and instructors regularly practice mindfulness training in order for it to be effective in inpatient treatment.

Although clinical experience suggests that in general there are no particular contraindications in providing mindfulness-based treatment for severe and challenging problems, specific methods, strategies, exercises and meditation styles, e.g., the way in which mindfulness practice is proposed, should be used for various forms of severe pathology and psychological problems (psychosis, BPD, dissociative disorders, etc.). The success and/or failure of these should be analyzed in order to understand which strategies work best for which patients in which conditions. Implementing mindfulness-based group work with challenging inpatients often requires gradual progress regarding the difficulty of the exercises proposed. This can be done by passing from exteroceptive to interoceptive exercises, from shorter to longer exercises, and from informal to formal meditation (Didonna, 2008).

As far as actual outcomes are concerned, to date there are few randomized and controlled studies (Bach & Hayes, 2002; Katz et al., 2000) that have evaluated the effectiveness of acceptance and mindfulness-based interventions in inpatient treatment. This is because the application of this approach is in a relatively early stage and also because it is notoriously difficult to demonstrate the effectiveness of one therapeutic intervention (such as mindfulness training) within an inpatient setting, separating it from the rest of the numerous specific and non-specific therapeutic variables which characterize a hospitalized treatment program. For example, it is quite difficult to differentiate the effect of the ward milieu from the specific effect of the therapy and differentiate the impact of each intervention on the outcome. Nevertheless, there are several encouraging qualitative studies (Barley et al., 1993; Bohus et al., 2000; Gaudiano & Herbert, 2006; Katz et al., 2002; York, 2007) whose results suggest that patients value mindfulness-based intervention and find it beneficial at discharge and that mindfulness can be a key component in a therapeutic inpatient program.

Further investigation is clearly required to establish whether or not the benefits are maintained at follow-up and to understand how clinical improvement at discharge can be associated with changes in mindfulness skills.

Mindfulness-based interventions are not an array of therapeutic techniques, but they do attempt to offer patients a new cognitive style, a "way of being" and a general approach to life and suffering. For this reason, mindfulness can be effectively used even for individuals with high levels of suffering, such as hospitalized patients, if we are able to transmit to them not only the meditation techniques, but above all the core and basic principles of the mindfulness-based perspective (acceptance, compassion, here and now, non-judgement, etc.), which are aimed at understanding the causes of and reducing individual suffering.

References

Bach, P., & Hayes, S. C. (2002). The use of Acceptance and Commitment Therapy to prevent the rehospitalization of psychotic patients: A randomized controlled trial. *Journal of Consulting and Clinical Psychology, 70,* 1129–1139.

Baer, R. (2003). Mindfulness training as a clinical intervention: A conceptual and empirical review. *Clinical Psychology: Science and Practice, 10*(2), 125–143.

Barley, W. D., Buie, S. E., Peterson, E. W., Hollingsworth, A. S., Griva, M., Hickerson, S. C., et al. (1993), The development of an inpatient cognitive-behavioral treatment program for borderline personality disorder. *Journal of Personality Disorder, 7,* 232–240.

Bohus, M., Haaf, B., Stiglmayer, C., Pohl, U., Bohme, R. & Linehan, M. (2000), Evaluation of inpatient dialectical-behavioral therapy for borderline personality disorder-A prospective study. *Behaviour Research and Therapy, 38,* 875–887.

Didonna, F. (2008). Mindfulness and its clinical applications for severe psychological problems: conceptualization, rationale and hypothesized cognitive mechanisms of change (submitted for publication).

Gaudiano, B., & Herbert, J. (2006). Acute treatment of inpatients with psychotic symptoms using Acceptance and Commitment Therapy: Pilot results. *Behaviour Research and Therapy, 44*(3), 415–437.

Katz, L. Y., Gunasekara, S., & Miller, A. L. (2002). Dialectical behavior therapy for inpatient and outpatient parasuicidal adolescents. Adolescent Psychiatry

Katz, L. Y., Gunasekara, S., Cox, B. J. & Miller, A. L. (2000). A controlled trial of dialectical behavior therapy for suicidal adolescent inpatients. Presented at annual meeting of the American Academy of Child and Adolescent Psychiatry, New York.

Linehan, M. M. (1993). *Cognitive-behavioural treatment of borderline personality disorder.* New York: Guilford Press.

Linehan, M. M., Armstrong H., Suarez A., Allmonn D., & Heard H. (1991). Cognitive-behavioural treatment of chronically parasuicidal borderline patients. *Archives of General Psychiatry, 48,* 1060–1064.

Mason O. J., & Hargreaves I. (2001). A qualitative study of Mindfulness-Based Cognitive Therapy for depression. *British Journal of Medical Psychology, 74,* 197–212.

Segal, Z. V., Williams, J. M., & Teasdale, J. D. (2002). *Mindfulness-based cognitive therapy for depression: A new approach to preventing relapse.* New York: The Guilford Press.

Singh, N. N., Singh, S. D., Sabaawi, M., Myers, R. E., & Wahler, R. G. (2006). Enhancing treatment team process through mindfulness-based mentoring in an inpatient psychiatric hospital. *Behavior Modification, 30*(4), 423–441.

York, M. (2007). A qualitative study into the experience of individuals involved in a mindfulness group within an acute inpatient mental health unit. *Journal of Psychiatric and Mental Health Nursing, 14*(6), 603–608.

25

Training Professionals in Mindfulness: The Heart of Teaching

Susan Lesley Woods

"The most practical thing we can achieve in any kind of work is insight into what is happening inside of us as we do it. The more familiar we are with our inner terrain, the more surefooted our teaching – and living – becomes."

Parker Palmer

There is currently substantial interest in the use of mindfulness-based approaches in clinical practice. This raises a number of interesting questions regarding the training of health professionals. There are a number of treatment modalities utilizing mindfulness but not as yet collective agreement as to the components and characteristics of mindfulness as they relate to the clinical setting. Furthermore, some mindfulness-based clinical programs employ mindfulness practice as the key to their approach, while others use mindfulness as a set of skills. The heart of mindfulness, however, is more than a clinical method or skill set, and because of this presents some atypical challenges for professional training. This chapter will outline the ways in which some mindfulness-based trainings are distinctive from other professional training programs.

Health care professionals are used to being instructed in particular theories and techniques and then gaining direct experience from the application of those techniques in clinical practice. And, indeed, some aspects of mindfulness can be taught through our usual ways of communicating knowledge via the transmission of concepts and through intellect. But there is a large part of mindfulness that can only be truly discovered and communicated when the clinician/instructor embodies this approach whole-heartedly. By this, we mean going beyond method to connect to heart, "meaning *heart* in its ancient sense, as the place where intellect and emotion and spirit will converge in the human self" (Palmer & Parker, 1998). This places a different emphasis on clinical learning because it means delivering mindfulness from a position that resonates with an authenticity about what the practice brings to the life of the clinician. Unfortunately, it is beyond the scope of this chapter to comment on every clinical program that incorporates aspects of mindfulness-based practices. So, the focus will be on just two, mindfulness-based stress reduction (MBSR) (Kabat-Zinn, 1990) and mindfulness-based cognitive therapy (MBCT) (Segal, Williams, & Teasdale, 2002). Because these two programs emphasize the practice of formal and informal mindfulness, it allows us to discuss elements of mindfulness as they are taught in the MBSR and MBCT programs and how these are embodied by the teacher. Through embodiment, the teacher models a way of communicating a sense of unity and integration about the experience of mindfulness and her/his relationships in the world; one that offers an genuine presence. From this position, we can address key questions about training.

MBSR is the foundational program upon which many other clinical approaches have been based. MBSR and MBCT are fundamentally the same but are different in the clinical groups they are intended for and the way in which learning is targeted. These two programs, delivered in a group format, provide a rigorous training in formal daily mindfulness meditation and how to integrate its practice into daily living. MBSR works with patients who present with a broad range of medical, psychological and stress related diagnoses. MBCT, targets a specific clinical population, those who are vulnerable to a relapse of depression and adds an additional component, elements of a traditional psychological treatment, cognitive behavior therapy.

The Heart of the Matter

Mindfulness originates from the Buddhist contemplative tradition. It has been described as an, "awareness that emerges through paying attention on purpose, in the present moment, and nonjudgmentally to the unfolding of experience moment by moment." (Kabat-Zinn, 2003; Baer, 2003). Dimidjian and Linehan have posited that key components of mindfulness can be categorized into "(1) observing, noticing, bringing awareness; (2) describing, labeling, noting; and (3) participating." They also identify three characteristics embedded in the way one engages with these activities, "(1) nonjudgmentally, with acceptance, allowing; (2) in the present moment, with beginner's mind; and (3) effectively" (Dimidjian & Linehan, 2003). This constructive description of what constituent components and characteristics might be embedded in mindfulness is helpful in bringing some clarity to the factors we are practicing with and engaging in when teaching mindfulness.

The practice of mindfulness offers a means to directly observe the nature of thoughts, emotions, and physical sensations and the ways in which they either contribute to happiness, or to suffering. Attention is directed to the examination of all experience as it arises in the present moment. It is not a passive process but rather a kindhearted and intentional engagement of wakefulness. With sustained practice, it is possible to see the many ways we get hijacked by wishing things to be different from what is actually present. As a result of continuing effort, energy and patience, this "awareness" presents the possibility of less reliance on self-absorbed thinking, emotions and behaviors and wider choices especially when presented with stressful situations or difficulties.

Until recently, in the west, little emphasis has been placed on the study of the human mind in understanding the role of positive mental states and emotions. Instead psychology has paid attention to negative mood and thought disorders and to the development of a range of psychological interventions that are designed to work with unhelpful modes of mind. Directing attention towards investigating those mental states that engender happiness, loving-kindness, compassion, joy, generosity, and equanimity has been largely neglected. Also ignored, until recently, have been methods of teaching such positive mind states as kindness and compassion in the establishment and development of the therapeutic relationship. Instead the focus has tended to rely on a sense of constructive neutrality informed by a particular theoretical technique or a blend of various methods as a way to work through material presented in therapy (Freedberg, 2007).

In both Western psychology and Buddhist contemplative tradition, emotions and mental constructs are seen as strong influences in how people think and behave. Several schools of Buddhism teach that some qualities of mind are more helpful than others for creating long lasting happiness and transformation (Goleman, 2003). Craving, hatred, holding onto a sense of "I," "me," or "mine" are seen as harmful states of mind, whereas expending effort on strengthening and developing attention, concentration, and mindfulness lead to equanimity and wisdom based on an understanding of conditions leading to happiness and unhappiness (Ekman, Davidson, Ricard, & Wallace, 2005). When the Dalai Lama was asked what might contribute to healthy states of mind, he responded, "cultivating positive mental states like kindness and compassion definitely leads to better psychological health and happiness." (Dalai Lama & Cutler, 1998).

Although compassion is a central theme in psychotherapy it is not clearly defined or understood and yet it is considered to be a core component of moving toward health and healing (Glaser, 2005). Compassion is most generally understood as a sense of sympathy and concern for the suffering or misfortune of another along with an ability to resonate with that sorrow. It is not to be confused with feeling sorry for someone, which carries with it a sense of superiority. Instead, a pre-cursor for the establishment of compassion is empathy, the appreciation for the feeling experience of another and the understanding that as human beings we will all encounter difficulties from time to time. Kindness and compassion when extended toward oneself and directed outwards toward others, tend to relax the judgments we have of ourselves and of others and is characterized by a deep state of caring.

Caring and compassion play important roles in our work as clinicians. It has been suggested that taking care of oneself, as well as caring for clients, is particularly relevant in carrying out effective therapy (Gilbert, 2006). Evidence suggests that when health care professionals are dissatisfied with their jobs and are experiencing psychological distress, patient care suffers (Shanafelt, Bradley, Wipf, & Black, 2002). Working as a health professional brings its own unique stressors, particularly for those whose work consistently involves them working with clinical populations with high levels of suffering. When Shapiro et al., facilitated an eight week MBSR program for therapists in training, the results indicated a reduction in perceived stress. In addition, participants in this study demonstrated higher levels of positive affect and self-compassion (Shapiro, Brown, & Biegel, 2007). These preliminary results appear to offer health professionals a way to develop a healthier response to the effects of stressors in their own lives and when working with clients.

Elements of teaching in MBSR/MBCT

A. Embodied Awareness

Early on in the MBSR and MBCT programs an exploration of body sensations is highlighted. This is not usual territory in psychological treatment. The body as a container and resource of information and wisdom is often neglected. In the MBSR and MBCT programs, the intuitive intelligence of the body is re-discovered, emphasized and supported not only through what is being encountered in meditation practice but also through the mindful movement aspects of the programs. Too often the body is only noticed when physical pain or discomfort is present. Simple mindful movements can remind us that we can move for the joy of being in motion for its own sake and can help ground us in our bodies. Incorporating specific attention and awareness to movement as a vehicle of knowledge provides a reservoir of information. This can alert us to somatic connections before we are made aware of them cognitively which in turn can identify proactive ways of taking care of ourselves . Those who wish to teach the MBSR and MBCT programs will need to have a personal system of mindful movement like yoga, tai chi, qigong.

When the teacher of MBSR and MBCT communicates a stance of open-hearted awareness towards all that is being encountered in the moment through the practice of mindfulness, including body sensations, a different relationship to pain and suffering emerges. In reinforcing the relevance of each moment rather than seeking to change or dispute what is arising or trying to make sense of the past or predict the future, a different frame of reference is highlighted. In traditional psychological approaches, interventions typically assume that something is amiss which needs to be fixed or adjusted. Mindfulness posits the opposite that by being curious about all inner sensorial experiences, (body, emotions, cognitions) an uncovering of intrinsic health occurs, and in this insight lies the recognition of being a part of a greater whole (Kabat-Zinn, 1996). This has important implications for those mental health illnesses that present with excessive attachment to egocentric thinking.

Awareness in Dialogue

Mindfulness stays firmly in the present moment. Its focus is on what is here right now; what is present. This stance has a different center from many psychological methods, where examination of past history as it relates to current difficulties is a critical focus. A central and important theme in the MBSR and MBCT programs is allowing awareness and attention to be directed toward the inner exploration of the unfolding nature of physical, emotional and cognitive sensations in the present, and also the outward articulation of that process. This requires a special kind of responsiveness on the part of the teacher.

The word "inquiry," often used to describe this process, can sometimes convey a sense of looking for something in particular, and has its derivation in the Latin, "quaerere" and "inquirere" to seek (Concise Oxford Dictionary, 2004. Eleventh Edition). This suggestion that there is something to find can create a more narrowly focused framework for what is unfolding in the MBSR and MBCT groups. Using the word "dialogue" to describe the unfolding meaning of the process of inquiry allows for a more spacious frame of reference which supports a sense of discovery and "exploration of a subject" (Concise Oxford Dictionary, 2004. Eleventh Edition.) rather than looking for answers.

To some extent the instruction and delivery of the mindfulness practices in MBSR and MBCT can be learned through modeling and repetition until the basic language of instruction is committed to memory. But the teacher who operates solely from a position of rote learning and intellect will find it difficult to facilitate the discussion and exploration of mindfulness practice, which comprises a significant portion of the classes. The teacher who relies primarily on technique will be challenged to learn to sit with and be with the comments, questions and experiences arising from mindfulness practice. To respond from a mind solely orientated toward the concepts of patient, diagnosis, illness, or disease is to leave out what mindfulness has the potential to offer.

Instead the MBSR/MBCT teacher encourages the group participants to encounter a place of "not-knowing." Where meaning is uncovered moment by moment without moving to "fix" or shape the essence of what is being experienced. The teacher offers and invites open-ended conversations that can reveal the unfolding nature of what is present in the room rather than a quest for answers, closure, or even requiring anything to be found. The conversations open up into the possibility of rediscovering and befriending empirical connections to meaning. This requires from the teacher a gentle and compassionate attentiveness and steadiness, an understanding born of her/his own encountering of what comes up in personal practice. Otherwise there is a tendency to rationalize this observed learning. This is where the instructor's personal practice becomes central to working with the material presented by the participants. It is where Segal et al. noticed, when observing the MBSR instructors at the Center for Mindfulness (Appendix B) "the remarkable way they were able to embody a different relationship to the most intense distress and emotion in their patients. And we had seen the MBSR instructors going further in their work with negative affect than we had been able to do in the group context, by staying within our therapist roles." (Segal et al., 2002).

Experiential Engagement

Both MBSR and MBCT emphasize that the instructor teach from an experiential engagement with mindfulness rather than through a cognitive process. The reasons for this are described by the developers of MBCT when they articulate their own learning process in Segal et al. (2002). Their initial view was that mindfulness-based interventions could be taught in very much the same way as any other therapy, through learning about the rationale for the techniques and then applying them. However as they continued to observe the MBSR teachers at the Center for Mindfulness, they came to appreciate the qualitative difference it made to the teaching when the instructor spoke from a place of personal experience with the practice of mindfulness. As they noted, "A vital part of what the MBSR instructor conveyed was his or her own embodiment of mindfulness in interactions with the class...Participants in the MBSR program learn about mindfulness in two ways: through their own practice, and when the instructor him- or herself is able to embody it in the way issues are dealt with in the class." (Segal et al., 2002).

The transformational potential of mindfulness practice can only be available to participants and teachers alike if one is living with the practice by actively employing the attitudinal foundations within the fabric of one's own life. It is this quality that is referred to in the reference manual of the Center for Mindfulness. "In order for a class or for the program as a whole to have any meaning or vitality, the person who is delivering it must make every effort to embody the practice in his or her own life and teach out of personal experience and his or her own wisdom, not just in a cookbook fashion out of theory and out of the thinking mind. Otherwise, the instruction becomes a mechanical didactic exercise at best and the true virtues of the mindfulness approach will be lost. We never ask anything of our patients that we are not asking of ourselves to a greater degree, moment to moment and day by day." (Kabat-Zinn & Santorelli, 1996). In teaching MBSR and MBCT, the teacher is embracing a specific way of being with and engaging in experience, by paying deliberate attention to it with an attitude of kindly interest. There is nothing foreign about awareness and paying attention for it is an innate human ability, but mindfulness illuminates and reinforces this faculty in a clearly defined and organized manner. This is because there are specific aspects within the attending – that of non-striving, compassionate listening, deepening self-inquiry and self-acceptance – which require an ongoing and sustained focus. The intention is that nothing is pushed away, chased after or tuned out. Eventually, more difficult mind states such as anger, hatred, hopelessness and helplessness can be seen for what they are – the proliferation of unconstructive qualities of mind created by contact with an unpleasant moment.

Often it is our reactions to difficult and stressful situations, or from wanting to hold onto and find ways to replicate pleasurable experiences, which lead to much "thinking," problem solving and "doing." Sometimes this method of processing the emotional, cognitive and feeling material born out of experience works well. But at times it can lead to an impasse. Then it is as though thinking takes over and we become engaged in creating a potent narrative about what we are going to do, what we could have done and what we should have been able to do.

The MBSR/MBCT teacher will encounter this type of thinking many times from the group participants as they struggle to make sense of their relationship to difficulties, disappointments and pain. It is here, at this intersection that mindfulness (and the teacher's manner of embodying this) offers the possibility to step out of all this "doing" mode, and into "being" mode, by moving toward all sensations just as they are in this moment. It is an insightful process of attending to and allowing for what is here. In acknowledging what is present, observation of the sensations can include a narrow focus of attention or a broader frame of awareness. This is not easy and requires concentration and effort that kindly notices when the attention has moved away from the present moment. It involves a gentle mindful intention to return back to a commitment to be present for each moment along with patience and a quality of friendliness and openness. This requires practice over time because it needs remembering and reinforcement. It is difficult to see how this process can be revealed and acknowledged by the teacher in any other form than from a deep sense of having encountered these moments many times in one's own practice.

It is when meeting suffering in its entirety and in the present moment that a quality of awareness and self-kindness, directed toward the unwanted, is embodied by the teacher through the discovery in personal meditation practice of being able to be with her/his own unconstructive and difficult modes of mind. Over time and with practice, aversive states (a need to create distance from negative affect and to remove and reject difficulty and suffering) are lessened. This is not a passive stance but rather one of receptivity, acknowledgment and compassionate action. A "willingness to embrace in awareness and nonjudgmentally those aspects of oneself that one is most highly defended against, are essential qualities for the successful pursuit of this work" (Kabat-Zinn & Santorelli, 1996). It is only through the instructor's own experience with mindfulness practice, that she/he improves the possibilities of representing these qualities of acceptance, nonjudgment, kindness, continuing investigation, self-inquiry and compassion in their fullness.

Relevance of Personal Practice

Directing awareness through personal mindfulness practice toward strengthening such positive mind states as loving-kindness and compassion requires attention, receptivity, patience, and trust, all attributes of a practical engagement with mindfulness. This takes practice and time. By working regularly and directly with what arises from her/his experience of mindfulness practice, and cultivating such attitudinal modes of mind as nonjudgment, patience, beginner's mind, trust, non-striving, acceptance and letting go, the teacher conveys the possibility to MBSR and MBCT participants of developing a different relationship to difficulties and stress (Kabat-Zinn, 1990). These attitudinal elements of mindfulness become very much a part of what the teacher embodies in instruction and can also be seen as important features of psychotherapy.

Highlighting the efficacy of continuous personal work in this particular way is a somewhat unusual approach in the delivery of clinical training programs, although there is a similar association in of undergoing personal therapy when training as a psychodynamic therapist. The difference here is that embedded in the practice of mindfulness is the assumption that continuing to practice in this way provides an authentic way of being that adds a richness for living in the world.

By sustaining effort, patience and friendliness to the contents of our own mind/body, particularly those aspects of thinking and feeling that we have the most difficulty with, understanding grows about hearing, receiving and being with all the reactions and responses presented by the MBSR and MBCT group participants. Curiosity and compassion are conveyed by the clinician's ability to authentically present the process of returning to the present moment. This is the platform the instructor can offer to the participants, originating as it does from having met oneself again and again in personal practice with a sense of nonjudgment, self-acceptance and compassion.

Professional Training Programs in MBSR and MBCT

Combining an emphasis on the clinician's personal mindfulness practice alongside her/his development of knowledge and theory requires careful consideration when designing professional training for MBSR and MBCT teachers. At a basic level, professional training in MBSR and MBCT will develop and advance teaching skills for the practice of mindfulness. It will foster the enhancement of group process as it relates to mindfulness, encourage and support interpersonal skills, such as warmth, acceptance, compassion and respect alongside appropriate professional and personal boundaries. In the case of MBCT, it will also include the understanding, placement and implementation of the cognitive behavioral segments embedded in the program. Additionally, there is a responsibility to convey intention and meaning to the unfolding nature of mindfulness practice and the various ways that this can be communicated by the clinician.

Training programs will also need to carefully identify the underlying principles of mindfulness practices and their implications for either the general medical population, or for a targeted clinical diagnosis. We can remember that the practice of mindfulness is more than a skill set; more than a behavioral intervention and more than a clinical method developed as a way to work with health care issues. Insight into the application of and implications for mindfulness grows with the experience of practicing and teaching it. So, finding ways within each training program to support and reinforce the instructor's ongoing personal commitment to practice will be as important as the presentation of the intellectual material. This is why at a later stage, after gaining some experience in facilitating MBSR and MBCT groups, additional training and supervision can offer incremental opportunities for gaining deeper perspectives.

In the Buddhist tradition, the engagement with mindfulness is practiced through long-term personal practice and under the supervision of teachers. There are a number of centers worldwide that offer teacher-led silent retreats for those wishing to deepen their practice by engaging in sustained practice for specific lengths of time. MBSR and MBCT teachers need to find ways of sustaining their personal practice as well as obtaining supervision of their teaching with experienced mindfulness-based teachers. Both these processes can take place within supervision, or by having supervision separate from personal mindfulness practice being experienced through recognized mindfulness teaching centers or with an experienced mindfulness practitioner. As mindfulness-based approaches in clinical settings grows, more seasoned practitioners with both a personal mindfulness practice and the experience of facilitating mindfulness-based interventions will develop. This will provide a useful and practical support system for training purposes. This is where having a method of identifying/certifying those clinician/instructors who have undergone a recognized process of training and who can then provide supervision and mentorship will be an important contribution to the field.

Representative Training Routes

Mindfulness-Based Stress Reduction Trainings

There are a number of well established training programs in the USA and Europe that stress the importance of personal mindfulness practice in order to teach MBSR. In fact the relevance of a continuing mindfulness practice is emphasized from the foundation programs to full certification as an instructor in MBSR. One of the best known of these centre is the training programs offered by the Center For Mindfulness (CFM) in Worcester, MA (Appendix B). In the CFM trainings, the establishment of a daily mindfulness meditation practice and attendance at silent, teacher-led retreats is a prerequiste for entry to teacher trainings after the initial 7-day residential training retreat. An additional requirement is to have trained in a professional field at the graduate level that encompasses an intellectual knowledge of the scientific and medical underpinnings for MBSR. Personal psychological development is encouraged, as well as the experience of body centered movement such as mindful yoga, tai chi, qigong.

The CFM offers a 7-day residential training retreat. This program is an intense education in the teaching of MBSR. The retreat provides an opportunity to explore the practice of mindfulness, the structure of the program, how to teach and guide others, as well as examine research supporting the efficacy of the program. The CFM also offers a practicum in MBSR, which provides the opportunity to attend an MBSR class at the CFM where all the sessions of the eight-week program are taught by senior instructors. The practicum offers a rich experiential learning through being a participant in the group and in observing the instructor teaching. After the group has ended, practicum participants meet with the teacher for discussion and instruction.

A further layer of teacher training provided by the CFM is the Teacher Development Intensive, an advanced eight-day teacher training retreat. This program is a highly interactive and collaborative learning where MBSR teaching skills are clarified and refined and the structural underpinnings of the MBSR program are examined. There is an in-depth exploration of the intersection between personal mindfulness practice and the teaching of mindfulness itself, along with time devoted to exploring those moments of challenge when teaching. An important component in this training is recognizing how our modes of mind effect our actions and how they inform our teaching. Ongoing supervision and consultation is also provided by the CFM.

Mindfulness-Based Cognitive Therapy Trainings

There are also a diverse and growing number of MBCT training programs currently available in the USA and Europe but referencing them all would be impracticable. Instead a focus on some generic methods of delivery will be reviewed by examining MBCT training in North America and the UK. In North America, MBCT professional training programs are currently delivered in one or two-day introduction seminars, a five-day training retreat program (Level 1) and an eight-day advanced teaching and study retreat program (Level 2) (Appendix B). An additional layer of training is also provided by supervision and consultation from experienced teachers. From the onset, teaching revolves around the intersection of didactic material and the experiential. In the one and two-day seminars, exposure to some of the mindfulness meditation practices that patients will be taken through is as much a part of the teaching as discussion of the structure and rationales for MBCT.

The five-day professional training program in MBCT (Level 1) is an intense course that introduces the clinician/instructor to the structure and themes of MBCT and also provides periods of time devoted to personal mindful practice alongside the teaching of didactic instruction material. It offers an opportunity to work with the application of mindfulness and the placement of the cognitive behavioral elements through a course of instructive, experiential, large and small group teachings. A deliberate focus is placed on the intersection of the intellectual grasp of the materials and the experience of the practice of mindfulness. This emphasis highlights the ways in which as clinicians we tend to be more comfortable and used to being taught a method. By returning to silence and the practice of mindfulness at the end of the day during the first few days of the program, the clinician/instructor discovers what it is to be with thoughts/emotions/body sensations that arise from what is being taught and experienced.

It is not that the power of the intellect is being discouraged, rather what is being encouraged, is to meet the nature of mind with openness, receptivity and patience. In this way the MBCT program is being explored not simply as a series of techniques, but also as a learning that is taking place on the inside. This is similar to the experience that will be encountered by MBSR and MBCT group participants. The domain is one of going back and forth between experiential awareness and intellectual thought.

As a way to reinforce the efficacy of ongoing learning there are different entry requirements for attendance in the Level 1 and Level 2 trainings. The eight-day level 2 training, is intended for those professionals who have an established personal mindfulness practice, are aware of the necessity of personal practice as a platform from which to teach and have attended teacher-led silent meditation retreats. It is for those clinicians who have already taught MBCT groups. Much is learned from the experience of facilitating MBCT groups, not only from the perspective of the practicalities involved but also from what is being elicited in the instructor during the teaching. Learning to return to the landscape of mindfulness, rather than be drawn into the territory of psychologically based interventions is where much of the instructional nature of this training is placed.

Opening days of silence support the process of mindfulness practice, a reminder to re-enter mindful awareness as place to be, and from which to teach. From this place of remembering a focus is held on the intention and integrity of mindfulness-based experiential learning alongside the understanding of the intention and sequencing of the cognitive behavioral elements. Learning is fostered by the use of large and small groups, dyads and teacher supervision as well as the return to silent mindfulness practice at the end of the day through breakfast the following day.

In the UK, there are now a number of avenues for training in MBCT at the introductory level as well as the more advanced and these are based in several centers around the country. The trainings at The Center for Mindfulness Research and Practice at Bangor University, in Wales, are wide-ranging and similar in ideology to the programs outlined for North America. However, in addition Bangor offers a master's degree in mindfulness-based approaches, which provides two directions for learning; an MSc or an MA. The MSc is available to those who are interested in scientific research and the MA follows a more experiential methodology (Appendix B).

The University of Oxford in Oxford offers a master's of studies degree in MBCT (Appendix B). It is a part-time program open to mental health professionals with psychotherapy experience and is taught over two years. It is structured around ten three-day teaching blocks and two residential retreats, five days in the first year and seven days in the second. It includes instruction in MBCT, an understanding of germane clinical and cognitive psychology as well as aspects of Buddhist psychology and philosophy. Placing residential mindfulness retreats within an academic curriculum highlights the importance of the clinician's own experiential practice alongside intellectual learning.

Another avenue of training includes a one-year certificate or two-year diploma program. The University of Exeter offers such a program (Appendix B). These training programs provide trainees with both the ability to participate in an MBCT group as well as facilitate a group under supervision. Trainees have the opportunity to learn the theory and research reinforcing MBCT and be instructed in Buddhist psychology. Once enrolled in these programs, attendance at a teacher-led silent retreats is expected.

Conclusion and Future Directions

Training in mindfulness-based approaches for clinicians is evolving with increased understanding and knowledge of what mindfulness actually offers in a clinical setting. This chapter has focused on just two of the clinical programs that utilize mindfulness, MBSR and MBCT, because at their core, they provide a sustained and systematic instruction in mindfulness meditation practice which has important and novel implications for training health professionals. Mindfulness is not a quick fix or a time limited intervention for the amelioration of pain and suffering. It is an approach that concentrates on the study of direct experience and consciousness and is a commitment over time to nurture the mind toward the possibility of insight and wisdom.

There are many questions in the future about the role of mindfulness in health care settings. We are at the beginning of our understanding about the efficacy of mindfulness as a clinical treatment. We are only just starting to learn about what aspects of mindfulness make a difference in clinical settings. We do not really know what are the elements of competency for its instruction. Bringing a scientific lens to understanding the various components in mindfulness and how best to convey and instruct those elements in clinical settings will be the subject of further studies (Baer, 2003; Baer, Smith, Hopkins, Krietemeyer, & Toney, 2006). There is empirical evidence that mindfulness practiced over time and regularly, contributes to happiness and alleviates suffering. There is also preliminary scientific evidence that the Buddhist practice of meditation can shape the way the brain processes certain aspects of emotion and thought (Davidson & Harrington, 2002; Davidson, Kabat-Zinn, Schumacher, Rosenkranz, et al., 2003).

MBSR and MBCT employ mindfulness practice as the core to their programs intervention. Other clinical programs focus on teaching specific components of mindfulness as a skill set, a way to address suffering alongside the use of Western therapies. Further clinical studies are needed to better study these two ways of applying mindfulness-based interventions. MBCT constructs a platform for the delivery of what cognitive behavior therapy understands to be the thought and mood patterns contributing to relapse in depression and what the rigorous practice of mindfulness offers in developing a different relationship to those experiences. MBSR offers the systematic exploration of the effects of stress as a potent component in our relationship to healing and health and works with generic medical and psychological problems. Both offer an opportunity for the group participants to enhance experiential understanding about a more universal arena of health and well-being, one that is heart centered in its fullest sense by connecting to a deep core of wisdom; a profound feeling of being at home regardless of where we are and what is happening.

Mindfulness is a way to remember how to re-discover the experience of the moment. Its practice takes us deeply into the way the mind/body works. It is only by meeting our minds over and over again in practice that we can hope to convey a sense of insight bathed in compassion and embark on the journey of embodying what is being asked in teaching. For this reason professional teaching programs need to encompass both intellectual and experiential learning in mindfulness, otherwise what the practice has to offer will lose its heart centered approach to working with suffering.

References

Baer, R. (2003). Mindfulness training as a clinical intervention: A conceptual and empirical review. *Clinical Psychology: Science and Practice, 10*, 125–143.

Baer, R., Smith, G. T., Hopkins, J., Krietemeyer, J., & Toney, L. (2006). Using self-report assessment methods to explore facets of mindfulness. *Assessment, 13*(1), March, 27–45.

Concise Oxford Dictionary (2004). Eleventh Edition

Dalai Lama & Cutler, H. C. (1998). *The art of happiness*. New York: Riverhead Books, 41.

Davidson, R. J. & Harrington, A. (Eds.) (2002). *Visions of compassion*. New York. Oxford University Press.

Davidson, R. J., Kabat-Zinn, J., Schumacher, J., Rosenkranz, M., et al. (2003). Alterations in brain and immune function produced by mindfulness meditation. *Psychosomatic Medicine, 65*, 564–570.

Dimidjian, S., & Linehan, M. (2003). Defining an agenda for future research on the clinical application of mindfulness practice. *Clinical Psychology: Science and Practice, 10*(2), 166.

Ekman, P., Davidson, R. J., Ricard, M., & Wallace, B. A. (2005). Buddhist and psychological perspectives on emotions and well-being. *Current Directions in Psychological Science, 14*(2), 59–63.

Freedberg, S. (2007). Re-examining empathy: A relational-feminist point of view. *Social Work, 52*(3), 251–259.

Gilbert, P. (2006). *Compassion: Conceptualizations, research and use in psychotherapy*. New York: Routledge.

Glaser, A. (2005). *A call to compassion*. York Beach, ME: Nichols-Hayes, Inc.

Goleman, D. (2003). *Destructive emotions*. New York: Bantam

Kabat-Zinn, J. (1990). *Full catastrophe living.* New York: Bantam Doubleday Dell.

Kabat-Zinn, J. (2003) Mindfulness-based Interventions in context: Past, present and future. *Clinical Psychology: Science and Practice, 10*(2), 145.

Kabat-Zinn, J., & Santorelli, S. (1996). *A teaching mandala. Mindfulness-based stress reduction professional training resource manual.* Massachusetts: Center for Mindfulness in Medicine, Health Care, and Society.

Palmer, & Parker J. (1998). *The courage to teach.* San Francisco: John Wiley & Sons, 6, 11

Segal, Z., Williams, J., & Teasdale, J. (2002). *Mindfulness-based cognitive therapy for depression: A new approach to preventing relapse.* New York: Guildford Press.

Shanafelt, T. D., Bradley, K. A., Wipf, J. E., & Black, A. L. (2002). Burnout and self-reported patient care in an internal medicine residency program. *Annals of Internal Medicine, 136*, 358–367.

Shapiro, S. L., Brown, K. W., & Biegel, G. M. (2007). Teaching Self-Care to Caregivers: Effects of Mindfulness-Based Stress Reduction on the Mental Health of Therapists in training. *Training and Education in Professional Psychology, 1*(2), 105–115.

Appendix A: Mindfulness Practice

Thomas Bien and Fabrizio Didonna

Traditional Buddhist teaching says there are 84,000 dharma doors. In essence, that means there are lots of ways to practice. Here are some that we consider useful as a foundation for mindfulness.

A Word About Posture

In the practice of formal meditation the first step is finding a correct physical posture. Our body posture has a very direct and powerful effect on our state of mind. We know that body and mind are interrelated, and for this reason the mindful state arises naturally when physical posture and mental attitude support each other. So, a correct and upright posture helps one's mind naturally come to rest in a state of calm and presence. The best meditation posture is one in which you feel yourself at once comfortable, relaxed, alert, and grounded one that you can maintain comfortably for some time. A correct posture reduces obstacles to concentration such as physical pain, distractions, sleepiness, and wandering mind. We can achieve this if the body finds balance, stillness, stability, and wakefulness. As Tibetan Buddhist teacher Sogyal Rinpoche said (1994): "The whole point of correct posture is to create a more auspicious environment for meditation".

When we meditate it is helpful to wear loose clothing, with nothing constricting the waist, and no shoes or, better yet, barefoot.

There are several postures that can allow you to establish the best conditions for meditation. In the *sitting position* you may choose to settle on a straight-backed chair or on a soft surface on the floor, with your buttocks supported by a cushion such as the traditional *zafu* or kneeling bench. Whether you sit on the floor or on a chair, the key element is to keep your back straight; not rigid, but simply erect or uplifted, with the back of the neck aligned with your spine. Adopt a dignified, noble and upright posture. According to noted mindfulness teacher, Jon Kabat-Zinn (2005), "a dignified sitting posture is itself an affirmation of freedom, and of life's harmony, beauty, and richness, and the posture itself is the meditation." A useful instruction is to imagine you are being pulled up through the top of the head by a string. If sitting on a chair, you may choose to sit away from the back of the chair so that your back is self-supporting. Let your feet rest flat on the floor. Sitting on a chair is a very good way to practice meditation, and should not be considered less valuable than sitting on the floor. You may also choose to sit in the *kneeling position* ("*Seiza*" or "*Japanese*") sitting on a bench, or a cushion that is used as a saddle, with your knees resting on the floor.

Remember that while sitting it is fine to change positions if you feel pain. It is important to be gentle with yourself.

Allow your hands to find a stable support. You may choose to rest your hands in your lap, just below the navel, or rest your left hand inside the right hand, palms facing upwards and thumbs lightly touching. Relax your shoulders. You may keep your eyes open, or gently close them to prevent external distractions. However you sit, it is important to find the most balanced, relaxed and grounded position, one that allows your mind to go deeply into the process of meditation.

Mindfulness of Breathing

The breath lies at the intersection between the voluntary and involuntary nervous systems. For this reason, mindfulness of breathing offers a unique opportunity to bring body and mind together. When we are agitated, we often catch our breath and breathe shallowly. Because the breath is shallow, we then feel even more anxious, creating a negative feedback loop: We are upset or anxious, so we breathe in a tight way. Then because we are breathing in such a way, we start to feel even more anxious.

Fortunately, the reverse is also true. When we let our attention settle on the breath, calming it by just letting it be itself and not forcing it to go any particular way, the breathing calms down, and with it, the mind. It is as if mindful breathing sends a message to the brain, saying, "Everything is okay, no need to worry," and this helps us to feel more at ease.

Mindful breathing is foundational to many mindfulness exercises. It need not take a lot of time, and is very enjoyable and refreshing when done properly. In fact, the definition of doing it properly is that you enjoy the process.

Mindfulness of breathing can be done sitting, standing, or lying down. Let your awareness drop down into the abdomen, away from all the thinking, and simply let your body breathe in and out exactly as it wants to. You can notice the flow of the air in and out, the rise and fall of the abdomen, the onset of the breath, the inflection point just before you begin to exhale, and the length of the pause before your body begins another cycle. Focusing on what is interesting or pleasant about these sensations greatly facilitates concentration. Cultivate the sense that with each breath you are nourishing every cell in your body. When your thinking pulls you away, notice this without recrimination, and come back to the breath. Smile a gentle Buddha smile. Continue for a comfortable period of time.

Sitting Meditation

There are many different styles of meditation. Each style has somewhat different methods, different goals, and different results. The style of meditation most related to mindfulness is *vipassana*, sometimes called insight meditation. Descriptions of this technique vary somewhat, but all styles of vipassana meditation include an object of focus (most often, the breath), and the cultivation of accepting awareness when the mind wanders from that focus. While concentration is helpful, it is not necessarily the goal of this type of meditation to attain perfect concentration on the breathing. More important is that, when the mind wanders, one notices this wandering in a kindly way, without self-recrimination, and returns gently to the breath. If one continues to do this, this is correct vipassana. It does not matter whether your mind wanders one hundred times during the course of a meditation session, or only once. If you notice each time and bring the mind back, not struggling against the mind's natural tendency to wander, but simply observing it, that is good practice.

In vipassana practice, there is no struggle to identify the thoughts, or to try to correct them. Rather, one simply notes the thoughts, as much as possible without getting caught up in their content or debating their validity, and then returns to the breath. By the endless repetition of this process, the meditator becomes aware of the *process* of consciousness, coming to know and accept how the mind works, without struggling against it. One cannot emphasize enough that the central characteristic is precisely this observing without struggling.

Here are some specific steps for this practice:

1. Choose a quiet place.
2. As described above, sit in a way that helps you to be both alert and relaxed.
3. Allow time for the transition from whatever you've been doing to the meditative state, adopting an unhurried attitude. Take a moment or two to open to the environment around you, the sounds, smells, whatever is present. Note the sensations present in your body. Feel your skin as that which *connects* you with everything else rather than that which divides you from it.
4. Gently allow the focus of your awareness to settle onto the abdomen, to a point about two finger breadths below the navel. (Alternatively, you can focus on the point where the air makes contact with your nostrils.) From there, notice the body breathing in and breathing out, letting the breath unfold of its own accord, not forcing in any way. Attend clearly to the *pleasantness* of this process.
5. As soon as you notice that your mind has wandered away from the breath, briefly note what you have been thinking about, or just say to yourself "thinking, thinking", and return to your breathing. The most important thing to remember is that such wandering is completely natural and acceptable. So do not engage in accusations against yourself for this. (Or, if you do, note that also as just more thinking, in the same spirit in which you observe other thoughts). This practice is called *mere recognition*, and the essence of it is to simply notice and return, notice and return, without much involvement with content.
6. Repeat this process for a comfortable period of time, gradually lengthening your meditation periods to at least 30 or 40 minutes. The Latin motto, *propera lente*, is highly pertinent: hasten slowly. Do not attempt to do more than you are ready for, but accept yourself as you are. Your capacity to sit will gradually increase. If you like, you can do this in a methodical way. For example, if 5 minutes is the most you can do to begin with, practice daily for 5 minutes for a week or so, then try 10 minutes for a week, then 15, and so on. If you try to force yourself to do things you are not ready to do, you may give up altogether.

7. When you finish your sitting meditation, take your time coming out of it. See about bringing the same attitude of clear, accepting awareness into your daily life. During the day, return frequently to your meditation by practicing a few mindful breaths. There are many opportunities for this — while waiting in line at the bank or store, while waiting for your computer to boot up or finish a task, while you are on hold on the telephone, while you are paused in traffic or at a red light, and so on.

Metta Meditation

Metta means loving-kindness. There are many reasons to cultivate feelings of kindness toward ourselves and others. Traditional Buddhist teaching lists the following benefits of such practice: (1) sleeping well, (2) waking up feeling well and light in heart, (3) having no unpleasant dreams, (4) being liked by others and at ease with them, especially children, (5) being dear to animals, (6) being supported and protected by gods and goddesses, (7) protection from fire, poison, and sword, (8) being able to attain meditative concentration easily, (9) one's face becomes bright and clear, (10) mental clarity at the time of death, (11) being reborn in the Brahma Heaven (Nhat Hanh, 1997). One need not take this literally to understand how much value Buddhist tradition places on this practice.

Such a practice is foundational to the kind of empathy that the work of therapy requires (Bien, 2006). In one demonstration (cited in Barasch, 2005) a Tibetan-trained monk who practiced loving-kindness meditation was able to discriminate subtle changes in facial expression of emotion to a level two standard deviations above the mean, a capacity that would stand any therapist in good stead. There is also evidence that compassion is good for us. In one study (McClelland, 1986), students who watched a film of Mother Teresa performing acts of compassion showed an elevation in S-Iga in their saliva, indicating improved immune functioning. This occurred even for students who disapproved of Mother Teresa and her work.

All forms of meditation are already a practice of kindness, to oneself, and by extension, to other people. But it is also helpful at times to make this aspect more explicit. To practice loving-kindness meditation, begin with yourself. Sit quietly, enjoying your breathing. As you continue to breathe in and out, dwell gently with simple phrases such as:

May I be happy.
May I have ease of well-being.
May I be free from negative emotions.
May I be safe.
Take your time with each one. Do not rush the process.
Then, when you are ready, perhaps when you have begun to feel the effect of the practice, widen the circle outward to include someone else, beginning with the person closest to you, breathing in and out, dwelling with the same phrases, but now for her sake, (placing her name in the blanks):
May ____ be happy.
May ____ have ease of well-being.
May ____ be free from negative emotions.
May ____ be safe.

Then the practice can be extended in the same way to a friend, a "neutral" person (someone you don't know well), and more challengingly, to an enemy – someone whom you find disturbing to even think about. Finally, in the last step, radiate the same intentions toward all beings.

There is no need for each practice session to include all the levels (self, dearest person, friend, neutral person, enemy, and all beings). What is most important is that the practice be done in a deep, leisurely way. At times, a whole meditation session may be used simply to generate lovingkindness toward self or toward one other person. Each level is as valuable as the other.

Physiologically, anger is a very expensive, destructive emotion, triggering the release of hormones such as epinephrine, norepinephrine, and cortisol that are implicated in heart disease and other health problems. Metta meditation can help here, since under the principle of reciprocal inhibition, one cannot feel both love and anger at the same time. If you are angry with someone, and wish to take care of this emotion by replacing it with kindness, it is helpful to begin with yourself rather than immediately trying to cultivate kindness toward the person you are angry with. Once you are feeling kindly toward yourself, you may be able to take that additional step more easily.

At times, you may be able to just sit and generate feelings of kindness toward all beings, envisioning yourself as emitting rays of love and compassion to everyone, bathing your mind in this feeling. But if that becomes too diffuse or abstract, return to the more concrete form described above.

Mindfulness of the Body

Every teacher knows that students love attention. Sometimes students will even act disruptively in the classroom in order to get it, especially if they feel they cannot seem to get it any other way.

Your body also loves attention. It loves it when you simply appreciate it, stopping to attend to exactly how things are with it.

While mindfulness of the body can be practiced in different postures, it is often enjoyable to practice lying down when this is possible. As you lie on your back on the floor or mat, spend a few moments enjoying your breathing. Note how the floor is supporting you, holding you up.

After a little while, begin with your feet. On an inbreath, say to yourself silently, "Breathing in, I am aware of my feet." On the outbreath, say, "Breathing out I smile to my feet." After the first time, you can shorten the words to just "feet" on the inbreath, and "smiling" on the outbreath. Notice just exactly what sensations are present in your feet. Note any sensations on the surface, such as temperature, or the feel of socks or shoes, or of the floor against your heels, as well as sensations within the feet, such as any tiredness or discomfort, or feelings of pleasant relaxation. Whatever is there, positive or negative, embrace it with accepting awareness. Contemplate how valuable your feet are, how many things are possible because of having two good feet. Send your feet kindness and appreciation.

When you are ready, taking your time and not rushing, move up to your legs.

"Breathing in, I am aware of my legs. Breathing out, I smile to my legs." Note with some precision the exact sensations that are present in your legs. Remember how valuable your legs are, and send them love and appreciation.

After several minutes, do the same with: your hands, your arms, your neck and shoulders, the muscles in your face, your back, and your chest and stomach, again taking your time with each part of the body. Then finally, embrace your body as a whole in the same way, "Breathing in, I am aware of my body. Breathing out, I smile to my body." Note exactly how the body is feeling right now, and send appreciation and love to your body.

It is possible to get much more detailed with this practice. For example, you can take each foot, hand, or leg, one at a time. You can differentiate upper and lower arms and legs, and even focus on each digit individually. You can also specifically send kindness to the organs and parts of the body, such as your blood, your bones, your skin, your heart, your eyes, and so on. Keep in mind, though, that when we try to do too much, we risk becoming impatient. If we become compulsive about the practice, this can generate anxiety. So only practice to the extent that helps you to feel calm and light.

Mindful Eating

The essence of eating meditation is to know that you are eating when you are eating, to be aware of the vast array of sensory experiences that are available when you eat. One way to begin this is to sit mindfully in front of your food, and rather than diving right in, pause to breathe in and out a few times. Notice what you hear and see and around. Look deeply at your food. Consider all the conditions required for this food to be in front of you. If you are looking, say, at a simple piece of bread, the wheat had to grow in the fields, receiving the sun, the rain, and nutrients of the soil. The farmer had to take care of it, water it, fertilize, and harvest it. The raw wheat had to be milled. The baker had to bake it and send it on to the store where you purchased it, and so on. In this way you can begin to see the piece of bread more truly for what it is, a miraculous manifestation of the entire cosmos.

When you are ready, lift the bread to your mouth, noting the movements of your hands and the action of your teeth as you bite into it. Note the grinding motion, the work of your tongue, and the release of saliva. Note how the flavor changes as you begin to chew slowly, chewing each bite well and thoroughly. Note the activity of swallowing, and any lingering taste. In short, notice everything. It is amazing how much there is to notice in the "simple" act of eating a piece of bread. If you tend to eat quickly, try taking three mindful breaths between bites. Alternatively, chew each bite at least thirty times, doing this in a relaxed, non-compulsive way.

When you feel too busy, and your mind is too active to eat a whole meal in this way, modifications are easy. It is always possible to at least take a few mindful breaths and contemplate your food before beginning to eat, and then perhaps at least eat the first bite in a deep and mindful way.

A simple meal can be a wonderful experience if we are mindful. It is a shame if we miss it.

Mindfulness of Sight and Sound

During our daily life, we normally see and hear on automatic pilot. This informal exercise aims at opening our senses to establish a deep connection with our visual and auditory awareness in the present moment. Practicing this exercise reveals how often we fail to really see and hear the things around us in a vivid way, perceiving only a small fraction of what is going on around us. Frequently, rather than perceiving things freshly in themselves, we perceive only the categories we normally use to make sense of our world (Segal, Williams, & Teasdale, 2002). We do not see the flower but only our concept of "flower." We do not hear the actual sound made by a passing car, but only the concept "car noise." We also immediately categorize each percept as positive, negative, or neutral and uninteresting. Mindful seeing and hearing frees us of the shallow and automatic perceptions that render us deaf and blind to the world around us.

Seeing Meditation

The duration of this practice normally ranges from 5 to 15 minutes.

To begin with, you can stand in front of a window or in a chosen a location outdoors. When you feel ready, begin to carefully observe an object of your choice, close or distant, on which you will focus all your awareness. While observing, try to avoid naming or categorizing the object (for example *a tree*), but instead try to describe it through its physical and sensory characteristics – the shape, the color, areas of light and shadow, whether it is rough or smooth, the distance between it and you, its movement or stillness, the differences and relationships between various parts of the object. If the object is one you can hold, you might even take it in your hands to observe it more closely. During the observation, the mind may wander and thoughts may take you away from your visual awareness. When this happens simply notice that the mind is wandering – acknowledge this event – and as soon as possible, simply go back intentionally to seeing with clarity and depth. Stay with the object until you feel you have made deep contact with it. After some time you can choose to move your attention to another object and observe it in the same way.

Imagine yourself seeing way a dog sitting in a park might do so.. Everything around you is interesting and full of life. No categories, concepts, or labels stand between you and what you see. Your seeing is direct and fresh, full of openness and curiosity. No thoughts interfere with the wonder of the act of seeing.

Along these lines, it is reported of Zen master Thich Nhat Hanh that one day, as he was walking in the forest with some children, one of them asked him what color the bark of a tree was. He wanted to avoid giving an answer that would interfere with the freshness of really seeing by providing a conceptual kind of answer, as would have been the case if he'd simply said something like "brown." Instead, he told the child, "It is the color that you see," pointing the child back in the direction of his own experience.

Hearing Meditation

When you are ready, listen to the sounds around you, wherever you may be.

Let go of naming and categorising the origin and source of the sounds, and just note their physical features; volume, tone, pitch, continuity or discontinuity, their distance from you, the spaces between sounds, the silence out of which sound arises. If you notice that your mind is wandering, be aware for a moment of where your mind is going, and then gently, bring your attention back to the sounds in the here and now.

You might also choose to listen to a piece of music. Listen to the patterns of sounds and instruments, staying in touch with the how the music changes from moment to moment. Note the interplay between the various instruments. Hear the airiness of the flute, the specific and concrete tension and grittiness of violin strings, rather than labeling the instruments. If someone is singing, note the exact quality of this particular human voice. Try to hear these sounds as if you were from another planet and had never heard such things before. It doesn't matter if you like or dislike the music. Even sounds of distortion in the speakers can be interesting if you hear without judgment and with a gentle sense of curiosity.

Mindful Walking (Walking Meditation)

Mindful walking is a form of meditation in action. People who find it difficult to stay still for a long time in sitting meditation may find it easier to develop attention and mindful awareness by practicing this form of meditation. For some people the bodily experience of walking provides a more clear and vivid subject for meditation than meditation while sitting or lying. In walking meditation we focus on the sensations of walking. Unlike sitting meditation, during walking meditation we keep our eyes open and are more aware of the outside world (natural or human sounds, visual stimuli, the wind, the weather, the sun, etc.). Mindful walking is a meditation that can be practiced in a more *formal way* – for example by practicing for a specified length of time (15–20 minutes, or even more) and walking very slowly (see description below), or in a more *informal way* each time we move from one place to another. Informal walking meditation is available to us many times a day. In informal walking meditation, we walk at our normal pace, simply becoming aware of our walking. This allows us to develop more meditative awareness in our daily lives. If possible, practice this meditation for the first time outdoors. Find a quiet place, a park or open space, where you will be able to walk for fifteen or twenty minutes without encountering too many distractions.

Begin by cultivating a correct standing posture. This can be considered a meditation in itself. In the upright position, known as the *mountain posture*, the back is straight but not stiff, shoulders and torso are relaxed, the head is aligned with the spine, with feet parallel and shoulder-width apart (about 15–20 cm or 5–10 inches). Knees are soft and slightly bent. You may notice that when you bend the knees slightly, you feel more grounded. Become aware of gravity keeping you connected to the earth moment by moment.

Let arms and hands rest along the body, clasping your hands either behind your back or in front.

Body awareness is the first *foundation of mindfulness*, so bring all your attention to the sensations in your body, in particular to the sensations in the soles of your feet. Be aware of your weight being transferred through the soles of your feet to the earth. You can also be aware of all the subtle movements you continuously make with your feet and legs, and other parts of the body, in order to keep balanced and upright. Notice the constant adjustments you make in order to maintain balance. Normally we take the ability to be able to stand upright completely for granted. But once you pay close attention, you will appreciate why it took several years to learn how to do this! Let your gaze fall a moderate distance in front of you, looking slightly downwards, perhaps meeting the ground a few meters or yards ahead.

Note the moment when you feel ready to start walking. To begin with, it may be helpful to walk at a very slow pace, as if you were walking in slow motion. Chose a short path to walk back and forth on. First, bring your feet together and begin walking by lifting the heel of the first foot from the ground. As the foot begins to lift off the ground, notice how the weight of your body begins to shift onto the other foot and leg. When the foot has been completely lifted, notice that the entire weight of the body is on the opposite foot and leg, and also note the sensations in the forward foot while it travels through the air. Bring the foot forward until it gently reaches the ground, letting the heel touch first followed by the rest of the foot. At the same time bring your awareness to the other foot as it begins to lift from the ground in the same manner as the first. Notice also any sensation that may arise in the body, and any emotion (joy, serenity, boredom, curiosity etc.) you may feel – moment by moment.

There are three important moments to notice during walking meditation: the moment in which we lift one foot off the ground, the phase in which the foot is suspended and moves through the air, and the moment in which the foot rests on the ground once again. Try saying the words "lifing," "moving," and "placing" to yourself in order to focus your attention on these three phases.

When you reach the end of your path, slowly turn around and begin again, becoming aware of the different sensation resume your walk. It is very useful to try to maintain an attitude of gentle curiosity during the walking meditation, as if you were a child taking your first steps. Every step is a discovery, an accomplishment, a new experience.

You can introduce some variations while walking and observe how these increase or decrease your awareness. For example, try changing the pace and rhythm of your walk. How does the experience change if you go from a very slow mindful walking to mindful running? Or you can chose to take some steps with eyes closed or partially closed, and notice how your sense of balance changes. See about bringing a half smile to your lips as you walk, even if this does not come spontaneously to you, and notice how it is to walk with a smile. A smile can facilitate a sense of presence, serenity, and of walking just to enjoy the walking, without goal or purpose.

As with the other exercises, if the mind wanders, simply try to notice it and, as soon as possible, do your best to bring it gently back to the present moment and to all the physical sensations created by walking, step by step.

Experience these sensations rather than to *thinking* about them. Thinking can lead to judgments and negative mental states such as anxiety, boredom, or sadness. Instead see about staying with the direct sensations themselves.

Just as mindful breathing unites body and mind, so that our attention is not lost in a cloud of worry about the future or regret about the past, walking meditation also creates an integration of mind and body in the present moment, as you continue to just notice what is happening and nothing else.

When you finish walking, take a few moments to feel and integrate the effects of the practice, noticing any differences, particularly in regards to physical sensations and emotional and mental states, between the beginning and the end of the meditation.

Lake Meditation

Lake Meditation uses guided imagery. Unlike the previous forms of meditation which are based on the here and now, for this meditation we imagine a particular scene or landscape which expresses the nature of mindfulness.

A lake embodies the receptivity of water, the capacity to stay in touch with all the changes on its surface. It expresses both the impermanence of the flow of momentary experience, and the calm and quiet of its depths. Even though on the surface there may be rain, wind, or snow, the lake receives it acceptingly, letting whatever happens happen, moment by moment, without resistance or struggle (Kabat-Zinn, 1994).

During this meditation we try to embody these aspects of the lake, nurturing our own lake-like properties. This meditation can help us discover our inner nature, recognize our intrinsic stability, and find balance. It offers an image of strength and depth, the capacity to deal in peace and tranquillity with the challenging events of life, finding within ourselves the capacity to become like the undisturbed waters of a lake.

We suggest taping the text of this meditation and listening to it on a stereo or with earphones when practicing. The words should be spoken slowly, pausing between each phrase.

Find a comfortable position. It may be best to lie down, as this posture resembles the form of the lake. But if lying down is difficult or uncomfortable you may choose to sit on the mat or on a chair. If you have one, use a mat or a rug and lie comfortably, releasing any tension in the body. Let arms and legs rest freely on the mat or floor.

After you have settled in your position, begin to focus on the sensations in your body. Allow yourself to drop into a sense of calmness and tranquillity, maintaining a sense of presence and grounding, of contact with the earth.

Bring your attention to your breathing and hold it there for some time. Simply observe the phases of the breath, noticing the changing sensations during inspiration and expiration. It is not necessary to breathe in any particular way. Simply stay connected with your breathing, allowing the body to breathe just as it wants and needs.

When you feel ready, picture the most beautiful lake you can imagine, one that is very quiet. It's a late summer day . . . the water is pure and clear, and you feel nourished and soothed by this beautiful stretch of crystal clear, blue or emerald green water . . . There are no people around. The temperature in and out of the water is pleasantly warm, and you can sense the cool depth of the lake's waters. Luscious green vegetation surrounds the lake, with tall, ancient trees all around the shore.

You feel comfortable and safe, and looking at the beauty of this place you experience a sense of great peace and calm. The windless surface of the lake is smooth, without ripples, and the water is like a great mirror reflecting everything around it. The lake, like all water, is profoundly receptive, containing and receiving everything it encounters without disturbance, without changing its essential nature. As your practice of meditation deepens, you too learn to welcome and contain every internal event (thoughts, emotions, sensations) or external event without disturbance, as though reflecting off the surface of the lake.

You can see the lake reflecting the sky, the clouds, the mountain, the trees, the birds, but also reflecting your own mind. Imagine your mind taking on the attributes of the lake. Thoughts may ripple and trouble your mind, like a sudden breeze that ripples the surface of the lake, but deep within you remain unaffected. You see these thoughts as unimportant and passing, impermanent and fleeting mental facts. You become quiet, still, clear, and at rest.

Now let yourself go even further, and imagine you are floating safely and effortlessly on your back on the water. Your mind is very quiet and you feel at peace. Thoughts arise and try to capture your attention, but you simply let them drift away, like the impermanent reflections of birds flying over the lake and departing. Whatever arises, you remain aware that you are floating on the calm surface of the water. You float comfortably and effortlessly, safe and at ease. The clear, clean water embraces you and you merge with it.

When you feel ready, bring the image of the lake inside of you so that you *become* the lake, so that your body lying down and the lake become one. Feel its body as your body. Breathe together with the lake, moment by moment. Let your mind be open, reflecting anything that arises in your inner or outer experience. You may experience moments of complete stillness, as when the lake is calm and clear, and moments of restlessness, as when the water is troubled and cloudy.

Above you the sky is blue and light. You are alone, and your aloneness is filled with peace. Stay like this for a while. Feel how much peace surrounds you. Feel the tranquillity. Your entire being is permeated by water. You feel safe. . . .

The warmth of the sun is relaxing and calming and very pleasant. Stay in touch with these sensations and nourish them with the calm and tranquillity the lake transmits to you. The winds on the lake may cause ripples or waves on the surface, yet you know that its depth, the vastest part of it, is untouched and unperturbed. Your problems are like ripples on the lake, not changing the essence of who you are. The water lets everything pass through it, with no resistance, its essence remaining in tact. In the end, the lake always returns to its own essence of calmness and tranquillity.

In this moment, as you sit or lie down, embrace all the qualities of your mind and your body as the earth holds and encircles the lake The lake is a mirror of water, and since it yields, it need not break, but instead renews itself continuously, moment by moment.

References

Barasch, M. I. (2005). *Field notes on the compassionate life: A search for the soul of kindness.* New York: Rodale.

Bien, T. (2006). *Mindful therapy: A guide for therapists and helping professionals.* Boston: Wisdom.

Kabat-Zinn, J. (1994). *Wherever you go, there you are: Mindfulness meditation in everyday life.* New York: Hyperion.

Kabat-Zinn, J. (2005). Coming to our senses. London: Piatkus Books Ltd

McClelland, D. C. (1986). Some reflections on the two psychologies of love. *Journal of Personality, 54*(2) June, 344–349.

Nhat Hanh, Thich (1997). *Teachings on love* (Esp. pp. 1–19.). Berkeley: Parallax.

Rinpoche, S. (1994). *The tibetan book of living and dying.* New York: Harper-Collins

Segal, Z., Williams, J., & Teasdale, J. (2002). *Mindfulness-based cognitive therapy for depression: A new approach to preventing relapse.* New York: Guilford Press.

Appendix B: Resources

Here, readers may find a number of resources in several countries worldwide, helpful for those who wish to train himself/herself in mindfulness-based approaches or maintain and deepen his/her own meditation practice.

United States

Center for Mindfulness in Medicine, Health Care, and Society

University of Massachusetts Worcester Campus,

55 Lake Avenue North Worcester, Massachusetts 01655

Tel: 508-856-2656

Email: mindfulness@umassmed.edu

Website:http://www.umassmed.edu/cfm

Website:http://www.umassmed.edu/Content.aspx?id=41252&linkidentifier
    =id& itemid=41252

Institute for Meditation and Psychotherapy

35 Pleasant St.,

Newton Center, MA, USA, 02459

Website:www.meditationandpsychotherapy.org

Website:http://meditationandpsychotherapy.org/

Insight Meditation Society

www.dharma.org

1230 Pleasant St.,

Barre, MA USA 01005

978-355-4378

Barre Center for Buddhist Studies

149 Lockwood Rd.,

Barre, MA USA 01005

978-355-2347

Website: www.dharma.org/bcbs

New York Insight Meditation Center

28 West 27th Street, 10th floor,

New York, New York 10001

Tel: 212-213-4802

Website: www.nyimc.org

Insight LA,

2633 Lincoln Blvd, #206, Santa Monica, CA 90405

The Center for Mindfulness and Psychotherapy

2444 Wilshire Blvd. Suite 202,

Santa Monica, CA 90403

(310) 712-1948

Website:http://www.mindfulnessandpsychotherapy.org/

Mindful Awareness Research Center (MARC)

UCLA Semel Institute for Neuroscience and Human Behavior

760 Westwood Plaza, Rm. 47-444 Box 951759,

Los Angeles, CA 90095-1759

Tel: 310 206 7503

Fax: 310 206 4446

Email: marcinfo@ucla.edu

Website:www.marc.ucla.edu

Spirit Rock Meditation Centre

PO Box 169,

Woodacre, CA 94973

Tel: (415) 488-0164

Fax: (415) 488-1025

Email: SRMC@spiritrock.org

Website: http://www.spiritrock.org/

Mindfulness-Based Stress Reduction Program

Duke Integrative Medicine,

Duke University Medical Center,

DUMC Box 102904

Durham, NC 27710

Tel: 919-680-6826

Email: info@dukeintegrativemedicine.org

Website:http://www.dukeintegrativemedicine.org/

Awareness and Relaxation Training

Santa Cruz, CA 95065

Website: http://www.mindfulnessprograms.com/

Phone: 831/469-3338

Email Bob Stahl: bob@mindfulnessprograms.com

Mindfulness-Based Stress Reduction

University of Wisconsin Hospital

Madison, WI 53705

Website:

http://www.uwhealth.org/alternativemedicine/mindfulnessbasedstressreduction/11454

E-mail: ka.bonus@hosp.wisc.edu

Phone: 608-265-8325

For Training and workshop on Acceptance and Commitment Therapy

Association for Contextual Behavioral Science,
Website:http://www.contextualpsychology.org

For Training and workshop on Dialectical Behavior Therapy

Website:http://www.behavioraltech.com/index.cfm?CFID=2517201&
   CFTOKEN=90613839
http://depts.washington.edu/brtc/
http://faculty.washington.edu/linehan/

Europe
United Kingdom

Oxford Cognitive Therapy Centre

Provides training in cognitive therapy, also sells resource materials. Hosts
workshops in mindfulness-based approaches for therapists.

Oxford Cognitive Therapy Centre,
Warneford Hospital,
Oxford,
OX3 7JX
England
Tel: +44 (0)1865 223986
Fax: +44 (0)1865 223740
http://www.octc.co.uk/index.html"
with
Oxford Mindfulness Centre Wellcome Building   University of Oxford
Dept. of
Psychiatry Warneford Hospital   Oxford · OX3 7JX   United Kingdom
Tel: 01865 226468 Fax: 01865 223948
http://www.oxfordmindfulness.org/ http://www.mbct.co.uk/

The Centre for Mindfulness Research and Practice
University of Wales, Bangor, UK.
Centre for Mindfulness Research and Practice
School of Psychology,
Dean St Building,
Bangor University,
Bangor LL57 1UT
Tel: 01248 382939
Fax: 01248 383982
Email: mindfulness@bangor.ac.uk

Website: http://www.bangor.ac.uk/imscar/mindfulness/uk_profs.php

Gaia House
West Ogwell,
Newton Abbot,

Devon, TQ12 6EN - England

Tel: +44 (0)1626 333613

Fax: +44 (0)1626 352650

Email: generalenquiries@gaiahouse.co.uk
Website: http://www.gaiahouse.co.uk/

Italy
Istituto Italiano per la Mindfulness (IS.I.MIND)
For training in MBCT and Mindfulness-Based Meditation
Director: Dr. Fabrizio Didonna
Email: info@istitutomindfulness.com
Website: http://www.istitutomindfulness.com
Istituto di Scienze Cognitive
Via Fiume, 13/b – 58100 Grosseto – Italy
Tel and Fax: +39 0564 416672
Email: isc@istitutodiscienzecognitive.it
Website: http://www.istitutodiscienzecognitive.it/

AMECO (Associazione di Meditazione di Consapevolezza)
Website: http://digilander.libero.it/Ameco/

Istituto Lama Tzong Khapa (ILTK)
The main Buddhist Center in Italy
Mahayana Vipassana Tradition
Via Poggiberna, 9,
Pomaia 56040 (Pisa) Italy
Tel: +39 050.685654
Fax: 050.685695
Email: iltk@iltk.it

Website:http://www.iltk.it/it/L1_homepage.htm

France
Plum Village (Zen Master Thich Nhat Hanh)
Lower Hamlet,
Meyrac 47120,
Loubes-Bernac, France
Tel: +(33) 5.53.94.75.40
Fax: +(33) 5.53.94.75.90
E-mail: LH-office@plumvillage.org
E-mail: PVlistening@plumvill.net -
Website: http://www.plumvillage.org/
For training in MBCT
Claude Penet et Stéphane Roy
virtualroys@aol.com

Switzerland

For workshops and professional training in Mindfulness-Based Cognitive Therapy

Dr Guido Bondolfi MD.& Dr Lucio Bizzini Ph.D.
Hôpitaux Universitaires de Genève,
Département de psychiatrie,
Programme Dépression,
6-8, rue du 31-décembre,
CH – 1207 Genève - Switzerland
Tel: +41 22 718 45 11
Fax: +41 22 718 45 80

Association Suisse de Psychotherapie Cognitive
(ASPCO) features both workshops and professional training in Mindfulness-Based Cognitive Therapy.
Website: http://www.aspco.ch/

Centre Vimalakirti

Charles Genoud & Patricia Feldman-Genoud,
Genève – Switzerland

Email: info@vimalakirti.org

Website: www.vimalakirti.org
Meditation Center Beatenberg - Meditationszentrum Beatenberg
Waldegg

CH-3803 Beatenberg,
Schweiz
Tel: ++41 (0)33 841 21 31
Fax: ++41 (0)33 841 21 32

Email: info@karuna.ch

Belgium
For the French speaking part, Wallonie
Site Francophone sur la Pleine Conscience (Mindfulness) en Psychothérapie
French site for Mindfulness and Psychotherapy.
Includes downloadable guided mindfulness meditations in French (mp3 format).
Website: www.ecsa.ucl.ac.be/mindfulness

For The Dutch (Flemish) speaking part, Vlaanderen

Dr. Edel Maex
Antwerpen
Voor informatie over de trainingen gegeven in de Stresskliniek van het Ziekenhuis Netwerk Antwerpen bel 03 280 3505 of mail naar Dr Edel Maex:
edel.maex@zna.be
Voor trainingen voor jongeren kan je mailen naar Jen
Bertels:bertels.jen@skynet.be Patrice Van

Huffel:patricevanhuffel@skynet.beWebsite:
http://www.levenindemaalstroom.be/Stress.html

Dr. Johan Vandeputte
Universitary Hospital of Gent,
Department of Mood and Anxiety disorders
tel 32-9-332 21 11
website: http://www.wakkerworden.org/

Instituut voor Aandacht & Mindfulness
Dr. David Dewulf
Universitary Hospital in Gent
dd@mindbody.be
website: http://www.aandacht.be/

Portugal
Associação Portuguesa Para O Mindfulness - Portuguese Association
for Mindfulness
Núcleo de Estudos e Intervenção Cognitivo-Comportamental,
Faculdade de Psicologia e Ciâncias da Educação da Universidade de
Coimbra,
Rua do Colégio Novo, Apartado 6153, 3001-802 Coimbra
Phone: 0035 1239851464
e-mail: a.p.mindfulness@gmail.com

Germany
MBSR-Institut Freiburg
Konradstrasse 32
79100 Freiburg
Phone : 0761 - 40119895
http://www.mbsr-institut-freiburg.de
Email:info@mbsr-institut-freiburg.de
For training in MBCT and MBSR
Institute for Actsamkeit and Stressbewaltigung,
Kirchstr. 45,
50181 Bedburg,
Germany,
Tel: 0049-172-2186681
EMail: MBSR2002@aol.com
Website: http://www.institut-fuer-achtsamkeit.de/homepage.html
Holland/Nederland
For MBCT training in Holland
MBCT Trainingen,
Ger Schurink,
Grotestraat 209-B,
7622GH Borne,
074-2666090,

Website: http://www.mbcttrainingen.nl/

For MBSR training in Holland

Tinge Training & Therapie

Johan Tinge,
Oosterveld 14,
9451 GX Rolde,
Tel: 0592 - 24 36 48
Bank: 32 18 03 558

Website:http://www.aandachttraining.nl/

Argentina

Mindfulness Argentina
Araoz 1942
Buenos Aires
Phone : Oo54 -11-1551476688 Or - 47478870
Web : http://www.mindfulnessvision.com.ar
E-Mail: clara@visionclara.com.ar

Australia
Sydney
Stress Reduction Centre in Australia Limited
Mailing address: Suite 7, 2 Redleaf Avenue, Wahroonga, New South Wales
2076, AUSTRALIA
Phone: (61-2) 94878030
Website: http://stressreductioncentreinaustralia.com/
E-mail: Charleskhong@yahoo.com.au

Melbourne
Health, Wellbeing and Development
Building 10, Campus Centre
Monash University
Clayton
Melbourne
VICTORIA 3168
AUSTRALIA
Phone: 61 3 99053156
Website: http://www.adm.monash.edu.au/community-services/
E-mail: sally.trembath@adm.monash.edu.au

South Africa
Institute for Mindfulness South Africa
Phone: (021) 465-6318
Website: http://www.mindfulness.org.za
e-mail: vzaacks@gmail.com
Mindfulness–Based Stress Reduction (MBSR) center in Cape Town
Website:http://www.mbsr.co.za/
Main Web site on MBCT
http://www.mbct.com/Index.htm
http://www.mbct.co.uk

Main Web site on MBSR

http://www.umassmed.edu/Content.aspx?id=41252&linkidentifier=
    id&itemid=41252

Tapes and CDs for Mindfulness Meditation Practice

CDs of the MBSR Programme by Jon Kabat-Zinn:

http://www.stressreductiontapes.com

CDs used in Oxford's MBCT Programme by Mark Williams:

http://www.octc.co.uk/html/mindfulness.html

CDs used in the Centre for Mindfulness Research and Practice – Bangor

by Rebecca Crane, Sarah Silverton, Cindy Cooper and Judith Soulsby:

http://www.bangor.ac.uk/mindfulness

CDs of the MBCT programme in Italian language by Fabrizio Didonna

Email: info@istitutomindfulness.com

Website: http://www.istitutomindfulness.com

Index

Printed in the United States
133135LV00006BA/5-20/P